Assessment in Occupational Therapy and Physical Therapy

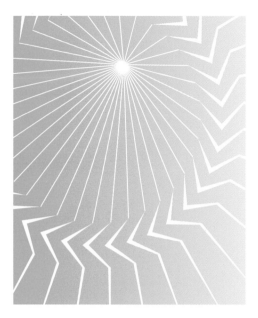

Julia Van Deusen, PhD, OTR/L, FAOTA
Professor
Department of Occupational Therapy
College of Health Professions
Health Science Center
University of Florida
Gainesville, Florida

Denis Brunt, PT, EdD
Associate Professor
Department of Physical Therapy
College of Health Professions
Health Science Center
University of Florida
Gainesville, Florida

Assessment in Occupational Therapy and Physical Therapy

W.B. SAUNDERS COMPANY
A Division of Harcourt Brace & Company

Philadelphia London Toronto Montreal Sydney Tokyo

W.B. SAUNDERS COMPANY
A Division of Harcourt Brace & Company

The Curtis Center
Independence Square West
Philadelphia, Pennsylvania 19106

Library of Congress Cataloging-in-Publication Data

Assessment in occupational therapy and physical therapy / [edited by]
Julia Van Deusen and Denis Brunt.

    p.   cm.

    ISBN 0-7216-4444-9

    1. Occupational therapy.   2. Physical therapy.   I. Van Deusen,
Julia. II. Brunt, Denis.
    [DNLM: 1. Physical Examination—methods. 2. Physical Therapy—
    methods. 3. Occupational Therapy—methods. WB 205 A847 1997]

RM735.65.A86 1997   616.07'54—dc20

DNLM/DLC   96-6052

Assessment in Occupational Therapy and Physical Therapy   0-7216-4444-9

Printed in the United States of America

Last digit is the print number: 9   8   7   6   5   4   3   2   1

*To those graduate students everywhere
who are furthering their careers
in the rehabilitation professions*

Contributors

ELLEN D. ADAMS, MA, CRC, CCM
Executive Director, Physical Restoration Center, Gainesville, Florida
Work Activities

JAMES AGOSTINUCCI, ScD, OTR
Associate Professor of Physical Therapy, Anatomy & Neuroscience, Physical Therapy Program, University of Rhode Island, Kingston, Rhode Island
Motor Control: Upper Motor Neuron Syndrome

MELBA J. ARNOLD, MS, OTR/L
Lecturer, Department of Occupational Therapy, University of Florida, College of Health Professions, Gainesville, Florida
Psychosocial Function

FELECIA MOORE BANKS, MEd, OTR/L
Assistant Professor, Howard University, Washington, DC
Home Management

IAN KAHLER BARSTOW, PT
Department of Physical Therapy, University of Florida, Gainesville, Florida
Joint Range of Motion

JULIE BELKIN, OTR, CO
Director of Marketing and Product Development, North Coast Medical, Inc., San Jose, California
Prosthetic and Orthotic Assessments: Upper Extremity Orthotics and Prosthetics

JERI BENSON, PhD
Professor of Educational Psychology— Measurement Specialization, The University of Georgia, College of Education, Athens, Georgia
Measurement Theory: Application to Occupational and Physical Therapy

STEVEN R. BERNSTEIN, MS, PT
Assistant Professor, Department of Physical Therapy, Florida International University, Miami, Florida
Assessment of Elders and Caregivers

DENIS BRUNT, PT, EdD
Associate Professor, Department of Physical Therapy, College of Health Professions, Health Science Center, University of Florida, Gainesville, Florida
Editor; Gait Analysis

PATRICIA M. BYRON, MA
Director of Hand Therapy, Philadelphia Hand Center, P.C., Philadelphia, Pennsylvania
Prosthetic and Orthotic Assessments: Upper Extremity Orthotics and Prosthetics

SHARON A. CERMAK, EdD, OTR/L, FAOTA
Professor, Boston University, Sargent College, Boston, Massachusetts
Sensory Processing: Assessment of Perceptual Dysfunction in the Adult

BONNIE R. DECKER, MHS, OTR
Assistant Professor of Occupational Therapy, University of Central Arkansas, Conway, Arkansas; Adjunct Faculty, Department of Pediatrics, University of Arkansas for Medical Sciences, Little Rock, Arkansas
Pediatrics: Developmental and Neonatal Assessment; Pediatrics: Assessment of Specific Functions

ELIZABETH B. DEVEREAUX, MSW, ACSW/L, OTR/L, FAOTA
Former Associate Professor, Director of the Division of Occupational Therapy (Retired), Department of Psychiatry, Marshall University School of Medicine; Health Care and Academic Consultant, Huntington, West Virginia
Psychosocial Function

JOANNE JACKSON FOSS, MS, OTR
Instructor of Occupational Therapy, University of Florida, Gainesville, Florida
Sensory Processing: Sensory Deficits; Pediatrics: Developmental and Neonatal Assessment; Pediatrics: Assessment of Specific Functions

ROBERT S. GAILEY, MSEd, PT
Instructor, Department of Orthopaedics, Division of Physical Therapy, University of Miami School of Medicine, Coral Gables, Florida
Prosthetic and Orthotic Assessments: Lower Extremity Prosthetics

JEFFERY GILLIAM, MHS, PT, OCS
Department of Physical Therapy, University of Florida, Gainesville, Florida
Joint Range of Motion

BARBARA HAASE, MHS, OTR/L
Adjunct Assistant Professor, Occupational Therapy Program, Medical College of Ohio, Toledo; Neuro Clinical Specialist, Occupational Therapy, St. Francis Health Care Centre, Green Springs, Ohio
Sensory Processing: Cognition

EDWARD J. HAMMOND, PhD
Rehabilitation Medicine Associates P.A., Gainesville, Florida
Electrodiagnosis of the Neuromuscular System

CAROLYN SCHMIDT HANSON, PhD, OTR
Assistant Professor, Department of Occupational Therapy, College of Health Professions, University of Florida, Gainesville, Florida
Community Activities

GAIL ANN HILLS, PhD, OTR, FAOTA
Professor, Occupational Therapy Department, College of Health, Florida International University, Miami, Florida
Assessment of Elders and Caregivers

CAROL A. ISAAC, PT, BS
Director of Rehabilitation Services, Columbia North Florida Regional Medical Center, Gainesville, Florida
Work Activities

SHIRLEY J. JACKSON, MS, OTR/L
Associate Professor, Howard University, Washington, DC
Home Management

PAUL C. LaSTAYO, MPT, CHT
Clinical Faculty, Northern Arizona University; Certified Hand Therapist, DeRosa Physical Therapy P.C., Flagstaff, Arizona
Clinical Assessment of Pain

MARY LAW, PhD, OT(C)
Associate Professor, School of Rehabilitation Science; Director, Neurodevelopmental Clinical Research Unit, McMaster University, Hamilton, Ontario, Canada
Self-Care

KEH-CHUNG LIN, ScD, OTR
National Taiwan University, Taipei, Taiwan
Sensory Processing: Assessment of Perceptual Dysfunction in the Adult

BRUCE A. MUELLER, OTR/L, CHT
Clinical Coordinator, Physical Restoration Center, Gainesville, Florida
Work Activities

KENNETH J. OTTENBACHER, PhD
Vice Dean, School of Allied Health Sciences, University of Texas Medical Branch at Galveston, Galveston, Texas
Foreword

ELIZABETH T. PROTAS, PT, PhD, FACSM
Assistant Dean and Professor, School of Physical Therapy, Texas Woman's University; Clinical Assistant Professor, Department of Physical Medicine and Rehabilitation, Baylor College of Medicine, Houston, Texas
Cardiovascular and Pulmonary Function

A. MONEIM RAMADAN, MD, FRCS
Senior Hand Surgeon, Ramadan Hand Institute, Alachua, Florida
Hand Analysis

ROBERT G. ROSS, MPT, CHT
Adjunct Faculty of Physical Therapy and Occupational Therapy, Quinnipiac College, Hamden, Connecticut; Clinical Director, Certified Hand Therapist, The Physical Therapy Center, Torrington, Connecticut
Clinical Assessment of Pain

JOYCE SHAPERO SABARI, PhD, OTR
Associate Professor, Occupational Therapy Department, New York, New York
Motor Control: Motor Recovery After Stroke

BARBARA A. SCHELL, PhD, OTR, FAOTA
Associate Professor and Chair, Occupational Therapy Department, Brenau University, Gainesville, Georgia
Measurement Theory: Application to Occupational and Physical Therapy

MAUREEN J. SIMMONDS, MCSP, PT, PhD
Assistant Professor, Texas Woman's University, Houston, Texas
Muscle Strength

JULIA VAN DEUSEN, PhD, OTR/L, FAOTA
Professor, Department of Occupational Therapy, College of Health Professions, Health Science Center, University of Florida, Gainesville, Florida
Editor; Body Image; Sensory Processing: Introduction to Sensory Processing; Sensory Processing: Sensory Defects; An Assessment Summary

JAMES C. WALL, PhD
Professor, Physical Therapy Department; Adjunct Professor, Behavioral Studies and Educational Technology, University of South Alabama, Mobile, Alabama
Gait Analysis

Foreword

In describing the importance of interdisciplinary assessment in rehabilitation, Johnston, Keith, and Hinderer (1992, p. S-5) note that "We must improve our measures to keep pace with the development in general health care. If we move rapidly and continue our efforts, we can move rehabilitation to a position of leadership in health care." The ability to develop new assessment instruments to keep pace with the rapidly changing health care environment will be absolutely critical to the future expansion of occupational therapy and physical therapy. Without assessment expertise, rehabilitation practitioners will be unable to meet the demands for efficiency, accountability, and effectiveness that are certain to increase in the future. An indication of the importance of developing assessment expertise is reflected in recent publications by the Joint Commission on Accreditation of Health Care Organizations (JCAHO). In 1993 the JCAHO published *The measurement mandate: On the road to performance improvement in health care.* This book begins by stating that "One of the greatest challenges confronting health care organizations in the 1990's is learning to apply the concepts and methods of performance measurement." The following year, the JCAHO published a related text titled *A guide to establishing programs and assessing outcomes in clinical settings* (JCAHO, 1994). In discussing the importance of assessment in health care, the authors present the following consensus statement (p. 25):

"Among the most important reasons for establishing an outcome assessment initiative in a health care setting are:

- to describe, in quantitative terms, the impact of routinely delivered care on patients' lives;
- to establish a more accurate and reliable basis for clinical decision making by clinicians and patients; and
- to evaluate the effectiveness of care and identify opportunities for improvement."

This text, *Assessment in Occupational Therapy and Physical Therapy,* is designed to help rehabilitation practitioners achieve these objectives. The text begins with a comprehensive chapter on measurement theory that provides an excellent foundation for understanding the complexities of assessing impairment, disability, and handicap as defined by the World Health Organization (WHO, 1980).

The complexity of defining and assessing rehabilitation outcome is frequently identified as one of the reasons for the slow progress in developing instruments and conducting outcome research in occupational and physical therapy. Part of the difficulty in developing assessment procedures and outcome measures relevant to the practice of rehabilitation is directly related to the unit of analysis in research investigations (DeJong, 1987). The unit of analysis in rehabilitation is the individual and the individual's relationship with his or her environment. In contrast, the unit of analysis in many medical specialties is an organ, a body system, or a pathology. In fact, DeJong has argued that traditional medical research and practice is organized around these pathologies and organ systems; for example, cardiology and neurology. One consequence of this organizational structure is a focus on assessment procedures and outcome measures that emphasize an absence of pathology or the performance of a specific organ or body system; for instance, the use of an electrocardiogram to evaluate the function of the heart. In contrast to these narrowly focused medical specialties, the goal of rehabilitation is to improve an individual's ability to function as independently as possible in his or her natural environment. Achieving this goal requires measurement instruments and assessment skills that cover a wide spectrum of activities and environments. Julia Van Deusen and Denis Brunt have done an admirable job of compiling current information on areas relevant to interdisciplinary assessment conducted by occupational and physical therapists. The chapters cover a wide range of assessment topics from the examination of muscle strength (Chapter 2) to the evaluation of work activities (Chapter 20). Each chapter provides detailed information concerning evaluation and measurement protocols along with research implications and their clinical applications.

Assessment in Occupational Therapy and Physical Therapy will help rehabilitation practitioners to achieve the three objectives of outcome assessment identified by the JCAHO. In particular, the comprehensive coverage of assessment and measurement procedures will allow occupational and physical therapists to achieve the final JCAHO outcome assessment objective; that is, to evaluate the effectiveness of care and identify opportunities for improvement (JCAHO, 1994, p. 25).

In today's rapidly changing health care environment, there are many variables related to service delivery and cost containment that rehabilitation therapists cannot control. The interpretation of assessment procedures and the development of treatment programs, however, are still the direct responsibility of occupational and physical therapists. Information in this text will help therapists meet this professional responsibility. In the current bottom-line health care environment, *Assessment in Occupational Therapy and Physical Therapy* will help ensure that the consumers of rehabilitation services receive the best possible treatment planning and evaluation.

REFERENCES

DeJong, G. (1987). Medical rehabilitation outcome measurement in a changing health care market. In M. J. Furher (Ed.), *Rehabilitation outcomes: Analysis and measurement* (pp. 261–272). Baltimore: Paul H. Brookes.

Johnston, M. V., Keith, R. A., & Hinderer, S. R. (1992). Measurement standards of interdisciplinary medical rehabilitation. *Archives of Physical Medicine and Rehabilitation, 73,* 12-S.

Joint Commission on Accreditation of Healthcare Organizations (1994). *A guide to establishing programs for assessing outcomes in clinical settings.* Oakbrook Terrace, IL: JCAHO.

Joint Commission on Accreditation of Healthcare Organizations (1993). *The measurement mandate: On the road to performance improvement in health care.* Oakbrook Terrace, IL: JCAHO.

World Health Organization. (1980). *International classification of impairment, disability, and handicap.* Geneva, Switzerland: World Health Organization.

KENNETH OTTENBACHER

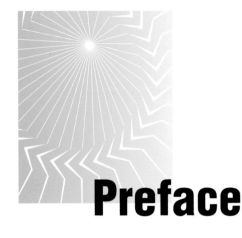

Preface

Our professions of occupational therapy and physical therapy are closely linked by our mutual interest in rehabilitation. We interact through direct patient service activities, and students in these fields frequently have courses together in the educational setting. Because of their common core and the fact that joint coursework is cost effective, it is probable that in the future more, rather than fewer, university courses will be shared by occupational and physical therapy students. One type of content that lends itself well to such joint study is that of assessment. *Assessment in Occupational Therapy and Physical Therapy* is well suited as a text for graduate students in these joint courses.

Although designed as a text for graduate students in occupational therapy, physical therapy, and related fields, this book will also meet the needs of advanced clinicians. *Assessment in Occupational Therapy and Physical Therapy* is intended as a major resource. When appropriate, certain content may be found in more than one chapter. This arrangement minimizes the need to search throughout the entire volume when a specialist is seeking a limited content area. It is assumed that the therapists using this text will have a basic knowledge of the use of clinical assessment tools. Our book provides the more extensive coverage and research needed by health professionals who are, or expect to be, administrators, teachers, and master practitioners. *Assessment in Occupational Therapy and Physical Therapy* is not intended as a procedures manual for the laboratory work required for the entry-level student who is learning assessment skills. Rather, this book provides the conceptual basis essential for the advanced practice roles. It also provides a comprehensive coverage of assessment in physical therapy and in occupational therapy. After a general overview of measurement theory in Unit One, Unit Two covers component assessments such as those for muscle strength or chronic pain. Unit Three thoroughly addresses the assessment of motor and of sensory processing dysfunction. In Unit Four, age-related assessment is covered. Finally, in Unit Five, activities of daily living are addressed.

The contributing authors for this book have been drawn from both educational and service settings covering a wide geographic area. Although the majority of authors appropriately are licensed occupational therapists or physical therapists, contributors from other health professions have also shared their expertise. Such diversity of input has helped us reach our goal of providing a truly comprehensive work on assessment for occupational therapists and for physical therapists.

JULIA VAN DEUSEN
DENIS BRUNT

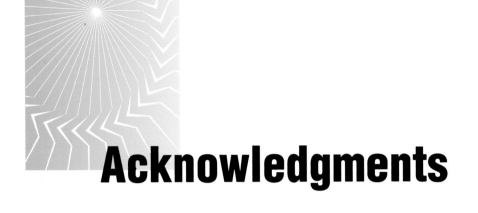

Acknowledgments

We wish to express our sincere thanks to all those who have helped contribute to the success of this project, especially

The many contributors who have shared their expertise

The staff in the Departments of Occupational Therapy and Physical Therapy, University of Florida, for their cooperation

The professionals at W. B. Saunders Company who have been so consistently helpful, particularly Helaine Barron and Blair Davis-Doerre

The special reviewers for the chapter on hand assessment, especially Kristin Froelich, who viewed it through the eyes of an occupational therapy graduate student, JoAnne Wright, and Orit Shechtman, PhD, OTR

And the many, many others.

JULIA VAN DEUSEN
DENIS BRUNT

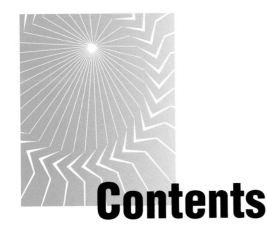

Contents

UNIT FIVE

Assessment of Activities of Daily Living 419

Overview of Measurement Theory

Measurement Theory: Application to Occupational and Physical Therapy

Jeri Benson, PhD

Barbara A. Schell, PhD, OTR, FAOTA

SUMMARY This chapter begins with a conceptual overview of the two primary issues in measurement theory, validity and reliability. Since many of the measurement tools described in this book are observationally based measurements, the remainder of the chapter focuses on several issues with which therapists need to be familiar in making observational measurements. First, the unique types of errors introduced by the observer are addressed. In the second and third sections, methods for determining the reliability and validity of the scores from observational measurements are presented. Since many observational tools already exist, in the fourth section we cover basic guidelines to consider in evaluating an instrument for a specific purpose. In the fifth section, we summarize the steps necessary for developing an observational tool, and, finally, a discussion of norms and the need for local norms is presented. The chapter concludes with a brief discussion of the need to consider the social consequences of testing.

The use of measurement tools in both occupational and physical therapy has increased dramatically since the early 1900s. This is due primarily to interest in using scientific approaches to improve practice and to justify each profession's contributions to health care. Properly developed measures can be useful at several levels. For clinicians, valid measurement approaches provide important information to support effective clinical reasoning. Such measures help define the nature and scope of clinical problems, provide benchmarks against which to monitor progress, and serve to summarize important changes that occur as a result of the therapy process (Law, 1987). Within departments or practice groups, aggregated data from various measures allow peers and managers to both critically evaluate the effectiveness of current interventions and develop directions for ongoing quality improvement.

Measurement is at the heart of many research endeavors designed to test the efficacy of therapy approaches (Short-DeGraff & Fisher, 1993; Sim & Arnell, 1993). In addition to professional concerns with improving practice, measurement is taking on increased importance in aiding decision-making about the allocation of health care resources. At the health policy level, measurement tools are being investigated for their usefulness in classifying different kinds of patient groups, as well as justifying the need for ongoing service provision (Wilkerson et al., 1992). Of particular concern in the United States is the need to determine the functional outcomes patients and clients experience as a result of therapy efforts.

Most of the measures discussed in the remaining chapters of this book can be thought of as being directed at quantifying either impairments or disabilities (World Health Organization, 1980). Impairments are problems that occur at the organ system level (e.g., nervous system, musculoskeletal system). Impairments typically result from illness, injury, or developmental delays. Impairments may or may not result in disabilities. In contrast to impairment, disability implies problems in adequately performing usual functional tasks consistent with one's age, culture, and life situation. Different psychometric concerns are likely to surface when considering the measurement of impairments versus functional abilities. For instance, when rating impairments, expectations are likely to vary as a function of age or gender. For example, normative data are needed for males and females of different ages for use in evaluating the results of grip strength testing. Alternatively, a major concern in using functional assessments to assess disability is how well one can predict performance in different contexts. For example, how well does being able to walk in the gym or prepare a light meal in the clinic predict performance in the home? Therefore, before evaluating a given tool's validity, one must first consider the purpose for testing. Thus, whether a therapist is assessing an impairment or the degree of disability, the purpose for testing should be clear.

The objective of this chapter is to provide occupational and physical therapy professionals with sufficient theoretical and practical information with which to better understand the measurements used in each field. The following topics are addressed: the conceptual basis of validity and reliability; issues involved in making observational measurements, such as recent thinking in assessing the reliability and validity of observational measures; guidelines for evaluating and developing observational measurement tools (or any other type of tool); and, finally, the need for local norms. Clinicians should be able to use this information to assess the quality of a measurement tool and its appropriate uses. Such understanding should promote valid interpretation of findings, allowing for practice decisions that are both effective and ethical. Educators will find this chapter useful in orienting students to important measurement issues. Finally, researchers who develop

and refine measures will be interested in the more recent procedures for studying reliability and validity.

CONCEPTUAL BASIS OF VALIDITY AND RELIABILITY

Psychometric theory is concerned with quantifying observations of behavior. To quantify the behaviors we are interested in studying, we must understand two essential elements of psychometric theory: reliability and validity. Therefore, a better understanding of the conceptual basis for these two terms seems a relevant place to start.

Validity

Validity is the single most important psychometric concept, as it is the process by which scores from measurements take on meaning. That is, one does not validate a scale or measuring tool; what is validated is an interpretation about the scores derived from the scale (Cronbach, 1971; Nunnally, 1978). This subtle yet important distinction in terms of what is being validated is sometimes overlooked, as we often hear one say that a given measurement tool is "valid." What is validated is the score obtained from the measurement and not the tool itself. This distinction makes sense if one considers that a given tool can be used for different purposes. For example, repeated measures of grip strength could be used by one therapist to assess a patient's consistency of effort to test his or her apparent willingness to demonstrate full physical capacity and to suggest his or her motivation to return to work. Another therapist might want to use the same measure of grip strength to describe the current level of strength and endurance for a hand-injured individual. In the former situation, the grip strength measurement tool would need to show predictive validity for maximum effort exertion, whereas in the latter situation, the tool would need to show content validity for the score interpretation. It is obvious then that two separate validity studies are required for each purpose, as each purpose has a different objective. Therefore, the score in each of the two above situations takes on a different meaning depending on the supporting validity evidence. Thus, validity is an attribute of a measurement and not an attribute of an instrument (Sim & Arnell, 1993).

A second aspect of validity is that test score validation is a matter of degree and not an all-or-nothing property. What this means is that one study does not validate or fail to validate a scale. Numerous studies are needed, using different approaches, different samples, and different populations to build a body of evidence that supports or fails to support the validity of the score interpretation.

Thus, validation is viewed as an continual process (Messick, 1989; Nunnally, 1978). Even when a large body of evidence seems to exist in support of the validity of a particular scale (e.g., the Wechsler Intelligence Scales), validity studies are continually needed, as social or cultural conditions change over time and cause our interpretation of the trait or behavior to change. Thus, for a scale to remain valid over time, its validity must be reestablished periodically. Later in this chapter, the social consequences of testing (Messick, 1989) are discussed as a reminder of the need to reevaluate the validity of measures used in occupational and physical therapy as times change and the nature of the professions change. Much more is said about the methods used to validate test scores later in the chapter in the context of the development and evaluation of observational measurement tools.

Reliability Theory

Clinicians and researchers are well aware of the importance of knowing and reporting the reliability of the scales used in their practice. In understanding conceptually what is meant by *reliability*, we need to introduce the concept of *true score*. A true score is the person's actual ability or status in the area being measured. If we were interested in measuring the level of "functional independence" of an individual, no matter what scale is used, we assume that each individual has a "true" functional independence score, which reflects what his or her functional abilities are, if they could be perfectly measured. An individual's true score could be obtained by testing the individual an infinite number of times using the same measure of functional independence and taking the average of all of his or her test scores. However, in reality it is not possible to test an individual an infinite number of times for obvious reasons. Instead, we estimate how well the *observed score* (often from one observation) reflects the person's true score. This estimate is called a reliability coefficient.

While a true score for an individual is a theoretical concept, it nonetheless is central to interpreting what is meant by a reliability coefficient. A reliability coefficient is an expression of how accurately a given measurement tool has been able to assess an individual's true score. Notice that this definition adds one additional element to the more commonly referred to definition of reliability, usually described as the accuracy or consistency of the measurement tool. By understanding the concept of true score, one can better appreciate what is meant by the numeric value of a reliability coefficient. In the next few paragraphs, the mathematic logic behind a reliability coefficient is described.

In an actual assessment situation, if we needed to obtain a measure of a person's functional independence, we likely would take only one measurement. This one measurement is referred to as an individual's *observed score*. The discrepancy between an individual's true score and his or her observed score is referred to as the *error score*. This simple relationship forms the basis of what is referred to as "classical test theory" and is shown by Equation 1–1:

$$\text{observed score (O)} = \text{true score (T)} + \text{error score (E)}$$
$$[1]$$

Since the concept of reliability is a statistic that is based on the notion of individual differences that produce variability in observed scores, we need to rewrite Equation 1–1 to represent a group of individuals who have been measured for functional independence. The relationship between observed, true, and error scores for a group is given by Equation 1–2:

$$\sigma^2_O = \sigma^2_T + \sigma^2_E \qquad [2]$$

where σ^2_O is the "observed score" variance, σ^2_T is the "true score" variance, and σ^2_E is the "error score variance." The variance is a group statistic that provides an index of how spread out the observed scores are around the mean "on the average." Given that the assumptions of classical test theory hold, the error score drops out of Equation 1–2, and the reliability coefficient (ρ_{xx}) is defined as

$$\rho_{xx} = \sigma^2_T / \sigma^2_O \qquad [3]$$

Therefore, the proper interpretation of Equation 1–3 is that a reliability coefficient is the proportion of observed score variance that is attributed to true score variance. For example, if a reliability coefficient of 0.85 were reported for our measure of functional independence, it would mean that 85% of the observed variance can be attributed to true score variance, or 85% of the measurement is assessing the individual's *true* level of functional independence, and the remaining 15% is attributed to measurement error.

The observed score variance is the actual variance obtained from the sample data at hand. The true and error score variance cannot be calculated in classical test theory because they are theoretical concepts. As it is impossible to test an individual an infinite number of times to compute his or her true score, all calculations of reliability are considered estimates. What is being estimated is a person's true score. The more accurate the measurement tool is, the closer the person's observed score is to his or her true score. With only one measurement, we assume that O = T. How much confidence we can place in whether the assumption of O = T is correct is expressed by the reliability coefficient. (For the interested reader, the derivation of the reliability coefficient, given that the numerator of Equation 1–3 is theoretical, is provided in many psychometric theory texts, e.g., Crocker & Algina, 1986, pp. 117–122. Also,

Equation 1–3 is sometimes expressed in terms of the error score as $1 - (\sigma^2_E / \sigma^2_O)$.)

In summary, the conceptual basis of reliability rests on the notion of how well a given measurement tool is able to assess an individual's true score on the behavior of interest. This interpretation holds whether one is estimating a stability, equivalency, or internal consistency reliability coefficient. Finally, as discussed earlier with regard to validity, reliability is not a property of the measurement tool itself but of the score derived from the tool. Furthermore, as pointed out by Sim and Arnell (1993) the reliability of a score should not be mistaken for evidence of the validity of the score.

Measurement Error

The study of reliability is integrally related to the study of how measurement error operates in given clinical or research situations. In fact, the choice of which reliability coefficient to compute depends on the type of measurement error that is conceptually relevant in a given measurement situation, as shown in Table 1–1.

The three general forms of reliability shown in Table 1–1 can be referred to as classical reliability procedures because they are derived from classical test theory, as shown by Equation 1–1. Each form of reliability is sensitive to different forms of measurement error. For example, when considering the measurement of edema it is easy to recognize that edema has both trait (dispositional) and state (situational) aspects. For instance, let us say we developed an edema battery, in which we used a tape measure to measure the circumference of someone's wrist and fingers, fol-

lowed by a volumetric reading obtained by water displacement and a clinical rating based on therapist observation. Because an unimpaired person's hand naturally swells slightly at different times or after some activities, we would expect some differences if measurements were taken at different times of day. Because these inconsistencies are expected, they would not be attributed to measurement error, as we expect all the ratings to increase or decrease together. However, inconsistencies among the items within the edema battery would suggest measurement error. For example, what if the tape measure indicated an increase in swelling, and the volumeter showed a decrease? This would suggest some measurement error in the battery of items. The internal consistency coefficient reflects the amount of measurement error due to internal differences in scores measuring the same construct.

To claim that an instrument is a measure of a trait that is assumed to remain stable over time for noninjured individuals (excluding children), such as coordination, high reliability in terms of consistency *across time* as well as *within time points across items or observations* is required. Potential inconsistency over measurement time is measured by the stability coefficient and reflects the degree of measurement error due to instability. Thus, a high stability coefficient and a high internal consistency coefficient are required of tools that are attempting to measure traits. It is important to know how stable and internally consistent a given measurement tool is before it is used to measure the coordination of an injured person. If the measurement is unstable and the behavior is also likely to be changing due to the injury, then it will be difficult to know if changes in scores are due to real change or to measurement error.

TABLE 1–1

OVERVIEW OF CLASSICAL APPROACHES FOR ESTIMATING RELIABILITY

Reliability Type	Sources of Error	Procedure
Stability (test-retest) For tools monitoring change over time (e.g., Functional Independence Measure)	Change in subject situation over time (e.g., memory, testing conditions, compliance) Any change treated as error, as trait expected to be stable	Test, wait, retest with the same tool and same subjects Use PPM; results will range from –1 to 1, with negatives treated as 0. Time intervals should be reported. Should be > 0.60 for long intervals, higher for shorter intervals
Equivalency (parallel forms) For multiple forms of same tool (e.g., professional certification examinations)	Changes in test forms due to sampling of items, item quality Any change treated as error, as items thought to be from same content domain	Prepare parallel forms, give forms to same subjects with no time interval Use PPM; results will range from –1 to 1, with negatives treated as 0. Should be > 0.80
Internal consistency (how will items in tool measure the same construct) For tools identifying traits (e.g., Sensory Integration and Praxis Test)	Changes due to item sampling or item quality Any change treated as error, because items thought to be from same content domain	A. **Split half:** Test, split test in half. Use PPM, correct with Spearman-Brown. Should be > 0.80 B. **Covariance procedures:** Average of all split halves. KR20, KR 21 (dichotomous scoring: right/wrong, multiple choice), Alpha (rating scale). Should be > 0.80

Issue of Sample Dependency

The classical approaches to assess scale reliability shown in Table 1–1 are sample-dependent procedures. The term *sample dependent* has two different meanings in measurement, and these different meanings should be considered when interpreting reliability and validity data. Sample dependency usually refers to the fact that the estimate of reliability will likely change (increase or decrease) when the same scale is administered to a different sample from the same population. This change in the reliability estimate is primarily due to changes in the amount of variability from one sample to another. For example, the reliability coefficient is likely to change when subjects of different ages are measured with the same scale. This type of sample dependency may be classified within the realm of "statistical inference," in which the instrument is the same but the sample of individuals differs either within the same population or between populations. Thus, reliability evidence should be routinely reported as an integral part of each study.

In terms of interpreting validity data, sample dependency plays a role in criterion-related and construct validity studies. In these two methods, correlational-based data are frequently reported, and correlational data are highly influenced by the amount or degree of variability in the sample data. Thus, a description of the sample used in the validity study is necessary. When looking across validity studies for a given instrument, we would like to see the results converging for the different samples from the same population. Furthermore, when the results converge for the same instrument over different populations, even stronger validity claims can be made, with one caution: Validity and reliability studies may produce results that fail to converge due to differences in samples. Thus, in interpreting correctly a test score for patients who have had cerebrovascular accidents (CVAs), the validity evidence must be based on CVA patients of a similar age. Promising validity evidence based on young patients with traumatic brain injury will not necessarily generalize.

The other type of sample dependency concerns "psychometric inference" (Mulaik, 1972), where the items constituting an instrument are a "sample" from a domain or universe of all potential items. This implies that the reliability estimates are specific to the subdomain constituting the test. This type of sample dependency has important consequences for interpreting the specific value of the reliability coefficient. For example, a reliability coefficient of 0.97 may not be very useful if the measurement domain is narrowly defined. This situation can occur when the scale (or subscale) consists of only two or three items that are slight variations of the same item. In this case, the reliability coefficient is inflated since the items differ only in a trivial sense. For example, if we wanted to assess mobility and used as our measure the ability of an individual to ambulate in a 10-foot corridor, the mobility task would be quite narrowly defined. In this case, a very high reliability

coefficient would be expected. However, if mobility were more broadly defined, such as an individual's ability to move freely throughout the home and community, then a reliability coefficient of 0.70 may be promising. To increase the 0.70 reliability, we might increase the number of items used to measure mobility in the home and community. Psychometric sample dependency has obvious implications for validity. The more narrowly defined the domain of behaviors, the more limited is the validity generalization. Using the illustration just described, being able to walk a 10-foot corridor tells us very little about how well the individual will be able to function at home or in the community. Later in the chapter, we introduce procedures for determining the reliability and validity of a score that are not sample dependent.

Numerous texts on measurement (Crocker & Algina, 1986; Nunnally, 1978) or research methods (Borg & Gall, 1983; Kerlinger, 1986) and measurement-oriented research articles (Benson & Clark, 1982; Fischer, 1993; Law, 1987) have been written; these sources provide an extensive discussion of validity and the three classical reliability procedures shown in Table 1–1.

Given that the objective of this chapter is to provide applications of measurement theory to the practice of occupational and physical therapy, and that most of the measurement in the clinic or in research situations involves therapists' observations of individual performance or behavior, we focus the remaining sections of the chapter on the use of observational measurement. Observational measurements have a decided advantage over self-report measurements. While self-report measurements are more efficient and less costly than observational measurements, self-report measures are prone to faking on the part of the individual making the self-report. Even when faking may not be an issue, some types of behaviors or injuries cannot be accurately reported by the individual. Observational measures are favored by occupational and physical therapists because they permit a direct measurement of the behavior of the individual or nature and extent of his or her injury. However, observational measurements are not without their own sources of error. Thus, it becomes important for occupational and physical therapists to be aware of the unique effects introduced into the measurement process when observers are used to collect data.

In the sections that follow, we present six issues that focus on observational measurement. First, the unique types of errors introduced by the observer are addressed. In the second and third sections, methods for determining the reliability and validity of the scores from observational measurements are presented. Since many observational tools already exist, in the fourth section we cover basic guidelines one needs to consider in evaluating an instrument for a specific purpose. However, sometimes it may be necessary to develop an observational tool for a specific situation or facility. Therefore, in the fifth section, we summarize the steps necessary for developing an observational tool along with the need for utilizing standardized procedures. Finally, the procedures for developing local norms to guide decisions of therapists and health care managers in evaluating treatment programs are covered.

ERRORS INTRODUCED BY OBSERVERS

Observer effects have an impact on the reliability and the validity of observational data. Two distinct forms of observer effects are found: 1) the observer may fail to rate the behavior objectively (observer bias) and 2) the presence of the observer can alter the behavior of the individual being rated (observer presence). These two general effects are summarized in Table 1–2 and are discussed in the following sections.

Observer Bias

Observer bias occurs when characteristics of the observer or the situation being observed influence the ratings made by the observer. These are referred to as systematic errors, as opposed to random errors. Systematic errors usually produce either a positive or negative bias in the observed score, whereas random errors fluctuate in a random manner around the observed score. Recall that the observed score is used to represent the "true score," so any bias in the observed score has consequences for how reliably we can measure the true score (see Equation 1–3). Examples of rater characteristics that can influence observations range from race, gender, age, or social class biases to differences in theoretical training or preferences for different procedures.

In addition to the background characteristics of observers that may bias their observations, several other forms of systematic observer biases can occur. First, an observer may tend to be too lenient or too strict. This form of bias has been referred to as either *error of severity* or *error of leniency*, depending on the direction of the bias. Quite often we find that human beings are more lenient than they are strict in their observations of others. A second form of bias is the *error of central tendency*. Here the observer tends to rate all individuals in the middle or average category. This can occur if some of the behaviors on the observational form were not actually seen but the observer feels that he or she must put a mark down. A third type of systematic bias is called the *halo effect*. The halo effect is when the observer forms an initial impression (either positive or negative) of the individual to be observed and then lets this impression guide his or her subsequent ratings. In general, observer biases are more likely to occur when observers are asked to rate high-inference or evaluation-type variables (e.g., the confidence with which the individual buttons his or her shirt) compared with very specific behaviors (e.g., the person's ability to button his or her shirt).

To control for these forms of systematic observer bias, one must first be aware of them. Next, to remove their potential impact on the observational data, adequate training in using the observational tool must be provided. Often, during training some of these biases come up and can be dealt with then. Another method is to have more than one observer present so that differences in rating may reveal observer biases.

Observer Presence

While the "effect" of the presence of the observer has more implications for a research study than in clinical practice, it may be that in a clinical situation, doing

TABLE 1-2		
OBSERVER EFFECTS AND STRATEGIES TO MANAGE THEM		
Influences	**Definition**	**Strategies to Control**
Observer biases		
Background of observer	Bias due to own experiences (e.g., race, gender, class, theoretical orientation, practice preferences)	Increase observer awareness of the influence of his or her background
Error of severity or leniency	Tendency to rate too strictly or too leniently	Provide initial and refresher observer training Provide systematic feedback about individual rater tendencies
Error of central tendency	Tendency to rate everyone toward the middle	Do coratings periodically to detect biases Minimize use of high-inference items where possible
Halo effect	Initial impression affects all subsequent ratings	
Observer presence	Changes in behavior as a result of being measured	Spend time with individual before evaluating to desensitize him or her to observer Discuss observation purpose after doing observation
Observer expectation	Inflation or deflation of ratings due to observer's personal investment in measurement results	Do routine quality monitoring to assure accuracy (e.g., peer review, coobservations)

something out of the ordinary with the patient can alter his or her behavior. The simple act of using an observational form to check off behavior that has been routinely performed previously may cause a change in the behavior to be observed.

To reduce the effects of the presence of the observer, data should not be gathered for the first few minutes when the observer enters the area or room where the observation is to take place. In some situations, it might take several visits by the observer before the behavior of the individual or group resumes to its "normal" level. If this precaution is not taken, the behavior being recorded is likely to be atypical and not at all representative of normal behavior for the individual or group.

A more serious problem can occur if the individual being rated knows that high ratings will allow him or her to be discharged from the clinic or hospital, or if in evaluating the effect of a treatment program, low ratings are initially given and higher ratings are given at the end. This latter situation describes the concept of observer expectation. However, either of these situations can lead to a form of systematic bias that results in *contamination* of the observational data, which affects the validity of the scores. To as much an extent as possible, it is advisable not to discuss the purpose of the observations until after they have been made. Alternatively, one can do quality monitoring to assure accuracy of ratings.

ASSESSING THE RELIABILITY OF OBSERVATIONAL MEASURES

The topic of reliability was discussed earlier from a conceptual perspective. In Table 1–1, the various methods for estimating what we have referred to as the classical forms of reliability of scores were presented. However, procedures for estimating the reliability of observational measures deserve special attention due to their unique nature. As we noted in the previous section, observational measures, compared with typical paper-and-pencil measures of ability or personality, introduce additional sources of error into the measurement from the observer. For example, if only one observer is used, he or she may be inconsistent from one observation to the next, and therefore we would want some information on the *intrarater* agreement. However, if more than one observer is used, then not only do we have intrarater issues but also we have added inconsistencies over raters, or *interrater* agreement problems. Notice that we have been careful not to equate intrarater and interrater agreement with the concept of reliability. Observer disagreement is important only in that it reduces the reliability of an observational measure, which in turn reduces its validity.

From a measurement perspective, percentage of observer agreement is not a form of reliability (Crocker & Algina, 1986; Herbert & Attridge, 1975). Furthermore,

research in this area has indicated the inadequacy of reporting observer agreement alone, as it can be highly misleading (McGaw et al., 1972; Medley & Mitzel, 1963). The main reason for not using percentage of observer agreement as an indicator of reliability is that it does not address the central issue of reliability, which is how much of the measurement represents the individual's true score. The general lack of conceptual understanding of what the reliability coefficient represents has led practitioners and researchers in many fields (not just occupational and physical therapy) to equate percentage of agreement methods with reliability. Thus, while these two concepts are not the same, the percentage of observer agreement can provide useful information in studying observer bias or ambiguity in observed events, as suggested by Herbert and Attridge (1975). Frick and Semmel (1978) provide an overview of various observer agreement indices and when these indices should be used prior to conducting a reliability study.

Variance Components Approach

To consider the accuracy of the true score being measured via observational methods, the single best procedure is the variance components approach (Ebel, 1951; Frick & Semmel, 1978; Hoyt, 1941). The variance components approach is superior to the classical approaches for conducting a reliability study for an observation tool because the variance components approach allows for the estimation of multiple sources of error in the measurement (e.g., same observer over time, different observers, context effects, training effects) to be partitioned (controlled) and studied. However, as Rowley (1976) has pointed out, the variance components approach is not well known in the disciplines that use observational measurement the most (e.g., clinical practice and research). With so much of the assessment work in occupational and physical therapy being based on observations, it seems highly appropriate to introduce the concepts of the variance components approach and to illustrate its use.

The variance component approach is based on an analysis of variance (ANOVA) framework, where the variance components refer to the mean squares that are routinely computed in ANOVA. In an example adapted from Rowley (1976), let us assume we have $n \geq 1$ observations on each of p patients, where hand dexterity is the behavior to be observed. We regard the observations as equivalent to one another, and no distinction is intended between observations (observation five on one patient is no different than observation five on another patient). This "design" sets up a typical one-way repeated-measures ANOVA, with p as the independent factor and the n observations as replications. From the ANOVA summary table, we obtain MSp (mean squares for patient) and MSw (mean squares within patients, or the error term). The reliability of a *score* from a single observation of p patients would be estimated as:

$$r_{ic} = \frac{MS_p - MS_w}{MS_p + (n - 1)MS_w} \qquad [4]$$

Equation 1–4 is the intraclass correlation (Haggard, 1958). However, what we are most interested in is the *mean* score observed for the p patients over the n > 1 observations, which is estimated by the following expression for reliability:

$$r_{xx} = \frac{MS_p - MS_w}{MS_p} \qquad [5]$$

Generalizability Theory

Equations 1–4 and 1–5 are specific illustrations of a more generalized procedure that permits the "generalizability" of observational scores to a universe of observations (Cronbach et al., 1972). The concept of the universe of observational scores for an individual is not unlike that of true score for an individual introduced earlier. Here you can see the link that is central to reliability theory, which is how accurate is the tool in measuring true score, or, in the case of observational data, in producing a score that has high generalizability over infinite observations. To improve the estimation of the "true observational score," we need to isolate as many sources of error as may be operating in a given situation to obtain as true a measurement as is possible.

The variance components for a single observer making multiple observations over time would be similar to the illustration above and expressed by equations 1–4 and 1–5, where we corrected for the observer's inconsistency from each time point (the mean squares within variance component). If we introduce two or more observers, then we can study several different sources of error to correct for differences in background, training, and experience (in addition to inconsistencies within an observer) that might adversely influence the observation. All these sources of variation plus their interactions now can be fit into an ANOVA framework as separate variance components to adjust the mean observed score and produce a reliability estimate that takes into account the background, level of training, and years of experience of the observer.

Roebroeck and colleagues (1993) provide an introduction to using generalizability theory to estimate the reliability of assessments made in physical therapy. They point out that classical test theory estimates of reliability (see Table 1–1) are limited in that they cannot account for *different* sources of measurement error. In addition, the classical reliability methods are sample dependent, as mentioned earlier, and as such cannot be generalized to other therapists, situations, or patient samples. Thus, Roebroeck and associates (1993) suggest that generalizability theory (which is designed to account for multiple

sources of measurement error) is a more suitable method for assessing reliability of measurement tools used in clinical practice. For example, we might be interested in how the reliability of clinical observations is influenced if the number of therapists making the observations were increased or if more observations were taken by a single therapist. In these situations, the statistical procedures associated with generalizability theory help the clinical researcher to obtain reliable ratings or observations of behavior that can be generalized beyond the specific situation or therapist.

A final point regarding the reliability of observational data is that classic reliability procedures are group-based statistics, where the between-patient variance is being studied. These methods are less useful to the practicing therapist than the variance components procedures of generalizability theory, which account for variance within individual patients being treated over time. Roebroeck and coworkers (1993) illustrate the use of generalizability theory in assessing reliably the change in patient progress over time. They show that in treating a patient over time, what a practicing therapist needs to know is the "smallest detectable difference" to determine that a real change has occurred rather than a change that is influenced by measurement error. The reliability of change or difference scores is not discussed here, but the reliability of difference scores is known to be quite low when the pre- and postmeasure scores are highly correlated (Crocker & Algina, 1986; Thorndike & Hagen, 1977). Thus, generalizability theory procedures account for multiple sources of measurement error in determining what change in scores over time is reliable. For researchers wanting to use generalizability theory procedures to assess the reliability of observational data (or measurement data in which multiple sources of error are possible), many standard "designs" can be analyzed using existing statistical software (e.g., SPSS or SAS). Standard designs are one-way or factorial ANOVA designs that are crossed, and the sample size is equal in all cells. Other nonstandard designs (unbalanced in terms of sample size, or not all levels are crossed) would required specialized programs. Crick and Brennan (1982) have developed the program GENOVA, and a version for IBM-compatible computers is available (free of charge), which will facilitate the analysis of standard and nonstandard ANOVA-based designs.

It is not possible within a chapter devoted to "psychometric methods in general" to be able to provide the details needed to implement a generalizability study. Our objective was to acquaint researchers and practitioners in occupational and physical therapy with more recent thinking on determining the reliability of observers or raters that maintains the conceptual notion of reliability, i.e., the measurement of true score. The following sources can be consulted to acquire the details for implementing variance components procedures (Brennan, 1983; Crocker & Algina, 1986; Evans, Cayten & Green, 1981; Shavelson & Webb, 1991).

ASSESSING THE VALIDITY OF OBSERVATIONAL MEASURES

Validity tells us what the test score measures. However, since any one test can be used for quite different purposes, we need to know not just "is the test score valid" but also "is the test score valid for the purpose for which I wish to use it?" Each form of validity calls for a different procedure that permits one type of inference to be drawn. Therefore, the purpose for testing an individual should be clear, since being able to make predictions or discuss a construct leads to very different measurement research designs.

Several different procedures for validating scores are derived from an instrument, and each depends on the purpose for which the test scores will be used. An overview of these procedures is presented in Table 1–3. As shown in the table, each validation procedure is associated with a given purpose for testing (column 1). For each purpose, an illustrative question regarding the interpretation of the score is provided under column 2. Column 3 shows the form of validity that is called for by the question, and column 4, the relevant form(s) of reliability given the purpose of testing.

Law (1987) has organized the forms of validation around three general reasons for testing in occupational therapy: descriptive, predictive, and evaluative. She indicates that an individual in the clinic might need to be tested for several different reasons. If the patient has had a stroke, then the therapist might want "to compare [him or her] to other stroke patients (descriptive), determine the probability of full recovery (prediction) or assess the effect of treatment (evaluative)" (p. 134). For a tool used descriptively, Law suggests that evidence of both content and construct validation of the scores should exist. For prediction, she advises that content and criterion-related data be available. Finally, for evaluative, she recommends that content and construct evidence be reported. Thus, no matter what the purpose of testing is, Law feels that all instruments used in the clinic should possess content validity, as she includes it in each reason for testing.

Given that validity is the most important aspect of a test score, we shall discuss the procedures to establish each form of validity noted in Table 1–3 for any measurement tool. However, we focus our illustrations on observational measures. In addition, we point out the issues inherent in each form of validation so that the practitioner and researcher can evaluate whether sufficient evidence has been established to ensure a correct interpretation of the test's scores.

Construct Validation

Construct validation is required when the interpretation to be made of the scores implies an explanation of the behavior or trait. A construct is a theoretical conceptualization of the behavior developed from observation. For example, functional independence is a construct that is operationalized by the Functional Independence Measure (FIM). However, for a construct to be useful, Lord and Novick (1968) advise that the construct must be defined on two levels: operationally and in terms of how the construct of interest relates to other constructs. This latter point is the heart of what Cronbach and Meehl (1955) meant when they introduced the term *nomological network* in their classical article that defined construct validity. A nomological network for a given construct, functional independence, stipulates how functional independence is influenced by other constructs, such as motivation, and in turn influences such constructs as self-esteem. To specify the nomological network for functional independence or any construct, a strong theory regarding the construct must be available. The stronger the substantive theory regarding a construct, the easier it is to design a validation study that has the potential for providing strong empirical evidence. The weaker or more tenuous the substantive theory, the greater the likelihood that equally weak empirical evidence will be

TABLE 1–3			
OVERVIEW OF VALIDITY AND RELIABILITY PROCEDURES			
Purpose of the Test	**Validity Question**	**Kind of Validity**	**Reliability Procedures**
Assess current status	Do items represent the domain?	Content	a) Internal consistency within each subarena b) Equivalency (for multiple forms) c) Variance components for observers
Predict behavior or performance	How accurate is the prediction?	Criterion-related: concurrent or predictive	a) Stability b) Equivalency (for multiple forms) c) Variance components for observers
Infer degree of trait or behavior	How do we know a specific behavior is being measured?	Construct	a) Internal consistency b) Equivalency (for multiple forms) c) Stability (if measuring over time) d) Variance components for observers

gathered, and very little advancement is made in understanding the construct.

Benson and Hagtvet (1996) recently wrote a chapter on the theory of construct validation in which they describe the process of construct validation as involving three steps, as suggested earlier by Nunnally (1978): 1) specify the domain of observables for the construct, 2) determine to what extent the observables are correlated with each other, and 3) determine whether the measures of a given construct correlate in expected ways with measures of other constructs. The first step essentially defines both theoretically and operationally the trait of interest. The second step can be thought of as internal domain studies, which would include such statistical procedures as item analysis, traditional factor analysis, confirmatory factor analysis (Jreskog, 1969), variance component procedures (such as those described under reliability of observational measures), and multitrait-multimethod procedures (Campbell & Fiske, 1959). A relatively new procedure to the occupational and physical therapy literature, Rasch modeling techniques (Fischer, 1993) could also be used to analyze the internal domain of a scale. More is said about Rasch procedures later in this chapter. The third step in construct validation can be viewed as external domain studies and includes such statistical procedures as multiple correlations of the trait of interest with other traits, differentiation between groups that do and do not possess the trait, and structural equation modeling (Jöreskog, 1973). Many researchers rely on factor analysis procedures almost exclusively to confirm the presence of a construct. However, as Benson and Hagtvet (1996) pointed out, factor analysis focuses primarily on the internal structure of the scale only by demonstrating the convergence of items or similar traits. In contrast, the essence of construct validity is to be able to discriminate among different traits as well as demonstrate the convergence of similar traits. The framework provided by Benson and Hagtvet for conducting construct validity studies indicates the true meaning of validity being a process. That is, no one study can confirm or disconfirm the presence of a construct, but a series of studies that clearly articulates the domain of the construct, how the items for a scale that purports to measure the construct fit together, and how the construct can be separated from other constructs begins to form the basis of the evidence needed for construct validation.

To illustrate how this three-step process would work, we briefly sketch out how a construct validity study would be designed for a measure of functional independence, the FIM. First, we need to ask, "How should the theoretical and empirical domains of functional independence be conceptualized?" To answer this question, we would start by drawing on the research literature and our own informal observations. This information is then summarized to form a "theory" of what the term *functional independence* means, which becomes the basis of the construct, as shown in Figure 1–1 above the dashed line.

A construct is an abstraction that is inferred from behavior. To assess functional independence, the construct must be operationalized. This is done by moving from the

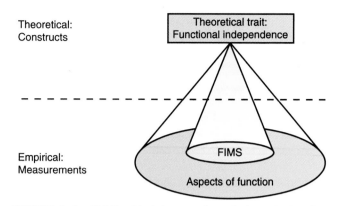

FIGURE 1–1. Relationship between a theoretical construct and an empirical measurement.

theoretical, abstract level to the empirical level, as shown in Figure 1–1 below the dashed line, where the specific aspects of function are shown. Each construct is assumed to have its own empirical domain. The empirical domain contains all the possible item types and ways to measure the construct (e.g., nominal or rating items, self-report, observation, performance assessment). Finally, shown within the empirical domain in Figure 1–1 is our specific measure of functional independence, the FIM. The FIM operationalizes the concept of functional independence in terms of an individual's need for assistance in the areas of self-care, sphincter management, mobility, locomotion, communication, and social cognition (Center for Functional Assessment Research, 1990). A number of other possible aspects of function are not included in the FIM (such as homemaking, ability to supervise attendants, or driving) because of the desire to keep the assessment tool as short as possible and still effectively reflect the degree of functional disability demonstrated by individuals.

Figure 1–2 illustrates how others have operationalized the theoretical construct of functional independence for rehabilitation patients, such as the Level of Rehabilitation Scale (LORS) (Carey & Posavac, 1978) and the Barthel (Mahoney & Barthel, 1965). It is expected that the LORS and Barthel would correlate with the FIM because they operationalize the same construct and their items are a subset of the aspects of function domain (see large shaded circle in Figure 1–2). However, the correlations would not be perfect because they do not operationalize the construct of functional independence in exactly the same way (e.g., they include some different aspects of functional independence).

In our hypothetical construct validity study, we now have selected a specific measurement tool, so we can move on to step 2. In the second step, the internal domain of the FIM is evaluated. An internal domain study is one in which the items on the scale are evaluated. Here we might use factor analysis to determine how well the items on the FIM measure a single construct or whether the two dimensions recently suggested by Linacre and colleagues (1994) can be empirically verified. Since the developers of the FIM (Granger et al., 1986) suggest that the items be summed to total score, which implies one dimension, we can test two

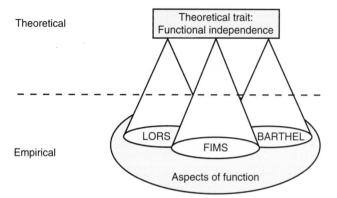

FIGURE 1–2. Several empirical measures of the same theoretical construct.

competing conceptualizations of what the FIM items seem to measure.

For the third step in the process of providing construct validity evidence for the FIM scores, we might select other variables that are assumed to influence one's level of functional independence (e.g., motivation, degree of family support) and variables that functional independence is thought to influence (e.g., self-esteem, employability). In this third step, we are gathering data that will confirm or fail to confirm our hypotheses about how functional independence as a construct operates in the presence of other constructs. To analyze our data, we could use multiple regression (Pedhazur, 1982) to study the relation of motivation and degree of family support to functional independence. A second regression analysis might explore whether functional independence is related to self-esteem and employability in expected ways. More advanced statistical procedures combine the above two regression analyses in one analysis. One such procedure is structural equation modeling (Jöreskog, 1973). Benson and Hagtvet (1996) provide an illustration of using structural equation modeling to assess construct validation in a study similar to what was just described. The point of the third step is that we expect to obtain results that confirm our hypotheses of how functional independence as a construct operates. If we do happen to confirm our hypotheses regarding the behavior of functional independence, this then becomes one more piece of evidence for the validity of the FIM scores. However, the generalization of the construct beyond the sample data at hand would not be warranted (see earlier section on sample dependency). Thus, for appropriate use of the FIM scores with individuals other than those used in the hypothetical study described here, a separate study would need to be conducted.

Content Validation

To determine the content validity of the scores from a scale, one would need to specify an explicit definition of the behavioral domain and how that domain is to be operationally defined. This step is critical, since the task in content validation is to ensure that the items adequately assess the behavioral domain of interest. For example, consider Figure 1–1 in thinking about how the FIM would be evaluated for content validity. The behavioral domain is the construct of functional independence, which needs to be defined in its broadest sense, taking into account the various perspectives found in the research literature. Then functional independence is operationally defined as that set of behaviors assessed by the FIM items (e.g., cognitive and motor activities necessary for independent living). Once these definitions are decided on, an independent panel of experts in functional independence would rate whether the 5 cognitive items and the 13 motor items of the FIM adequately assess the domain of functional independence. Having available a table of specifications (see section on developing an observational form and Table 1–5) for the experts to classify the items into the cells of the table facilitates the process. The panel of experts should be: 1) independent of the scale being evaluated (in this case, they were not involved in the development of the FIM) and 2) undisputed experts in the subject area. Finally, the panel of experts should consist of more than one person.

Crocker and Algina (1986) provide a nice framework for conducting a content validity study along with practical considerations and issues to consider. For example, an important issue in assessing the content validity of items is what exactly the expert rates. Does the expert evaluate only the content of the items matching the domain, the difficulty of the task for the intended examinee that is implied in the item plus the content, the content of the item and the response options, or the degree of inference the observer has to make to rate the behavior? These questions point out that the "task" given to the experts must be explicitly defined in terms of *exactly* what they are to evaluate so that "other item characteristics" do not influence the rating made by the experts. A second issue pertains to how the results should be reported. Crocker and Algina (1986) point out that different procedures can lead to different conclusions regarding the match between the items and the content domain.

The technical manual for an assessment tool is important for evaluating whether the tool has adequate content validity. In the technical manual, the authors need to provide answers to the following questions: "Who were the panel of experts?" "How were they sampled?" "What was their task?" Finally, the authors should indicate the degree to which the items on the test matched the definition of the domain. The results are often reported in terms of percentage of agreement among the experts regarding the classification of the items to the domain definition. Content validation is particularly important for test scores used to evaluate the effects of a treatment program. For example, a therapist or facility manager might be interested in determining how effective the self-care retraining program is for the patients in the spinal cord injury unit. To draw the conclusion that the self-care treatment program was effective in working with rehabilitation patients with spinal cord injuries, the FIM scores must be content valid for measuring changes in self-care skills.

Criterion-Related Validity

There are two forms of criterion-related validation: concurrent and predictive. Each form is assessed in the same manner. The only difference between these two forms is when the criterion is obtained. Concurrent validation refers to the fact that the criterion is obtained at approximately the same time as the predictor data, whereas predictive validation implies that the criterion was obtained some time after the predictor data. An example of concurrent validation would be if the predictor is the score on the FIM taken in the clinic and the criterion is the observation made by the therapist on visiting the patient at home the next day, then the correlation between these two "scores" (for a group of patients) would be referred to as the concurrent validity coefficient. However, if the criterion observation made in the home is obtained 1 or 2 months later, the correlation between these scores (for a group of patients) is referred to as the predictive validity coefficient. Thus, the only difference between concurrent and predictive validation is the time interval between when the predictor and criterion scores are obtained.

The most important consideration in evaluating criterion-related validity results is "what is the criterion?" In a criterion-related validity study, what we are actually validating is the predictor score (the FIM in the two illustrations just given) based on the criterion score. Thus, a good criterion must have several characteristics. First, the criterion must be "unquestioned" in terms of its validity, i.e., the criterion must be considered the "accepted standard" for the behavior that is being measured. In the illustrations just given, we might then question the validity of the therapist's observation made at the patient's home. In addition to the criterion being valid, it must also be reliable. In fact, the upper bound of the validity coefficient can be estimated using the following equation:

$$r_{yx}' = \sqrt{(r_{xx}) \cdot (r_{yy})} \qquad [6]$$

where r_{yx}' is the upper bound of the validity coefficient, r_{xx} is the reliability of the predictor, and r_{yy} is the reliability of the criterion. If the reliability of the predictor is 0.75 and the reliability of the criterion is 0.85, then the maximum validity coefficient is estimated to be 0.80, but if the reliability of the predictor is 0.60 and criterion is 0.70, then maximum validity coefficient is estimated to be 0.42. Being able to estimate the maximum value of the validity coefficient prior to conducting the validity study is critical. If the estimated value is too low, then the reliability of the predictor or criterion should be improved prior to initiating the validity study, or another predictor or criterion measure can be used.

The value of the validity coefficient is extremely important. It is what is used to evaluate the accuracy of the prediction, which is obtained by squaring the validity coefficient (r_{xy}^2). In the illustration just given, the accuracy of the prediction is 36% when the validity coefficient is 0.60 and 18% when the validity coefficient is 0.42. The accuracy of the prediction tells us how much variance the predictor is able to explain of the criterion out of 100%. Given the results just presented, it is obvious that the choice of the predictor and criterion should be made very carefully. Furthermore, multiple predictors often improve the accuracy of the prediction. To estimate the validity coefficient with multiple predictors requires knowledge of multiple regression, which we do not go into in this chapter. A readable reference is Pedhazur (1982).

Since criterion-related validation is based on using a correlation coefficient (usually the pearson product-moment correlation coefficient if the predictor and criterion are both continuous variables), then the issues to consider with this form of validity are those that impact the correlation coefficient. For example, the range of individual scores on the predictor or criterion can be limited, the relationship between the predictor and criterion may not be linear, or the sample size may be too small. These three factors singly or in combination lower the validity coefficient. The magnitude of the validity coefficient also is reduced, influenced by the degree of measurement error in the predictor and criterion. This situation is referred to as the validity coefficient being attenuated. If a researcher wants to see how high the validity coefficient would be if the predictor and criterion were perfectly measured, the following equation can be used:

$$r_{yx}' = r_{xy}/\sqrt{(r_{xx}) \cdot (r_{yy})} \qquad [7]$$

where r_{xy}' is the corrected or *disattenuated* validity coefficient, and the other terms have been previously defined. The importance of considering the disattenuated validity coefficient is that it tells us whether it is worth it to try and improve the reliability of the predictor or criterion. If the disattenuated validity coefficient is only 0.50, then it might be a better strategy to select another predictor or criterion.

One final issue to consider in evaluating criterion-related validity coefficients is that since they are correlations, they can be influenced by other variables. Therefore, correlates of the predictor should be considered to determine if some other variable is influencing the relationship of interest. For instance, let us assume that motivation was correlated with the FIM. If we chose to use the FIM to predict employability, the magnitude of the relationship between the FIM and employability would be influenced by motivation. We can control the influence of motivation on the relationship between the FIM and employability by using partial correlations. This allows us to evaluate the magnitude of the actual relationship free of the influence of motivation. Crocker and Algina (1986) provide a discussion of the need to consider partial correlations in evaluating the results of a criterion-related validity study.

Now that the procedures for assessing reliability and validity have been presented, it would be useful to apply them by seeing how a therapist would go about evaluating a measurement tool.

EVALUATION OF OBSERVATIONAL MEASURES

Numerous observational tools can be used in occupational and physical therapy. To assist the therapist in selecting which observational tool best meets his or her needs, a set of guidelines is provided in Table 1–4. These guidelines are designed to be helpful in evaluating any instrument, not just observational tools. We have organized the guidelines into five sections (descriptive information, scale development, psychometric properties, norms and scoring, and reviews by professionals in the field). To respond to the points raised in the guidelines, multiple sources of information often need to be consulted.

To illustrate the use of the guidelines, we again use the FIM as a case example because of the current emphasis on outcome measures. Due to the FIM being relatively new, we need to consult multiple sources of information to evaluate its psychometric adequacy. We would like to point out that a thorough evaluation of the FIM is beyond the scope of this chapter and, as such, we do not comment on either the strengths or the weaknesses of the tool. Rather, we wanted to sensitize the therapist to the fact that a given

TABLE 1–4

GUIDELINES FOR EVALUATING A MEASUREMENT TOOL

	Manual	Grant Reports	Book Chapter	Articles
Descriptive Information				
Title, author, publisher, date	X	X		X
Intended age groups			X	
Cost	X			
Time (train, score, use)			X	
Scale Development				
Need for instrument	X	X	X	X
Theoretical support			X	X
Purpose	X	X	X	X
Table of specifications described?				
Item development process			X	
Rationale for number of items				
Rationale for item format	X	X	X	
Clear definition of behavior	X			
Items cover domain	X			
Pilot testing		X	X	X
Item analysis		X	X	X
Psychometric Properties				
Observer agreement			X	X
Reliability				
Stability				
Equivalency	NA			
Internal-consistency		X		X
Standard error of measurement				
Generalizability approaches		X	X	
Validity				
Content				
Criterion related				
Construct				X
Sample size and description		X	X	X
Norms and Scoring				
Description of norm group	NA			
Description of scoring	X			
Recording of procedures	X			
Rules for borderline	X			
Computer scoring available				
Standard scores available				
Independent Reviews	NA	NA		X

NA = nonapplicable; X = information needed was found in this source.

tool can be reliable and valid for many different purposes; therefore, each practitioner or researcher needs to be able to evaluate a given tool for the purpose for which he or she intends to use it.

Numerous sources may need to be consulted to decide if a given tool is appropriate for a specific use. Some of the information needed to evaluate a measurement tool may be found in the test manual. It is important to recognize that different kinds of test manuals, such as administration and scoring guides and technical manuals, exist. In a technical manual, you should expect to find the following points addressed by the author of the instrument (at a minimum):

- Need for the instrument
- Purpose of the instrument
- Intended groups or ages
- Description of the instrument development procedures
- Field or pilot testing results
- Administration and scoring procedures
- Initial reliability and validity results, given the intended purpose
- Normative data (if relevant)

Sometimes the administration and scoring procedures and the normative data are a separate document from the technical manual. Book chapters are another source of information and are likely to report on the theoretical underpinnings of the scale and more extensive reliability, validity, and normative results that might include larger samples or more diverse samples. The most recent information on a scale can be found in journal articles, which are likely to provide information on specific uses of the tool for specific samples or situations. Journal articles and book chapters written by persons who were not involved in the development of the instrument offer independent sources of information in terms of how useful the scale is to the research community and to practicing therapists. Finally, depending on the popularity of a given scale, independent evaluations by experts in the field may be located in test review compendiums such as Buros' *Mental Measurement Yearbooks* or *Test Critiques* found in the reference section of the library.

As shown in Table 1–4, we consulted four general types of sources (test manual, grant reports, book chapters, and journal articles) to obtain the information necessary to evaluate the FIM as a functional outcome measure. The FIM, as part of the Uniform Data System, was originally designed to meet a variety of objectives (Granger & Hamilton, 1988), including the ability to characterize disability and change in disability over time, provide the basis for cost-benefit analyses of rehabilitation programs, and be used for prediction of rehabilitation outcomes. To evaluate the usefulness of the FIM requires that the therapist decide for what specific purpose the FIM will be used. A clear understanding of your intended use of a measurement tool is critical to determining what form(s) of reliability and validity you would be looking to find ad-

dressed in the manual or other sources. In our example, we assume the reason for using the FIM is to determine its usefulness as an outcome measure of "program effectiveness of an inpatient rehabilitation program." Such outcomes would be useful in monitoring quality, meeting program evaluation guidelines of accrediting bodies, and helping to identify program strengths useful for marketing services. In deciding whether the FIM is an appropriate tool for our purposes, the following questions emerge:

Does it measure functional status?

Should single or multiple disciplines perform the ratings?

How sensitive is the FIM in measuring change from admission to discharge of inpatients?

How well does it capture the level of human assistance required for individuals with disabilities in a variety of functional performance arenas?

Does it work equally well for patients with a range of conditions, such as orthopedic problems, spinal cord injury, head injury, and stroke?

Most of these questions are aimed at the reliability and validity of the scores from the FIM. In short, we need to know how the FIM measures functional status and for what groups, as well as how sensitive the measurement is.

According to Law (1987, p. 134), the form of validity called for in our example is evaluative. Law describes evaluative instruments as ones that use "criteria or items to measure change in an individual over time." Under evaluative instruments, Law suggests that the items should be responsive (sensitive), test-retest and observer reliability should be established, and content and construct validity should be demonstrated. Given our intended use of the FIM, we now need to see if evidence of these forms of reliability and validity exists for the FIM.

In terms of manuals, the only one available is the *Guide for the Use of the Uniform Data Set for Medical Rehabilitation Including the Functional Independence Measure (FIM) Version 3.1*, which includes the FIM (Center for Functional Assessment Research, 1990). Stated in the Guide is that the FIM was found to have "face validity and to be reliable" (p. 1), with no supporting documentation of empiric evidence within the *Guide*. Since the FIM was developed from research funding, we needed to consult an additional source, the final report of the grant (Granger & Hamilton, 1988). In the final report is a brief description of interrater reliability and of validity. Interrater reliability was demonstrated through intraclass correlations of 0.86 on admission and 0.88 on discharge, based on the observations of physicians, occupational and physical therapists, and nurses. The interrater reliability study was conducted by Hamilton and colleagues (1987). In a later grant report, Heinemann and colleagues (1992) used the Rasch scaling technique to evaluate the dimensionality of the FIM. They found that the 18 items do not cluster into one total score but should be reported separately as motor (13 items) and cognitive (5 items) activities. Using this formulation, the authors reported internal consistency estimates of 0.92 for motor and 0.83 for cognitive activities. The Rasch scaling technique also indicated where specific items are in need of revision and that others could be eliminated due to redundancy. The Rasch analysis indicated that the FIM items generally do not vary much across different patient subgroups, with the exception of pain and burn patients on the motor activities and patients with right and bilateral stroke, brain dysfunction, and congenital impairments on the cognitive activities (Heinemann et al., 1992). This implies that the FIM items do not fit well for these disability groups and should be interpreted cautiously. The authors indicate that further study of the FIM in terms of item revision and item misfit across impairment groups was needed. In sum, the reliability data reported in the sources we reviewed seem to indicate that the FIM does produce reliable interrater data, and that the FIM is composed of two internally consistent subscales: motor and cognitive activities.

The information provided in the grant under the heading of validity related primarily to scale development and refinement (e.g., items were rated by clinicians as to ease of use and apparent adequacy), to which the authors refer as *face* validity. In the face validity study conducted by Hamilton and associates (1987), clinical rehabilitation therapists (with an average of 5.8 to 6.8 years of experience) rated the FIM items on ease of use, redundancy, and other factors. However, the results from the face validity study do not address whether the scale possesses content validity. In fact, psychometricians such as Crocker and Algina (1986), Nunnally (1978), and the authors of the *Standards for Educational and Psychological Testing* (1985) do not recognize face validity as a form of scale validation. Therefore, if face "validity" is to be used, it would be more appropriately placed under instrument development procedures. (The procedures for determining the content validity of scores from an instrument were described previously under the section on validity of observational measures.)

In terms of construct validity of the FIM for our intended purpose, we wanted to see whether the FIM scores can discriminate those with low levels of functional independence from those with high levels of independence. It was necessary to consult journal articles for this information. Several researchers reported the ability of the FIM to discriminate levels of functional independence of rehabilitation patients (Dodds et al., 1993, Granger et al., 1990).

From a partial review of the literature, we can say that the FIM was able to detect change over time and across patients (Dodds et al., 1993; Granger et al., 1986). While the interrater agreement appears adequate from reports by the test authors, some researchers report that when ratings are done by those from different disciplines or by untrained raters, reliability decreases (Adamovich, 1992; Chau et al., 1994; Fricke et al., 1993). From a validity perspective, recent literature strongly suggests that the FIM may be measuring several different dimensions of functional ability

(Dodds et al., 1993; Linacre et al., 1994). Based on this evidence, questions have been raised about the appropriateness of using a total FIM score, as opposed to reporting the separate subscale scores.

As was already mentioned, more literature about the FIM exists than has been referenced here, and a thorough review of all the relevant literature would be necessary to fully assess the FIM. The intent here is to begin to demonstrate that effective evaluation of measurement tools requires a sustained effort, using a variety of sources beyond the information provided by the test developer in the test manual. However, even this cursory review suggests that observer agreement studies should be undertaken by the local facility to check the consistency among therapists responsible for rating patient performance (see section on reliability of observation measures). This is but one example of the kinds of responsible actions a user of measurement tools might take to assure appropriate use of measurement scores.

DEVELOPMENT OF OBSERVATIONAL MEASURES

Quite often an observational tool does not exist for the required assessment, or a locally developed "checklist" is used (e.g., prosthetic checkouts or homemaking assessments, predriving assessments). In these situations, therapists need to be aware of the processes involved in developing observational tools that are reliable and valid. The general procedures to follow in instrument construction have been discussed previously in the occupational therapy literature by Benson and Clark (1982), although their focus was on a self-report instrument. We shall adjust the procedures to consider the development of observational instruments that basically involve avoiding or minimizing the problems inherent in observational data. To illustrate this process, we have selected the evaluation of homemaking skills. The purpose of this assessment would be to predict the person's ability to safely live alone.

There are two major problem areas to be aware of in using observational data: 1) attempting to study overly complex behavior and 2) the fact that the observer can change the behavior being observed. The second point is not directly related to the development of an observational measure but relates more to the reliability of the measure. The first point is highly relevant to the development of an observational measure and is addressed next.

Often when a therapist is interested in making an observation of an individual's ability to perform a certain task, the set of behaviors involved in the task can be overly complex, which creates problems in being able to accurately observe the behavior. One way to avoid this problem is to break down the behavior into its component parts. This is directly analogous to being able to define the behavior, both conceptually and empirically. This relationship was illustrated in Figures 1–1 and 1–2, in which a conceptual definition of the trait *functional independence* was given above the dashed line. It should be recognized that several conceptual definitions based on different theoretical positions regarding our understanding of what functional independence means could exist. Each conceptual definition of a trait could in turn lead to different ways to operationalize the trait at the empirical level (see the area below the dashed line in Figure 1–2). First, let us consider how conceptual and operational definitions are developed for the behavior to be observed. A conceptual or theoretical definition begins most often with unsystematic observations or hunches about a particular behavior from working in the clinic. For instance, therapists may be aware that meal planning and preparation, cleaning, and washing clothes are typical behaviors that people must do to live alone. Therapists often have to make predictions about how well a person would do at home, based on patient performances observed in the clinic. For instance, a therapist may feel that by observing a patient in the simple act of making a cup of instant coffee, a prediction could be made about that person's safety in preparing meals at home. These thoughts are then abstracted up to a more theoretical level where they are fit into a complex of behavior patterns, and a theory regarding the behavior of interest begins to be formed. Theories are used to explain behavior and in this case are only useful if they can be empirically verified. Therefore, it is important to be able to test a theory, which is where the operational definition comes in. To test a theory we must move from the conceptual level to the empirical level, at which the actual data are collected. To collect data regarding a particular theory of behavior, we must operationally define the behavior to be studied. An operational definition then makes concrete what is implied in the conceptual definition. For example, the concept of kitchen safety might be operationalized as the person's ability to verbalize kitchen safety concerns; demonstrate safe use of the stove; and safely obtain supplies, prepare food, and clean up afterward.

The conceptual definition of the behavior is important because it attempts to define the boundary of the domain covered by the behavior. For instance, a narrow definition of kitchen safety might be operationalized as the ability to safely heat meals in a microwave. A broader definition would include obtaining groceries, preparing three meals a day, and cleaning up after meal preparation. Also, the domain may consist of one or more dimensions. For each dimension, each act or task must be explicitly and sequentially described. That is, within each dimension are potentially several "behavior units" that comprise the behavior to be observed, and each must be detailed. For instance, the concept of "kitchen safety" can include cognitive as well as motor aspects. A person can verbalize safe procedures but act unsafely, or a person may not even be aware of safety concerns. Further, the scope of safety issues can vary. For instance, a person may be safe in routine situations but unable to respond to emergency situations, such as a fire on the stove. This lack of safety can be due to cognitive problems (e.g., lack of immediate recognition of problem and timely response), motor problems (e.g., moves too slowly to respond to the emergency), or affective problems (e.g., does not care about safety).

In thinking about the behavior units and dimensions of the behavior to be observed, Borg and Gall (1983) have suggested that to be able to observe the behavior reliably, one should use descriptive or low-inference variables or items. In general, "observer inference refers to the degree of observer judgement intervening between the actual data observed and the subsequent coding of that data on observational instruments." (Herbert & Attridge, 1975, p. 10). A descriptive or low-inference variable is one that can be clearly defined and easily observed (e.g., turns on the stove). While many behaviors in occupational or physical therapy are of the low-inference variety, on some occasions a therapist may be called on to observe high-inference behaviors. A high-inference variable is one that involves a series of events, where the behaviors are more global or where the therapist must draw a conclusion about the behavior being observed. Examples of high-inference variables might be items such as "how well will the person respond to kitchen emergencies?" or more globally, "How well does the individual respond to household emergencies?" Being able to respond to emergencies represents a series of behaviors. How should the therapist rate the behavior if all behaviors related to emergency responses are not successful, such as when the person can dial 911 but cannot describe what to do next for a fire? Even more difficult to reliably observe are evaluative variables. An evaluative variable requires an inference regarding the behavior, plus the therapist must make a judgment about the behavior as well. For example, an evaluative item might be, "Rate how safe the person is likely to be living alone." Not only does this type of item or variable require an inference, but the therapist must make a qualitative judgment to respond to the item.

Borg and Gall (1983) have warned that high-inference and evaluative variables often lead to less-reliable observations. To counter this reliability problem, Medley and Mitzel (1963, p. 252) have espoused a very strong position, stating that the observer should use the least amount of judgment possible, only a judgment "needed to perceive whether the behavior has occurred or not." Herbert and Attridge's (1975) position on the level of inference is more balanced, calling for the level of inference that is demanded by the complexity of the behavior studied. If it is essential to the behavior being observed that high-inference or evaluative variables are necessary, then to produce reliable observational data, a great deal of attention must be given to training observers to be able to "see" and then rate the high-inference and evaluative types of variables consistently. This point is addressed more in the section on training observers.

To organize the behavior units and dimensions of the behavior as specified in the conceptual and operational definitions, a table of specifications is often used. A table of specifications guides instrument construction to ensure that 1) all dimensions and behavior units are considered and 2) a sufficient number of items is written to cover each dimension. Later, if content validation is required for the type of test score interpretation, the table of specifications again is used in classifying the instrument's items by a panel of experts.

An example of a table of specifications is shown in Table 1–5 for measuring the behavior of kitchen safety. In the table, the column headings indicate important components of the construct of kitchen safety. The rows reflect different dimensions of each of these behavior units. At each intersection of the rows and columns, we would make a judgment about the relative importance of this cell and the number of items to be included. It is common to use experts as resources in identifying the degree of importance of each part of the assessment. Assuming we wanted to keep the tool brief, we might start by limiting ourselves to 20 items total, and then apportion them, based on our predetermined percentages. For example, the first row-by-column cell, "verbalize safety and cognitive," we show as being somewhat less important (10%, or two items) then the second row-by-column cell, "obtain supplies and sensorimotor" (20%, or four items). The number of items depends on many factors, such as the level of complexity of the behavior to be measured, the number of dimensions and behavior units that were operationally defined, and the amount of time available to observe the behavior.

The Observational Form

Once the behavior to be observed has been fully defined (both theoretically and operationally) and the number of items has been decided on, the next step is to produce the observational form. The observational form is used to record or score the behavior. If each behavior unit under each dimension has been described, then it is just a matter of transferring those descriptions, which then become the items, to the observational form. If each behavior is well defined and involves low-inference behaviors, the form can be quite easy to use, as shown in Table 1–6.

It may be important to have several high-inference or evaluation items, such as those shown in the lower part of Table 1–6. It should be obvious that these items require a higher level of observation skill and are much more difficult to measure objectively. To increase the level of reliability for the high-inference and evaluative items, one can opt to have fewer categories to record the behavior. That is, a three-point scale is easier to use and produces more reliable ratings than a seven-point scale. Borg and Gall (1983) suggest that most human observations cannot be reliably rated on a continuum with more than five points. While it is a well-known fact that if you increase the observation points (all other factors held constant), the amount of variance increases, which in turn increases the reliability of a scale. However, the increase in variance and, hence, reliability may be spuriously inflated and represent more

TABLE 1–5				
EXAMPLE OF TABLE OF SPECIFICATIONS FOR KITCHEN SAFETY*				
	Verbalize Safety	**Obtain Supplies**	**Prepare Food**	**Clean Up**
Cognitive	10%/2	10%/2	15%/3	5%/1
Sensorimotor	—	20%/4	20%/4	10%/2
Affective	10%/2	—	—	—

Percentage indicates percent of items allocated per cell, followed by actual number of items. A blank cell indicates that the component/dimension represented by that cell is not relevant.

error variance than systematic variance. Therefore, we agree with Borg and Gall that using three to five observation points per item should be sufficient to rate most behaviors and improves the reliability of the observations of high-inference and evaluative items.

Finally, when the observational form is developed, it is important to field test the instrument. Field testing (or pilot testing) allows one to be sure all aspects of the behavior have been included, determine whether each behavior unit is sufficiently described to be able to rate it, and assess how easy the form is to use. In addition, instructions on how to use the form should be developed and field tested. Any revisions to the form or instructions should be made and field tested again to see how the revisions work. Once the form has been sufficiently field tested, we then turn to the training of observers to use the form.

Rasch Scaling Procedures

Often the items on the observational form are arranged hierarchically. That is, some behaviors are presumed to be easier than others, or some behaviors precede others. For instance, many therapists would suggest that getting on and off a chair is easier than getting in and out of a bathtub. From a theoretical perspective, it is important to be able to validate this hierarchy. The Rasch measurement models (Fischer, 1993) are procedures that are currently being used in the development of assessment tools in occupational therapy that have the potential to validate hierarchically based assessments. Rasch measurement models are, in part, scaling procedures that permit a test developer to rank order the items on a scale from easiest to hardest. This ordering of items in turn allows the ordering of individuals in terms of their ability on the trait being measured. For example, the FIM motor and cognitive items could be hierarchically ordered such that an individual can be placed on a continuum from less independent to more independent. More importantly, Rasch scaling converts the ordinal response that the observer marks on the FIM (7 = complete independence to 1 = total assistance) to an interval scale of measurement. Interval measurements have more desirable properties than ordinal measurements, e.g., the

TABLE 1-7

OVERVIEW OF STEPS IN DEVELOPING OBSERVATIONAL MEASURES

Develop conceptual definition of behavior to be observed
Develop operational definitions of behaviors to be observed
Develop table of specifications
    Percentage weights of relative behaviors within domain
    Number of items
Develop observation form
    Pilot
    Define and repilot as needed
    Finalize form
Train observers to use form
Assess rater agreement
    Intrarater
    Interrater
Assess reliability appropriate to purpose
    Classical procedures
    Variance components procedures
    Rasch-based procedures
Assess validity appropriate to purpose
    Content
    Criterion referenced
    Construct
Assess any ethical issues
    Unintended effects of measurement
    Social consequences

help to prevent "rater drift" (Borg & Gall, 1983) and ensure the reliability of the observational data. An overview of the steps we have presented in developing an observational measure is given in Table 1–7.

DEVELOPING LOCAL NORMS FOR OBSERVATIONAL MEASURES

Before addressing the need for local norms and how to gather them, it might be useful to consider the topic of norms in general. Norms refer to the scores obtained from the individuals who were tested during standardization of the scale. For many commercially available measurement tools, normative data have already been collected and summarized in the test manual for use in evaluating an individual's score. These types of tools are more commonly referred to as standardized measurements. Standardized means that the measurement has been taken under a specific set of guidelines for administration and scoring. When data are collected in a systematic standardized fashion, the scores for all the individuals tested can be combined and summarized. The data are typically summarized by reporting means, standard deviations, percentiles, and various forms of standard scores. The summarized data then are reported as norms in the manual accompanying the test. Norms should not be confused with standards, which are predetermined levels used to make decisions. Rather, norms are just the summarized data for the sample tested. If a different sample is tested, the norms can change. Given that norms are sample dependent, a thorough description of the individuals in the norm group is essential for score interpretation.

In describing the norm group, attention should be paid to how relevant, representative, and recent the norm group is. *Relevant* refers to whether the norm group has similar characteristics to those of individuals to be evaluated. For example, if your practice involves mostly children and you see that in the norm group, the youngest age represented is 16, the norms will not be relevant. Representative refers to whether the population was sampled in a way that adequately reflects your patients or clients. For example, were appropriate percentages of ages, genders, and ethnic groups included? Finally, recency of norms refers to when the normative data were gathered. If the normative data are a few years old and no changes have occurred in our understanding of the trait or behavior being tested, then recency of norms is not an issue. However, if our understanding of the trait changes, like the FIM comprising three dimensions (and therefore three scores) and not one, then normative data on the FIM would have to be recollected to ensure adequate interpretation of the three new scores.

Normative data are very useful for therapists to compare an individual's level of functioning with the typical expectations for an unimpaired person. In some cases, a treatment facility might want to develop local norms. For instance, if a commercially developed tool is used frequently by the facility for which normative data are already available, collection of local norms would enable a comparison of the type of individuals seen at the facility to the commercial norms. One might find differences in the characteristics of individuals served by your own facility and the sample that was used to develop the norms in the test manual. Additionally, many tools used in practice do not have normative data; therefore, compiling local norms would help in clinical decision-making.

To develop local normative data, one must be sure that the measurement tool is used in a standardized manner; that is, all therapists are trained in using the tool, administering it in the same time frame, and scoring it in the same manner. Under these conditions, the data collected on the tool at the facility can be combined and basic descriptive statistics computed (e.g., means, standard deviations, percentiles). From the descriptive statistics, standard scores can be computed to use in comparing individual scores (e.g., T-scores, where the mean is set at 50 and the standard deviation is 10). In this way, a person's raw score can be converted to a percentile and to a T-score for comparison. While percentiles are useful in that most people can understand them, they are not appropriate for statistical analyses. For example, a manager at the treatment facility might want to see what the "average" intake score is on the patients who have a diagnosis of head injury and their "average" exit scores. Percentiles should not be averaged; therefore, some form of standard score could be used. By compiling data on the tool over time, the manager could look at cost-to-benefit relationships, such as the differences in outcomes associated with different lengths of stay, and different kinds of therapy services. In fact, the need for such information has been an important motivator for the development of tools such as the FIM and the Uniform Data System (Center for Functional Assessment Research, 1990).

SUMMARY AND CONCLUSIONS

This chapter began with a conceptual overview of the two primary issues in measurement theory, validity and reliability. Since many of the measurement tools described in this book are observationally based measurements, we focused much of the chapter around the issues therapists need to be familiar with in making observational measurements. This overview should set the stage for a better understanding of observational measurement encountered in later chapters in this book. Finally, the chapter ends with the use of local norms to enable therapists and facility managers to make comparisons of individuals or groups of individuals at their facility.

A chapter on measurement theory would not be complete without attention to the ethics involved in testing human beings. We are reminded of the seminal work of Messick (1989), in which he asserts that one should not interpret the meaning of any score without consideration of the social consequences of that test score.

Because it is common to use tools to assess individuals, we must be careful that the label of the tool does not take on more meaning than the validity evidence can support. That is, many traits such as competence, self-esteem, and functional independence have value implications that may not be a part of their validity evidence. Thus, careful test score interpretation is called for. Finally, we must constantly be aware of the potential and actual social consequences of testing, e.g., the risks of a self-fulfilling prophecy operating when the assumption is that identified impairments necessarily result in disability. Since no "statistically based approaches" exist to evaluate the value implications of test use or the social consequences of test interpretation, it becomes important to raise and openly discuss these concerns in a variety of forums. In summary, responsible testing requires that the measurement community understand that "validity and values are one imperative, not two, and test validation implicates both science and the ethics of assessment" (Messick, 1994, p.8).

GLOSSARY

Attenuated—Measurement error has influenced the result.

Disattenuated—Measurement error removed.

Local norms—Normative data collected at a specific facility or site.

Nomological network—A representation of how different constructs are interrelated.

Norms—Summarized scores from group tested during standardization of a scale.

Observer bias—When characteristics of the observer or the situation being observed influence the ratings made by the observer.

Observer presence—When the presence of the observer alters the behavior of the individual being tested.

Reliability coefficient—An expression of how accurately a given measurement tool has been able to assess an individual's true score.

Sample dependency—Has two forms: a) inferential, when the statistic of interest fluctuates from sample to sample and b) psychometric, when the items constituting an instrument are a "sample" from a universe of all potential items.

Standardized—Measurement taken under a specific set of guidelines for administration and scoring.

Table of specifications—Grid used to lay out the dimensions of a scale.

Validity—The process by which scores from measurements take on meaning.

Validity coefficient—Correlation between a predictor and the criterion.

REFERENCES

*Adamovich, B. L. B. (1992). Pitfalls in functional assessment: A comparison of FIM ratings by speech-language pathologists and nurses. *Neurorehabilitation, 2*(4), 42–51.

Andrich, D. (1988). *Rasch models of measurement. Sage University Paper Series on Quantitative Applications in the Social Sciences, 07-068.* Beverly Hills: Sage Publications.

Benson, J., & Clark, F. (1982). A guide for instrument development and validation for occupational therapists. *American Journal of Occupational Therapy, 36,* 789–800.

Benson, J., & Hagtvet, K. (1996). The Interplay Between Design and Data Analysis in the Measurement of Coping. In M. Zeidner & N. Ender (Eds.), *Handbook of coping: Theory, research applications.* New York: Wiley.

Borg, W., & Gall, M. (1983). *Educational research: An introduction* (4th ed.). New York: Longman.

Brennan, R. (1983). *Elements of generalizability theory.* Iowa City, IA: American College Testing Program.

Campbell, D., & Fiske, D. (1959). Convergent and discriminant validation by the multitrait-multimethod matrix. *Psychological Bulletin, 56,* 81–105.

Carey, R. G., & Posavac, E. J. (1978). Program evaluation of a physical medicine and rehabilitation unit: A new approach. *Archives of Physical Medicine and Rehabilitation, 59, 145–154.*

*Center for Functional Assessment Research. (1990). Guide for the use of the uniform data set for medical rehabilitation including the functional independence measure (FIM) version 3.1. Buffalo, NY: Research Foundation—State University of New York.

*Chau, N., Daler, S., Andre, J. M., & Patris, A. (1994). Inter-rater agreement of two functional independence scales: The Functional Independence Measure (FIM) and a subjective uniform continuous scale. *Disability and Rehabilitation, 16*(2), 63–71.

_____

* Indicates the source was used to evaluate the FIM.

Crick, G., & Brennan, R. (1982). GENOVA: *A generalized analysis of variance system (Fortran IV computer program and manual.)* Dorchester, MA: University of Massachussets at Boston, Computer Facilities.

Crocker, L. J., & Algina, J. (1986). Introduction to classical and modern test theory. New York: Holt.

Cronbach, L. J. (1971). Test validation. In R. L. Thorndike (Ed.), *Educational measurement* (2nd ed.) (pp. 443–507). Washington DC: American Council on Education.

Cronbach, L. J., Gleser, R., Nanda, H., & Rajaratnam, N. (1972). *The dependability of behavioral measurements: Generalizability of scores and profiles.* New York: Wiley.

Cronbach, L. J., & Meehl, P. E. (1955). Construct validity of psychological tests. *Psychological Bulletin, 52,* 281–302.

*Dodds, A., Martin, D. P., Stolov, W. C., & Deyo, R. A. (1993). Validation of the Functional Independence Measurement and its performance among rehabilitation inpatients. *Archives of Physical Medicine, 74,* 531–536.

Ebel, R. (1951). Estimation of the reliability of ratings. *Psychometrika, 16,* 407–424.

Evans, W. J., Cayten, D. G., & Green, P. A. (1981). Determining the generalizability of rating scales in clinical settings. *Medcare, 19,* 1211–1220.

Fischer, A. (1993). The assessment of IADL motor skills: An application of many faceted Rasch analysis. *American Journal of Occupational Therapy, 47,* 319–329.

Frick, T., & Semmel, M. (1978). Observer agreement and reliabilities of classroom observational measures. *Review of Educational Research, 48,* 157–184.

*Fricke, J., Unsworth, C., & Worrell, D. (1993). Reliability of the Functional Independence Measure with occupational therapists. *Australian Occupational Therapy Journal, 40*(1), 7–15.

*Granger, C. V., Cotter, A. C., Hamilton, B. B, Fiedler, R. C., & Hens, M. M. (1990). Functional assessment scales: A study of persons with multiple sclerosis. *Archives of Physical Medicine and Rehabilitation, 71,* 870–875.

*Granger, C. V., & Hamilton, B. B. (1988). *Development of a uniform national data system for medical rehabilitation 1984–1987.* (Grant Number G008435062). Washington DC: National Institute on Disability and Rehabilitation Research, Office of Special Education and Rehabilitation Services, Department of Education.

*Granger, C. V., Hamilton, B. B., Keith, R. A., Zielezny, M., & Sherwin, F. S. (1986). Advances in functional assessment for medical rehabilitation. *Topics in Geriatric Rehabilitation, 1*(3) 59–74.

Haggard, E. (1958). *Intraclass correlation and the analysis of variance.* New York: Dryden Press.

*Hamilton, B. B., Granger, C. V., Sherwin, S. S., Zielezny, M., & Tashman, J. S. (1987). A uniform national data system for medical rehabilitation. In M. J. Fuhrer (Ed.), *Rehabilitation outcomes: Analysis and measurement* (pp. 137–146). Baltimore, MD: Paul H. Brookes Publishing Co.

*Heinemann, A., Hamilton, B., Granger, C., Linacre, M., & Wright, B. (1992). *Rehabilitation efficacy for brain and spinal injured: Final report.* (Grant Number R49/CCR503609). Atlanta, GA: Center for Disease Control.

Herbert, J., & Attridge, C. (1975). A guide for developers and users of observation systems and manuals. *American Educational Research Journal, 12,* 1–20.

Hoyt, C. (1941). Test reliability estimated by the analysis of variance. *Psychometrika, 6,* 153–160.

Jöreskog, K. G. (1969). A general approach to maximum likelihood factor analysis. *Psychometrika, 34,* 183–202.

Jöreskog, K. G. (1973). A general method for estimating a linear structural equation system. In A. Goldberger & D. Duncan (Eds.). *Structural equation models in the social sciences* (pp. 85–112). New York: Academic Press.

Kerlinger, F. (1986). *Foundations of behavioral research* (3rd ed.). New York: Holt.

Law, M. (1987). Measurement in occupational therapy: Scientific criteria for evaluation. *Canadian Journal of Occupational Therapy, 54*(3), 133–138.

*Linacre, J. M., Heinemann, A. W., Wright, B. D., Granger, C. V., & Hamilton, B. B. (1994). The structure and stability of the Functional Independence Measure. *Archives of Physical Medicine, 75,* 127–132.

Lord, F., & Novick, M. (1968). *Statistical theories of mental test scores.* Reading, MA: Addison-Wesley.

Mahoney, F. I., & Barthel, D. W. (1965). Functional evaluation: The Barthel index. *Maryland State Medical Journal, 14,* 61–65.

McGaw, B., Wardrop, J., & Bunda, M. (1972). Classroom observation schemes—Where are the errors? *American Journal of Educational Research, 9,* 13–27.

Medley, D., & Mitzel, H. (1963). Measuring classroom behavior by systematic observation. In N. Gage (Ed.). *Handbook of research on teaching.* Skokie, IL: Rand McNally.

Messick, S. (1994). Foundations of validity: Meaning and consequences in psychological assessment. *European Journal of Psychological Assessment, 10,* 1–9.

Messick, S. (1989). Validity. In R. Linn (Ed.)., *Educational measurement* (3rd ed.). Washington DC: American Council on Education.

Mulaik, S. (1972). *The foundations of factor analysis.* New York: McGraw Hill.

Nunnally, J. (1978). *Psychometric theory* (2nd ed.). New York: McGraw Hill.

Pedhazur, E. (1982). *Multiple regression in behavioral research* (2nd ed.). New York: Holt.

Roebroeck, M., Harlaar, J., & Lankhorst, G. (1993). The application of generalizability theory reliability assessment: An illustration using isometric force measurements. *Physical Therapy, 73,* 386–395.

Rowley, G. (1976). The reliability of observational measures. *American Journal of Educational Research, 13,* 51–60.

Shavelson, R., & Webb, N. (1991). *Generalizability theory: A primer.* Newbury Park: Sage.

Short-DeGraff, M., & Fisher, A. G. (1993). Nationally speaking–A proposal for diverse research methods and a common research language. *American Journal of Occupational Therapy, 47,* 295–297.

Sim, J., & Arnell, P. (1993). Measurement validity in physical therapy research. *Physical Therapy, 73,* 102–115.

Spool, M. (1978). Training programs for observers of behavior: A review. *Personnel Psychology, 31,* 853–888.

Standards for Educational and Psychological Testing. (1985). Washington DC: American Psychological Association.

Thorndike, R., & Hagen, E. (1977). *Measurement and evaluation in psychology and education* (4th ed.). New York: Wiley & Sons.

Wilkerson, D. L., Batavia, J.D., & DeJong, G. (1992). The use of functional status measures for payment of medical rehabilitation services. *Archives of Physical Medicine, 74,* 111–120.

World Health Organization (1980). *International classification of impairments, disabilities, and handicaps.* Geneva: World Health Organization.

Component Assessments of the Adult

CHAPTER 2

Muscle Strength

Maureen J. Simmonds, MCSP, PT, PhD

SUMMARY One of the most frequent physical assessment tests used in rehabilitation is the testing of muscle strength. Strength measurements are used for diagnostic and prognostic purposes. Changes in strength are also used to assess changes in a patient's condition and to determine the effectiveness of exercise programs. Although *strength* is a frequently used term, it is not universally used for the same measurement. Strength may be used when *muscle torque, force, power,* or *work* would be a more appropriate term. A myriad of anatomic, physiologic, biomechanical, psychological, pathologic and other factors contribute to muscle performance. Knowledge of these factors is important if tests of muscle strength are to be carried out and interpreted in a meaningful manner. Clinical assessment of muscle strength involves measuring the force exerted against an external force or resistance. This force may include the effect of gravity and that exerted by a therapist or a muscle testing device. Manual muscle tests (MMTs) without instrumentation have a long history of clinical use but have been subjected to little scientific scrutiny. MMTs are limited by the strength of the examiner and are of limited value because of their unproven reliability and lack of responsiveness. Instrumented MMTs with hand-held dynamometry improve the reliability and responsiveness of testing muscle strength but are also limited by the strength of the examiner. Isokinetic and isoinertial devices are now frequently used to assess muscle performance in static and dynamic modes. The devices are mechanically reliable and are reasonably reliable in measuring the forces exerted by muscles, although this depends on the conditions of testing. Most reliability studies have been conducted on normal, healthy individuals. The validity of muscle strength tests has not been tested. They appear to have face validity for measuring the force exerted by a muscle. The validity of muscle strength tests as diagnostic or prognostic tools has not been established. Muscle strength tests are in frequent use despite the paucity of information about the reliability of strength tests in populations for whom the test is designed, rather than in healthy individuals. It is essential that the relationship between the patient's problems with function and clinical tests of muscle strength is established.

OVERVIEW OF MUSCLE STRENGTH

The measurement of muscle strength is a fundamental component of a physical assessment. Strength measurements are used in clinical practice for diagnostic purposes, to examine the improvement or deterioration of a patient's status over time, and as a predictive or prognostic tool. Strength tests are also used to determine the extent of strength loss by comparing the results of strength tests between opposite limbs or against normative data.

In addition, strength tests are used in clinical research as outcome measures. The results of strength tests can be used to describe a population and examine the effects of exercise programs or some other therapy. Measurements of static and dynamic muscle performance (torque output, fatigue, work, or power) can be related to the histochemistry, biochemistry, and electromyographic activity of muscle to better understand the physiologic bases of muscle function and to determine the relationship between static and dynamic strength tests and functional activities.

The major function of the muscular system is to stabilize and support the body and allow movement to occur. Muscle function is the product of a myriad of contributing subsystems. The biologic subsystems include sensory, motor, and cognitive systems. In addition, muscle function is influenced by the environment, the task, and the time and effort required to complete the task.

Many different techniques purport to measure strength. Some are very simple, such as manual muscle tests (MMTs), and others use complex equipment and computerized technology and provide a plethora of information. Is one method of testing better or more reliable than the other? What do these tests tell us? Do either of these methods of testing have anything to do with function? Clinicians and researchers test muscle strength regularly, but what do we really know about the psychometric characteristics of the tests in common clinical use? Are the tests reliable, valid, sensitive, and specific? Have the tests been tested? If so, under what conditions? Finally, what is known about the factors that influence the test? To address these and other questions, it is necessary to discuss strength testing in a comprehensive manner. Thus, the purpose of this chapter is to critically review the theoretical and practical bases of muscle strength and the clinical methods of muscle strength testing.

Historical Perspective of Strength Tests

MANUAL MUSCLE TESTS

Early clinical tests of muscle strength involved the use of manual resistance by the therapist. The tests were, and still are, considered useful diagnostic and prognostic tests (Lamb, 1985), although they have been subjected to little scientific scrutiny. The initial development and documentation of MMTs occurred about 80 years ago and are attributed to Lovett, an orthopedic surgeon (Daniels and Worthingham, 1986; Kendall et al., 1993). The principles of MMT have changed little since that time, although some modifications have been made, especially in regard to the grading system used.

The bases of MMTs are simple and essentially reflect anatomic and biomechanical principles. Thus, they are measures of impairment rather than function, and while their use is most common for persons with disorders of the muscle or peripheral neural systems (Daniels and Worthingham, 1986), these tests have been used for patients with central nervous system problems, including those with brain injury (Riddle et al., 1989).

Fundamental to MMT is the notion that muscles, either individually or as a group, have a specific action on a joint. Based on this premise and utilizing the effects of gravity and manual resistance provided by the therapist as external forces, a patient is positioned in such a way that one muscle or group of muscles is primarily responsible for moving a joint through a specific range of motion. Grading of muscle strength is then based on the arc of movement produced by the muscle and the amount of external resistance to the motion. The muscle or tendon is palpated by the therapist to ensure that the muscle of interest is contracting and no substitution of muscle activity is responsible for the specific movement tested.

INSTRUMENTED TESTS OF MUSCLE STRENGTH

Although the criteria for grading muscle strength are quite specific, manual grading does not provide quantitative data about the force or torque generated by the muscle. Thus, instrumented strength testing (IST) was developed. Instrumented strength testing allows one to quantify more precisely the force generated by a muscle or a group of muscles. Early IST devices consisted of cable tensiometers, strain gauges, or hand-held load cells that measured isometric strength at some point in the range. Hand-held dynamometers (HHDs) are in regular clinical use and are discussed later in this chapter.

The second generation of IST devices were those that measured dynamic muscle strength. Such devices can be categorized as isokinetic, i.e., constant velocity, or isoinertial, i.e., constant resistance. The Cybex II (Lumex Inc., Bay Shore, NY), Kin-Com (Chattecx Corp., Chattanooga, TN), and Lido (Loredan Biomedical Inc., Davis, CA) are examples of isokinetic devices that can be used to measure muscle strength in the limbs or the trunk. The B-200 (Isotechnologies, Inc., Hillsborough, NC) back testing device is an example of an isoinertial device that measures trunk strength. These devices provide quantitative information about muscle function. They can provide information about muscle strength, endurance, power, and coordination. The technological sophistication of these devices has advanced and moved ahead of the scientific evaluation of the technology, due, in part, to successful marketing.

Terms and Issues Related to Strength Testing and Measurement

Mayhew and Rothstein (1985) have noted that *strength* is a vague, nonscientific term that needs to be operationally defined if it is to be of value. They base their argument on the fact that reported tests of muscle strength have utilized many different ways of determining strength, a fact that is indicative of the imprecise use of the word. A dictionary definition of strength highlights the problem. *Muscular strength* is defined as *muscular force or power.* Yet these are different terms with different meanings. It is therefore imperative that operational definitions are used.

Strength is defined as the force or torque produced by a muscle during a maximal voluntary contraction. It is a measure of the maximal force or torque required to resist an isometric or isotonic contraction. *Torque* is a more precise term. It is the degree to which a force tends to rotate an object about a specified fulcrum. *Torque* is not a commonly used term in lay usage, which may explain why it is a less ambiguous term than *strength.*

Quantified strength values may be reported in absolute terms or in relative values. For example, the strength of one muscle group may be expressed as a ratio with the torque of another muscle group. The agonist-to-antagonist ratio is most frequently used, but strength may also be expressed in terms of body weight.

Another measurement term is *power. Power* is work per unit time. The temporal factor indicates that the muscle is working over a period of time. This time period may be long or short. One example of such a period is the time taken by the muscle to move a limb through a range of motion. Alternatively, the time may be the total duration of a purposefully fatigue-inducing endurance activity. *Endurance* is the ability to maintain torque over a period of time or a set number of contractions. Conversely, *fatigue* is the inability to maintain torque over a period of time or a set number of contractions. Fatigue is described as either the amount of power that is lost or that which is maintained. Thus, a 30% loss of power is equivalent to the maintenance of 70% of power. These terms apply to all types of muscle contractions.

An *isometric contraction* is when the muscle generates an internal force or tension, but no movement of a joint occurs. The term *isometric* is a misnomer. It means constant length, but clearly the muscle does change shape and the protein filaments within the muscle certainly shorten (Gordon et al., 1966). An *isotonic contraction* is when the internal force generated by a muscle results in movement of a joint. Again, the term *isotonic* is a misnomer. *Isotonic* means same tension or force through the motion, yet this is clearly not the case.

Isotonic contractions are further described as concentric and eccentric. A *concentric contraction* is a shortening contraction. It occurs when the internal force produced by the muscle exceeds the external force of resistance. An *eccentric contraction* is one in which the muscle lengthens while it continues to maintain tension.

Cogent discussion of the measurement of muscle performance requires consideration of the principles of measurement as well as the principles of muscle activity. Measurement principles are discussed in depth elsewhere in this book. Some fundamental principles are now briefly presented.

Reliability is the degree to which repeated measurements of a stable phenomenon fall closely together. These measurements can be taken by the same person (intratester or within-tester reliability) or by different testers (intertester or between-tester reliability). Devices that measure the same phenomenon may also be compared (concurrent, parallel-forms reliability). The notion of reliability is illustrated in Figure 2–1. Reliability of measures is important, but it is not the only criterion to be considered. A reliable measure is not useful if it does not measure what it is supposed to measure. If the measure misses the target, it is not a true or valid measure.

Validity is the accuracy of the measurement. It is the degree to which the measurement corresponds to the true state of affairs. It is *the* most important consideration when selecting a test. A measure is validated by accumulating evidence that supports logical inferences made from the measure (Johnston et al., 1992).

The types of validity in most frequent use include face, construct, and criterion validity. *Face validity* is the lowest

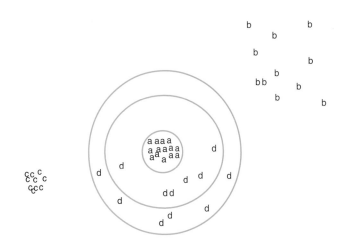

Graphic representation of the concepts of reliability and validity

a Scores are both reliable and valid
b Scores are neither reliable nor valid
c Scores are reliable but not valid
d Scores are valid but not reliable

FIGURE 2–1. Graphic representation of reliability and validity.

level of validity. A measure has face validity if it simply appears to measure what it is supposed to measure. *Construct validity* is the degree to which the scores obtained are in agreement with the theoretical construct of that which is measured. *Criterion validity* concerns the extent to which the measure is related to other measures that are regarded as a "gold standard" of measurement. Another property that any clinical measurement tool needs is responsiveness or sensitivity to change. *Responsiveness* is the ability of a test to measure clinically important change.

Variability and error are factors in all measurements. A number of sources contribute to the variability of test measurements. Knowledge of the sources of variability is necessary for appropriate interpretation of test results.

The *measurement device* may be a source of variability. The device may be reliable, in that under the same conditions it always provides a similar reading. However, the device may *systematically* over- or underestimate the measurement. This is one reason why devices such as an HHD are not necessarily interchangeable.

The *observer* is another source of variability in a test measurement. Generally, less variability occurs within than between observers. The variability may be more systematic within than between observers but may differ depending on the test; therefore, it needs to be measured.

The *subject* can be a source of variability. Strength measurements may change within a testing session due to fatigue or discomfort. They may change between sessions depending on the stability of the condition, intervening activities, and other stresses.

Psychometric factors obviously influence the measurement of muscle strength. In addition, a myriad of biologic and motivational characteristics contribute to the muscle tension, muscle strength, and muscle performance that is being measured. These factors are now discussed.

Biologic Factors Influencing Muscle Strength

At the most basic level, movement and force are produced by the contraction of the sarcomeres (Ghez, 1991). The amount of contractile force that a muscle can produce depends on its absolute size, i.e., its length and cross-sectional area, the cytoarchitecture, the phenotype, and the vascularity of the muscle. These factors influence not only the magnitude of force that the muscle can generate but also how quickly that force can be generated and the duration for which it can be maintained.

The amount of force generated by a muscle is controlled through the recruitment order and the firing rate of the motor neuron. Motor units are recruited in a fixed order from weakest to strongest. The weakest input controls the SF (slow fatigable) fibers, which are resistant to fatigue but generate the least force. The FFR (fast fatigue-resistant) units are recruited next and, finally, the FF (fast fatigable)

units which can exert the most force, but which are prone to fatigue. In humans, muscles are composed of many different types of motor fibers; however, the fibers supplied by each motor neuron are homogenous. Some pathologic or injury conditions, e.g., low back problems, result in selective atrophy of FF (Mattila et al., 1986; Rissanen et al., 1995; Zhu et al, 1989). However, this loss can be reversed with training at maximal or submaximal effort (Rissanen et al., 1995).

The endurance performance of a muscle is influenced by a number of factors. The morphologic characteristics of the muscle, muscle mass, capilliary density, and percentage of SF fibers are all related to efficiency of activity (Coyle, 1995). The recruitment of a larger muscle mass and the spread of power output over a large area, including the recruitment of different muscles, all potentially enhance endurance or limit fatigue.

Biomechanical factors are also important in muscle function. These factors are linked to anatomic structure and play a role in the muscles' ability to generate force and cause movement. Cytoarchitectural factors that influence muscle performance include the arrangement of muscle fibers and the angle of pull of the muscle.

At the macro muscle level, aponeuroses and tendons can both store energy and redirect force, thus improving the efficiency of muscle action. Passive tension of a muscle contributes to the total tension that a muscle generates. Shorter muscles have relatively high levels of passive tension earlier in the range than longer muscles. This fact contributes to the differences in length-tension relationships between muscles.

Another factor that influences muscle performance is elastic energy. Elastic energy can be stored and transformed into kinetic energy (Soderberg, 1992). Passive tension and elastic energy are important because they influence measurements of muscle strength. Application of a stretch prior to a measurement can increase the amount of force generated by the muscle.

At the micro level, the generation of force is influenced by the arrangement of muscle fibers (Trotter et al., 1995). If the fibers of the motor unit are in series rather than parallel, then the capacity of the motor unit to develop force is hindered. This is because the total force that can be developed by a motor unit is related to the sum of forces generated by fibers lying in parallel, not in series, to each other. Thus, forces would be smaller in a series-fibered muscle, such as sartorious, compared with a muscle with parallel fibers, such as soleus (Edgerton et al., 1989).

Based on the work of several researchers, Soderberg (1992) has illustrated how muscles with the same mass, angle of pull, and fiber type, but with different cross-sectional areas and length differ in the magnitude of force that they can generate and the velocity with which they can generate this force. All other factors being equal, the larger the muscle's cross-sectional area, the larger is the muscle's force-generation capacity. Within this same muscle paradigm, it is clear that the shorter the muscle fibers, the greater the velocity with which the peak force can be achieved (Soderberg, 1992).

The force-velocity relationships of a muscle are also important considerations. Essentially, lower forces are associated with faster velocities. Conversely, higher forces are associated with slower velocities. However, this relationship holds true only for concentric contractions. Eccentric contractions are associated with higher forces at higher velocities. The magnitude of force generated isometrically is lower than that generated eccentrically but higher than that generated concentrically (Komi, 1973).

It is clear that many factors influence the force that a muscle can exert and the duration for which it can do so. The physical factors discussed above are doubtless related to function. Some of the functional implications, such as the preponderance of SO (slow oxidative) muscle fibers in endurant muscles, are obvious. It also seems obvious that the method of testing muscles should provide information about their functional ability. This is not always the case. For instance, is an isometric test of muscle strength the best way to test a muscle whose primary function is one that involves rapid motion? Also, isolated tests of individual muscles may not give much indication of their ability to function in a coordinated pattern of activity.

PAIN AND MUSCLE PERFORMANCE

Perhaps one of the most important but least studied factors that influences muscle performance is the presence of pain. Pain and the fear of pain and injury influence the measure of muscle strength. This invalidates the measure as one of true strength. The presence of pain during an MMT is cause to discontinue the test (Daniels and Worthingham, 1986). But testing of muscle strength is done and needs to be done in patients with chronic pain. In such cases, the influence of pain on the measure of muscle strength has to recognized.

Pain has been oversimplified, which is why it has remained enigmatic, problematic, and a frequent cause of frustration for patient and clinician alike. A few erroneous beliefs about pain exist: 1) in the acute pain state, tissue injury and pain are related; and 2) in the chronic pain state, the tissue has healed and no physiologic reason exists for the pain to persist. The assumption, then, is that the pain is psychological or at least exaggerated.

In truth, pain and injury are not always well correlated. Nociceptive activity contributes to the physiologic dimension of pain, but pain is multidimensional and has cognitive and affective dimensions as well as physiologic components. Even the physiologic component of pain has been oversimplified. Unfortunately, a review of pain mechanisms is beyond the scope of this chapter. However, in measuring the muscle strength of patients that have had, or do have pain, clinicians and researchers should be aware that:

1. *Any* innervated tissue can be a source of pain
2. Tissue injury leads to the release of a *cascade* of biochemical mediators that are both neurogenic and nonneurogenic in origin
3. These biochemical mediators sensitize nociceptive nerve endings directly and indirectly (Coderre et al, 1993)

The presence of pain, the anticipation of pain, and the fear of injury can influence the performance of the person being tested. This influence can be at both a conscious and an unconscious level. Research is needed to examine the effect of pain on measures of muscle strength, both during test sessions and over time. Simplistic interpretations about a patient's "real pain" or lack of effort during muscle strength testing should be recognized as a reflection of the personal biases of the clinician. Although some workers have suggested that strength testing can provide evidence of pain and malingering, this is not true. No empirical evidence supports this biased opinion. Furthermore, the notion is flawed from a theoretical perspective because it assumes that pain mechanisms are stable and that a simple relationship exists between pain and motion or pain and muscle contraction. None of these assumptions are correct.

DEMOGRAPHIC FACTORS INFLUENCING MUSCLE STRENGTH

Conventional wisdom suggests that females are weaker than males and older individuals are weaker than younger individuals. This notion is reasonable and true for group comparisons of young versus old or male versus female *but* only as long as confounding variables such as height, weight, health status, and usual activity level are controlled. Several authors have reported that the strength of females is about 60 to 70 percent that of males (Backman et al., 1995; Kumar et al., 1995a; Kumar et al., 1995b; Newton et al, 1993a). This appears to be true across different muscle groups and for both isometric and dynamic methods of testing. However, Backman and colleagues (1995) reported that differences in measures of muscle strength between genders almost disappeared when the subjects' weight was considered. One fact that is evident from the literature is that a large range of individual variability exists in measures of muscle strength. Endurance measures are characterized by even greater variability. It is possible that psychosocial factors, including motivational factors, contribute to the high variability in endurance performance, which is a test of tolerance. Certainly, measures of pain tolerance are strongly influenced by psychosocial rather than physiologic factors (Harris and Rollman, 1983). Endurance is associated with the ability to tolerate discomfort and pain.

Significant losses in maximal force production occur with aging, although substantial variability can be seen in the rate of loss, both between individuals and between muscles (Rogers and Evans, 1993). The decline in muscle can be attributed to loss of muscle mass or an altered capacity of the muscle to generate force. Recent research has shown that dynamic strength declines earlier and more rapidly than isometric strength (Pentland, et al., 1995). Thus, the method of testing influences the results between different age groups.

Although a decline of muscle mass occurs in the elderly, this loss of strength is greater than that accounted for by cross-sectional area alone (Vandervoort and McComas, 1986). The loss of muscle mass is due to a decline in both the number and the size of muscle fibers and in the degree of vascularization (Rogers and Evans, 1993). Differential loss of fiber type may account for the differential decline in isokinetic, compared with isometric, strength (Pentland et al., 1995).

All of the previously discussed factors are influenced by inactivity and by cardiovascular fitness, as well as by aging. Thus, it is difficult to tease out causes and consequences of aging, inactivity, and cardiovascular fitness on measures of muscle strength. Furthermore, these changes can be reversed through training of sufficient intensity and duration. Thus, although normative data must account for gender and age, individual variability is paramount. Individual variability in muscle strength testing is even more crucial when tests of muscle strength are conducted clinically. In a clinical population, the physiologic and psychosocial impact of an injury or disease enhances this individual variability.

Cognitive Factors Influencing Muscle Strength

The capability for intentional and purposeful human action is rooted in cognitive activity (Bandura and Cervone, 1983). Tests of muscle strength are learned psychomotor skills for the tester and the testee. The contributory role of learning must be considered when strength tests are administered and interpreted. More practice over a longer time is necessary to learn a complex motor skill. If the test movement for strength testing is an unfamiliar movement or skill, then optimal performance cannot occur before the movement is learned. This results in a series of strength tests that show an increase in the magnitude of measured force over a period of time. This increase in force is the result of a learning effect, as well as an increase in muscle strength capability. (See section on trunk testing for more discussion on learning). A distinction must be made between an increase in muscle torque due to a true change in muscle strength and an increase in muscle torque due to learning the motor skill of the test.

Motivation and self-perception of abilities influence the measurement of strength. Self-efficacy is one's belief in personal capabilities to perform a specific action. Estlander and colleagues (1994) found that the patients' belief in their ability to endure physical activities was the most powerful predictor of isokinetic performance. Perhaps more importantly, these authors showed that a patient's fear of reinjury was also a pertinent factor in strength testing.

The patient's ability to focus on the strength test and to screen out distractions influences the measurement. This can be facilitated through instructions by the tester. Distractions have been shown to have a negative influence on test results. They influence the planning of the activity as well as the activity itself (Pratt and Abrams, 1994). Thus, strength testing conditions should be focused on the test in a consistent manner so that the truest measure of muscle strength is obtained.

Summary

Figure 2–2 summarizes the preceding information. It is clear from this overview section that many factors contribute to what would appear to be a simple muscle contraction. Clinicians must be aware that a myriad of factors contribute to muscle strength and that assessment of muscle strength is more than a mere test of the muscle. Although it is necessary to know *how* to test muscle strength, it is also necessary to know what the results of the test mean. The interpretation of the test results must be made in the context of all relevant factors.

CLINICAL STRENGTH TESTING

Muscle strength tests are indicated in the majority of patients who have pathology or injury that results in movement impairment. Tests of muscle strength are the most frequently used tests in physical rehabilitation (Cole et al., 1994). This is not surprising. The modus operandi of therapists involved in physical rehabilitation is to assist patients in attaining their optimum level of physical and occupational function. Muscles play a fundamental role in function, and loss of function is the primary reason that patients are referred to therapy.

It is clear from the previous section that many factors along the neuromuscular pathway, as well as cognitive and motivational factors, influence muscle performance. It is also clear that muscles contract and work in different ways depending on their usual function. It seems obvious, therefore, that if muscles are to be assessed, they should be assessed using tests that provide useful information regarding the muscle's ability to function. Secondly, the tests should provide objective, reliable information in the clinical population for which the tests are designed. Thirdly, the tests should be simple to use and simple to interpret; otherwise the tests will not be used, or if they are, then they are subject to misinterpretation. The following section discusses specific tests and the instruments used to assess

Subject factors

Healthy
Patients
  Injury
  Pathology
  Comorbidity
  Pain
Gender
Age
Height
Weight
Usual activity level
  Active
  Sedentary
General health status

Psychological factors

Motivation
Learning
Level of skill
Self-efficacy
Fear of injury
Distress
Depression
Perceived effort
Expectation

Methodologic factors

Manual
Instrumented
Individual vs. group muscles
Position of subject
Joint position of test
Stabilization
Warm-up
Prestretch
Previous practice
Rest periods
Encouragement
Order of testing
Static vs. dynamic
Concentric vs. eccentric
Velocity of testing
Isokinetic
Isoinertial
Criterion values
  Average
  Peak
Absolute or relative values
Position in range
Force/torque
Work
Power
Device
Device settings
Gravity correction
Tester skill
Tester expectation
Tester strength

STRENGTH

Muscle factors

Fiber type
  Fast fatigable
  Fast fatigue resistant
  Slow fatigable
Cytoarchitecture
  Angle of pull
  Length of lever
  Parallel vs. series fibers
Size of muscle
  Length
  Cross-sectional area
Vascularity
Innervation ratio

Measurement factors

Operational definition
Reliability
  Intratester
  Intertester
  Test-retest
Validity
  Face
  Construct
  Discriminative
  Predictive
Responsiveness

FIGURE 2–2. Summary of factors influencing the measure of muscle strength.

muscle strength and endurance. Issues of validity, reliability, and utility are addressed within this section.

Strength Test Protocol Documentation

No matter what the type or the purpose of the strength test, the testing protocol must be well described. Strength tests, as with any other measurement test, must be reproduced as exactly as possible so that measurement errors and artifacts are minimized. Thus, test protocol descriptions should include the following:

1. *Warm-up procedure.* The length of time or number of contractions prior to the test, as well as whether the warm-up contractions were maximal or submaximal.
2. *Previous practice sessions.* Motor skills are learned and improve with practice. Does the test measure a change in strength or an improvement in skill?
3. *The method of stabilization.* Can the subject stabilize himself or herself by holding on with hands? Are stabilization straps used? If so, where are the straps placed, and how many are there? The better the stabilization, the higher the torque.
4. *Rest periods.* What is the length of the rest period between contractions and set of contractions?
5. *Position of the subject.* Include the relation of the muscle to gravity. Is the position easily reproducible? Does the subject have back support? What are

the angles of the hip or knee? What is the effect of gravity?

6. *Order of testing.* Include the type of contractions (isometric, concentric, or eccentric), the muscle groups, and the velocity of testing.
7. *Commands and vocal encouragement.* Standardized commands should be used. Vocal encouragement should be standardized as much as possible.
8. *Test range of motion.* At what point in the range was the strength test conducted?
9. *Criterion measure.* Are peak or average values of torque or force used? Is work or power used? What was the number of repetitions, and were absolute or relative values used? For example, with absolute values, are the torques expressed as angle specific or the angles at peak torque? If relative values are used, relative to what?
10. *Instrument and settings.* What instrument was used, and how was it used? What were the settings on the machine, e.g., damping, lever arm, pause, or minimum force?

Isometric Tests

MANUAL MUSCLE TESTS

Probably the most common tests in general use are MMTs. These tests have a long history of use, require no equipment, and are generally regarded as basic clinical skills. These facts no doubt contribute to the frequency with which MMTs are used. Manual muscle tests are well described by Kendall and colleagues (1993) and by Daniels and Worthingham (1986). Both groups of authors stress the importance of attention to detail when using MMTs. Kendall and coworkers suggest that precision in MMT is necessary to preserve the "science" of muscle testing (p. 4). In fact, MMT has been subjected to little scientific scrutiny. That is not to suggest that the techniques are not sound, but merely that they have not been systematically tested. Proponents of techniques have the responsibility to test the techniques that they describe so well.

Nevertheless, some important points must be kept in mind regarding the use of MMT. Both Kendall and associates (1993) and Daniels and Worthingham (1986) describe standardized positions that attempt to isolate muscle function. Resistance to the motion is applied throughout the range of motion (Daniels and Worthingham, 1986) or at a specific point in the range (Kendall et al., 1993). In addition to applying resistance through the range of motion (the "make test"), Daniels and Worthingham also use a "break test" at the end of range. In the break test, the patient is instructed to "hold" the limb as the therapist applies a gradual increasing resistance. Pain or discomfort should not occur, and if it does then the test should be discontinued (Daniels and Worthingham, 1986, p. 3). Make and break tests are not equivalent and should not be used interchangeably. Using dynamometry, Bohannon (1988, 1990) has shown that significantly greater strength values occur with the break test compared with the make test in both healthy subjects and in patients.

Grading systems for MMT have included letter grades, numeric grades, percentage grades, and descriptive criteria. Pluses and minuses have also been utilized (Table 2–1). The methods of Kendall and colleagues and of Daniels and Worthingham have obvious similarities and some differences (e.g., grading system). Neither method has a proven advantage. Neither method has been subjected to much critical scrutiny. Based on the weight of the limited evidence available, the reliability of MMT is low (Beasley, 1961; Frese et al., 1987; Wadsworth et al., 1987). It is obvious that the reliability of the test would depend on which muscle was being tested, the strength of that muscle, and whether other confounding factors such as, but not limited to, the presence of spasticity, were present. The confounding impact of spasticity on the results of muscle strength tests is not surprising. It is surprising that the examiners' designation of "normal" is somewhat idiosyncratic.

In a study by Bohannon (1986), one third of the normal subjects were graded as "normal minus." Bohannon examined muscle strength of the knee extensors in a controlled trial. He compared knee extension "make" forces in 60 healthy adults and 50 patients with a variety of neuromuscular diagnoses. The MMT grades were contrasted with forces measured with an HHD. The author calculated dynamometer percentage scores for the patients, based on the dynamometer scores measured on the

TABLE 2–1

GRADING SYSTEMS USED IN MANUAL MUSCLE TESTING

Grading Symbols				Criteria for Muscle Grading
Normal	10	5	5.0	100%	Can move or hold against gravity and maximum resistance
Good +	9	4+	4.5	80%	Can raise part against
Good	8	4	4.0		gravity and an external
Good –	7	4–	3.66		resistance
Fair +	6	3+	3.33	50%	Can raise part against
Fair	5	3	3.0		gravity
Fair –	4	3–	2.66		
Poor +	3	2+	2.33	20%	Produces movement with
Poor	2	2	2.0		gravity eliminated
Poor –	1	2–	1.5		
Trace	T	1	1.0	5%	A flicker or feeble contraction
Zero	0	0	0.0	0%	No contraction

healthy subjects. These calculated scores were then compared with the measured scores. Essentially, the results revealed that the MMT and HHD scores were correlated but significantly different. Bohannon also reported that the MMT percentage scores overestimated the extent to which the patient was "normal." However, Bohannon seems to have trouble with the designation *normal,* since a third of his normal subjects were designated as "normal minus." Problems with this study are evident. One of the more pertinent concerns relates to the different starting positions used in testing muscle strength with HHD compared with MMT. All HHD testing was conducted in sitting positions, whereas MMT tests were conducted in side-lying positions. The author did not correct for effect of gravity even though it would have had a significant impact. Finally, Bohannon did not report reliability in this study.

Reliability differs depending on the strength of the muscle and its anatomic characteristics. It seems obvious that it is easier to palpate a contraction in a large superficial muscle like the quadriceps than in a small deep muscle such as the piriformis. Thus, reliability would be higher for an MMT in the quadriceps. Conversely, it would be difficult to determine whether the contraction of the quadriceps was good (80%) or normal (100%) in a large athletic individual because the therapist would have difficulty challenging the muscle with manual resistance.

This problem of relatively weak therapist strength was reported by Deones and colleagues (1994). These investigators measured quadriceps strength in a healthy population using the Kin-Com and HHD. They reported poor correlations in strength measured with each device, which they attributed to the examiner not being able to resist the force of the quadriceps.

In a review of MMT, Lamb (1985) noted that in MMT, the patient responds to the amount of force applied by the examiner. Different examiners no doubt apply a different amount of force, and the same examiner may apply a different amount of force at different times. Force application by therapists has been reviewed and tested and is a significant source of variability (Simmonds and Kumar, 1993a; Simmonds et al., 1994). Although the application of the testing technique can be standardized in terms of patient position and the point at which the examiner applies resistance to the muscle, the amount of applied resistance is still variable. The examiner also has to compare the muscle with "normal," but the concept of normal and the expectation of how a muscle should perform is somewhat idiosyncratic. In addition to problems with reliability, MMT grading scales are not responsive to change (Griffen et al., 1986). A large change in muscle strength is necessary before such variation is reflected in a change of grade on an MMT scale. For example, a muscle may be conferred a grade of "good" because it can move a joint through a full range of movement against gravity and an external force applied by the examiner. Although repeated testing over time would reveal an increase in the muscle's functional ability, this improvement could not be measured using the zero-normal grading system. The use of "pluses" and "minuses" to the grading system may have been instituted in an effort to improve the responsiveness of the test but probably only leads to lower levels of reliability.

The lack of reliability and responsiveness of MMT is problematic because the test is supposed to measure change in a patient's muscle strength. This may not be a problem clinically if other more responsive tests are used to measure change in the patient's function. The other tests may provide more useful information in regard to how the muscle is functioning; they could also help to validate MMTs. But one must ask, if MMTs are not useful, why use them?

The main value of the MMTs is in their *apparent* ability (which needs to be tested) to isolate and to test the contractability and "strength" of individual muscles and groups of muscles that are weak. The use of MMTs is less useful in stronger muscles because it is limited by the ability and strength of the therapist to provide resistance to the muscle while adequately stabilizing the patient. MMTs have limited usefulness in recording improvement or deterioration in a patient's condition because they have poor reliability and lack responsiveness. It could be argued that, if the reliability and responsiveness of MMTs is poor, then validity is moot. However, different types of validity exist.

The lowest level of validity is face validity. Face validity asks, does the test appear to measure what it is supposed to measure? So, is an MMT supposed to measure the ability of a muscle to contract, to move a limb through a range of motion, or to function normally? Manual muscle tests measure the ability of a muscle to contract and to move a limb through a range of motion. They do not measure the ability of a muscle to function. Function is much more complex than an isolated muscle contraction. Although one can infer that function will be impaired if a muscle or

group of muscles cannot contract, MMTs do not test muscles in a functional manner, and the relationship between muscle impairment and functional deficit is certainly not clear. The patient's motivation, determination, ability to problem-solve and substitute alternative motor patterns has far more to do with function than with the isolated ability of a muscle to contract.

Although the MMT has a long history and is entrenched in clinical education and practice, it is a technique that needs to be systematically and scientifically scrutinized. It is necessary to determine which specific MMT tests are reliable, under what conditions, and in what patient group. It is also necessary to determine which MMTs are not useful, and they should be discarded. Finally, it is necessary to determine the diagnostic and prognostic and discriminative validity of MMTs and to determine what can be reasonably inferred from the results of specific MMTs.

INSTRUMENTED MUSCLE TESTING

The problems of poor reliability and responsiveness are alleviated somewhat with the use of instrumented MMTs (Bohannon, 1986; Currier, 1972; Riddle et al., 1989; Stratford and Balsor, 1994; Trudelle-Jackson et al., 1994). However, instrumented hand-held MMTs are still limited by the therapist's ability to adequately resist muscle strength.

Instrumented muscle testing has increased the level of accuracy and the reliability of strength testing and has contributed significantly to the body of knowledge about muscle performance. One of the first devices to be used in measuring muscle strength was the cable tensiometer. As the name implies, cable tensiometers measure tension in a cable. To use this device to test muscle performance, one end of the cable is attached to a limb segment and the other to a fixed object. The tensiometer is then placed on the cable, and a gauge on the meter measures the amount of tension. Calibration is necessary to convert the gauge reading into a measure of force. This is usually done by suspending known weights from the cable, reading and recording the measurement from the gauge, and converting these units into units of force. A key procedural factor for using the cable tensiometer is that the cable must be positioned along the line of muscle action. A second procedural point to consider (because it facilitates computation) is that the cable should make a 90-degree angle with the point of attachment to the body.

Cable tensiometers have been used in research (Beasley, 1961; Currier, 1972), are fairly reliable, and provide the quantitative data needed for research and clinical applications. However, they have never been widely used in the clinic. The same is true for strain gauges. A strain gauge is a device that has electroconductive material incorporated in it. The application of a load to this device results in deformation of the electroconductive material, which changes the electrical resistance and thus the electrical output to a display device. Again, calibration is necessary to convert the electrical output into force. These devices are not discussed further here because they have not been utilized by clinicians in the past and are unlikely to be so in the future.

In contrast, HHD has been widely adopted in clinical practice. A few reasons probably account for the adoption of these instruments.

1. The need to document the results of clinical tests in a quantitative manner. This is a prerequisite so that treatment efficacy can be established and optimal treatment regimens can be defined.
2. The technique of HHD is the same as that used during the MMT, and therapists are very familiar with MMT techniques.
3. The devices are inexpensive, simple to understand, and simple to use.

Two devices are described and discussed in this section: the modified sphygmomanometer (Fig. 2–3) and the HHD (Fig. 2–4).

A *modified sphygmomanometer* (SM) can be used to quantify the resistance offered during a manually resisted isometric contraction (Giles, 1984; Helewa et al., 1981; Helewa et al., 1990). Sphygmomanometers are usually available in the clinic and are easily modified to measure muscle strength. Essentially, the MS is a regular sphygmomanometer from which the bladder has been removed from the cuff. The bladder is folded into three sections and placed in a cotton bag. Alternatively, the cuff may simply be rolled up. A baseline pressure is set within the MS, and the device is then placed between the body part and the therapist's hand, as if an MMT was being carried out. The patient then performs a resisted contraction against the MS cuff, and the pressure is noted. Conversion from units of pressure to units of force necessitates calibration.

The MS has one advantage over the HHD, and thus is related to its softness and compressibility of the material.

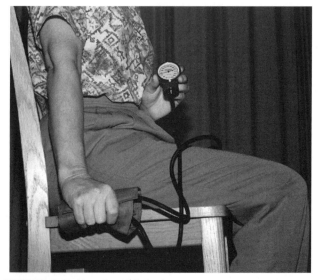

FIGURE 2–3. Use of modified sphygmomanometer to measure grip strength.

Thus, the MS can be applied against bony surfaces without causing discomfort (the experience of pain or discomfort during a test would confound the results of the test).

The HHD is a hand-held device that incorporates spring scales or strain gauges to measure applied force. The HHD measures the applied force in kilograms or pounds; thus, no conversion of measurement units is required. The HHD is used in the same way as the MMT and the MS. Thus, it is subject to some of the same limitations of MMT, especially that regarding the strength of the examiner. Bohannon (1986) suggests that this limitation may lessen as the examiner becomes more experienced. Beasley (1956) showed that examiners were able to hold against higher forces with practice. A learning effect exists for the examiner as well as for the patient. The learning effect results in a greater amount of force being recorded, but the force difference is obviously not reflective of a change in muscle strength.

The HHD has been tested for intrarater, interrater and interdevice reliability for different muscles and in different population groups (Bohannon, 1990; Riddle et al., 1989; Trudelle-Jackson et al., 1994) and for quantitative comparisons between make and break tests (Stratford and Balsor, 1994). This device has also been compared with other, more technically sophisticated, devices such as the Kin-Com isokinetic testing unit (Deones et al, 1994; Stratford and Balsor, 1994; Trudelle-Jackson et al, 1994).

In a nonblinded trial, Bohannon (1988) used an HHD to measure intratester and intrasession reliability of measures of force in the elbow flexors of 31 healthy subjects. He reported good reliability (ICC = 0.995). Trudelle-Jackson and colleagues (1994) tested interdevice reliability and did not demonstrate such high levels of reliability. These authors also tested a healthy population. They compared two different HHDs and measured hamstring force. Intraclass correlation coefficients between the two devices was low (ICC = 0.58). These results suggest that different devices cannot be used interchangeably to measure a patient's progress. These authors also compared the force measured with the HHDs to that measured with the Kin-Com (parallel forms of concurrent reliability). The ICCs calculated between the Kin-Com and each HHD were reasonable (ICCs = 0.83 and 0.85), but an analysis of variance between the Kin-Com and the HHDs revealed a significant difference between the Kin-Com and one of the HHDs. The mean force measured with each HHD was 7.5 kg and 12.5 kg; the mean force measured with the Kin-Com was 13 kg. This suggests that the difference in values is clinically significant as well as statistically significant. It also shows that calibration should be checked periodically, and that HHD devices are not interchangeable.

Riddle and colleagues (1989) tested the strength of several muscle groups within and between sessions in a sample of patients with brain damage. They measured the muscle forces on the paretic and nonparetic limbs. To their surprise, they obtained higher levels of reliability on the nonparetic limb compared with the paretic limb

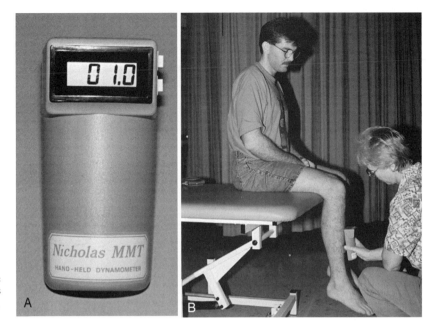

FIGURE 2-4. *A*, Hand-held dynamometer. *B*, Use of hand-held dynamometer to measure quadriceps force. (*A* and *B*, Courtesy of Lafayette Instrument, Lafayette, IN.)

(ICC = 0.90–0.98 and 0.31–0.93, respectively). This was a repeated measures design with strength measures taken more than 2 days apart. The lower level of reliability obtained on the nonparetic side may be due to the difficulty associated with applying adequate resistance to strong muscles.

The HHD dynamometer can be used to assess isometric strength in many muscle groups relatively easily. Its reliability is lower when it is used to test relatively large and relatively strong muscles. Although isometric measurement of force has face validity, it is not clear how much force is necessary to perform specific functional tasks. Also, HHD is not useful for testing trunk strength or hand strength.

For hand strength testing, two devices are in common clinical use: grip strength dynamometers (Fig. 2–5) and pinch meters (Fig. 2–6). Both of these devices measure force, which is recorded in pounds or kilograms on a gauge. Computerized versions of these devices are available but are not always necessary or advantageous, depending on the mathematic algorithms used in the software. Standardized testing protocols are included with the devices. Both intra- and interrater reliability of the grip strength dynamometer is good in normals (Neibuhr et al, 1994; Stratford et al, 1987; Stratford, 1989) and patients (Stegnick Jansen, 1995).

The influence of the position of the elbow joint during testing of normal subjects is not clear. Mathiowetz and associates (1985) showed that elbow joint position influenced the magnitude of grip force, but the results were not replicated by Balogun and colleagues (1991). Stegnick Jansen (1995) contrasted grip force in a patient and control

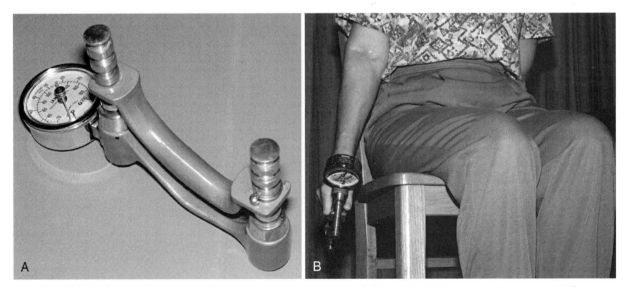

FIGURE 2-5. *A*, Grip dynamometer. (Sammons Preston, Burr Ridge, IL.) *B*, Use of grip dynamometer to measure grip force.

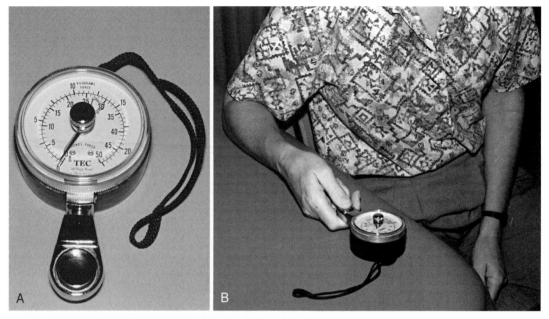

FIGURE 2–6. *A,* Pinch meter. *B,* Use of pinch meter to measure pinch force.

group with the elbow in flexed compared with extended position. Twenty-two subjects with lateral epicondylitis and 15 normal subjects participated. Excellent reliability coefficients were reported (ICCs ≥ 0.95). Noteworthy was the fact that elbow position did not influence grip strength in the normal group but did influence grip strength in the patient group. In the patient group, grip strength was greater with the elbow flexed on both the involved and the uninvolved sides. The magnitude of difference was much greater on the involved side. This work highlights the problems inherent in testing normal subjects and generalizing those findings to patient populations. Patients and nonpatients are different.

To summarize, it can be stated that reliability of instrumented MMT is reasonable and appears to be primarily limited by the strength of the examiner, standardization of technique is important, and instruments are not interchangeable. The validity of instrumented MMT is subject to the same issues and questions posed for noninstrumented MMT. The validity needs to be assessed.

Dynamic Tests

Isometric measurements provide some information about muscle strength that is important to clinicians. But because muscles usually function in a dynamic manner, it makes sense to measure muscle performance in a dynamic manner (Fig. 2–7). Although dynamic testing appears to be more functional, the relationship between function and dynamic testing has not been established (Rothstein et al., 1987). One of the first papers to appear in the physical therapy literature about isokinetic exercise was by Hislop and Perrine (1967). These authors differentiated between isotonic (constant load) and isokinetic (constant speed) exercise. They suggested that isotonic exercise involves

muscular contractions against a mechanical system that provides a constant load, such as when lifting a free weight. In fact, the load of a free weight is not constant because changes in the angulation of the limb lever influence the effect of gravity on the load. A consequence of this is that the muscle could be working at its greatest mechanical advantage when the resistance of the load has its least effect (Hislop and Perrine, 1967), and the muscle would not be challenged throughout its range. Theoretically, isokinetic exercise challenges the muscle throughout its range.

Isokinetic testing uses an electromechanical device that prevents a moving body segment from exceeding a preset angular speed. The axis of the device is aligned with the anatomic axis of the joint that will be moving. The lever arm of the device is attached to the subject's limb, and the subject is instructed to move as fast as possible. The device does not initiate motion, nor does it provide any resistance to motion until the preset speed is reached. However, as soon as the subject's limb moves as fast as the preset speed, the device exerts an opposing force against the moving body. As the subject tries to accelerate, the machine resists the movement. The harder the subject pushes against the device, the greater is the resistance provided by the device. This resistance is measured by the machine throughout the range of motion and torque curves are plotted using range of motion and torque (Fig. 2–8). The earliest machines used a strip chart recorder, but most machines are now computerized. Algorithms within the software compute measures such as average and peak values of torque, power, and work in addition to the position within the range at which peak torque was generated. The output is usually presented in tabular and graphic form (Fig. 2–8).

Much of the research in isokinetic testing has been conducted on the knees of normal subjects, but researchers have examined the machines, muscle groups other than quadriceps, and patient groups. Most devices have different attachments that allow an examiner to test different muscle groups, including those of the trunk. Trunk testing machines are discussed separately.

There is no doubt that the ability to test muscle performance in a dynamic quantitative manner has contributed to the body of knowledge about muscle performance. Isometric tests provide information about the ability of a muscle to

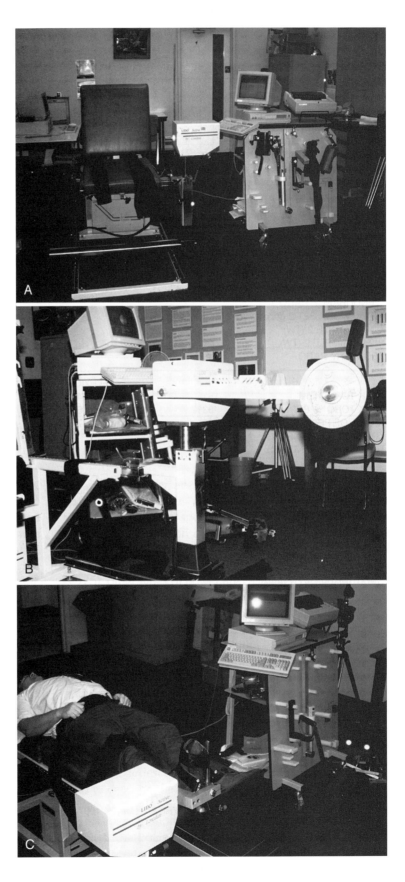

FIGURE 2–7. *A*, Lido isokinetic device. *B*, Calibration of the Lido isokinetic device using weights. *C*, Subject in position for the measurement of ankle dorsi- and plantarflexion. (*A–C*, Courtesy of Loredan Biomedical, Inc., Davis, CA.)

persist because they have an aura of credibility and technologic sophistication that does not invite questioning—critical or otherwise. This facilitates the adoption of erroneous terms into accepted dogma.

Appropriate terms or measures obtained with dynamic strength testing devices usually include such measurements as isometric torque or force and isokinetic force or torque throughout the range of joint motion and at different velocities. Power and work can be computed from torque and velocity data using the equations noted previously. Test factors that can influence these measures are as follows.

Velocity. The velocity at which the isokinetic test is conducted makes a significant difference to the torque output and the position in range at which peak torque output occurs (Chen et al., 1987; Gehlsen et al., 1984; Hsieh et al., 1987; Osternig et al., 1977; Rothstein et al., 1983; Tredinnick and Duncan, 1988; Watkins et al., 1984). It is well known that a force velocity relationship exists in dynamic muscle contractions. This relationship is essentially linear (Rothstein et al., 1983). An increase in the load on a dynamically contracting muscle causes the velocity of the contracting muscle to decrease. Similarly, as the velocity of the muscle contraction increases, the torque generated by the muscle decreases, and peak torque occurs later in the range. These findings are robust between different muscle groups and between normal subjects and patient groups.

Experience and Repetitions. Isokinetic tests are not only a test of strength but also a test of motor skill. Learning is involved in this skill, which is reflected in torque increases, and of course influences the reliability of the test. Based on their study of knee extensor torque in 40 healthy women, Johnson and Seigel (1978) recommended that a mean of three repetitions provides the highest level of reliability (0.93–0.99). Their protocol included a warm-up of three submaximal and three maximal contractions, and strength tests conducted at 180 degrees per second. In another study, Mawdsley and Knapik (1982) tested 16 subjects with no warm-up, in three sessions across 6 weeks, at 30 degrees per second. They reported no significant difference in torque values across the 6-week time period. The results from the within-session testing were interesting. In the first trial, the first test produced the highest torque, whereas in the second and third sessions, the first trial produced the lowest torque. It is difficult to explain why torque values increased with each repetition within the first test session but decreased with each repetition in the second and third sessions. Based on the information reported, any interpretation would be entirely speculative. However, the fact that no significant difference was seen between the averaged values across the 6-week period suggests that under the conditions of testing used in the study, a reasonable level of reliability can be expected over a relatively long time period (6 weeks).

Calibration and Equipment. The manufacturers of isokinetic devices usually supply the calibration protocol for use with their machine. For the Lido isokinetic device, weights of known value are applied to the load arm at a known distance from the point of rotation. Because the weight values and arm length are known, the torque applied to the shaft is also known. This torque value is then compared with that torque value recorded by the machine. This calibration procedure tests in the isometric mode. Isokinetic calibration is not specifically tested, which is problematic when strength testing is conducted in the isokinetic mode. The manufacturers claim that their device has long-term stability and accuracy, but whether this has been tested with the machine in clinical use is not clear. Cybex II calibration protocol uses known weights applied at a single speed. But based on extensive testing of the device, Olds and associates (1981) have suggested that the Cybex should be tested daily and at every test speed. Essentially, the calibration protocol needs to simulate the clinical testing situation as much as possible. This includes testing the machine with the settings that are used during clinical testing, eg, the damp setting on the Cybex II.

Damp is a means of reducing signal artifacts in electrical systems. An undamped eletric signal results in "overshoot" or an erroneously high torque reading. Sapega and colleagues (1982) showed that the overshoot was due to inertial forces rather than muscular torque. The Cybex II has five damp settings (0–4). Increasing the value of the damp setting results in a decrease in the peak torque and a shift of the curve to the right, which implies that peak torque occurred later in the range (Sinacore et al., 1983). The important point is that all the machine settings must be documented, and clinical evaluations must be retested using the same settings.

Another factor that affects torque output is gravity. The effect of gravity obviously varies with the position of the limb. If gravity is not corrected for, then the torque generated, and thus the power and work calculated, would be subject to error (Winter et al., 1981). The error would be systematic and therefore would not affect the reliability of the isokinetic tests, but the validity of the measurements would be compromised. Fillyaw and coworkers (1986) tested peak torques of the quadriceps and hamstrings in 25 soccer players. They computed the effect of gravity and added this value to the quadriceps torque and subtracted it from the hamstring torque. Depending on the speed of testing, the effect of gravity correction on mean peak torques was approximately 6 ft-lb in the quadriceps and 8 ft-lb in the hamstrings.

One other equipment consideration that affects isokinetic muscle testing relates to the center of rotation of the equipment and its alignment with the center of rotation of the joint axis. This is an especially important issue in measuring muscle strength in multijoint areas, such as the trunk.

Testing Protocol. Potentially many factors within the specific testing protocols could influence the measurement of muscle strength. Factors such as length and type of warm-up activity, the number and length of rest periods, and the type and order of muscle contractions could all influence muscle strength. Differences in testing protocols make it difficult to compare the results from different studies. But these factors have not been specifically tested, so the extent of the influence is really not known and these factors should be tested.

The mechanical aspects of isokinetic machines appear to be reliable. But how reliable is the device for measuring muscle strength? And is the level of reliability different in patient populations compared with normals and at different testing speeds? A reasonable level of reliability appears to exist in testing muscle strength, as long as standard protocols are adhered to. Standardization is crucial because so many factors can influence the test measurement. The validity of the tests and of the interpretation of the output has received less scrutiny.

The reliability of specific isokinetic devices in measuring muscle strength has been examined to a limited extent testing different muscle groups. In a recent review of isokinetic testing of the ankle musculature, Cox (1995) concluded that isokinetic testing was generally reliable. However, he noted that reliability was higher for the plantar- and dorsiflexors than for the inverters and everters. It was apparent from the review that most studies were conducted on normals. Frisiello et al. (1994) examined the test-retest reliability of the Biodex isokinetic dynamometer (Biodex Medical Systems, Shirley, NY) on medial and lateral rotation of the shoulder. He tested eccentric peak torque of both shoulders in 18 healthy adults at 90 and 120 degrees per second. He reported ICC values between 0.75 and 0.86, with medial rotation being slightly less reliable than lateral rotation.

It appears from the literature that isokinetic devices are mechanically reliable within themselves, but comparisons between devices have not been conducted. It also appears that isokinetic devices measure muscle torque reliably. Many reliability studies have been conducted measuring peripheral muscle strength in normal subjects. The "normal" subjects are frequently well educated, well motivated, and free from pain and dysfunction. Typical patients may also be well educated and well motivated, but they usually have some discomfort and dysfunction, which may influence their performance and thus the reliability of the strength measure. Therefore, the assumption of similar levels of reliability in patients is not appropriate. Reliability needs to be established in the specific populations that are to be tested under the conditions of testing that are used in that population.

Trunk Testing

Finally, an area of testing that has evolved rapidly in the last decade is the use of isokinetic and isoinertial devices to measure isometric and dynamic muscle strength in the trunk. Spinal problems are complex problems that are difficult to prevent, difficult to diagnose, and difficult to treat. The tendency for spinal problems to recur is a source of frustration to all. Low back problems are highly prevalent and very costly in financial and personal terms. They can lead to a great deal of distress and demand on the health care system. Many patients in rehabilitation are patients with low back problems. The trunk is a complex multisegmental system with multiple joints, multiple axes of motion, and multiple complex musculature. It is more difficult to measure range of motion and muscle strength in the trunk than it is in peripheral joints because of the trunk's complexity. The perceived need to quantitatively measure trunk function coupled with the availability of new technology has led to the development of trunk testing devices. There is now a great deal of use, and unfortunately misuse, of trunk testing devices.

Functional strength tests of trunk musculature have been used as a preemployment screening tool, as a measure of progress in rehabilitation, and as a "malingerer detector." Use of functional muscle testing as a screening device is based on some epidemiologic data that suggest that manual materials handling leads to back injuries. However, the supporting evidence for this notion is not strong. Most studies are retrospective; do not distinguish between back injuries, reports of back injuries, and time lost from work; and do not account for confounding psychosocial variables (Pope, 1992).

This knowledge has not stemmed the tide of technology or the inappropriate use of isodevices. Recent critical reviews on trunk strength testing with isodevices conclude that no evidence has been found to support the use of these devices for preemployment screening, medicolegal evaluation, or even clinical evaluation (Andersson, 1992; Mooney et al., 1992; Newton and Waddell, 1993; Pope, 1992). The strength of this criticism may be a reaction to overclaims by manufacturers and overinterpretation of results by those with a vested interest in the device or in the results of the test. Inappropriate interpretation of results may also be due to an incomplete understanding of biopsychosocial factors that contribute to a person's performance on an isodevice. Medicolegal issues and clinicians' suspicions have complicated the use of trunk testing machines to a shameful degree. However, on the positive side, these machines do provide information that is not otherwise available. Systematic research is now necessary to determine the validity of the information that these devices do provide about trunk function.

Trunk testing devices have contributed to the body of knowledge on trunk performance, including isometric and dynamic trunk strength. Isomachines for trunk testing were introduced about 10 years ago. They now include the Cybex back testing system, the Lido, the Kin-Com, and the B-200 (Fig. 2–9), which is an isoinertial (constant resistance) device, most trunk testing machines are isokinetic. All the isokinetic devices operate on similar principles to each other and to the isokinetic devices that measure peripheral muscle strength. The main difference between the devices is in the test positions (lying, sitting, semistanding, or standing) and the

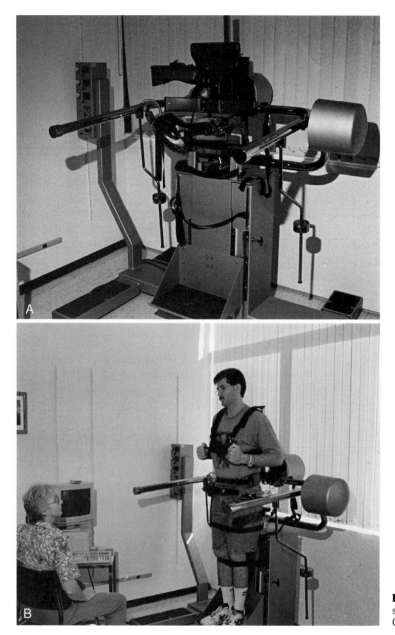

FIGURE 2–9. *A,* B-200 isoinertial back testing unit. *B,* Shows subject in the B-200 isoinertial back testing device. (*A* and *B,* Courtesy of Isotechnologies, Inc., Hillsborough, NC.)

degree of stabilization and constraints to motion. Some of the machines can measure strength in all directions of trunk motion simultaneously and with the person in the same device, eg, the B-200. Other devices have different machines for different motions. For example, the Cybex system has one device that measures trunk flexion and extension and another that measures axial rotation.

All of the factors that need to be considered in isokinetic testing in peripheral muscles, such as warm-up protocol and standardization of instructions, need to be considered in trunk testing. There are, however, some factors that are unique to strength testing of the trunk because of its biomechanical complexity.

The amount of torque generated by a muscle is the product of force and the length of the lever arm from the axis of motion. Determining the axis of motion in a multiaxial system is obviously problematic. The hip joint (Hasue et al., 1980), the L5-S1 joint (Davies and Gould,

1982), and the iliac crest (Suzuki and Endo, 1983) have all been used as a designated axis of motion. It is not clear whether any axis has more validity than another. However, regardless of which axis is intended for selection, an error of plus or minus one spinal level exists between the segment that is intended for selection and that which is actually selected (Simmonds and Kumar, 1993b). The important points for testing are that the specific axis should be documented and that the same axis should be used for repeated testing.

In peripheral joints, isometric strength was shown to be greater than dynamic strength. Moreover, as the velocity of testing increased, the magnitude of torque decreased and it occurred later in the range. The same phenomenon is present in trunk masculature, and this holds for all directions of movement (Kumar et al., 1995a; Kumar et al., 1995b).

The position of testing trunk performance influences the

results because of differential biomechanical advantages of the musculature and because of the differential effects of gravity on the trunk. Cartas and colleagues (1993) evaluated the effect of subject position on isometric and isoinertial muscle performance. They tested 25 healthy male subjects with the B-200 isoinertial dynamometer on two different occasions. The first test involved isometric measurements in three directions and in three positions; sitting (hip in 90 degrees flexion), semistanding (hip at 135 degrees flexion), and standing. The second session involved dynamic testing in three directions against 50 percent resistance. Isometric flexion strength was highest in standing and lowest in semistanding, whereas isometric extension strength was not influenced by position. Dynamic muscle performance was highest in standing for all directions. These results give an indication of the importance of posture to muscle strength and suggest that one particular posture is not optimal for all muscle performance. Unfortunately, these tests were conducted in normal, pain-free individuals. The results cannot be generalized to the patient population because patients have different pathophysiologic constraints on their posture and on their muscle performance.

Several investigators have used isomachines to compare muscle performance between patients and pain-free subjects (Cassisi et al., 1993; Gomez, 1994; Newton et al., 1993). Newton and colleagues (1993) tested 70 normal subjects and 120 patients using the Cybex II device. They considered the reliability of the device and the learning effect of the subjects. They evaluated whether isokinetic measures could discriminate between patients and controls. They also examined the relationship between clinical and isokinetic measures.

Similar to other reports, the device was found to be reliable and a learning effect was noted. It was interesting to find that the magnitude of the learning effect was greater in the patients than in the controls. A couple of factors can account for this.

First, the magnitude of difference was calculated as a percentage change in mean torque. The torque output was lower in the patient group compared with the control group; thus, patients are at a mathematical advantage. For example, it can be seen from Table 2–2 that the magnitude of change between the first and second test of trunk extension at 120 degrees per second was 14.6 ft-lb in the normal group and 18.3 ft-lb in the patients, a negligible difference between groups. However, when this difference is presented as a *percentage* learning increase, the apparent learning effect is much more significant in the patient group (28%, compared with 15% in the normal group). All data should be scrutinized, and this example shows why.

Cooke and colleagues (1992) examined isokinetic performance in 45 subjects with low back pain. They acknowledged a learning effect between the first and second tests but found no significant difference in strength measures between the second and third test. They conducted isokinetic tests at 2 and 4 weeks following therapy and measured an improvement in muscle strength beyond that

which would have occurred with learning. This implies that isokinetic devices can be useful for measuring clinical change. Studies that have compared males and females and patients and controls are consistent in their findings. Muscle strength is lower in a group of females compared with a group of males. Furthermore, muscle strength is lower in a group of patients compared with a group of healthy subjects. However, within all groups, a high level of variability is seen between individual subjects. This variability compromises the ability of the isokinetic test results to discriminate between *individual* patients and *individual* controls. In attempting to classify subjects as patients or controls, Newton and colleagues (1993) found that isokinetic scores were not useful. Using two standard deviations as the cut-off criteria, 80 percent of patients were designated "normal." This figure was reduced to 56 percent using one standard deviation as the cutoff criterion. The data from this study did not provide much support for the ability of isokinetic tests to discriminate between normal subjects and those with spinal problems. Mean torque scores are not useful in discriminating between patients and control subjects. Is it possible that evaluation of the ratio between flexor to extensor strength is more useful? Although some authors have suggested that this is the case (Mayer et al., 1985; McNeill et al., 1980; Suzuki and Endo, 1983), no consensus as to the normative ratio has been reached. This lack of consensus can be explained by recent work of Kumar and colleagues (1995a, 1995b). They showed that the ratio of flexion to extension strength varies as a function of trunk position and speed of testing.

Other difficulties in attempting to use isokinetic scores to discriminate between patients and controls are reported by Gomez (1994). Gomez tested 168 normal subjects and 120 patients using the B-200, specifically to look at

| TABLE 2–2 |

SHOWS HOW USE OF PERCENTAGE CHANGE SCORES TO DEMONSTRATE A LEARNING EFFECT IS BIASED IN FAVOR OF PATIENTS*

Velocity of Test (degrees per sec)	Test 1 (ft-lb)	Test 2 (ft-lb)	Magnitude of Change	Learning % Increase
Normal Group (n = 21)				
60	122.6	142.9	20.3	16
90	116.9	132.4	15.5	13
120	98.8	113.4	14.6	15
Patient Group (n = 20)				
60	93.5	122.0	28.5	30
90	88.3	100.9	12.6	14
120	63.4	81.7	18.3	28

* Based on data from Newton, M., Thow, M., Somerville, D., Henderson, I., & Waddell, G. (1993). Trunk strength testing with iso-machines. Part 2: Experimental evaluation of the Cybex II back testing system in normal subjects and patients with chronic low back pain. *Spine, 18*(7), 812–824.

asymmetry of trunk strength and range of motion. He found that asymmetric motion and strength was present in the subjects with low back pain. However, the asymmetry did not discriminate between patients and normal subjects. This was because *ALL* subjects were asymmetric and moved asymmetrically.

The magnitude of variability of isokinetic test data both within and between groups argues against the value of using normative isokinetic data. Comparing the magnitude of force exerted by a patient against a normative database is probably less useful than using the patient as his or her own control and measuring the *change* in performance. The tremendous variability in the magnitude of muscle strength is due to the myriad of factors that influence strength and that influence the measurement of muscle strength. It is difficult for normative databases to control for the considerable number of relevant factors.

It is obvious from the previous discussion that many issues regarding trunk testing with isomachines are unresolved. These issues will only be resolved through systematic research. They will not be resolved through anecdotal evidence or patient or clinician testimonials. It can be stated that these machines are mechanically reliable and appear to measure muscular torque reliably. The validity of the devices in terms of measuring trunk function has not been established.

CONCLUSIONS

This chapter shows how complex the measurement of muscle strength is. The strength of a muscle is dependent on a variety of factors in different domains (see Fig. 2–2). Measures of muscle strength are dependent on the strength of the muscle but on many other factors too. The reliability of muscle strength varies with the methodology of testing. Reliability and responsiveness have not been adequately demonstrated with MMTs. The reliability of instrumented muscle testing is reasonable, at least in normal subjects, but devices are not interchangeable. The greatest shortcoming in tests of muscle strength lies in their lack of proven diagnostic and prognostic validity when they are used for this purpose.

Systematic research is necessary. Priorities of research include

1. Establishing the reliability of strength tests in populations for whom the test is intended
2. Establishing whether and how isometric and dynamic tests of muscle strength can be used for diagnostic and prognostic purposes
3. Demonstrating the relationship of isometric and dynamic tests of muscle strength to function

Finally, before using any measurement test, clinicians should ask themselves why they are using the test and what they hope to learn from the results of that test. What are the factors that influence the test? They should also ask whether the measurement has any relationship with the patient's problem as the patient perceives it.

I would like to leave the reader with the following point to ponder: We sometimes measure what we measure because we can measure it, it is easy to measure, and we have been taught to measure it. We do not measure what we should measure because it is more difficult and more complex. We then use the easy measure to infer things about the difficult measure.

Isolated and constrained tests of muscle strength on their own do not provide an adequate indication of coordinated discomfort-free functional muscle activity.

GLOSSARY*

Concentric—A shortening muscle contraction.

Eccentric—An eccentric muscle contraction is one in which the muscle lengthens as it continues to maintain tension.

Endurance—The ability to maintain torque over a period of time or a set number of contractions.

Fatigue—The inability to maintain torque over a period of time or a set number of contractions. What you lose or what you maintain, ie, 30 percent loss of power equals maintenance of 70 percent power.

Isoinertial—Constant resistance to a movement.

Isokinetic—Constant velocity of the joint, not a constant shortening or lengthening of the muscle.

Isometric—An isometric contraction is when the muscle generates an internal force or tension but no movement of a joint occurs.

Isotonic—An isotonic contraction is when the internal force generated by a muscle results in movement of a joint.

Moment arm—The perpendicular distance from the line of action of the force to the fulcrum.

Power—Work per unit time.

Reliability—The degree to which repeated measurements of a stable phenomenon fall closely together.

Responsiveness—The ability of a test to measure clinical change.

Sensitivity—The ability of a test to correctly identify *all* subjects with the condition of interest.

Specificity—The ability of a test to identify *only* subjects with the condition of interest.

Strength—1) Force or torque produced by a muscle during a maximal voluntary contraction; 2) measurement of force output at the end of a lever; or 3) maximal force or torque required to resist an isometric or isotonic contraction.

---

*The definitions given here are operational definitions.

Torque—The degree to which a force tends to rotate an object about a specified fulcrum.

REFERENCES

Andersson, G. B. J. (1992). Methods and application of functional muscle testing. In J. N. Weinstein (Ed.), *Clinical efficacy and outcome in the diagnosis and treatment of low back pain.* (pp. 93–99). New York: Raven Press.

Backman, E., Johansson, V., Hager, B., Sjoblom, P., & Henriksson, K. G. (1995). Isometric muscle strength and muscular endurance in normal persons aged between 17 and 70 years. *Scandinavian Journal of Rehabilitation Medicine, 27,* 109–117.

Balogun, J. A., Alkamolafe, C., & Amusa, L. O. (1991). Grip strength: Effects of testing posture and elbow position. *Archives of Physical Medicine and Rehabilitation, 72,* 280–283.

Bandura, A., & Cervone, D. (1983). Self-evaluative and self-efficacy mechanisms governing the motivational effects of goal systems. *Journal of Personality and Social Psychology, 5,* 1017–1028.

Battie, M. C., Bigos, S. J., Fisher, L., Hansson, T. H., Jones, M. E., & Wortley, M. D. (1989). Isometric lifting strength as a predictor of industrial back pain. *Spine, 14*(8), 851–856.

Beasley, W. C. (1956). Influence of method on estimates of normal knee extensor force among normal and post polio children. *Physical Therapy Review, 36,* 21–41.

Beasley, W. C. Quantitative muscle testing: Principles and applications to research and clinical services. *Archives of Physical Medicine and Rehabilitation, 42,* 398–425.

Bohannon, R. W. (1988). Make tests and break tests of elbow flexor muscle strength. *Physical Therapy, 68,* 193, 194.

Bohannon, R. W. (1990). Make versus break tests for measuring elbow flexor muscle force with a hand-held dynamometer in patients with stroke. *Physiotherapy, Canada, 42,* 247–251.

Bohannon, R. W. (1986). Manual muscle test scores and dynamometer test scores of knee extension strength. *Archives of Physical Medicine and Rehabilitation, 67,* 390–392.

Cartas, O., Nordin, M., Frankel, V. H., Malgady, R., Sheikhzadeh, A. (1993). Quantification of trunk muscle performance in standing, semistanding and sitting postures in healthy men. *Spine, 18*(5), 603–609.

Cassisi, J. E., Robinson, M. E., O'Conner, P., MacMillan, M. (1993). Trunk strength and lumbar paraspinal muscle activity during isometric exercise in chronic low-back pain patients and controls. *Spine, 18*(2), 245–251.

Chen, W.-Y., Pierson, F. M., & Burnett, C. N. (1987). Force-time measurements of knee muscle functions of subjects with multiple sclerosis. *Physical Therapy, 67*(6), 934–940.

Coderre, T. J., Katz, J., Vaccarino, A. L., Meizak, R. (1993). Contributions of central neuroplasticity to pathological pain: Review of clinical and experimental evidence. *Pain, 52,* 259–285.

Cole, B., Finch, E., Gowland, C., & Mayo, N. (1994). The heart of the matter. In J. Basmajian (Ed.), *Physical rehabilitation outcome measures.* Toronto, Canada: Canadian Physiotherapy Association, Health and Welfare.

Cooke, C., Menard, M. R., Beach, G. N., Locke, S. R., Hirsch, G. H. (1992). Serial lumbar dynamometry in low back pain. *Spine, 17*(6), 653–662.

Cox, P. D. Isokinetic testing of the ankle: A review. *Physiotherapy (Canada), 47,* 97–106, 1995.

Coyle, E. F. (1995). Integration of the physical factors determining endurance performance ability. *Exercise and Sports Sciences Reviews, 23,* 25–64.

Currier, D. P. (1972). Maximal isometric tension of the elbow extensors at varied positions. *Physical Therapy, 52*(10), 1043–1049.

Daniels, L., Worthingham, C. (1986). *Muscle testing: Technique of manual examination* (5th ed.). Philadelphia: W. B. Saunders.

Davies, G. L., & Gould, J. A. (1982). Trunk testing using a prototype Cybex II isokinetic dynamometer stabilization system. *Journal of Orthopaedic and Sports Physical Therapy, 3,* 164–170.

Deones, V. L., Wiley, S. C., Worrell, T. (1994). Assessment of quadriceps muscle performance by a hand-held dynamometer and an isokinetic dynamometer. *Journal of Orthopaedic and Sports Physical Therapy, 20*(6), 296–301.

Edgerton, V. R., Roy, R. R., & Gregor, R. J. (1989). Motor unit architecture and interfiber matrix in sensorimotor partitioning. *Behavioral and Brain Science, 12,* 651, 652.

Estlander, A.-M., Vanharanta, H., Moneta, G. B., Kaivanto, K. (1994). Anthropometric variables, self-efficacy beliefs, and pain and disability ratings on the isokinetic performance of low back pain patients. *Spine, 19,* 941–947.

Fillyaw, M., Bevins, T., & Fernandez, L. (1986). Importance of correcting isokinetic peak torque for the effect of gravity when calculating knee flexor to extensor muscle ratios. *Physical Therapy, 66*(1), 23–31.

Frese, E., Brown, M., & Norton, B. J. (1987). Clinical reliability of manual muscle testing. *Physical Therapy, 67*(7), 1072–1076.

Frisiello, S., Gazaille, A., O'Halloran, J., Palmer, M. L., & Waugh, D. (1994). Test-retest reliability of eccentric peak torque values for shoulder medial and lateral rotation using the biodex isokinetic dynamometer. *Journal of Orthopaedic and Sports Physical Therapy, 19*(6), 341–344.

Gehlsen, G. M., Grigsby, S. A., & Winant, D. M. (1984). Effects of an aquatic fitness program on the muscular strength and endurance of patients with multiple sclerosis. *Physical Therapy, 64*(5), 653–657.

Ghez, C. (1991). Muscles: Effectors of the motor systems. In E. R. Kandel, J. H. Schwartz, & T. M. Jessel (Eds.), *Principles of neural science* (3rd ed.) (pp. 548–563). New York: Elsevier.

Giles, C. (1984). The modified sphygmomanometer: An instrument to objectively assess muscle strength. *Physiotherapy (Canada), 36,* 36–41.

Gomez, T. L. (1994). Symmetry of lumbar rotation and lateral flexion range of motion and isometric strength in subjects with and without low back pain. *Journal of Orthopaedic and Sports Physical Therapy, 19*(1), 42–48.

Gordon, A. M., Huxley, A. F., Julian, F. T. (1966). The variation in isometric tension with sarcomere length in vertebrate muscle fibres. *Journal of Physiology (London), 184,* 170–192.

Griffen, J. W., McClure, M. H., & Bertorini, T. E. (1986). Sequential isokinetic and manual muscle testing in patients with neuromuscular disease. *Physical Therapy, 66*(1), 32–35.

Harris, G., Rollman, G. (1983). The validity of experimental pain measures. *Pain, 17,* 369–376.

Hasue, M., Fujiwara, M., & Kikuchi, S. (1980). A new method of quantitative measurement of abdominal and back muscle strength. *Spine, 5*(2), 143–148.

Helewa, A., Goldsmith, C., Smythe, H. (1981). The modified sphygmomanometer: An instrument to measure muscle strength: A validation study. *Journal of Chronic Disease, 34,* 353–361.

Helewa, A., Goldsmith, C., Smythe, H., & Gibson, E. (1990). An evaluation of four different measures of abdominal strength: patient, order and instrument variation. *Journal of Rheumatology, 17*(7), 965–969.

Hislop, H. J. & Perrine, J. J. (1967). The isokinetic concept of exercise. *Physical Therapy 47*(2), 114–117.

Hsieh, L.F., Didenko, B., Schumacher, R., Torg, J. S. (1987). Isokinetic and isometric testing of knee musculature in patients with rheumatoid arthritis with mild knee involvement. *Archives of Physical Medicine and Rehabilitation, 68,* 294–297.

Ivy, J. L., Costill, D. L., Maxwell, B. D. (1980). Skeletal muscle determinants of maximum aerobic power in man. *European Journal of Applied Physiology, 44,* 1–8.

Johnson, J:, & Seigel, D. (1978). Reliability of an isokinetic movement of the knee extensors. *The Research Quarterly 49*(1), 88–90.

Johnston, M. V., Keith, R. A., Hinderer, S. R., (1992). Measurement standards for interdisciplinary rehabilitation. *Archives of Physical Medicine and Rehabilitation, 73,* S3–S23.

Kannus, P. (1994). Isokinetic evaluation of muscle performance: Implications for muscle testing and rehabilitation. *International Journal of Sports Medicine, 15,* S11–S18.

Kendall, F. P., McCreary, E. K., Provance, P. G. (1993). *Muscle testing and function* (4th ed.). Baltimore: Williams & Wilkins.

Komi, P. V. (1973). Measurement of the force-velocity relationship in human muscle under concentric and eccentric contractions. In S. Cerquiglini (Ed.), *Biomechanics III* (pp. 224–229). Basel: Karger.

Kumar, S., Dufresne, R. M., Van Schoor, T. (1995a). Human trunk strength profile in flexion and extension. *Spine, 20*(2), 160–168.

Kumar, S., Dufresne, R. M., Van Schoor, T. (1995b). Human trunk strength profile in lateral flexion and axial rotation. *Spine, 20*(2), 169–177.

Lamb, R. L. Manual muscle testing. In J. M. Rothstein (Ed.), *Meas-*

urement in physical therapy (pp. 47–55). New York: Churchill Livingstone.

Mathiowetz, V., Rennels, C., & Donahoe, L. (1985). Effect of elbow position on grip and key pinch strength. *Journal of Hand Surgery, 10A,* 694–697.

Mattila, M., Hurme, M., Alaranta, H., et al. (1986). The multifidus muscle in patients with lumbar disc herniation. A histochemical and morphometric analysis of intraoperative biopsies. *Spine, 11,* 732–738.

Mawdsley, R. H., Knapik, J. J. (1982). Comparison of isokinetic measurements with test repetitions. *Physical Therapy 62*(2), 169–172.

Mayer, T., Smith, S., Keeley, J., & Mooney, V. (1985). Quantification of lumbar function. Part 2: Sagittal trunk strength in chronic low back pain patients. *Spine, 10,* 765–772.

Mayhew, T. P., & Rothstein, J. M. (1985). Measurement of muscle performance with instruments. In J. M. Rothstein (Ed.), *Measurement in physical therapy* (pp. 57–102). New York: Churchill Livingstone.

McNeill, T., Warwick, D., Andersson, C., & Schultz, A. (1980). Trunk strength in attempted flexion, extension, and lateral bending in healthy subjects and patients with low back disorders. *Spine, 5,* 529–538.

Moffroid, M. T., Kusiak, E. T. (1975). The power struggle. Definition and evaluation of power of muscular performance. *Physical Therapy, 55*(10), 1098–1104.

Moffroid, M. T., Whipple, R., Hofkosh, J., Lowman, E., & Thistle, H. (1969). A study of isokinetic exercise. *Physical Therapy, 49*(7), 735–747.

Mooney, V., Andersson, G. B. J., Pope, M. H. (1992). Discussion of quantitative functional muscle testing. In J. N. Weinstein (Ed.), *Clinical efficacy and outcome in the diagnosis and treatment of low back pain* (pp. 115, 116). New York: Raven Press.

Murray, M. P., Baldwin, J. M., Gardner, G. M., Sepic, S. B., & Downs, J. W. (1977). Maximum isometric knee flexor and extensor muscle contractions. *Physical Therapy, 57*(6), 637–643.

Nachemson, A., & Lindh, M. (1969). Measurement of abdominal and back muscle strength with and without pain. *Scandinavian Journal Rehabilitation Medicine 1,* 60–65.

Neibuhr, B. R., Marion, R., Fike, M. L. (1994). Reliability of grip strength assessment with the computerized Jamar dynamometer. *Occupational Therapy Journal of Research 14*(1), 3–18.

Newton, M., Thow, M., Somerville, D., Henderson, I., & Waddell, G. (1993). Trunk strength testing with iso-machines. Part 2: Experimental evaluation of the Cybex II back testing system in normal subjects and patients with chronic low back pain. *Spine, 18*(7), 812–824.

Newton, M., Waddell, G. (1993). Trunk strength testing with iso-machines. Part 1: Review of a decade of scientific evidence. *Spine, 18*(7), 801–811.

Olds, K., Godfrey, C. M., & Rosenrot, P. (1981). Computer assisted isokinetic dynamometry. A calibration study. Fourth Annual Conference on Rehabilitation Engineering, Washington, DC, p. 247.

Osternig, L. R., Bates, B. T., James, S. L. (1977). Isokinetic and isometric force relationships. *Archives of Physical Medicine and Rehabilitation, 58,* 254–257.

O'Sullivan, S. B. (1994). Motor control assessment. In S. B. O'Sullivan & T. J. Schmitz (eds.), *Physical rehabilitation assessment and treatment* (3rd ed.) (pp. 111–131). Philadelphia: F. A. Davis.

Pentland, W. E., Vandervoort, A. A., & Twomey, L. T. (1995). Age-related changes in upper limb isokinetic and grip strength. *Physiotherapy Theory and Practice, 11,* 165–173.

Pope, M. H. (1992). A critical evaluation of functional muscle testing. In J. N. Weinstein (Ed.), *Clinical efficacy and outcome in the diagnosis and treatment of low back pain* (pp. 111–113). New York: Raven Press.

Pratt, J., & Abrams, R. A. (1994). Action-centered inhibition: Effects of distractors on movement planning and execution. *Human Movement Science, 13,* 245–254.

Riddle, D. L., Finucane, S. D., Rothstein, J. M., & Walker, M. L. (1989). Intrasession and intersession reliability of hand-held dynamometer measurements taken on brain damaged patients. *Physical Therapy, 69,*182–194.

Rissanen, A., Kalimo, H., & Alaranta, H. (1995). Effect of intensive training on the isokinetic strength and structure of lumbar muscles in patients with chronic low back pain. *Spine, 20,* 333–340.

Rogers, M. A., & Evan, W. J. (1993). Changes in skeletal muscle with aging: Effects of exercise training. *Exercise and Sports Sciences Reviews, 21,* 65–102.

Rothstein, J. M., Delitto, A., Sinacore, D. R., & Rose, S. J. (1983). Electromyographic, peak torque, and power relationships during isokinetic movement. *Physical Therapy, 63,* 926–933.

Rothstein, J. M., Lamb, R. L., & Mathew, T. P. (1987). Clinical uses of isokinetic measurements. *Physical Therapy 67*(12), 1840–1844.

Sapega, A. A., Nicholas, J. A., Sokolow, D, & Saraniti, A. (1982). The nature of torque ''overshoot'' in Cybex isokinetic dynamometry. *Medicine and Science in Sports Exercise, 14,* 368–375.

Simmonds, M. J., & Kumar, S. (1993a). Health care ergonomics. Part I. The fundamental skill of palpation: A review and critique. *International Journal of Industrial Ergonomics, 11,* 135–143.

Simmonds, M. J., & Kumar, S. (1993b). Health care ergonomics. Part II. Location of body structures by palpation: A reliability study. *International Journal of Industrial Ergonomics, 11,* 145–151.

Simmonds, M. J., Kumar, S, & Lechelt, E. (1994). Use of a spinal model to quantify the forces and resultant motion during therapists' tests of spinal motion. *Physical Therapy, 75,* 212–222.

Sinacore, D. R., Rothstein, J. M., Delitto, A., & Rose, S. J. (1983). Effect of damp on isokinetic measurements. *Physical Therapy, 63*(8), 1248–1250.

Soderberg, G. (1992). Skeletal muscle function. In D. P. Currier & R. M. Nelson (Eds.), *Dynamics of human biologic tissues* (pp. 74–96).

Stegnick Jansen, C. W. (1995). *An explorative study of immobilization and exercise for patients with lateral epicondylitis.* Doctoral dissertation, Texas Woman's University, Houston, Texas.

Stratford, P. W., & Balsor, B. E. (1994). A comparison of make and break tests using a hand-held dynamometer and the Kin-Com. *Journal of Orthopaedic and Sports Physical Therapy 19*(1), 28–32.

Stratford, P., Levy, D. R., Gauldie, S., Levy, K., & Miseferi, D. (1987). Extensor carpi radialis tendonitis: a validation of selected outcome measures. *Physiotherapy (Canada), 39*(4), 250–255.

Stratford, P. W., Norman, G. R., & McIntosh, J. M. (1989). Generalizability of grip strength measurements in patients with tennis elbow. *Physical Therapy 69*(4), 276–281.

Suzuki, N., & Endo, S. (1983). A quantitative study of trunk muscle strength and fatigability in the low back pain syndrome. *Spine 8*(1), 69–74.

Tredinnick, T. J., & Duncan, P. W. (1988). Reliability of measurements of concentric and eccentric isokinetic loading. *Physical Therapy 68*(5), 656–659.

Trotter, J. A., Richmond, F. J. R., & Purslow, P. P. (1993). Functional morphology and motor control of series-fibered muscles. *Exercise and Sports Science Reviews, 23,* 167–214.

Trudelle-Jackson, E., Jackson, A. W., Frankowski, C. M., Long, K. M., & Meske, N. B. (1994). Interdevice reliability and validity assessment of the Nicholas hand-held dynamometer. *Journal of Sports and Physical Therapy 20*(6), 302–306.

Vandervoort, A. A., & McComas, A. J. Contractile changes in opposing muscles of the human ankle joint with aging. *Journal of Applied Physiology, 61,* 361–367.

Wadsworth, C. T., Krishnan, R., & Sear, M. (1987). Intrarater reliability of manual muscle testing and hand-held dynametric muscle testing. *Physical Therapy, 67*(9), 1342–1347.

Watkins, M. P., Harris, B. A., & Kozlowski, B. A. (1984). Isokinetic testing in patients with hemiparesis. *Physical Therapy, 64*(2), 184–189.

Winter, D. A., Wells, R. P., & Orr, G. W. (1981). Errors in the use of isokinetic dynamometers. *European Journal of Applied Physiology, 46,* 397–408.

Zhu, X.-Y., Parnianpour, M., Nordin, M., & Kahanovitz, N. (1989). Histochemistry and morphology of erector spinae muscle in lumbar disc herniation. *Spine, 14,* 391–397.

CHAPTER 3

Joint Range of Motion

Jeffery Gilliam, MHS, PT, OCS

Ian Kahler Barstow, PT

SUMMARY Early measurement of joint range of motion (ROM) was initiated by the necessity to assess disability from postwar injuries. Measurements of joint ROM provide information designed to describe status, document change, explain performance, and predict outcome. It is critical to establish reliability in goniometric measurements to substantiate consistency over time. Some level of validity should always be demonstrated with measurements of ROM, correlating the measurements taken with the actual angles involved. While it is difficult to compare reliability studies, those methods with established standardized procedures demonstrate a higher degree of repeatability. The universal goniometer has been established as one of the most accurate and efficient instruments used in measuring joint ROM. Because of the enormous financial burden related to low back pathology, methods of measuring lumbar ROM for purposes of function and disability have come under scrutiny. To establish ''normal'' ROM measurements as a standard for reference, population differences such as age, sex, race and ethnic background, as well as vocation, clearly need to be considered before standards can be enforced stringently. Measurements related to functional ROM continue to be the key to providing meaningful information about the patient's progress.

Within this chapter, each section covers a specific joint, examining reliability and validity studies on ROM for that joint, describing the latest devices and methods for measuring joint ROM, as well as providing tables with ''norms'' for joint ROM and information regarding functional ROM.

The measurement of joint range of motion (ROM) has been a part of clinical assessment since the early 1920s and continues to be one of the most commonly used techniques for evaluation used by physical and occupational therapists today (Cobe, 1928; Hewitt, 1928; Smith, 1982; Miller, 1985). The necessity of taking joint ROM measurements has been an accepted part of the evaluation procedure and is often performed clinically without the understanding of its purpose and usefulness in providing information for the

clinician, as well as to the patient, regarding progress or lack thereof (Bohannon, 1989; Miller, 1985). Certainly the meaning of joint ROM and what it tells therapists, particularly with regard to patient function, has been persistently challenged, especially in the area of lumbar ROM (Waddell, 1992).

Therapists have also witnessed that the term *normal* ROM assures neither normalcy nor that a patient will return to normal functional activity, particularly when related to return to work status (Waddell et al., 1992). Despite the difficulties with which therapists are confronted, it is clear that they will continue to use assessment of ROM as a part of the evaluative process. When assessing joint ROM, therapists want to link the act with a measurement, converting their observations into quantitative information (Michels, 1982). This information in turn allows therapists to make decisions regarding the necessity of specific treatment for the patient, as well as approach and modification of treatment. It also gives some indication of progress, as well as anticipated functional status or disability (American Medical Association, 1969; Miller, 1985). Assessment of joint ROM is based on what are termed objective measurements, as distinguished from subjective measurements, e.g., visual estimation. Objective measurements are characterized by the relative independence of the examiner, providing reliability estimates that demonstrate the apparent subjective error (Bohannon, 1989; Rothstein, 1989). Realizing that clinical measurements are probably never completely objective, relying always to some extent on the examiner's judgment (Rothstein, 1989), it should be noted that objective measures can provide evidence of improvement (increases in ROM) often earlier than subjective measurements or measurements of function (Bohannon, 1989).

An ongoing goal should be to constantly make efforts toward reducing the amount of error of variance in measurement procedures and to provide an accurate representation of the changes displayed by the patient. Bohannon (1989) lists four basic purposes for objective measures: 1) to describe status, 2) to document change, 3) to explain performance, and 4) to predict outcome. A fifth reason should be to encourage the patient's interest and motivation in the treatment program (Palmer and Epler, 1990).

In assessing ROM, the therapist can determine the patient's status by comparing measurements with those of the uninvolved joint or with "normal" values. The ability to document change is made by the therapist's remeasurements made over time. By knowing a patient's measurements in relation to measurements necessary for functional ROM (e.g., climbing steps or combing hair), the therapist can determine the patient's ability to perform a specific task. By measuring the ROM of various joints acting along a kinetic chain, functional activities can be predicted to some extent (Bohannon, 1982).

The purpose of this chapter is to provide the clinician with a quick reference to reliability and validity of ROM measurements for various upper and lower extremity joints. Another goal is to introduce alternative methods that depict novel and insightful procedures and instrumentation designed to acquire information regarding changes in musculoskeletal joint position. The majority of the sections on specific joint ROM provide both a table of "normal" joint ROM measurements and information regarding functional ROM, with particular emphasis on the upper ex-

tremities. In addition, by the year 2000 it is estimated that 15 percent of the Gross National Product may be spent on the low back problem (Cats-Baril & Frymoyer, 1991). Therefore, a special section on ROM for the lumbar spine, which offers an in-depth review of commonly used techniques, has been included.

HISTORICAL PERSPECTIVE

The early beginnings of ROM measurements date back to the first decade of this century, when two French physiologists, Camus and Amar (Smith, 1982), designed and began to use protractor goniometers to measure the relationship between mensuration and disablement. Indeed, much of the earlier literature appears to be a consequence of the postwar era and the necessity of relating ROM to disability (Smith, 1982).

The nomenclature and much of the standardized methods for measuring range of motion have been established by the American Academy of Orthopedic Surgeons. The basis for this system was established by research performed by Cave and Roberts (1936) and has been widely accepted throughout the medical world (Smith, 1982). The progression of these standards to improve objectivity by looking both at inter- and intraobserver reliability and validity (Hellebrandt et al., 1949; Leighton, 1955) added considerably to the progression toward increased objectivity of measurements. Although a variety of instruments and methods have been used for measuring ROM, the universal goniometer has been recognized as an accurate and convenient instrument for measurements (Defibaugh, 1964; Moore, 1949a; Salter, 1955).

Even though the methods indicated by the American Academy of Orthopedic Surgeons have been widely cited, both the reliability of these methods and the certainty of what has been cited as "normal range" values are highly questionable given the paucity of research that would confirm these methodologies. However, ongoing research has continued to substantiate the reliability and validity of certain methods and instrumentation, as well as document normal ROM values (Boone & Azen, 1979; Elveru et al., 1988; Gogia et al., 1987; Riddle et al., 1987; Rothstein et al., 1983). Although goniometry has long been used for assessment in physical therapy, it was not until the late 1940s that formal studies were performed to determine the reliability of these measurement techniques (Hellebrandt et al., 1949; Moore, 1949b). Moore cited earlier researchers in recognizing the necessity of locating the "axis of motion," as well as appropriate placement of the two arms of the goniometer along definitive bony landmarks. (For a more in-depth historical account of methodology and instrumentation, see Moore's two-part work [1949a, 1949b], which was followed by that of Hellebrandt et al., 1949.) The determination that the transparent universal goniometer was superior to other varied instrumentation was confirmed by these studies.

RELIABILITY

Clinicians agree that measurement of ROM is an important part of the assessment process; it thus becomes paramount that these measurements are shown to be reliable, i.e., they can be reproduced over time. It can be said that objective measures are only as good as their repeatability, i.e., their ability to be reproduced accurately (Gajdosik & Bohannon, 1987; Low, 1976). Hellebrandt and associates (1949) defined good reliability for ROM as an agreement of measurements within 3 degrees of one another. To substantiate what determines a reliable measurement procedure is difficult at best. Because reliability of goniometric measurements have been demonstrated to vary between different joints of the body (Boone et al., 1978; Hellebrandt et al., 1949; Low, 1976; Rothstein et al., 1983), measurement error may be attributed to factors such as length and mass of a body segment and ability to identify bony landmarks. Other factors influencing variation are changes occuring over time (Atha & Wheatley, 1976; Bohannon, 1984), differences due to the time of day that measurements are taken (Russell et al., 1992), and levels of goniometric skills among raters (Fish & Wingate, 1985). These variations certainly leave the therapist with the sobering thought that any interpretation of the data on goniometric measurement must be performed with discretion.

Comparing two different forms of a test on the same subjects (parallel-forms reliability) indicates whether measurements obtained can be used interchangeably (Rothstein & Echternach, 1993). Youdas et al., (1993) demonstrate an example of this when comparing goniometric measurements with visual estimates of ankle joint ROM. A comparison of two methods of goniometry (Grohmann, 1983) demonstrated no difference between using the lateral and over-the-joint methods of goniometry for measuring the elbow joint. In examining methodology, Ekstrand and coworkers (1982) determined that a standardized method increased reliability in joint motions of the lower extremity. The use of different instruments to make measurements of the same joint angle was demonstrated as reliable by Hamilton and Lachenbruch (1969), who used three different devices to measure finger joint angle. In comparing three different-sized goniometers to measure knee and elbow ROM, Rothstein and colleagues (1983) demonstrated a high level of interdevice reliability. Greene and Wolf (1989) demonstrated a strong relationship between the Ortho Ranger (electronic goniometer; Orthotronics, Inc., Daytona Beach, FL) and a universal goniometer for shoulder internal and external ROM but a poor relationship for elbow movements. A comparative

study (Goodwin et al., 1992) of three different methods of goniometry (universal goniometer, fluid goniometer, and electrogoniometer) for measuring elbow ROM showed significant differences between the goniometers and suggested that interchangeable use of the different types is inadvisable. The varied results of these studies suggest that although a small amount of error may occur within the goniometer, the main source of variation is in the methodology, and that by standardizing procedures, improved reliability can be realized.

VALIDITY

It has been suggested that the goniometric error is negligible and that the source of errors is from poor methodology (Salter, 1955). Although some small amount of error may occur within the instrument used for measurement due to equipment fault, the accuracy of goniometers can be ascertained. To validate a measurement of unknown validity, researchers compare it with another measurement of known validity (criterion-based validity) (Rothstein & Echternach, 1993). An example of this would be to compare an instrument designed for measuring ROM with something that has a known angle (Crowell et al., 1994). Concurrent validity, a class of criterion-based validity, can be established by comparing two instruments of measurement, one of unknown validity and the other having demonstrated validity during measurement of a specific joint (Rheault et al., 1988).

When assessing the accuracy of goniometric measurements, realizing the limitation of the information received is paramount. The goniometric measurements give the examiner quantity in degrees concerning a joint being assessed (Michels, 1982). However, this does not give us information about a specific tissue or allow the examiner to make qualitative judgments concerning worth, usefulness, or value of the joint being assessed (Bohannon, 1987; Rothstein, 1989). For example, when assessing lumbar ROM, the therapist cannot interpret the results as information about the vertebrae, disks, or muscles; nor can the therapist determine the level of function of the patient from the measurements alone. Until the results of the ROM measurements can be highly correlated with the status of a specific tissue, functional movement, or activity, the therapist is limited in the interpretation to a measurement of quantity in degrees only.

While therapists have depended on their knowledge of anatomy and appropriate placement of the goniometer to ensure accurate measurements (content validity), difficulty in finding bony landmarks or in identifying the axis of rotation may jeopardize the results. Radiographic comparisons have long been referred to as the "gold standard" in terms of validity studies and have been used effectively in studies of ROM (Enwemeka, 1986). Other methods such as cinematography (Bohannon, 1982; Vander-Linden & Wilhelm, 1991), electrogoniometry (Chiarello & Savidge, 1993), as well as other motion analysis systems (Day et al., 1984; Pearcy et al., 1984; Petersen et al., 1994; Scholz, 1989), offer new directions in strengthening content validity by demonstrating criterion-based validity (Gadjosik & Bohannon, 1987).

NORMALCY IN JOINT RANGE OF MOTION

While it is imperative that reliability is demonstrated for an ROM measurement procedure and that some form of validity is indicated to confirm a "true" measurement, it is also recommended that normative data be available to which to compare the measures. A point of reference is helpful in giving information to the clinician about where the patient is in terms of "normal range." Standards that clinicians use to judge the progress of their patient may assist in determining the cause of functional deficits. Many medicolegal and disability evaluations use "norms" as a standard in determining the level of disability (American Medical Association, 1969).

Because many studies have demonstrated bilateral symmetry in ROM measurements (Boone & Azen, 1979; Mallon et al., 1991; Roaas & Andersson, 1982), it has been suggested that the uninvolved joint be used as a reference point to assess progress made in the involved joint. However, this rationale has been challenged (Miller, 1985) from the standpoint that compensatory mechanisms alter biomechanics, causing changes in movement patterns and ROM. This may be particularly true in chronic diseases or injury.

Although the message is clear that normal values of joint ROM are necessary as a standard to measure progress, the problem becomes specificity of standards. General standards for ROM can not be applied across the board for all populations. An early study by Clark (1920) that listed rough averages for various joint ROM measurements was followed by studies in which measurements of a more specified population (Cobe, 1928; Hewitt, 1928) demonstrated that females had on the average greater wrist motion than males. More recent studies (Boone & Azen, 1979) examined age differences in a group of male subjects, noting an overall reduction in joint ROM with increased age, specifically indicating a progressive reduction in hip abduction and rotation during the first two decades of life. Bell and Hoshizaki (1981) demonstrated in eight different joints a general decline in ROM with age (not clearly indicated in upper extremity joints) and that females have greater ROM than males throughout life. When measuring ROM in the hip, knee, and ankle of males 30 to 40 years of age, Roaas and Andersson (1982) found significant differences between measures found by previous studies (American Academy of Orthopedic Surgeons,

1965; Boone & Azen, 1979). In looking at normal values of digital ROM in young adults, Mallon and colleagues (1991) found females had greater total active motion at all digits.

While the above studies demonstrate some general trends in regard to gender and age, fewer studies are available with regard to ROM differences in race and ethnic backgrounds (Ahlberg, et al., 1988; Allender et al., 1974; Roach & Miles, 1991). These studies clearly point to the shortcomings of following a strict adherence to a given set of "normal" measurements of ROM rather than allowing specific patient characteristics to determine the optimal measurements for a given situation. Finally, while all of these studies of normal measurements improve our knowledge base, the therapist should not lose sight of the most important aspect, returning the patient to an ROM that is functional. Understanding the ROM that is necessary for functional movement patterns is paramount when measuring joint ROM. Miller (1985) suggests three advantages of using functional ROM over other methods: 1) goals of treatment are based on individual characteristics, such as gender, age, and activity level; 2) therapists are better assisted in understanding the problem and developing strategies for treatment; and 3) therapists are able to focus on relieving a problem rather than on achieving a set quantity that has been deemed "normal."

WRIST AND HAND

Many complicating factors must be considered when measuring the joints of the wrist and hand, including the large number of joints and the intricacy in the variation of joint surfaces, particularly within the wrist. The numerous joints and multiple muscle attachments may lead to increased variations in measurements of the wrist when compared with a more simple joint like the elbow (Low, 1976). The presence of scars, edema, large hypertrophy, and deformed joints, as in rheumatoid arthritis, may also make the wrist difficult to measure in terms of goniometer placement. It is important to stabilize the numerous joint segments, allowing for accurate alignment of the goniometer during ROM measurements of the hand and wrist (Hamilton & Lachenbruch, 1969). Because a substantial number of variables can add to measurement error when measuring the joints of the hand and wrist, the necessity for providing a reliable method of measurement and instrumentation is foremost.

An early study assessing the finger joint angle (Hamilton & Lachenbruch, 1969) demonstrated no significant variance when looking at three different goniometers for determining joint angle: a dorsum goniometer, a universal goniometer, and a pendulum goniometer. When measuring ROM for the wrist and hands in flexion and extension, the clinician is confronted with basically three techniques for measurement: 1) measurement utilizing volar and dorsal surfaces (American Medical Association, 1984; Fess & Moran, 1981); 2) the use of the ulnar surface (Moore 1984; Norkin & White, 1985); and 3) the use of the radial surface (Hamilton & Lachenbruch, 1969) (Fig. 3–1).

The use of these different methods in measuring wrist ROM has led to varied approaches with conflicting results (Horger, 1990; Solgaard et al., 1986). When comparing the three methods in measuring passive wrist ROM in a clinical setting, LaStayo and Wheeler (1994) found that the dorsal/volar alignment method had a higher reliability than either the radial or ulnar method.

Under controlled conditions, Hamilton and Lachenbruch (1969) found the lateral (radial) method of measure-

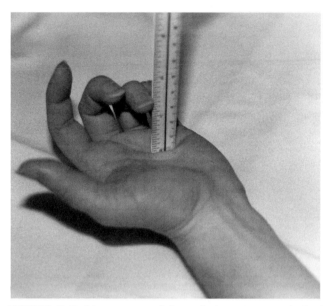

FIGURE 3–2. Measurement of finger flexion uses a method of measuring the distance between the pulp of the finger and the distal palmar crease.

ment was as reliable as the dorsal method when measuring finger ROM. Problems with good joint alignment secondary to joint deviation, edema, and enlarged joints make it apparent that appropriate selection of methods should be determined by the adaptability of the method to the specific clinical situation.

In estimating changes in ROM, the use of a standard error of measurement (SEM) in the wrist of ±4 to 6 degrees appears to be an acceptable figure for intratester reliability, while generally a slightly higher SEM, ±6 to 8 degrees, is characteristic of intertester reliability (Bear-Lehman & Abreu, 1989; Boone & Azen, 1979; Hamilton & Lachenbruch, 1969; Low, 1976), although this has not always been found to be the case, as LaStayo and Wheeler (1994) found a lower SEM and slightly higher intertester reliability during passive wrist measurement.

While the above studies present proven methods for measuring ROM in the wrist and hand, other methods have been presented in the literature that raise some interest, although with less substantial data confirming their reliability. Methods using a ruler to measure the distance between the finger and the palm of the hand (often a specific point, e.g., pulp of finger to distal palmar crease) (Fig. 3–2) to determine functional flexion of the digits (American Medical Association, 1988) have been used following tendon repair (Jansen & Watson, 1993). Dijkstra and associates (1994) present a method for measuring thumb apposition (distance between the thumb and wrist), demonstrating small intra- and interobserver variability (Fig. 3–3).

The importance of the thumb and the functional loss in its absence is difficult to quantify. The American Medical Association (1988) quantifies the loss of the thumb as a 40 percent loss of the total hand. Because of the unique structure and biaxial movement of the carpometacarpal

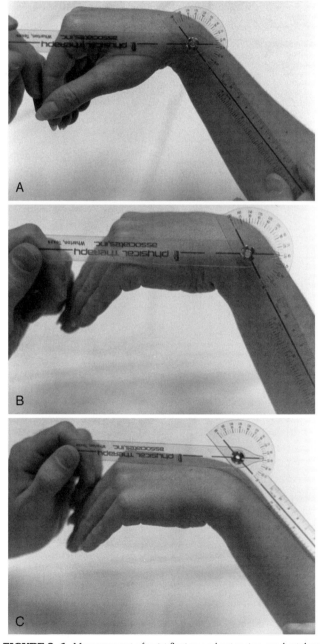

FIGURE 3–1. Measurement of wrist flexion and extension can be taken by using (A) the radial side of wrist and hand, (B) the ulnar side of hand, or (C) the suggested volar or dorsal side of hand.

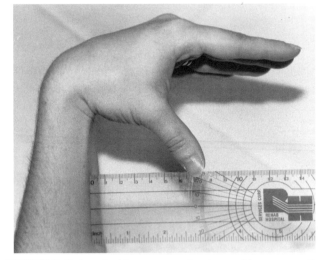

FIGURE 3–3. A method for measuring thumb apposition measures the distance between the pulp of the thumb and the wrist.

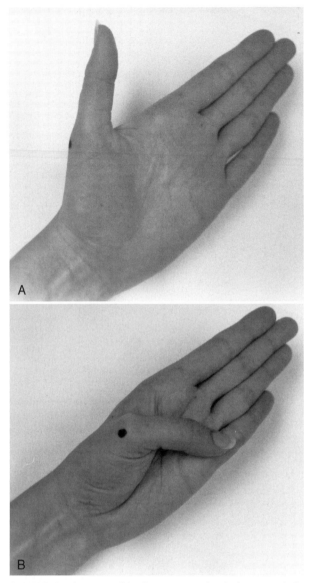

FIGURE 3–5. The range of the first metacarpal in the long axis. *A,* Start of movement. *B,* End of movement.

joint and the thumb's ability to move through a 360-degree arc, the ability to measure circumduction is of value to the therapist. Browne and coworkers (1979) present a method for measuring circumduction of the thumb by taking measurements of the axes of the ovoid-shaped design of circumduction (Fig. 3–4). An increased distance in measurements of the long axis (X-Z) (Fig. 3–5) and short axis (Y-Y′) (Fig. 3–6) give the therapist a quantifiable amount, indicating an increase in circumduction motion.

As previously mentioned, the intricacies of the joints of the hand and the complexity of the movement patterns most assuredly match the complexity of its function. However, a paucity of research on the measurement of digital ROM and effects of contiguous joints on ROM exists (Mallon et al., 1991). Digital ROM has often been left to a

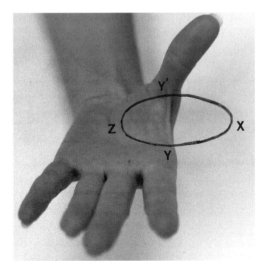

FIGURE 3–4. Circumduction motion of the metacarpal head about a long axis (X-Z), and a short axis (Y-Y′). (Adapted from Browne, E. Z., Teague, M. A., Gruenwald, C. [1979]. Method for measurement of circumduction of the thumb to evaluate results of opponensplasty. *Plastic and Reconstructive Surgery, 64,* 204–207.)

general concensus that the metacarpophalangeal joint (MCP) has 90 degrees of flexion and the proximal interphalangeal joint (PIP) has 100 degrees, while the distal interphalangeal joint (DIP) has 70 to 90 degrees (American Association Orthopedic Surgeons, 1965; American Medical Association, 1958). However, little has been done in the way of differentiating the values among the digits and quantifying these differences, as well as assessing the effects of adjacent joints in the finger and how they may affect ROM. Tables 3–1 and 3–2 give reported values provided by several researchers for "normal" ROM for the wrist and hand and for the digits of the hand.

While returning a patient to what would be considered a normal ROM is deemed important, a more critical measure is functional ROM, particularly in a clinical setting. In a 1985 study by Palmer and coworkers, 10 normal subjects performed 52 standardized tests, demonstrating a normal

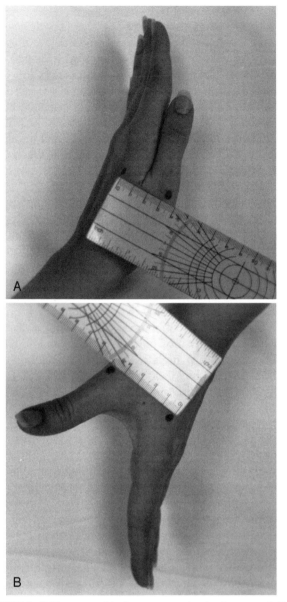

FIGURE 3–6. The range of the first metacarpal in the short axis. *A*, Start of movement. *B*, End of movement.

functional range of wrist motion to be 5 degrees flexion, 30 degrees extension, 10 degrees for radial deviation, and 15 degrees for ulnar deviation. In looking at ROM for joints of the hand (Hume et al., 1990), 11 activities of daily living were evaluated for functional ROM of the MCP and interphalangeal (IP) joints. Only a small percentage of the active ROM (AROM) of the joints was actually required for functional tasks. In this study, functional flexion averaged 61 degrees at the MCP joints, 60 degrees at the PIP joints, and 39 degrees at the DIP joints. The thumb demonstrated functional flexion averaging 21 degrees at the MCP joint and 18 degrees at the IP joint. This amount was 32 percent of the amount of flexion that was available. Ryu and colleagues (1991) demonstrated that a battery of activities of daily living could be performed with 70 percent of the maximal range of wrist motion, which was 40 degrees for wrist flexion and extension and 40 degrees of combined radial and ulnar deviation. This is somewhat more than that estimated previously by Palmer and associates (1985). Safaee-Rad and coworkers (1990), who looked at functional ROM in regard to three feeding tasks (eating with a spoon, eating with a fork, and drinking from a handled cup), found that 40 degrees forearm pronation to 60 degrees forearm supination, with 10 degrees wrist flexion to 25 degrees wrist extension and from 20 degrees wrist ulnar deviation to 5 degrees wrist radial deviation was required to perform tasks. Wrist rotation was found to be negligible. These estimates are more in line with earlier studies by Palmer and colleagues (1985). These measurements indicate ranges that are required to perform basic functional activities; however, when our goal is to return a patient to extracurricular activities, we clearly must assess the ROM necessary to realize a predetermined motor pattern.

ELBOW

Like other musculoskeletal joints, the elbow has received attention in the way of reliability studies. As a hingelike

TABLE 3–1

MEASUREMENTS WITHIN LIMITS OF "NORMAL" ROM IN DEGREES FOR THE HAND AND WRIST, REPORTED BY SEVERAL AUTHORS AND RESEARCHERS*

Joint	AAOS (1965)	Boone & Azen† (1979)	Dorinson & Wagner (1948)	Esch & Lepley (1974)	Gerhardt & Russe (1975)	AMA (1958)	Solgaard et al.‡ (1986)	Wiechec & Krusen (1939)
Wrist								
Flexion	80	76	80	90	60	70	77	60
Extension	70	75	55	70	50	60	73	55
Radial deviation	20	22	20	20	20	20	26	35
Ulnar deviation	30	36	40	30	30	30	40	75

* Studies not showing demographics in table did not include them in the original research.
† N = 109, 18–54 y, male.
‡ N = 31, 24–65 y, male and female.
AAOS = American Academy of Orthopedic Surgeons; AMA = American Medical Association.

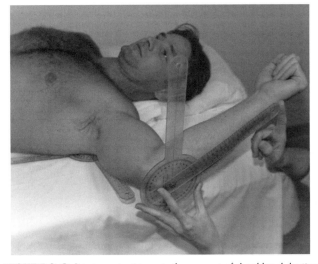

FIGURE 3–9. It is important to note the amount of shoulder abduction when measuring shoulder external and internal rotation.

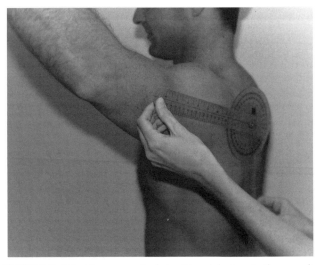

FIGURE 3–10. Measurement of shoulder abduction in the scapular plane. This position is the most functional position for elevation.

the scapula as the "moveable" reference point. Another method (Kibler, 1991) used a linear measurement from the nearest spinous process to the inferior angle of the scapula. When investigating various techniques used in previous studies, Gibson and coworkers (1995) demonstrated a high level of intra- and intertester reliability (intraclass correlation coefficient [ICC] = 0.95, 0.92) for the method of DeVita and coworkers (1990); however, they found low intertester reliability for the Kibler (1991) method. It has been suggested that these methods may provide results that prove to be somewhat difficult to interpret by the clinician, particularly the Kibler (1991) method.

When measuring shoulder ROM, the clinician needs to be aware of the contributions not only of shoulder flexion and abduction but also of accompanying motions, e.g., external and internal rotation. Accompanying motion that occurs during active shoulder flexion was ingeniously determined in a study by Blakely and Palmer (1984). In this study, a universal goniometer and a gravity-activated angle finder were utilized to determine that medial rotation of the humerus accompanied active and passive shoulder flexion movements. During measurements of shoulder internal and external rotation, the amount of shoulder abduction needs to be noted, as this may limit ROM measurements (Fig. 3–9). Also, the plane in which shoulder elevation is made should be recorded, as this too may limit the available ROM (Fig. 3–10). The plane of the scapula (30 degrees–45 degrees to the frontal plane) has been described as the most functional position for elevation because the capsule is not twisted on itself and the deltoid and supraspinatus are best aligned for shoulder elevation (Zuckerman & Matsen, 1989) (Fig. 3–11).

Riddle and colleagues (1987) examined both intertester and intratester reliability of shoulder passive range of motion (PROM), utilizing two different-sized universal goniometers. They demonstrated intratester reliability for

all motions ranging from ICC = 0.87 to 0.99, whereas intertester reliability for measurements of flexion, abduction, and lateral rotation ranged from ICC = 0.84 to 0.90. Intertester reliability for horizontal abduction and adduction, extension, and medial rotation was poor. The goniometric measurements of shoulder PROM appeared to be unaffected with different-sized goniometers in this study; however, reliability between testers appears to be specific to movements measured.

"Normal" ROM within the shoulder appears to be age specific, decreasing in all ranges slightly with increased age (Boone & Azen, 1979). A list of normal ROM measurements from several authors is provided in Table 3–4.

Functional ROM for the shoulder during three feeding tasks (eating with a spoon, eating with a fork, and drinking from a handled cup) required 5 degrees to 45 degrees

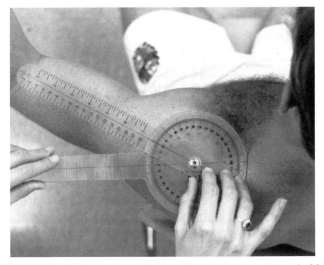

FIGURE 3–11. The plane of the scapula measures approximately 30 degrees to 45 degrees to the frontal plane.

TABLE 3-4

MEASUREMENTS WITHIN "NORMAL" LIMITS OF ROM FOR THE SHOULDER, REPORTED BY SEVERAL AUTHORS AND RESEARCHERS

Joint	AAOS (1965)	Boone & Azen* (1979)	Dorinson & Wagner (1948)	Esch & Lepley (1974)	Gerhardt & Russe (1975)	AMA (1958)	Wiechec & Krusen (1939)
Shoulder							
Flexion	180	167	180	170	170	150	180
Extension	60	62	45	60	50	40	45
Abduction	180	184	180	170	170	150	180
Internal rotation	70	69	90	80	80	40+	90
External rotation	90	104	90	90	90	90+	90
Horizontal abduction	—	45	—	—	30	—	—
Horizontal adduction	135	140	—	—	135	—	—

* N = 109, 18–54 y, male.
AAOS = American Academy of Orthopedic Surgeons; AMA = American Medical Association.

shoulder flexion, 5 degrees to 35 degrees shoulder abduction, and 5 degrees to 25 degrees shoulder internal rotation (Safaee-Rad et al., 1990). It has been demonstrated that restrictions in elbow joint ROM significantly increase the need for an increased arc of motion for both shoulder flexion and internal rotation during feeding tasks (Cooper et al., 1993).

CERVICAL SPINE

While the spinal segment is one of the most frequently treated areas of the body, it continues to be one of the most elusive areas in determining reliable measurements for ROM. Because of the difficulty in aligning the goniometer with a definitive axis of rotation, as well as the inability to locate standardized landmarks to act as points of reference (Cole, 1982), the cervical spine remains one of the least accurately yet most highly measured of all musculoskeletal joints. Having 23 points of contact at which motion occurs from the occiput to the first thoracic vertebra, cervical motion combines sliding and rotation with flexion (Kottke & Mundale, 1959). Because flexion and extension occur at each of the cervical vertebrae, the axis of rotation for flexion and extension movements is segmental in the sagittal plane with multiple axis; consequently, a single instantaneous axis of rotation (IAR) for the entire cervical spine cannot be isolated. Measuring the total movement of the head in any one plane approximates the change in the degrees occurring in the cervical spine. Anatomically, alignment of the goniometer's axis with the external auditory meatus has been used for measuring flexion and extension (Norkin and White, 1985). Due to the shift of the line of reference during flexion and extension, it becomes virtually impossible to maintain congruency with the reference point (Kottke & Mundale, 1959; Nordin & Frankel; 1989). Slight variations in alignment of the goniometer's

arms or placement of the axis may cause large variations in angular measurements (Robson, 1966). Much literature exists on various techniques that have been used over the years to try to determine more accurate and efficient ways to measure cervical ROM (Defibaugh, 1964; Hand, 1938; Loebl, 1967; Moore, 1978; Schenker, 1956). The tape measure is used to determine the distance between bony landmarks (e.g., chin to sternal notch, chin to acromion tip) in many of the methods tried over the years (Storms, 1955; Moll & Wright, 1976), with varying degrees of accuracy.

To avoid inaccuracies due to changing reference points, several early studies placed or attached a gravity-assisted device or an equivalent measurement device to the head and determined ROM by changes affected by gravity (Buck et al., 1959; Hand, 1938; Leighton, 1955; Schenker, 1956). This appears to have been one of the more accurate techniques for measurement described in the literature (Defibaugh, 1964b; Kadir, 1981; Tucci et al., 1986). An increased level of accuracy through increased standardization can be achieved by attaching a gravity goniometer to the subject's head and taking measurements from changes in head position. With the universal goniometer, a moderate to good level of accuracy was demonstrated with intratester reliability. However, intertester reliability proved to have only a marginal level of accuracy with extension and rotation, proving to offer a higher level of reliability than side-bending and cervical flexion (Tucci et al., 1986; Youdas et al., 1991). Improving on this method in terms of efficiency, accuracy, and ease of use, the cervical ROM instrument (CROM) has demonstrated a high level of intertester and intratester reliability (Capuano-Pucci et al., 1991) (Fig. 3–12).

Cinefluorography and the electronic digital inclinometer have contributed greatly to our knowledge of normal cervical ROM, demonstrating a high level of reliability when compared with radiographic measurements (Fielding, 1957; Kottke & Mundale, 1959; Mayer et al., 1993).

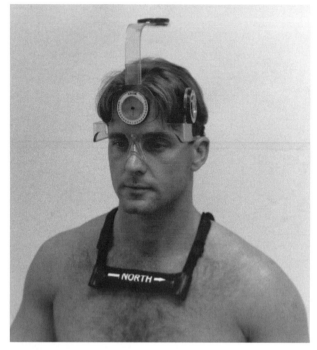

FIGURE 3–12. The use of the CROM instrument in measuring cervical ROM.

Table 3–5 lists normal ROM measurements provided by various contributors.

LUMBAR SPINE

Simple backache is the most disabling condition of people younger than 45 years of age and costs society an estimated 25 to 100 billion dollars a year (Frymoyer & Cats-Baril, 1991). The demand for scientific evidence in the management of this industrialized epidemic is becoming increasingly important (Helms, 1994). Objective mea-

surement of spinal ROM is thought to be of critical scientific importance in determining disability (American Medical Association, 1990), selecting appropriate therapeutic intervention (Maitland, 1986; McKenzie, 1981), and monitoring the patient's progress (Mayer and Gatchel, 1988). For example, disability ratings are largely based on the lumbar spine ROM measurements; i.e., they are based on lost ROM versus a mean value. Interestingly, many orthopedic surgeons (Davis, 1994) consider too much ROM, i.e., hypermobility leading to "instability," to be pathologic (Froning & Frohman, 1968; Frymoyer et al., 1979; Howes & Isdale, 1971). Thus, it is of critical importance that thorough, accurate documentation of mobility is undertaken to determine hypermobility (Burton et al., 1989), as well as hypomobility, through a chosen plane of motion.

In the appendicular skeleton, normal ROM can be determined by comparing ROM measurements both with normative data and with the uninvolved limb (American Academy of Orthopedic Surgeons, 1965; American Medical Association, 1990). In the axial skeleton, sagittal plane ROM is determined solely by comparison with normative data (Gilbert, 1993). Unfortunately, normative data, such as the mean value recommended by the American Medical Association, are inadequate (Sullivan et al., 1994), and a paucity of good, reliable, and valid data exists. Normal spinal ROM measurements are influenced to differing degrees by many factors. These variables are thought to include age (Moll & Wright, 1971; Sullivan et al., 1994; Tanz, 1953), gender (Batti'e et al., 1987; Burton & Tillotson, 1991; Moll & Wright, 1971), time of day (Russell et al., 1992), occupation (Russell et al., 1993), leisure activities (Burton & Tillotson, 1991), previous history of low back pain (Burton et al., 1989), sitting-to-standing height ratios (Batti'e et al., 1987), warming up (Keeley et al., 1986), obesity (Batti'e et al., 1987), and the techniques with which normative data are collected (Pearcy & Tibrewal, 1984).

TABLE 3–5

SEVERAL REPORTED VALUES FOR "NORMAL" ROM OF THE CERVICAL SPINE

Motion	AMA (1988)	Buck* (1959)	Defibaugh† (1964)	Capuano-Pucci et al.‡ (CROM) (1991)	Mayer et al.§ (Electronic Inclinometer) (1993)
Flexion	60	67	59	50	49
Extension	75	77	80	70	67
Rotation					
Right	80	73	85	70	87
Left	80	74	89	69	84
Lateral flexion					
Right	45	—	51	43	44
Left	45	—	49	44	39

* N = 100, 18–23 y, male and female.
† N = 30, 20–40 y, male.
‡ N = 20, x = 23.5 y, male and female.
§ N = 58, 17–62 y, male and female.

Generally, population studies agree that lumbar mobility declines with age (Moll & Wright, 1971; Russell et al., 1993; Sullivan et al., 1994; Tanz, 1953). With regard to gender, Moll and Wright (1971), using the modified Schöber technique, observed males to have greater ROM in the sagittal plane, but females were observed to have greater frontal plane motion. Russell and colleagues (1993), using the 3-Space Isotrak (Polhemus Navigation Sciences, UK), concurred that lateral bending was generally greater in females. Leisure activities have been proposed to influence lumbar mobility, and an increased exposure to adult sports has been shown to produce a reduction in spinal mobility when flexicurve techniques are used (Burton & Tillotson, 1991). Although it is generally accepted that a history of low back pain affects subsequent mobility (Burton et al., 1989; Russell et al., 1993), sobering is the work by Waddell and associates (1992); using a spinal inclinometer, they have shown that lumbar flexion in chronic low back pain patients was not restricted, as commonly believed. Batti'e and coworkers (1987) found ROM with distraction methods not only to be influenced by age and gender but also by obesity, height, and sitting-to-standing height ratio. With respect to height, Burton and colleagues (1989) could not find any clear correlation between sagittal mobility and trunk height. Russell and associates (1992) have demonstrated circadian variations and have further complicated the reliabilities of studies that did not control for time of day. For example, taking measurements at different times throughout the day can cause discrepancies of greater than 5 degrees. Of further consideration in obtaining reliable, normal values is the need for warm-up, as demonstrated by Keeley and coworkers (1986). Finally, both the reliability and validity of the methods used to gain normative values (e.g., distraction methods, inclinometry, flexicurve, and motion analysis techniques) must be scrutinized.

The most accurate spinal measurements rely on radiographic measures (Pearcy et al., 1985). Radiographic measures are thought to be the gold standard for validating methods and gaining normal ROM values. Due to ethical concerns regarding exposure, a large normative base using this gold standard is not available. Table 3–6 describes ROM in the sagittal and coronal plane and gives some insight considering age and gender (Bogduk, 1992).

Newer knowledge on lumbar spine motion reveals the importance of three-dimensional movement (Pearcy & Tibrewal, 1984; Pearcy et al., 1985; Pearcy et al., 1984). Normal-plane radiographs are limited to two-dimensional interpretations of three-dimensional information. "These two-dimensional measurements may be erroneous due to movements in the third dimension; and measurements of movements out of the planes of the radiographs are liable to large errors." (Pearcy, 1985). An exciting development is the 3-Space Isotrak, which gives three-dimensional motion analysis (Russell et al., 1993). It has been shown to be valuable not only in measuring the extremes of spinal motion but also, very importantly, in measuring the pattern of movement. It is of particular importance to note that large variations occur in normal ROM that have led researchers to question the usefulness of ascertaining normalcy (Hayes et al., 1989; Penning et al., 1984). Normal data are influenced by many variables besides age and gender, as has been illustrated. A very important consideration since the gold standard is of limited use is the objectivity of the methods to gain normal information.

The objective measurement of 15 joints encased in 18 cm of spine, inaccessible to the naked eye and moving in a coupled fashion, is a difficult task. In research, sophisticated, expensive equipment such as biplanar radiographs, vector stereography, and photographic methods have been used (Mayer & Gatchel, 1988). Clinically, the challenge of making objective measurements has been met by visual estimation (Nelson et al., 1979; Wolf et al., 1979), the goniometer (American Medical Association, 1971; Fitzgerald et al., 1983), flexible curves (Burton, 1986; Youdas et al., 1995), skin distraction methods (Macrae & Wright, 1969; Schöber, 1937; Williams et al., 1993), and the inclinometer (Loebl, 1967; Mayer et al., 1984).

The practice of estimating ROM by visual observation perseveres probably because it is time efficient and simple. It must be realized that all clinical examinations, even those thought to be irrefutably objective, are subject to observer bias and error (Deyo et al., 1994). Not surprising is the discrepancy of up to 30 percent that has been noted with

TABLE 3–6

RANGES OF SEGMENTAL MOTION IN MALES AGED 25 TO 36 YEARS*

| Level | Lateral Flexion | | Axial Rotation | | Flexion | Extension | Flexion and Extension |
	Left	Right	Left	Right			
L1-2	5	6	1	1	8 ± 5	5 ± 2	13 ± 5
L2-3	5	6	1	1	10 ± 2	3 ± 2	13 ± 2
L3-4	5	6	1	2	12 ± 1	1 ± 1	13 ± 2
L4-5	3	5	1	2	13 ± 4	2 ± 1	16 ± 4
L5-S1	0	2	1	0	9 ± 6	5 ± 4	14 ± 5

* Mean range (measured in degrees, with standard deviation).
From Bogduk, N., & Twomey, L. T. (1991). *Clinical anatomy of the lumbar spine* (2nd ed.). New York: Churchill Livingstone.

the use of such methods (Nelson et al., 1979; Wolf et al., 1979). Consequently, therapists should be hesitant in reaching important conclusions about facts such as progression based on these inadequate measures. Originally, the addendum to this procedure as advocated by the American Medical Association was the use of the goniometer (American Medical Association, 1971). The use of the uniaxial goniometer to measure multiaxial spinal movement is obviously problematic (Mayer & Gatchel, 1988). Fitzgerald and associates (1983) confirm these problems when they reported coefficients of variance (CVs) of up to 53 percent using the goniometer. (The use of CVs in determining reliability of measures is of questionable value [Williams et al., 1993], although they were commonly used in earlier research.)

Another method once described as promising (Merritt et al., 1986) and still prevailing is the finger-to-floor method. Interesting to note is that it has been long known that patients with multilevel stabilization involving more motion segments than merely the lumbar spine are able to touch their toes (Mayer et al., 1984). Advocates of this method are deceived not only by large amounts of accompanying hip movement but also by movements in the thoracic spine and, to a lesser degree, the amount of movement at the knee, ankle, and upper extremities. Merritt and colleagues (1986), in comparing three simple noninvasive methods, found the finger-to-floor method to be least reproducible.

Two methods that they found to be more promising and worthy of attention are the modified Schöber technique and the double inclinometer method. Both methods have the advantage of isolating the lumbar spine ROM. In 1937, Schöber used a simple tape measure to estimate lumbar ROM. This technique has been modified (Macrae & Wright, 1969) and remodified (Williams et al., 1993), and distraction techniques can be used to measure movement in the coronal plane as well. Fitzgerald and coworkers (1983), using the Schöber method, reported an interobserver reliability using the Pearson correlation coefficient of $r = 1.0$ for flexion and $r = 0.88$ for lumbar extension but had the disadvantage of using healthy, young subjects. Beattie and associates (1987) used both healthy subjects and subjects with low back pain and reported high reliability with the modified Schöber attraction method for measuring extension. Macrae and Wright (1969) attempted to validate both the modified Schöber and the Schöber techniques, comparing them with radiographic techniques. Pearson product-moment correlation coefficients of $r = 0.97$ for the modified Schöber and $r = 0.90$ for the Schöber technique were reported compared with radiography. Portek and colleagues (1983), however, demonstrated little collaboration between any of the commonly used clinical methods, including the modified Schöber technique and radiographs. Miller and associates (1992) have questioned the modified Schöber technique on both scientific merit due to the potential error (Table 3–7) and on clinical grounds. Clinically, these authors offer the double inclinometer (DI) as a validated technique that eliminates

TABLE 3–7
POTENTIAL ERRORS AFFECTING RELIABILITY OF THE MODIFIED SCHÖBER METHOD EVALUATED IN THIS STUDY

1. Presence or absence of "dimples of Venus."
2. Anatomic location of dimples of Venus.
3. Anatomic variability of location of 10-cm line (correlation among a skin mark 10 cm above the interdimple line, spinous process at that level, and the number of levels from T-12 to S-1 measured with the technique).
4. Problems introduced by skin distraction occurring in the absence of movement of underlying bony structures (e.g., the sacrum).
5. Problems engendered by expression of results of an essentially angular movement in linear terms (in centimeters, not degrees).
6. Problems in developing a normative database created by population variation in human height superimposed on a fixed-length test.

From Miller, S. A., Mayer, T., Cox, R., & Gatchel, R. J. (1992). Reliability problems associated with the modified Schöber technique for true lumbar flexion measurement. *Spine, 17,* 345–348.

many or all of the problems associated with the Schöber technique.

The DI is generally attributed to Loebl (1967). Reliability studies by Keeley and coworkers (1986) reported interrater reliability values of ICC = 0.92 for 9 subjects with chronic low back and 0.90 for 11 subjects without low back pain. Waddell and associates (1991), using the spinal inclinometer, showed an ICC of 0.91 for interobserver reproducibility of lumbar flexion. The landmarks used for measurement for both the Schöber and the DI methods are described in Table 3–8 and in the succeeding instructional on measurement of spinal ROM in the sagittal plane.

Today, electrogoniometers using these principles are offered. A more recent study concluded both the DI and the Cybex EDI (Cybex, Ronkonkoma, NY) to be substantially more reliable than observation (Chiarello & Savidge, 1993). Mayer and colleagues (1984), in a validation study, concluded that no significant difference existed between DI measures and radiographic measures

TABLE 3–8
REFERENCE POINTS ADVOCATED BY DIFFERENT AUTHORS WHEN MEASURING LUMBAR ROM

Technique	Inferior Landmark	Superior Landmark
Schöber	Lumbosacral junction	A point 10 cm above lumbosacral junction
Modified Schöber	5 cm below lumbosacral junction	A point 10 cm above lumbosacral junction
Modified-modified Schöber	Midline intersection of posterosuperior iliac spine	A point 15 cm above midline intersection

of ROM. An earlier study found little collaboration between the DI and radiography; therefore, validation of this technique is controversial (Portek et al., 1983). More recently, reliability studies have compared these two very promising methods. Merritt and associates (1986) suggested that to increase objectivity of spinal ROM measurements, the Schöber test should be used in routine clinical examinations. They showed that the modified Schöber method demonstrated high reproducibility (in flexion, CV = 6.3 percent for interexaminer reproducibility and 6.6 percent for intraexaminer reproducibility), whereas the inclinometer showed poorer reproducibility (in extension, CV = 65.4 percent for interexaminer reproducibility and 50.7 percent for intraexaminer reproducibility).

Gill et al., (1988) compared the repeatability of the modified Schöber, double inclinometer, finger-to-floor, and photographic methods. They concluded that the modified Schöber method was the most repeatable (CV = 0.9 percent for modified Schöber flexion and 2.8 percent for modified Schöber extension). An additional study (Williams et al., 1993) compared the modified-modified Schöber with the DI method. The authors found that the modified-modified Schöber method of measuring the lumbar ROM (ICC = flexion 0.72 and extension 0.76) was more reliable than the DI technique (lumbar flexion 0.60 and lumbar extension 0.68). No validation was given for this new method in the study. Problems with the DI technique may be attributed to palpation of bony landmarks, use of the flat surface of the inclinometer over the curvature of the flexing spine (i.e., offering many tangents), and technical skills.

Both techniques have both disadvantages and advantages. Either method is offered as a more reliable method than goniometric, eyeballing, or finger-to-floor measures. However, a problem common to both methods that should be considered is the starting position when standing (Keeley et al., 1986; Sullivan et al., 1994). To a large degree, the initial lordosis (not apparent lordosis) determines the amount of flexion or extension available. An obese person with increased lordosis has potentially less extension and a potential for an inflated flexion value. The American Academy of Orthopedic Surgeons (1965) advocates the use of tape measures when measuring lumbar spine flexion. The American Medical Association has revised its guidelines and now supports the use of the spinal inclinometer (Engelberg, 1988). The American Medical Association firmly states that an evaluation utilizing the spinal inclinometer takes precedence over an evaluation using an alternative measuring technique. Before 1988, the use of the goniometer was advocated by the American Medical Association, and it is questionable as to whether these measures, which have been shown to be notoriously unreliable, would have taken precedence over the Schöber techniques, which have been proven to be more reliable.

An area that is very controversial and of great importance to the manual therapist is the art of assessment of intervertebral ROM through passive spinal mobility tests. Clinicians trained in those specialized tests seem to be convinced of their reliability and validity (Grieve, 1987; Grimsby, 1990; Kaltenborn & Lindahlo, 1969; Maitland, 1986; Paris, 1987). In fact, a whole profession is based on the ability to reliably palpate intervertebral motion. Interesting to note is the discovery of the palpatory illusion (Lewit & Liebenson, 1993). Sobering is the scientific evidence that has proven these assessment techniques to be unreliable (Maher & Adams, 1994). Obviously, the opinion of many of these manual therapists must be scrutinized in light of the reliability studies.

Finally, the measurement of lumbar spine ROM is a clinical conundrum, especially when considering movement outside the sagittal plane. The measuring of normal values is inherently difficult and affected by many factors that are often overlooked. The usefulness of these measures to the clinician is not really clear. By using skin distraction, skin attraction, and double inclinometer methods, a therapist can improve the objectivity of lumbar spine ROM measurements in the sagittal plane. The low back problem threatens the health of the public, and it is only through becoming more scientific and thus more objective that clinicians move toward a solution.

Sagittal Spinal Range of Motion Measurement

To increase the reliability of lumbar flexion and extension, the double inclinometer method or versions of the Schöber method are recommended. The following procedure is suggested:

1. Accurate location of anatomic landmarks is critical. Helpful tips are that the dimples of Venus usually correspond to S-2, the iliac crests are approximately at the L-4,5 level, counting up the spinous processes will find T-12 and L-1, and the average length of the male lumbar column is 18 cm (Waddell et al., 1992; Williams et al., 1989).
2. A standardized starting position needs to be selected, e.g., bare feet, heels together, knees straight, equal weight-bearing, looking straight ahead, arms hanging at the side, relaxed (Waddell et al., 1992).
3. A "neutral" lumbopelvic position is required, e.g., midway between flexion and extension to eliminate troubles of differing lordosis (others have modified the standing starting position to eliminate this problem) (Sullivan et al., 1994).
4. Warm-up is necessary for reliable measures, e.g., flex and extend twice, left and right rotation twice, left and right lateral flexion twice, and one more flexion and extension (Keeley et al., 1986; Waddell et al., 1992).
5. The inclinometers or tape measures should be placed on the selected points and held in place (Figs. 3–13 and 3–14).
6. Instruct the patient to bend forward as far as possible (Figs. 3–15 and 3–16).

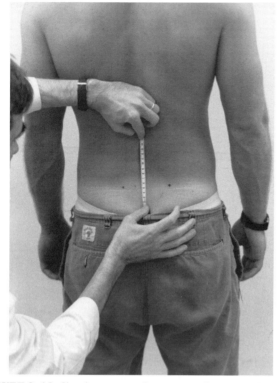

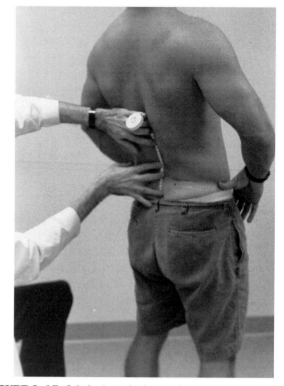

FIGURE 3–13. Skin distraction and attraction techniques are based on the fact that the distance between two points marked on the skin over the spine increases with flexion and decreases with extension. Demonstrated here is the modified Schöber's method. Initial measurement in neutral lumbar position.

FIGURE 3–15. Schöber's method using the attraction technique with trunk extension.

7. If the modified Schöber technique is being used, measure the length of the tape measure to the nearest millimeter. If the inclinometer method is being used, measure to the nearest degree.
8. Instruct the patient to return to neutral.
9. Ask the patient to bend backward as far as possible.

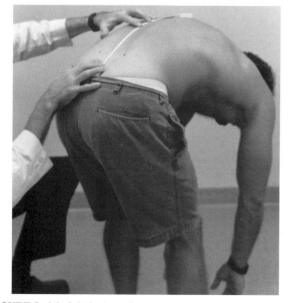

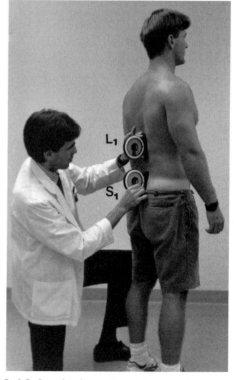

FIGURE 3–14. Schöber's method using the distraction technique with trunk flexion.

FIGURE 3–16. Spinal inclinometer methods require placement of the instruments over fixed points and taking tangential measurements. The superior inclinometer is fixed over T12-L1, and the inferior inclinometer is placed over the sacrum. Lumbar flexion and extension are derived from these simple measurements: total flexion (TF) = $L_1'-L_1$, pelvic flexion (PF) = $S_1'-S_1$, lumbar flexion = TF-PF.

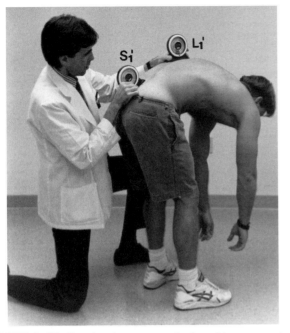

FIGURE 3–17. Spinal inclinometer method used to measure trunk flexion.

If the modified Schober technique is being used, measure the length of the tape measure to the nearest millimeter (Fig. 3–17). If the inclinometer method is being used, measure to the nearest degree (Fig. 3–18).

THORACIC SPINE

As with the lumbar spine, similar difficulties exist in measuring ROM through the thoracic spine. Difficulties in isolating pure planar movements due to coupling motions, as well as maintaining accurate contact with bony landmarks during measurement, are some of the problems clinicians are faced with. Although reliability studies for thoracic ROM have been elusive, recommendations from the literature indicate similar methods for measuring the thoracic spine as were incorporated with the lumbar spine, e.g., Loebl (DI). Placement of the inclinometer for sagittal flexion and extension should be on T-12/L-1, as well as on C-7/T-1, with the difference in the two beginning and end measurements giving the total thoracic ROM (American Medical Association, 1991).

HIP

During measurement of hip ROM, controlling for the movement of the pelvis is of paramount importance (Ashton et al., 1978; Gajdosik et al., 1993). The lumbar curve is often used as a reference point to alert the therapist

to any changes in pelvic position (Burdett et al., 1986; Day et al., 1984). The determination of degrees of true hip extension and flexion is probably one of the more complex measurements, as it is very difficult for the tester to delineate the obliteration of the normal lumbar curve during measurement, particularly in the presence of a hip flexion contracture (Gajdosik et al., 1993). To determine the amount of hip flexion deformity present, Ekstrand and colleagues (1982) utilized a rigid standardized procedure for measurement with identification and marking of the anatomic landmarks. The results showed coefficients of variation of 1.2 percent, 1.4 percent, and 2.5 percent for hip extension, hip flexion, and hip abduction, respectively. In this study, hip abduction was made with a double-protractor goniometer, whereas hip flexion and extension were determined by a gravity inclinometer attached to the patient's thigh. Table 3–9 lists norms for hip ROM according to individual researchers.

Using the universal goniometer, Boone and coworkers (1978) demonstrated a higher intratester reliability of r = 0.74 for hip abduction, as opposed to an intertester reliability of r = 0.55. Ashton and associates (1978) determined an overall relatively low level of reliability when giving specific procedural instructions (described by the American Academy of Orthopedic Surgeons, 1965) to an experimental group of therapists versus a control group of therapists, while measuring passive hip ROM in children with mild to moderate spastic cerebral palsy. With the exception of hip external rotation, which improved (r = 0.79 and 0.82) with specific instructions to the experi-

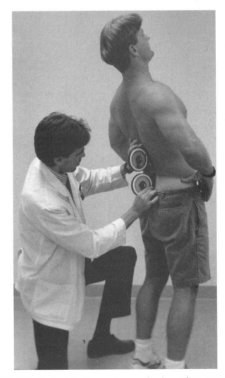

FIGURE 3–18. Spinal inclinometer method used to measure trunk extension.

TABLE 3–9

VALUES FOR "NORMAL" ROM FOR THE HIP, LISTED BY VARIOUS AUTHORS

Joint	AAOS (1965)	Boone & Azen* (1979)	Dorinson & Wagner (1948)	Esch & Lepley (1974)	Gerhardt & Russe (1975)	AMA (1958)	Roaas & Anderson† (1982)	Roach & Miles (NHANES 1) (1991)	Wiechec & Krusen (1939)
Hip									
Flexion	120	122	125	130	125	100	120	121	120
Extension	30	10	50	45	15	30	9	19	45
Abduction	45	46	45	45	45	40	39	42	45
Adduction	30	27	20	15	15	20	30	—	—
Internal rotation	45	47	30	33	45	40	33	32	—
External rotation	45	47	50	36	45	50	34	32	—

* N = 109, x = 22.4, male.
† N = 108, 30–40 y, male.
‡ N = 1683, 25–74 y, male and female.
AAOS = American Academy of Orthopedic Surgeons; AMA = American Medical Association.

mental group, the other measurements were inconsistent and had poor reliability. Hip extension measurements in particularly were low, even when the examiners made efforts to control for compensatory pelvic movement by flexion of the opposing hip (Fig. 3–19).

Straight-Leg Raise

Certainly one of the most measured ROMs has been for the straight-leg raise (SLR) (Fig. 3–20). However, this measurement has not been without its difficulties in ascertaining a standardized method in which reliability can be assured (Bohannon, 1984; Cameron et al., 1994; Gajdosik et al., 1985; Tanigawa et al., 1972). An early study

comparing three instruments (a standard plastic goniometer, a flexometer, and a tape measure) for measuring SLR (Hsieh et al., 1983) demonstrated a good level of intersession reliability for both the goniometer and the flexometer (r = 0.88) and for the tape measure (r = 0.74). In the same study, high intrasession reliability was found for all three (r = 0.94). To isolate the contribution of the lumbar spine, the pelvis was palpated during passive SLR to determine the point at which pelvic rotation began (Hsieh et al., 1983).

A review of the methods that might improve reliability has presented varied hip positions, active versus passive, and trial repetitions during SLR (Cameron et al., 1994). Cameron and coworkers determined that all of these factors made a difference in the amount of SLR experienced and recommended consistency of method during the performance and interpretation of the SLR. Other methods to determine SLR have included the knee extension method with the hips stabilized at 90 degrees of flexion

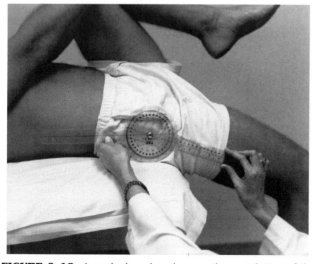

FIGURE 3–19. A method used to decrease the contribution of the lumbar spine to hip extension. Note that the lumbar spine is to stay in contact with the table during measurement.

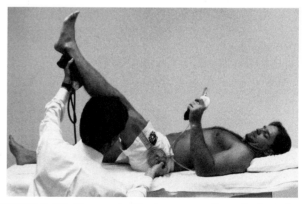

FIGURE 3–20. The use of a blood pressure cuff as a feedback device used to measure force placed against the posterior leg during SLR.

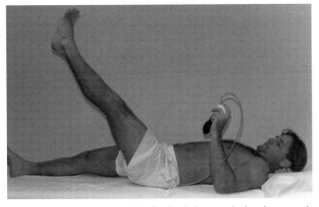

FIGURE 3–21. A pressurized biofeedback device, which indicates to the user changes in the position of the lumbar spine during SLR.

(Gajdosik & Lusin, 1983). Comparing the position of the ankle dorsiflexion versus plantar flexion during active and passive SLR (Gajdosik et al., 1985) showed significantly less ROM with dorsiflexion. The apparently critical aspect of SLR has been controlling pelvic rotation (Bohannon et al., 1985), which has been addressed using a method in which the opposite thigh is stabilized with straps versus the opposite thigh, slightly flexed to allow for low back flat position (Gajdosik et al., 1993). This particular study indicated increased ROM with low back flat position versus thigh stabilized with straps. The use of a passive versus an active method of measuring SLR does appear to influence straight-leg ROM, with greater increases apparent with passive ROM (Cameron et al., 1994; Gajdosik et al., 1993). An early study analyzing passive straight-leg raise demonstrated that the clinician should take into consideration the contribution of pelvic rotation to the angle of SLR when interpreting results. It should also be recognized that small increases in sequential multiple measurements of joint range may in fact be a normal occurrence of compliance of the viscoelastic tissues with repeated measurements (Atha & Wheatley, 1976; Bohannon, 1984; Cameron et al., 1994; McHugh et al., 1992). It has also been demonstrated that the accommodation to "stretch tolerance" level is a factor in measuring ROM during passive SLR (Halbertsma et al., 1994). In relation to measuring ROM of passive SLR, the necessity for controlling for the amount of force applied has often been overlooked (Bandy & Irion, 1994).

Conceivably, a method that might better control for force during SLR would be measuring force with a dynamometer (Bohannon & Lieber, 1986) or equivalent instrumentation (Helewa et al., 1993) (see Fig. 3–20). Perhaps a method that would better control for the contribution of the lumbar spine through pelvic rotation during SLR would be to use a stabilization device placed at the low back position, which would indicate when the lumbar curve began to flex (Jull et al., 1993) (Fig. 3–21).

PELVIC RANGE OF MOTION

Physical therapists are often involved with treatments that are designed to affect the position of the lumbopelvic region (Sal & Sal, 1991). Measuring the pelvic inclination allows therapists to monitor quantifiable changes in the position of the pelvis made during therapeutic intervention (Gilliam et al., 1994). A method (Alviso et al., 1988; Gajdosik et al., 1985), originally suggested by Sanders and Stavrakas (1981), uses trigonometric functions to measure pelvic ROM, achieving an overall intertester reliability of ICC = 0.87 and ICC = 0.90, respectively, when measuring posterior and anterior pelvic inclination. An early study (Day et al., 1984) measured both anterior and posterior pelvic tilt utilizing a computerized system with external markers over bony landmarks. A later technique introduced by Walker and colleagues (1987) utilized an inclinometer placed on the anterior superior iliac spine and the posterior superior iliac spine to determine the angle formed with the horizontal from a line drawn between the anterior-superior iliac spine and the posterior-superior iliac spine (Fig. 3–22). This method was later used (Gilliam et al., 1994), demonstrating a high level of both inter- and intraobserver reliability (ICC = 0.96, 0.95, respectively). This method, however, demonstrated poor validity compared with radiographic measurements. A modification to the inclinometer used by Gilliam and coworkers (1994) and Walker and colleagues (1987) provided two finger braces, allowing for palpation of the anterior-superior iliac spine and posterior-superior iliac spine while measurements are read (Crowell et al., 1994), demonstrating both good

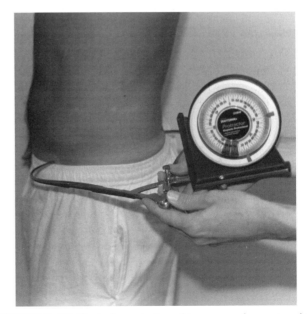

FIGURE 3–22. The inclinometer is used to measure changes in pelvic inclination, measured from an angle made by a line from the ASIS to the PSIS as it bisects the horizontal.

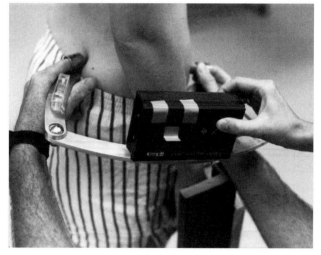

FIGURE 3–23. The use of an inclinometer utilizing finger braces, allowing for direct palpation of the ASIS and PSIS during inclinometer placement. (From Crowell, R. D., Cummings, G. S., Walker, J. R., & Tillman, L. J. [1994]. Intratester and intertester reliability and validity of measures of innominate bone inclination. *Journal of Orthopedic and Sports Physical Therapy, 20*[2], 88–97).

interrater reliability (ICC = 0.95) and validity (r = 0.93), (Fig. 3–23). This device should prove beneficial for measuring pelvic inclination in the sagittal plane.

KNEE

Few joints are exposed to measurements of ROM more than the knee. The movements of the knee joint are not those of a simple hinge joint but involve spinning, rolling, and gliding, often simultaneously (Nordin and Frankel, 1989; Smidt, 1973). Certainly in the medical age when total knee replacements and anterior cruciate ligament (ACL) repairs are common occurrences, associated goniometric readings of knee ROM during the rehabilitation process have added to the increased interest in the ROM of this joint.

An early study (Boone et al., 1978) using the universal goniometer demonstrated a high level of intratester reliability r = 0.87 while showing a significantly lower intertester reliability of r = 0.50 when measuring the knee. This study used standardized measurements described by the American Academy of Orthopedic Surgeons (1965) for knee AROM on 12 healthy volunteers. Investigations were later made into the reliability of various goniometers within a clinical setting in examining PROM at the knee (Rothstein et al., 1983). In this study, each individual was allowed to utilize his or her own technique in measuring the knee. The results showed high intertester and intratester ICC values of 0.99 and 0.97, respectively, but showed moderately low intertester ICC for knee extension (0.70), which was statistically shown to be related to the patient's test position. The use of various-sized goniometers did not

appear to affect the reliability of measurements, as indicated in this study (Rothstein et al., 1983). Universal and fluid-based goniometers have demonstrated good intertester reliability r = 0.87 and r = 0.83, whereas the fluid-based goniometer showed a concurrent validity of r = 0.82. However, statistical test differences between the instruments in this study suggest that the two instruments should not be used interchangeably (Rheault et al., 1988).

Goniometric measurements purport to give us an accurate account of the actual angle at the knee made by the universal goniometer; however, this is unsupported until a validity study can substantiate this claim. A radiographic study to verify the knee goniometry (Enwemeka, 1986) used the universal goniometer to measure six positions of the knee, 0 degrees to 90 degrees, comparing goniometric measurements with radiographic bone angle measurements. All goniometric measurements were comparable to the bone angle measurements, with the exception of the first 15 degrees, which were significantly different. In another study of goniometric measurements of the knee, both intertester reliability (ICC = 0.99) and validity (ICC = 0.98–0.99) were high when compared with roentgenograms (Gogia et al., 1987).

Many times, clinical situations lend themselves to visual estimations of ROM measurements at the knee. It has been suggested that visual estimation is more accurate than goniometric measurement when bony landmarks are not easily palpated (American Academy of Orthopedic Surgeons, 1965; Rowe, 1964). However, other sources have suggested that goniometry has proven to be more reliable than visual estimates of joint ROM (Moore, 1949a; Salter, 1955). An early study using a small subject size (20) demonstrated good intertester and intratester reliability when using visual estimates to determine ROM of knees affected by rheumatoid arthritis (Marks et al., 1978). A clinical study taken with a larger sample size (43) determined that PROM measurements were better determined goniometrically over visual estimation to minimize the error of measurement (Watkins et al., 1991). It has been traditionally suggested that a knee ROM of ≥90 degrees is necessary to negotiate elevated terrain, e.g., stairs, inclines.

Generally, normal ROM measurements for the knee are 0 to 135 or 140 degrees, decreasing with age. Studies of younger populations have shown that knee extension often measures less than 0 degrees. Normative measurements of the knee are presented in Table 3–10.

Measurement of anterior-posterior (A-P) translation (laxity) has been commonplace in knees suspected of being ACL deficient. As surgical procedures have progressed with ever-newer reconstructive techniques, the interest in evaluating the results of these techniques following operations has led to instruments specifically designed to measure the A-P motion. Understanding that the knee not only flexes and extends in the sagittal plane but also allows for A-P translation in the sagittal plane, as well as tibial rotation in the transverse plane (Nordin and Frankel, 1989), a

TABLE 3–10

VALUES FOR "NORMAL" ROM FOR THE KNEE, ACCORDING TO VARIOUS AUTHORS AND RESEARCHERS

Joint	AAOS (1965)	Boone & Azen* (1979)	Dorinson & Wagner (1948)	Ekstrand et al.† (1982)	Esch & Lepley (1974)	Gerhardt & Russe (1975)	AMA (1958)	Roaas & Anderson‡ (1982)	Roach & Miles (NHANES 1)§ (1991)	Wiechec & Krusen (1939)
Knee										
Flexion	135	143	140	144	135	130	120	144	132	135
Extension								–2		

* N = 109, 18–54 y, male.
† N = 25, 22–30 y, male.
‡ N = 108, 30–40 y, male.
§ N = 1683, 25–74 y, male and female.
AAOS = American Academy of Orthopedic Surgeons; AMA = American Medical Association.

method for determining the amount of translation has become important, particularly when the pathomechanics of an ACL deficient knee is under study. During the past 10 years, special measurement of A-P joint laxity during postreconstruction of knees with deficient ACLs has been measured via an arthrometer (Daniel et al., 1985) (Fig. 3–24). Earlier studies involving the KT-1000 (MEDmetrics Corps., San Diego, CA), an arthrometer designed to measure tibial translation, indicated that it was a useful tool for both confirming reduction and demonstrating a mean difference in laxity in normal and injured knees (Daniel et al., 1985). Hanten and Pace (1987) demonstrated measurements of ICC = 0.92 and 0.84, respectively, for inter- and intratester reliability when using the KT-1000 to test 43 healthy male subjects for A-P translation.

However, Forster and associates (1989) demonstrated significant inter- and intraexaminer variations in measurements of both absolute displacement of knees and side-to-side differences in pairs of knees. A more recent study (Graham et al., 1991) of the KT-1000 presented conflicting views, demonstrating a poor level of reliability (less than 50 percent) in determining laxity in the knee with a deficient ACL. Graham and colleagues (1991) indicated that the anterior drawer test and Lachmans test were found to be more accurate indicators of knees with deficient ACLs when compared with the KT-1000 (see Fig. 3–24). Another study (Holcomb et al., 1993) of A-P translation using the KT-1000 reported a high intratester reliability of ICC = 0.98–1.0, but a low intertester reliability of ICC = 0.53 was demonstrated. A more recent study (Rob-

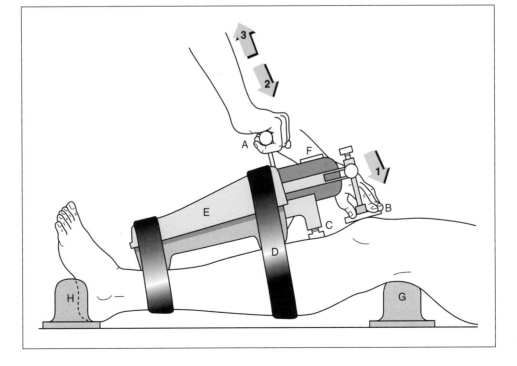

FIGURE 3–24. The use of an arthromometer for measurement of joint excursion (anterior or posterior translation) in the sagittal plane. A, force-sensing handle; B, patellar sensor pad; C, tibial tubercle sensor pad; D, Velcro strap; E, arthrometer case; F, displacement dial indicator (the data are sent via cable to an X-Y plotter as applied force versus joint displacement); G, thigh support; and H, foot support. 1, A constant pressure of 20 to 30 Newtons is applied to the patellar sensor pad to keep it in contact with the patella. 2, Posterior force is applied. 3, Anterior force is applied. (From Dale, D. M., et al. [1985]. Instrumented measurement of anterior laxity of the knee. *Journal of Bone and Joint Surgery, 67A*[5], 720–725.)

nett et al., 1995) demonstrated an intertester reliability of ICC = 0.67–0.75 for three different levels of force used with the KT-1000 and found that a change of > 5 mm must take place to indicate a true change in anterior tibial displacement. This may prove to be ineffective in demonstrating a possible ACL deficiency, as a difference of 3 mm in anterior tibial position between two knees of the same patient has been cited as diagnostic for ACL deficiency (Staubli & Jakob, 1991). Furthermore, validity studies have suggested the KT-1000 may underestimate A-P translation when compared with roentgen stereophotogrammetry in both operated and unoperated knees with deficient ACLs (Jonsson et al., 1993). In light of the conflicting results of these various studies, the reliability as well as the validity of this device in providing accurate measurements should be questioned.

ANKLE AND FOOT

The joints of the ankle and foot, because of their position and their necessity in locomotion, deserve more in the way of critical assessment in ROM, yet little research has substantiated reliability of methods or established normal ranges. This may be due in part to the significant complexity within each joint as well as to the multiple axes and planes of movement (Root et al., 1977) found within the ankle-foot complex. Because normal ambulation requires primary movements of ankle dorsiflexion and plantar flexion, these two motions have been the main focus of research on ROM of the ankle, followed by calcaneal inversion and eversion. It has been a long-held notion that 10 degrees of ankle dorsiflexion is necessary for normal locomotion (Root et al., 1977). Other authors have stated that only 5 degrees of dorsiflexion is necessary, whereas still others suggest that motion past a 90-degree angle to the lower leg is sufficient for normal gait (Downey, 1987; Tanz, 1960). During gait, the maximum amount of dorsiflexion occurs just before heel lift while the knee is in an extended position (Downey & Banks, 1989). Although the maximum amount of dorsiflexion occurs during the stance phase of gait, the clinician's evaluation of ankle dorsiflexion continues to be performed while the patient is in a non–weight-bearing position (Baggett and Young, 1993; Norkin and White, 1985). A study of ankle joint dorsiflexion by Baggett and Young (1993) measured the average amount of dorsiflexion available using the non–weight-bearing method as 8.25 degrees, while being substantially higher at 20.90 degrees with the weight-bearing technique (Fig. 3–25). The effect on measurements of ankle dorsiflexion with the knees flexed versus extended appears to make a difference. Using a gravity inclinometer, Ekstrand et al., (1982) determined the coefficient of variation of ±1.9, with mean ankle dorsiflexion of 22.5 degrees with knees straight and 24.9 degrees with knees flexed, mea-

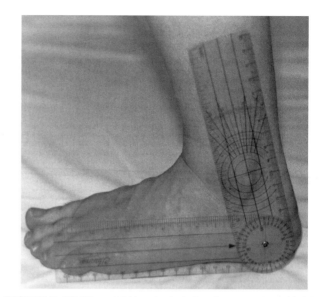

FIGURE 3–25. The weight-bearing technique for measuring ankle joint dorsiflexion. Alignment of one arm of the goniometer should be to the plane of the supporting surface, and the other arm is aligned to the lateral aspect of the fibula.

sured in weight-bearing position. Investigating three different methods in measuring ankle dorsiflexion, Bohannon and coworkers (1989) demonstrated that the majority (83.3 percent) had a high correlation; however, significantly different measurements between methods were found, demonstrating that the use of different landmarks can provide a reliable indication of ankle dorsiflexion. Although the universal goniometer appears to be the main mode used for measurement of ankle dorsiflexion and plantar flexion, Muwanga and associates (1985) introduced a new method for measuring ankle dorsiflexion and plantar flexion. The device allows the foot to rotate about an ankle pivotal point, assuring that the foot is held secure in a strapped position. These measurements described AROM measurements performed on normal volunteers. Both intratester and intertester reliability proved to have a difference of less than 3 degrees in 86 percent of the measurements.

Visual estimation continues to prove to be a poor method for determining ankle ROM when compared with the goniometer (Youdas et al., 1993). However, in a patient population, it has also been shown that with the universal goniometer, intertester reliability for active ankle joint measurement is poor for ankle dorsiflexion and plantar flexion (ICC = 0.25 and 0.28) (Youdas et al., 1993). Studies on PROM have found outcomes varying from good to poor in interrater reliability for ankle dorsiflexion (ICC = 0.74–0.87; Diamond et al., 1989) (ICC = 0.50; Elveru et al., 1988) and moderate reliability (ICC = 0.72) for plantar flexion (Elveru et al., 1988). Intrarater reliability has been shown to be more substantial in measuring ankle dorsiflexion for PROM (ICC = 0.90; Elveru et al., 1988) (ICC = 0.89–0.96 Diamond et al.,

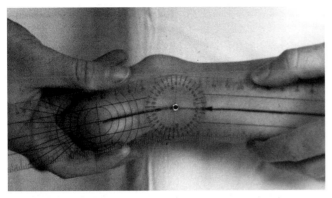

FIGURE 3–26. Measurement of hindfoot inversion and eversion performed with patient in prone-lying position.

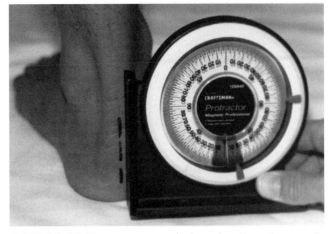

FIGURE 3–27. The measurement of calcaneal position using a gravity protractor. (From Sell, K. E., et al. [1994]. Two measurement techniques for assessing subtalar joint position: A reliability study. *Journal of Orthopedic and Sports Physical Therapy, 19*(3), 162–167.

1989), as well as PROM for ankle plantar flexion (ICC = 0.86) (Elveru et al., 1988). Intrarater reliability for AROM has been shown to be good for ankle dorsiflexion (ICC = 0.82) and plantar flexion (ICC = 0.86) (Youdas et al., 1993). Reliability differences in these studies appear to be associated with lengthy training periods incorporated prior to the experiment most probably improving the methodology for measurements taken (Diamond et al., 1989).

Just as measurements of ankle dorsiflexion and plantar flexion have demonstrated variations in weight-bearing versus non–weight-bearing measurements, Lattanza and coworkers (1988) determined that an increase in subtalar eversion position was greater in the weight-bearing position when examining subtalar neutral position. Of course since weight-bearing is the functional position of the ankle and foot, it should provide the necessary information as to position during gait. In the study by Elveru and colleagues (1988), measurement of hindfoot eversion and inversion and subtalar joint neutral (STJN) position has been shown

to have moderate intratester reliability (ICC = 0.75, 0.74, and 0.77, respectively) and poor intertester reliability (ICC = 0.17, 0.32, and 0.25) (Fig. 3–26). However, in a study of 31 diabetics, Diamond and associates (1989) measured ankle eversion and inversion and STJN position demonstrating moderate to good interrater and intrarater reliability. It has been purported that the subtalar joint motion is an important baseline indicator of the potential for excessive pronation versus supination during gait (Root et al., 1977). However, this supposition was based on research performed with an orthotic device designed as a mechanical analog of a subtalar and ankle joint system and was used during gait on only a few subjects (Wright et al., 1964). Techniques for assessing subtalar joint position have been conflicting. A reliability study (Picciano et al.,

TABLE 3–11

VALUES FOR "NORMAL" ROM FOR THE ANKLE AND FOOT, AS LISTED BY SEVERAL AUTHORS

Joint	AAOS (1965)	Baggett & Young* (1979)	Boone & Azen† (1948)	Dorinson & Wagner (1982)	Esch & Lepley (1974)	Gerhardt & Russe (1975)	Milgrom et al.‡ (1985)	AMA (1958)	Roaas & Andersson§ (1982)	Wiechec & Krusen (1939)
Plantar flexion	50		56	45	65	45	—	40	40	55
Dorsiflexion	20	8‖21¶	13	20	10	20	—	20	15	30
Subtalor joint										
Inversion	35		37	50	30	40	32	30	27	—
Eversion	15		26	20	15	20	4#	20	27	—

* N = 30, 18–66 y, male and female.
† N = 109, x = 22.4, male.
‡ N = 272, 18–20 y, males.
§ N = 96, 30–40 y, males.
‖ Non–weight-bearing.
¶ Weight-bearing.
# Hindfoot.
AAOS = American Academy of Orthopedic Surgeons; AMA = American Medical Association.

1993) of three methods for measuring STJN position (open kinetic chain, closed kinetic chain, and navicular drop test) demonstrated poor intra- and intertester reliability when measuring (n = 30 ft) with a goniometer (for the first two methods) and when measuring the distance change from the floor to the navicular mark on a marked index card (for the third method). However, a later study measuring STJN (Sell et al., 1994) using two measurement techniques (calcaneal position with an inclinometer [Fig. 3–27] and navicular drop test) in a weight-bearing position (n = 60) demonstrated moderate to high reliability.

Studies of normal ankle dorsiflexion demonstrated a reduction in mean values with increasing age (middle age to old age), decreasing from 20.0 degrees to 13.5 degrees in males, whereas in females these values decreased from 20.7 degrees to 10.1 degrees (Vandervorrt et al., 1992). Normal ROM for inversion and eversion of the subtalar joint using a method described by the American Academy of Orthopedic Surgeons (1965) was 35 degrees and 15 degrees, respectively. It has been suggested that 4 degrees to 6 degrees of inversion and eversion, for a minimal total range of 8 degrees to 12 degrees, is normal for locomotion (Root et al., 1977). Although norms have been cited for subtalar inversion and eversion and STJN (3 degrees varus) positions (Milgrom et al., 1985), the basis for "normal" STJN with regard to the stance phase of gait has been largely conjecture, without proven reliable or valid methods performed on any substantial-sized group during gait activities (Root et al., 1977; McPoil & Cornwall, 1994; Wright et al., 1964). Table 3–11 lists norms for ankle and foot ROM.

A measurement quite possibly offering the therapist increased information with regard to the biomechanical alignment and forces acting on the ankle and foot is measurement of tibia vara, which is the angle formed by the distal third of the leg to a horizontal line to the supporting stance surface (ground). Lohmann and associates (1987) demonstrated a mean absolute difference between measurements of tibia vara of 2 to 3 degrees (Fig. 3–28).

GLOSSARY

Attraction methods—Measuring procedure using a tape measure to record a decrease in distance between two points marked on the skin over the spine as it extends.

Coefficient of variation—Measure of variability in the measurements relative to the mean value. Depicts the variability of measurements within the subjects as well as the variability of the actual measurement. A ratio of the standard deviation and the mean in terms of a percentage.

Distraction methods—Measuring procedure using a tape measure to record an increase in distance between two points marked on the skin as the spine flexes.

Flexicurve techniques—Measuring procedures in which a tester manually molds a flexible curve to the midline contour of the subject's lumbar spine. The flexible curve is then traced onto paper, and either a tangential or a trigonometric method is used to calculate ROM.

Intraclass correlation coefficient (ICC)—Assesses common variance. Examines two or more sets of scores on the same variable.

Modified Schöber technique—Skin distraction-attraction method using a midline point 5 CM below the lumbosacral junction and a point 10 CM above it.

Pearson product-moment correlation coefficient—Generalized measure of linear association. Used in determining association concerning a bivariate distribution.

Pelvic inclinometer—Designed with calipers with a mounted gravity protractor. Able to measure the change in position of two separate points by the placement of either ends of the calipers over an identifable area used as a landmark.

Pendulum goniometer—Goniometer usually made of metal with two movement arms. One arm is allowed to move freely in accordance with the line of gravity and is used as a vertical reference.

Spinal inclinometer—A circular fluid-filled disk with a weighted needle indicator, which is maintained in the vertical, that is placed over the spine and used to measure ROM in degrees as the spine moves.

Subtalar joint neutral—The position in which the foot is neither pronated nor supinated. The position of inversion or eversion that the calcaneus assumes when the talus is congruent in relation to the tibia.

3-Space Isotrak—Electomagnetic device for the measurement of three-dimensional movements.

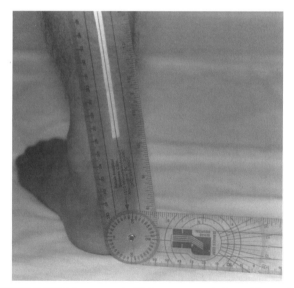

FIGURE 3–28. Measurement of tibia vara: an angle formed from a line parallel to the lower leg bisecting the horizontal (ground).

Universal goniometer—Clear plastic goniometer with 360-degree gauge with two moveable arms for placement on body segments. Used for measuring ROM in degrees.

REFERENCES

Ahlberg, A., Moussa, M., & Al-Nahdi, M. (1988). On geographical variations in the normal range of joint motion. *Clinical Orthopedics, 234,* 229–231.

Aho, A., Vortianinen, O., & Salo, O. (1933). Segmentary mobility of the lumbar spine in antero-posterior flexion. *Annales de Medecine Interne Fenniae, 44,* 275.

Allender, E., Bjornsson, O. J., Olafsson, O., Sigfusson, N., & Thorsteinsson, J. (1974). Normal range of joint movements in shoulder, hip, wrist, and thumb with special reference to side: A comparison between two populations. *International Journal of Epidemiology, 3*(3), 253–261.

Alviso, D. J., Dong, G. T., Lentell, G. L., (1988). Intertester reliability for measuring pelvic tilt in standing. *Physical Therapy, 68,* 1347–1351.

American Academy of Orthopedic Surgeons. (1965). *Joint motion method of measuring and recording.* Chicago: American Academy of Orthopedic Surgeons.

American Medical Association Committee on Rating of Disability and Physical Impairment (1969). *Guidelines to evaluation of permanent disability.* (pp. 584–589). Chicago: American Medical Association.

American Medical Association. (1958). A guide to the evaluation of permanent impairment of the extremities and back. *Journal of the American Medical Association* (special ed.), *166,* 1–109.

American Medical Association. (1990). *Guides to the evaluation of permanent impairment* (4th ed.) (pp. 78–101). Chicago: American Medical Association.

American Medical Association Committee on Rating of Mental and Physical Impairment (1971). *Guidelines to evaluation of permanent disability* (pp. 43–48). Chicago: American Medical Association.

American Medical Association. (1984). *Guides to the evaluation of permanent impairment* (2nd ed.) Chicago: American Medical Association.

American Medical Association. (1988). *Guides to the evaluation of permanent impairment* (3rd ed.). Chicago: American Medical Association.

Ashton, B. B., Pickles, B., & Roll, J. W. (1978). Reliability of goniometric measurements of hip motion in spastic cerebral palsy. *Developmental Medicine and Child Neurology.* 20, 87–94.

Atha, J., & Wheatley, P. W. (1976). The mobilising effects of repeated measurement on hip flexion. *British Journal of Sports Medicine, 10,* 22–25.

Baggett, B. D., & Young, G. (1993). Ankle joint dorsiflexion, establishment of a normal range. *Journal of the American Podiatric Medical Association, 83*(5) 251–254.

Baldwin, J., & Cunningham, K. (1974). Goniometry under attack: A clinical study involving physiotherapists. *Physiotherapy Canada, 26,* 74–76.

Bandy, W. D., & Irion, J. M. (1994). The effect of time on static stretch on the flexibility of the hamstring muscles. *Physical Therapy, 74,* 845–850.

Bartko, J. J., & Carpenter, W. T. (1976). On the methods and theory of reliability. *The Journal of Nervous and Mental Disease, 163*(5), 307–317.

Batti'e, M., Bigos, S., Sheely, A., & Wortley, M. (1987). Spinal flexibility and factors that influence it. *Physical Therapy, 67,* 653–658.

Bear-Lehman, J., & Abreu, B. C. (1989). Evaluating the hand: Issues in reliability and validity. *Physical Therapy, 69*(12), 1025–1033.

Beattie, P., Rothstein, J. M., & Lamb, R. L. (1987). Reliability of the attraction method for measuring lumbar spine backward bending. *Physical Therapy, 67,* 364–369.

Bell, R. D., & Hoshizaki, T. B. (1981). Relationships of age and sex with range of motion of seventeen joint actions in humans. *Canada Journal of Applied Sport in Science, 6,* 202–206.

Blakely, R. L., & Palmer M. L. (1984). Analysis of rotation accompanying shoulder flexion. *Physical Therapy, 64,* 1214–1216.

Bogduk, N., & Twoomey, L. T. (1991). *Clinical anatomy of the lumbar spine* (2nd ed.). Melbourne, Churchill Livingstone.

Bohannon, R. W. (1982). Cinematographic analysis of the passive straight-leg-raising test for hamstring muscle length. *Physical Therapy, 62,* 1269–1274.

Bohannon, R. W. (1984). Effect of repeated eight-minute muscle loading on the angle of straight-leg raising. *Physical Therapy, 64,* 491–497.

Bohannon, R. W. (1989). Objective measures. *Physical Therapy, 69*(7), 590–593.

Bohannon, R. W. (1987). Simple clinical measures. *Physical Therapy, 67*(12), 1845–1850.

Bohannon, R. W., Gajdosik, R. L., & LeVeau, B. F. (1985). Contribution of pelvic and lower limb motion to increases in the angle of passive straight leg raising. *Physical Therapy, 65,* 474–476.

Bohannon, R. W., & LeVeau, B. F. (1986). Clinician's use of research findings: A review of literature with implications for physical therapists. *Physical Therapy, 66,* 45–50.

Bohannon, R. W., & Lieber, C. (1986). Cybex II isokinetic dynamometer for passive load application and measurement: Suggestion from the field. *Physical Therapy, 66,* 1407.

Bohannon, R. W., Tiberio, D., & Zito, M. (1989). Selected measures of ankle dorsiflexion range of motion: Differences and intercorrelations. *Foot and Ankle, 10,* 99–103.

Boone, D. C., & Azen, S. P. (1979). Normal range of motion of joints in male subjects. *Journal of Bone and Joint Surgery, 61-A*(5), 756–759.

Boone, D. C., Azen, S. P., Lin, C., Spence, C., Baron, C., & Lee, L. (1978). Reliability of goniometric measurements. *Physical Therapy, 58* (11), 1355–1360.

Browne, E., Teague, M., & Gruenwald, C. (1979). Method for measurement of circumduction of the thumb to evaluate results of opponensplasty. *Plastic & Reconstructive Surgery, 64*(2), 204–207.

Buck, C. A., Dameron, F. B., Dow, M. J., & Skowlund, H. V. (1959). Study of normal range of motion in the neck utilizing a bubble goniometer. *Archives of Physical Medicine & Rehabilitation, 40,* 390–392.

Burdett, R. G., Brown, K. E., & Fall, M. P. (1986). Reliability and validity of four instruments for measuring lumbar spine and pelvic positions. *Physical Therapy, 66*(5), 677–684.

Burton, A. K. (1986). Regional lumbar sagittal mobility: Measurement by flexicurves. *Clinical Biomedical, 1,* 20–26.

Burton, A. K., & Tillotson, K. M. (1991). Does leisure sport activity influence lumbar mobility or the risk of low back trouble? *Journal of Spinal Disorders, 4,* 329–336.

Burton, A. K., Tilloston, K. M., & Troup, J. D. G. (1989). Variation in lumbar sagittal mobility with low back trouble. *Spine, 14,* 584–590.

Cameron, D. M., Bohannon, R. W., Owen, S. V. (1994). Influence of hip position on measurements of the straight leg raise test. *Journal of Orthopedic and Sports Physical Therapy, 19,* 168–172.

Capuano-Pucci, D., Rheault, W., Aukai, J., Bracke, M., Day, R., & Pastrick, M. (1991). Intratester and intertester reliability of the cervical range of motion device. *Archives of Physical Medicine and Rehabilitation, 72,* 338–339.

Cats-Baril, W. L., & Frymoyer, J. W. (1991). The economics of spinal disorders. In J. W. Frymoyer (Ed.), *The adult spine: Principles and practice* (pp. 85–105). Vol 1. New York: Raven Press.

Cave, E. F., & Roberts, S. M. (1936). A method for measuring and recording joint function. *Journal of Bone and Joint Surgery, 18,* 455–465.

Chiarello, C. M., & Savidge, R. (1993). Interrater reliability of the Cybex EDI-320 and fluid goniometer in normal patients with low back pain. *Archives of Physical Medicine and Rehabilitation, 74,* 32–37.

Clapper, M. P., & Wolf, S. L. Comparison of the reliability of the orthoranger and the standard goniometer for assessing active lower extremity range of motion. *Physical Therapy, 68*(2), 214–218.

Clark, W. A. (1920). A system of joint measurement. *Journal of Orthopedic Surgery, 2,* 687.

Crowell, R. D., Cummings, G. S., Walker, J. R., & Tillman, L. J. (1994). Intratester and intertester reliability and validity of measures of innominate bone inclination. *Journal of Orthopedic and Sports Physical Therapy, 20*(2), 88–97.

Cobe, H. M. (1928). The range of active motion at the wrist of white adults. *Journal of Bone and Joint Surgery, 26,* 763–774.

Cole, T. M. (1982). Measurement of musculoskeletal function: Goniometry. In F. J. Kottke, G. K. Stillwell, & J. F. Lehmann (Eds.), *Krusen's Handbook of Physical Medicine and Rehabilitation* (3rd ed.). Philadelphia: W.B. Saunders.

Cooper, J. E., Shwedyk, E., Quanbury, A. O., Miller, J., & Hildebrand, D.

(1993). Elbow restriction: effect on functional upper limb motion during performance of three feeding activities. *Archives of Physical Medicine and Rehabilitation, 74,* 805–809.

Currier, D. P. (1990). *Elements of research in physical therapy* (pp. 100, 160–177). Baltimore: Williams & Wilkins.

Daniel, D., Malcom, L., Losse, G., Stone, M. L., Sachs, R., & Burks, R. (1985). The measurement of anterior knee laxity after ACL reconstructive surgery. *Journal of Bone and Joint Surgery, 67*(5), 720–725.

Davis, H. (1994). Increasing rates of cervical and lumbar spine surgery in the United States, 1979–1990. *Spine, 19,* 1117–1124.

Day, J. W., Smidt, G. L., & Lehmann, T. (1984). Effect of pelvic tilt on standing posture. *Physical Therapy, 64*(2), 510–516.

Defibaugh, J. (1964a). Part I: Measurement of head motion. *Journal of the American Physical Therapy Association, 44,* 157–162.

Defibaugh, J. (1964b). Part II: An experimental study of head motion in adult males. *Journal of the American Physical Therapy Association, 44,* 163–168.

Delitto, A. (1989). Subjective measures and clinical decision making. *Physical Therapy, 69*(7), 585–589.

DeVita, J., Walker, M. L., & Skibinske, B. (1990). Relationship between performance of selected scapular muscles and scapular abduction in standing subjects. *Physical Therapy, 70*(8), 470–476.

Deyo, R. A., Haselkorn, J., Hoffman, R., & Kent, D. L. (1994). Designing studies of diagnostic tests for low back pain or radiculopathy. *Spine, 19* (185), 2057S–2065S.

Dhir, R., Ribera, V. A., & Jacobson, M. I. (1971). Gravity goniometer: A simple and multipurpose tool. *Clinical Orthopaedics and Related Research, 78,* 336–341.

Diamond, J. E., Mueller, M. J., Delitto, A., & Sinacore, D. R. (1989). Reliability of a diabetic foot evaluation. *Physical Therapy, 69,* 797–802.

Dijkstra, P. U., de Bont, L. G., van der Weele, L. T., & Boering, G. (1994). Joint mobility measurements: Reliability of a standardized method. *Cranio, 12*(1), 52–57.

Doody, S. G., Freedman, L., & Waterlan, J. C. (1970). Shoulder movements during abduction in the scapular plane. *Archives of Physical Medicine and Rehabilitation, 51,* 595–604.

Dorinson, S. M., & Wagner, M. L. (1948). An exact technic for clinically measuring and recording joint motion. *Archives of Physical Medicine, 29,* 468–475.

Downey, M. S., (1987). Ankle equinus. In E. McGlamry, (Ed.), *Comprehensive textbook of foot surgery.* Baltimore: Williams & Wilkins.

Downey, M. S., & Banks, A. S. (1989). Gastrocnemius recession in the treatment of nonspastic ankle equinus. A retrospective study. *Journal of American Podiatry Medical Association, 79,* 159–174.

Edwards, R. H. T., & McDonnell, M. (1974). Hand-held dynamometer for evaluating voluntary-muscle function. *Lancet, 757,* 758.

Ekstrand, J., Wiktorsson, M., Oberg, B., & Gillquist, J. (1982). Lower extremity goniometric measurements: A study to determine their reliability. *Archives of Physical Medicine and Rehabilitation, 63,* 171–175.

Elias, M. G., An, K., Amadio, P. C., Cooney, W. P., & Linscheid, R. (1989). Reliability of carpal angle determinations. *The Journal of Hand Surgery, 14-A*(6), 1017–1021.

Elveru, R. A., Rothstein, J. M., & Lamb, R. L. (1988). Methods for taking subtalar joint measurements. A clinical report. *Physical Therapy, 68,* 678–682.

Engelberg, A. L. (1988). *Guides to the evaluation of permanent impairment* (pp. 90–93). Chicago: American Medical Association.

Enwemeka, C. S. (1986). Radiographic verification of knee goniometry. *Scandanavian Journal of Rehabilitation and Medicine, 18,* 47–49.

Esch, D., & Lepley, M. (1974). *Evaluation of joint motion: Methods of measurement and recording.* Minneapolis: University of Minnesota Press.

Fess, E. E., & Moran, C. A. (1981). *Clinical Assessment Recommendations.* Garner, NC: American Society of Hand Therapists.

Fielding, W. (1957). Cineroentgenography of the normal cervical spine. *The Journal of Bone and Joint Surgery, 39-A*(6), 1280–1288.

Fish, D. R., & Wingate, L. (1985). Sources of goniometric error at the elbow. *Physical Therapy, 65,* 1666–1670.

Fitzgerald, G. K., Wynvenn, K. J., Rheault, W., & Rothschild, V. (1983). Objective assessment with established normal values for the lumbar spine range of motion. *Physical Therapy, 63,* 1776–1781.

Forster, I. W., Warren-Smith, C. D., & Tew, M. (1989). Is the KT-1000 knee ligament arthrometer reliable? *Journal of Bone and Joint Surgery, 71B*(5), 843–847.

Freedman, L., & Monroe, R., (1966). Abduction of arm in scapular plane: Scapular and glenohumeral movements. *Journal of Bone and Joint Surgery, 48A,* 1503–1510.

Froning, E. C., & Frohman, B. (1968). Motion of the lumbosacral spine after laminectomy and spinal fusion. *Journal of Bone and Joint Surgery, 50A,* 897–918.

Frymoyer, J. W., & Cats-Baril, W. L. (1991). An overview of the incidences and cause of low back pain. *Orthopedic Clinics of North America, 22,* 263–271.

Frymoyer, J. W., Hanley, E. N., Howe, J., Kuhlmann, D., & Matteri, R. E. (1979). A comparison of radiographic findings in fusion and non-fusion patients 10 or more years following lumbar disc surgery. *Spine, 4,* 435–439.

Gajdosik, R. L. (1985). Effects of ankle dorsiflexion on active and passive unilateral straight leg raising. *Physical Therapy, 65*(10), 1478–1482.

Gajdosik, R. L., & Bohannon, R. W. (1987). Clinical measurement of range of motion review of goniometry emphasizing reliability and validity. *Physical Therapy, 67*(12), 1867–1872.

Gajdosik, R. L., LeVeau, B. F., & Bohannon, R. W. (1985). Effects of ankle dorsiflexion on active and passive unilateral straight leg raising. *Physical Therapy, 65,* 1478–1482.

Gajdosik, R., & Lusin, G. (1983). Hamstring muscle tightness. *Physical Therapy, 63*(7), 1085–1088.

Gajdosik, R. L., Rieck, M. A., Sullivan, D. K., & Wightman, S. E. (1993). Comparison of four clinical tests for assessing hamstring muscle length. *Journal of Orthopedic and Sports Physical Therapy, 18,* 614–618.

Gajdosik, R., Simpson, R., Smith, R., & DonTigny, R. L. (1985). Intratester reliability of measuring the standing position and range of motion. *Physical Therapy, 65*(2), 169–174.

Gerhardt, J. J., & Russe, O. A. (1975). *International SFTR method of measuring and recording joint motion.* Bern: Huber.

Gibson, M. H., Goebel, G. V., Jordan, T. M., Kegerreis, S., & Worrell, T. W. (1995). A reliability study of measurement techniques to determine static scapular position. *Journal of Orthopedic and Sports Physical Therapy, 21,* 100–106.

Gilbert, P. J. (1993). Lumbar range of motion. In S. H. Hochsehuler, H. B. Cotler, & R. D. Guyer (Eds.), *Rehabilitation of the spine: Science & practice* (pp. 43–52). St. Louis: Mosby.

Gill, K., Krag, M. H., Johnson, G. B., et al. (1988). Repeatability of four clinical methods for assessment of lumbar spinal motion. *Spine, 13,* 50–53.

Gilliam, J., Brunt, D., MacMillan, M., Kinard, R., & Montgomery, W. J. (1994). Relationship of the pelvic angle to the sacral angle: Measurement of clinical reliability and validity. *Journal of Orthopedic and Sports Physical Therapy, 20*(4), 193–198.

Gogia, P. P., Braatz, J. H., Rose, S. J., & Norton, B. J. (1987). Reliability and validity of goniometric measurements at the knee. *Physical Therapy, 67,* 192–195.

Goodwin, J., Clark, C., Burdon, D., & Lawrence, C. (1992). Clinical methods of goniometry: A comparative study. *Disability and Rehabilitation, 14,* 10–15.

Graham, G. P., Johnson, S., Dent, C. M., & Fairclough, J. A. (1991). Comparison of clinical tests and the KT-1000 in the diagnosis of anterior cruciate ligament rupture. *British Journal Sports Medicine, 25*(2), 96, 97.

Greene, B. L., & Wolf, S. L. (1989). Upper extremity joint movement: Comparison of two measurement devices. *Archives of Physical Medicine and Rehabilitation, 70,* 288–290.

Gregerson, G. G., & Lucas, D. B. (1967). An in vivo study of axial rotation of the human thoracolumbar spine. *Journal of Bone and Joint Surgery, 49-A,* 247–262.

Grieve, G. P. (1987). *Common vertebral joint problems.* New York: Churchill Livingston.

Grimsby, O. (1990). Lumbar spine (Course notes).

Grohmann, J. E. L. (1983). Comparison of two methods of goniometry. *Physical Therapy, 63*(6), 922–925.

Halbertsma, J. P. K., & Goeken, L. N. (1994). Stretching exercises: Effect on passive extensibility and stiffness in short hamstrings of healthy subjects. *Archives of Physical Medicine and Rehabilitation, 75,* 976–981.

Hamilton, G., & Lachenbruch, P. (1969). Reliability of goniometers in assessing finger joint angle. *Physical Therapy, 49*(5), 465–469.

Hand, J. (1938). A compact pendulum arthrometer. *The Journal of Bone and Joint Surgery, 20,* 494, 495.

Hanten, W., & Pace, M. (1987). Reliability of measuring anterior laxity of the knee joint using a knee ligament arthrometer. *Physical Therapy, 67*(3), 357–359.

Hayes, M. A., Howard, T. C., Gruel, C. R., & Kopta, J. A. (1989). Roentgenographic evaluation of lumbar spine flexion-extension in asymptomatic individuals. *Spine, 14,* 327–331.

Helewa, A., Goldsmith, C. H., & Smythe, H. A. (1993). Measuring abdominal muscle weakness in patients with low back pain and matched controls: A comparison of 3 devices. *Journal of Rheumatology, 20,* 1539–1543.

Hellebrandt, F. A., Duvall, E. N., & Moore, M. L. (1949). The measurement of joint motion: Part III—Reliability of goniometry. *The Physical Therapy Review, 29,* 302–307.

Helms, S. (1994). Where to find real back pain relief. *Consumers Digest, July/August,* 29–75.

Hewitt, D. (1928). The range of active motion at the wrist of women. *Journal of Bone and Joint Surgery, 26,* 775–787.

Holcomb, K. R., Skaggs, C. A., Worrell, T. W., DeCarlo, M., & Shelbourne, K. D. (1993). Assessment of knee laxity following anterior cruciate ligament reconstruction. *Journal of Sports Rehabilitation, 2,* 97–103.

Hoppenfeld, S. (1976). *Physical examination of the spine and extremities* (pp. 247–249). New York: Appelton Century-Crofts.

Horger, M. M. (1990). The reliability of goniometric measurements of active and passive wrist motions. *American Journal of Occupational Therapy, 44,* 342–348.

Howes, R. G., & Isdale, I. C. (1971). The loose back. An unrecognized syndrome. *Rheumatology and Physical Medicine, 11,* 72–77.

Hsieh, C., Walker, J. M., & Gillis, K. (1983). Straight-leg raising test: Comparison of three instruments. *Physical Therapy, 63*(9), 1429–1433.

Hume, M. C., Gellman, H., McKellop, H., & Brumfield, R. H. (1990). Functional range of motion of the joints of the hand. *Journal of Hand Surgery of America, 15,* 240–243.

Jansen, C. W., & Watson, M. G. (1993). Measurement of range of motion of the finger after tendon repair in zone II of the hand. *The Journal of Hand Surgery, 18-A,* 411–417.

Jette, A. M. (1989). Measuring subjective clinical outcomes. *Physical Therapy, 69*(7), 580–584.

Jonsson, H., Karrholm, J., & Elmqvist, L. (1993). Laxity after cruciate ligament injury in 94 knees: The KT-1000 arthrometer vs. roentgen stereophotogrammetry. *Acta Orthopaedica Scandinavica, 64*(5), 567–570.

Jull, G., Richardson, C., Toppenberg, R., Comerford, M., & Bang, B. (1993). Towards a measurement of active muscle control for lumbar stabilization. *Australian Physiotherapy, 39*(3), 187–193.

Kadir, N., Grayson, M. F., Goldberg, A. A., & Swain, M. C. (1981). A new goniometer. *Rheumatology and Rehabilitation, 20,* 219–226.

Kaltenborn, F., & Lindahlo, O. (1969). Reproducibility of the results of manual mobility testing of specific intervertebral segments. *Swedish Medical Journal, 66,* 962–965.

Kaye, J. M., & Sorto, L. A. (1979). The K-square: A new biomechanical measuring device for the foot and ankle. *Journal of the American Podiatry Assocation, 69*(1), 58–64.

Keeley, J., Mayer, T. G., Cox, R., Gatchel, R. J., Smith, J., & Mooney, V. (1986). Quantification of lumbar function. Part 5: Reliability of range of motion measurements in the sagittal plane and an in vivo torso rotation measurement technique. *Spine, 11,* 31–35.

Kibler, W. B. (1991). Role of the scapula in the overhead throwing motion. *Contempory Orthopedics, 22,* 525–532.

Kottke, F. J., & Mundale, M. O. (1959). Range of mobility of the cervical spine. *Archives of Physical Medicine & Rehabilitation, 40,* 379–382.

LaStayo, P., & Wheeler, D. L. (1994). Reliability of passive wrist flexion and extension goniometric measurements: A multicenter study. *Physical Therapy, 74*(2), 162–176.

Lattanza, L, Gray, G. W., & Kantner, R. M. (1988). Closed versus open kinematic chain measurements of subtalar joint eversion: Implications for clinical practice. *Journal of Orthopedic and Sports Physical Therapy, 9,* 310–314.

Laupattarakasem, W., Sirichativapee, W., Kowsuwon, W., Sribunditkul, S., & Suibnugarn, C. (1990). Axial rotation gravity goniometer. *Clinical Orthopedics and Related Research, 251,* 271–274.

Leighton, J. R. (1955). An instrument and technic for the measurement of range of joint motion. *Archives of Physical Medicine & Rehabilitation, 36,* 571–578.

Lewit, K., & Liebenson, C. (1993). Palpation—problems and implica-tions. *Journal of Manipulative and Physiological Therapeutics, 16,* 586–590.

Loebl, W. (1967). Measurement of spinal posture and range of spinal movement. *Annals of Physical Medicine, 9,* 103–110.

Lohmann, K. N., Rayhel, H. E., Schneiderwind, W. P., & Danoff, J. V. (1987). Static measurement of tibia vara: Reliability and effect of lower extremity position. *Physical Therapy, 67*(2), 196–199.

Lovell, F. W., Rothstein, J. M., & Personius, W. J. (1989). Reliability of clinical measurements of lumbar lordosis taken with a flexible rule. *Physical Therapy, 69*(2), 96–105.

Low, J. L. (1976). The reliability of joint measurement. *Physiotherapy, 62*(7), 227–229.

Lumbsden, R. M., & Morris, J. M. (1968). An in vivo study of axial rotation and immobilization at the lumbosacral joint. *Journal of Bone and Joint Surgery, 50-A,* 1591–1602.

Macrae, I. F., & Wright, V. (1969). Measurement of back movement. *Annals in Rheumatic Diseases, 28,* 584–589.

Maher, C., & Adams, R. (1994). Reliability of pain and stiffness assessments in clinical manual lumbar spine examinations. *Physical Therapy, 74,* 801–809.

Maitland, G. D. (1986). *Vertebral manipulation* (5th ed.). London: Butterworth.

Mallon, W. J., Brown, H. R., & Nunley, J. A. (1991). Digital ranges of motion: Normal values in young adults. *Journal of Hand Surgery of America, 16-A,* 882–887.

Marks, J. S., Palmer, M. K., Burke, M. J., & Smith, P. (1978). Observer variation in the examination of knees joints. *Annals of the Rheumatic Diseases, 37,* 376, 377.

Mayer, T. G., Brady, S., Bovasso, E., Pope, P., & Gatchel, R. J. (1993). Noninvasive measurement of cervical tri-planar motion in normal subjects. *Spine, 18*(15), 2191–2195.

Mayer, T. G., & Gatchel, R. J. (1988). *Functional restoration for spinal disorders: The sports medicine approach* (pp. 124–138). Philadelphia: Lea & Febiger.

Mayer, T. G., Tencer, A. F., Kristoferson, S., & Mooney, V. (1984). Use of noninvasive techniques for quantification of spinal range of motion in normal subjects and chronic low back dysfunction patients. *Spine, 9*(6), 588–595.

Mayerson, N. H., & Milano, R. A. (1984). Goniometric measurement reliability in physical medicine. *Archives of Physical Medicine and Rehabilitation, 65,* 92–94.

McHugh, M. P., Magnusson, S. P., Gleim, G. W., & Nicholas, J. A. (1992). Viscoelastic stress relaxation in human skeletal muscle. *Medicine and Science in Sports and Exercise, 24,* 1375–1382.

McKenzie, I. A. (1981). *The lumbar spine. Mechanical diagnosis and therapy.* Waikanae, New Zealand: Spinal Publications Limited.

McPoil, T. G., & Cornwall, M. W. (1994). The relationship between subtalar joint neutral position and rearfoot motion during walking. *Foot and Ankle, 15,* 141–145.

McRae, R. (1983). *Clinical orthopaedic examination* (p. 51). Edinburgh, Scotland: Churchill-Livingstone.

Merritt, J. L., McLean, T. J., & Erikson, R. P. (1986). Measurement of trunk flexibility in normal subjects: Reproducibility of three clinical methods. *Mayo Clinic Proceedings, 61,* 192–197.

Michels, E. (1982). Evaluation and research in physical therapy. *Physical Therapy, 62,* 828–834.

Milgrom, C., Giladi, M., Simkin, A., Stein, M., Kashtan, H., Marguilies, J., Steinberg, R., & Aharonson, Z. (1985). The normal range of subtalar inversion and eversion in young males as measured by three different techniques. *Foot and Ankle, 6,* 143–145.

Miller, P. J. (1985). Assessment of joint motion. In J. M. Rothstein (Ed.), *Measurement in physical therapy* (pp. 103–136). New York: Churchill Livingstone.

Miller, S. A., Mayer, T., Cox, R., & Gatchel, R. J. (1992). Reliability problems associated with the modified Schöber technique for true lumbar flexion measurement. *Spine, 17,* 345–348.

Moll, J. M. H., & Wright, V. (1976). Measurement of joint motion. *Clinics in Rheumatic Diseases, 2,* 3–26.

Moll, J. M. H., & Wright, V. (1971). Normal range of spinal mobility. *Annals of Rheumatic Disease, 30,* 381–386.

Moore, M. L. (1949a). The measurement of joint motion: Part I—Introductory review of the literature. *Physical Therapy Review, 29,* 195–205.

Moore, M. L. (1949b). The measurement of joint motion: Part II—The technic of goniometry. *Physical Therapy Review, 29,* 256–264.

Moore, M. L. (1984). Clinical assessment of joint motion. In J. V. Basmajian (ed.), *Therapeutic exercise* (4th ed.) (pp. 194–224). Baltimore: William & Wilkins.

Morrey, B., & Chao, E. Y. S. (1976). Passive motion of the elbow joint. A biomechanical analysis. *Mayo Foundation, 58-A,* 501–508.

Muwanga, C. L., Dove, C. L., & Plant, G. R. (1985). The measurement of ankle movements—A new method. *Injury, 16,* 312–314.

Nelson, M. A., Allen, P., Clamp, S. E., & De Domball, F. T. (1979). Reliability and reproducibility of clinical findings in low back pain. *Spine, 4,* 97–101.

Nordin, M., & Frankel, V. H. (1989). *Basic biomechanics of the musculoskeletal system* (pp. 115–134). Philadelphia: Lea & Febiger.

Norkin, C. C., & White, D. J. (1985). *Measurement of joint motion: A guide to goniometry.* Philadelphia: F. A. Davis.

Palmer, A. K., Werner, F. W., Murphy, D., & Glisson, R. (1985). Functional wrist motion: A biomechanical study. *Journal of Hand Surgery of America, 10,* 36–39.

Palmer, L., & Blakely, R. L. (1986). Documentation of medical rotation accompanying shoulder flexion: A case report. *Physical Therapy, 66,* 55–58.

Palmer, M. L., & Epler, M. E. (1990). *Clinical assessment procedures in physical therapy* (pp. 2–13). Philadelphia: J. B. Lippincott Company.

Paris, S. (1987). The spine: etiology and treatment of dysfunction including joint manipulation (Course notes).

Payton, O. D. (1988). Research: The validation of clinical practice (2nd ed.) (pp. 108-110). Philadelphia: F. A. Davis.

Pearcy, M. J., (1985). Stereo radiography of lumbar spine motion. *Acta Orthopedica Scandinavica, 56,* 7.

Pearcy, M. J., Portek, I., & Shepherd, J. (1985). The effect of low back pain on lumbar spine movements measured by three dimensional x-ray analysis. *Spine, 10*(2), 150–153.

Pearcy, M. J., Portek, I., & Shepherd, J. (1984). Three dimensional x-ray analysis of normal movement in the lumbar spine. *Spine, 9*(3), 294–297.

Pearcy, M. J., & Tibrewal, S. B. (1984). Axial rotation and lateral bending in the normal lumbar spine measured by three dimensional radiography. *Spine, 9*(6), 582–587.

Penning, L., Wilmink, J. T., & vanWoerden, H. H. (1984). Inability to prove instability: A critical appraisal of clinical radiological flexion-extension studies in lumbar disc degeneration. *Diagnostic Imaging of Clinical Medicine, 53,* 186–192.

Petersen, C.M., Johnson, R.D, Schuit, D. & Hayes, K.W. (1994). Intraobserver and interobserver reliability of asymptomatic subjects' thoracolumbar range of motion using the OSI Ca6000 spine motion analyzer. *Journal of Orthopedic and Sports Physical Therapy, 20,* 207–212.

Petherick, M., Rheault, W., Kimble, S., Lechner, C., & Senear, V. (1988). Concurrent validity and intertester reliability of universal and fluid-based goniometers for active elbow range of motion. *Physical Therapy, 68,* 966–969.

Picciano, A. M., Rowlands, M. S., & Worrell, T. (1993). Reliability of open and closed kinetic chain subtalar joint neutral positions and navicular drop test. *Journal of Orthopedic and Sports Physical Therapy, 18,* 553–558.

Portek, I., Pearcy, M. E., Reader, G. P., & Mowatt, A. G. (1983). Correlation between cardiographic and clinical measurement of lumbar spine movement. *British Journal of Rheumatology, 22,* 177–205.

Pucci, D., Rheault, W., Aukai, J., Bracke, M., Day, R., & Pastrick, M. (1991). Intratester and intertester reliability of the cervical range of motion device. *Archives of Physical Medicine and Rehabilitation, 7,* 338–340.

Rheault, W., Miller, M., Nothnagel, P., Straessle, J., & Urban, D. (1988). Intertester reliability and concurrent validity of fluid-based and universal goniometers for active knee flexion. *Physical Therapy, 68*(11), 1676–1678.

Riddle, D. L., Rothstein, J. M., & Lamb, R. L. (1987). Goniometric reliability in a clinical setting. Shoulder measurements. *Physical Therapy, 67,* 668–673.

Roaas, A., & Andersson, G. B. J. (1982). Normal range of motion of the hip, knee, and ankle joints in male subjects, 30–40 years of age. *Acta Orthopaedica Scandinavica, 53,* 205–208.

Roach, K. E., Miles, T. P. (1991). Normal hip and knee active range of motion: The relationship to age. *Physical Therapy, 71*(9), 656–665.

Robnett, N.J., Riddle, D. L., & Kues, J. M. (1995). Intertester reliability of measurements obtained with the KT-1000 on patients with recon-

structed anterior cruciate ligaments. *Journal of Orthopedic and Sports Physical Therapy, 21,* 113–119.

Robson, P. (1966). *A method to reduce the variable error in joint range measurement* (pp. 262–265). London: Cerebral Palsy Physical Assessment Centre, Guy's Hospital Medical School.

Root, M. L., Orien, W. P., & Weed, J. H. (1977). *Clinical biomechanics Vol. II, normal and abnormal function of the foot.* Los Angeles: Clinical Biomechanics Corporation.

Rothstein, J. M. (1989). On defining subjective and objective measurements. *Physical Therapy, 69*(7), 577–579.

Rothstein, J. M., & Echternach, J. L. (1993). *Primer on measurement: An introductory guide to measurement issues.* (pp. 59-69). Alexandria, VA: American Physical Therapy Association.

Rothstein, J. M., Miller, P. J., & Roettger, R. F. (1983). Goniometric reliability in a clinical setting: Elbow and knee measurements. *Physical Therapy, 63*(10), 1611–1615.

Rowe, C. R. (1964). Joint measurement in disability evaluation. *Clinical Orthopedics, 32*(43), 43–52.

Russell, P., Pearcy, M. J., & Unsworth, A. (1993). Measurement of the range and coupled movements observed in the lumbar spine. *British Journal of Rheumatology, 32,* 490–497.

Russell, P., Weld, A., Pearcy, M. J., Hogg, R., & Unsworth, A. (1992). Variation in lumbar spine mobility measured over a 24 hour period. *British Journal of Rheumatology, 31,* 329–332.

Ryu, J. Y., Cooney, W. P., Askew, L. J., An, K. N., & Chao, E. Y. (1991). Functional ranges of motion of the wrist joint. *Journal of Hand Surgery of America, 16*(3), 409–419.

Safaee-Rad, R., Shwedyk, E., Quanbury, A. O., & Cooper, J. E. (1990). Normal functional range of motion of upper limb joints during performance of three feeding activities. *Archives of Physical Medicine and Rehabilitation, 71,* 505–509.

Saal, J. A., & Saal, J. S. (1991). Later stage management of lumbar spine problems. *Physical Medicine and Rehabilitation Clinics of North America, 2,* 205–221.

Salter, N. (1955). Methods of measurement of muscle and joint function. *The Journal of Bone and Joint Surgery, 37-B,* 474–491.

Sanders, G., & Stavrakas, P. (1981). A technique for measuring pelvic tilt. *Physical Therapy, 61*(1), 49, 50.

Schenker, A. W. (1956). Improved method of joint measurement. *New York State Journal of Medicine, 56,* 539–545.

Schöber, P. (1937). The lumbar vertebral column in backache. *Münchener Mevizinisdy Wodnerschrift, 84,* 336–338.

Scholz, J. P. (1989). Reliability and validity of the WATSMART™ three-dimensional optoelectric motion analysis system. *Physical Therapy, 69*(8), 679–689.

Scott, B. O. (1965). A universal goniometer. *Annals of Physical Medicine, 8*(4), 138–140.

Segal, D., Wiss, D., & Whitelaw, G. P. (1985). Functional bracing and rehabilitation of ankle fractures. *Clinical Orthopaedics and Related Research, 199,* 39–45.

Sell, K. E., Verity, T. M., Worrell, T. W., Pease, B. J., & Wigglesworth, J. (1994). Two measurement techniques for assessing subtalar joint position: A reliability study. *Journal of Orthopedic and Sports Physical Therapy, 19*(3), 162–167.

Smidt, G. L. (1973). Biomechanical analysis of knee flexion and extension. *Journal of Biomechanics, 6,* 79–92.

Smith, D. S. (1982). Measurement of joint range—An overview. *Clinics in Rheumatic Diseases, 8*(3), 523–531.

Snedecor, G. W., & Cochran, W. G. (1989) *Statistical methods* (pp. 37–39, 237–253). Ames, IA: Iowa State University.

Solgaard, S., Carlsen, A., Kramhoft, M., & Petersen, V. S. (1986). Reproducibility of goniometry of the wrist. *Scandinavian Journal of Rehabilitation Medicine, 18,* 5–7.

Staubli, H., & Jakob, R. P. (1991). Anterior knee motion analysis: Measurement and simultaneous radiography. *American Journal of Sports Medicine, 19*(2), 172–177.

Storms, H. (1955). A system of joint measurement. *Physical Therapy Review, 35,* 369–371.

Stratford, P., Agostino, V., Brazeau, C., & Gowitzke, B. (1984). Reliability of joint angle measurement: A discussion of methodology issues. *Physiotherapy Canada, 36*(1), 5–9.

Sullivan, M. S., Dickinson, C. E., & Troup, J. D. G. (1994). The influence of age and gender on the lumbar spine sagittal plane range of motion. *Spine, 19*(6), 682–686.

Tanigawa, M. C. (1972). Comparison of the hold-relax procedure and passive mobilization on increasing muscle length. *Physical Therapy, 52,* 725–735.

Tanz, S. S. (1953). Motion of the lumbar spine. A roentgenologic study. *American Journal of Roentgenology Radium Therapy and Nuclear Medicine, 69,* 399–412.

Tanz, S. (1960). The so-called tight heel cord. *Clinical Orthopedics, 16,* 184–188.

Task Force on Standards for Measurement of Physical Therapy. (1991). Standards for tests and measurements in physical therapy practice. *Physical Therapy, 71,* 589–622.

Tucci, S. M., Hicks, J. E., Gross, E. G., Campbell, W., & Danoof, J. (1986). Cervical motion assessment: A new, simple and accurate method. *Archives of Physical Medicine and Rehabilitation, 67,* 225–230.

Vander-Linden, D. W., & Wilhelm, I. J. (1991). Electromyographic and cinematographic analysis of movement from a kneeling to a standing position in healthy 5 to 7 year old children. *Physical Therapy, 71*(1), 3–15.

Vandervort, A. A., Chesworth, B. B., Cunningham, D. A., Peterson, D. H., Rechnitzer, P. A., & Koval, J. J. (1992). Age and sex effects on mobility of the human ankle. *Journal of Gerontology, 47,* M17–M21.

Waddell, G. (1992). Biopsychosocial analysis of low back pain. *Clinical Rheumatology, 6,* 523–555.

Waddell, G., Allan, D. B., & Newton, M. (1991). Clinical evaluation of disability in back pain. In J. W. Frymoyer (Ed.), *The adult spine: Principles and practice.* (pp. 155–168). New York: Raven Press.

Waddell, G., Somerville, D., Henderson, I., & Newton, M. (1992). Objective clinical evaluation of physical impairment in chronic low back pain. *Spine, 17,* 617–628.

Walker, M. L., Rothstein, J. M., Finucane, S. D., & Lamb, R. L. (1987). Relationships between lumbar lordosis, pelvic tilt, and abdominal muscle performance. *Physical Therapy, 67,* 512–516.

Watkins, M. A., Riddle, D. L., Lamb, R. L., & Personius, W. J. (1991). Reliability of goniometric measurements and visual estimates of knee range of motion obtained in a clinical setting. *Physical Therapy, 71,* 90–97.

White, A. A., & Panjabi, M. M. (1984). *Biomechanics of the spine.* Philadelphia: J. B. Lippincott.

Wiechec, F. J., & Krusen, F. H. (1939). A new method of joint measurement and a review of the literature. *American Journal of Surgery, 43,* 659–668.

Williams, P. L. (Ed.). (1989). *Gray's anatomy* (37th ed.). New York: Churchill Livingstone.

Williams, R., Binkley, J., Bloch, R., Goldsmith, C. H., & Minuk, T. (1993). Reliability of the modified-modified Schöber and double inclinometer methods for measuring lumbar flexion and extension. *Physical Therapy, 73,* 26–37.

Wolf, S. L., Basmajain, J. V., Russe, C. T. C., & Kutner, M. (1979). Normative data on low back mobility and activity levels. *American Journal of Physical Medicine, 58,* 217–229.

Wright, D. G., Desai, S. M., & Henderson, W. H. (1964). Action of the subtalar and ankle joint complex during the stance phase of walking. *Journal of Bone and Joint Surgery, 46*(A), 361–382.

Youdas, J. W., Bogard, C. L., Suman, V. J. (1993). Reliability of goniometric measurements and visual estimates of ankle joint active range of motion obtained in a clinical setting. *Archives of Physical Medicine and Rehabilitation,74,* 1113–1118.

Youdas, J. W., Carey, J. R., Garrett, T. R. (1991). Reliability of measurements of cervical spine range of motion—Comparison of three methods. *Physical Therapy, 71*(2), 98–106.

Youdas, J. W., Carey, J. R., Garrett, T. R., & Suman, V. J. (1994). Reliability of goniometric measurements of active arm elevation in the scapular plane obtained in a clinical setting. *Archives of Physical Medicine and Rehabilitation, 75,* 1137–1144.

Youdas, J. W., Suman, V. J., & Garrett, T. R. (1995). Reliability of measurements of lumbar spine sagittal mobility obtained with the flexible curve. *Journal of Orthopedic and Sports Physical Therapy, 21,* 113–120.

Zuckerman, J. D., & Matsen, F. A. (1989). Biomechanics of the shoulder. In M. Nordin, & V. H. Frankel (Eds.), *Basic biomechanics of the musculoskeletal system* (2nd ed.) (pp. 225–247). Philadelphia: Lea & Febiger.

CHAPTER 4

Hand Analysis

A. Moneim Ramadan MD, FRCS

SUMMARY   This chapter discusses the normal anatomy of the various structures of the hand, with emphasis on the anatomic, physiologic, and functional importance of each anatomic entity. Important factors about the functional and surgical anatomy of the hand are outlined. A short discussion of clinical examples and a comprehensive evaluation protocol follow.

The hand is involved in every aspect of our lives, from birth to death. It is hard to imagine a life without hands. Like any other organ in the human body, the hand has its own characteristics and functions and is uniquely equipped to perform its functions, to service, and to connect human beings with the outside world. It is an intricately structured and dynamic organ created with mathematic perfection and harmony between all its various parts. The ideal hand performs its function precisely and flawlessly. Disruption in any one of its parts interferes, in a major way, with its function. Problems of the hands rarely, if ever, affect the quantity of life, but they do drastically affect the quality of life.

Nothing in this chapter is new or revolutionary. The facts discussed are based on the experience of the author and the data obtained from other experts referenced. The only thing that might be unique is the emphasis the author places on the absolute necessity and need for any health care professional who will have the chance or the obligation to treat hands to be absolutely sensitive and attuned to the normal anatomy, the desired function, and the process of evaluation. There is no room for guess work and no place for luck. Without solid knowledge of the anatomy and function of this organ, very little will be able to be done. Medicine, at least from the anatomic point of view, is a science based on facts. When knowledge is not adequate, the professional must seek the help of colleagues and the literature.

The upper extremity is present to allow the hand to perform its functions. The length of the upper extremity and the position and the type of shoulder and elbow joints are primarily designed to allow the hand to function. Consequently, the shoulder, the arm, and the elbow, as much as they are not directly a part of the hand, are directly related to the hand. Anatomically, the hand starts from the wrist joint area. Functionally, however, the hand starts from the elbow.

ANATOMY

General Anatomy

SKIN

The skin is primarily the protective organ of the body, and it is unique in the hand (Barron, 1970). On the palmar or volar aspect, the skin is thicker, lighter in color, and more stably tethered in position when compared with the darker, thin, loose skin on the extensor aspect or the dorsal side. On the volar aspect, the skin is marked with creases or lines that are of utmost significance anatomically and functionally. The skin on the dorsum is more lax, is not directly attached to the bone structure underneath it, and also has wrinkles that allow the skin to stretch when one makes a fist (Fig. 4–1). If the skin on the dorsum of the hand were to be tight, then the wrinkles would disappear, and it would consequently become difficult to make a fist.

SUPERFICIAL FASCIA

The superficial fascia on the dorsal aspect of the hand is very thin. The superficial fascia in the palmar aspect has the fibrofatty tissue, the amount and the density of which vary from one location to the other. The palmar triangle in the center of the palm consists of the distal palmar crease as its base and the junction of the thenar and hypothenar eminence at the wrist as its tip (Fig. 4–2). It is the only area devoid of fat (Milford, 1988). In the areas where it is located, the fat acts as a pressure cushion. The absence of fat in the palmar triangle is significant, as it keeps the skin well tethered and consequently allows the cup of the hand to deepen when a fist is made. The fat extends to the web spaces to protect the vascular bundles, especially the veins.

DEEP FASCIA

Within the dorsal aspect, the deep fascia is arranged in two layers. The superficial layer covers the extensor tendons and continues into the extensor hood on the

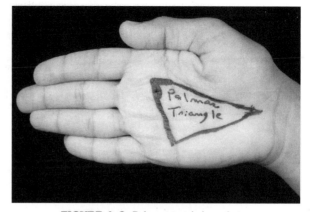

FIGURE 4–2. Palmar triangle boundaries.

extensor aspect of the fingers (Milford, 1988). The deep layer covers the interossei between the metacarpals. At the wrist level, the deep fascia is organized in the extensor retinaculum, which is divided into six compartments (Fig. 4–3). In the palmar aspect, the deep fascia is incorporated with the palmar aponeurosis.

Specialized parts of the deep fascia are the flexor retinaculum and the digital ligaments of Landsmeer and Clelland (Milford, 1988). This palmar fascia is a specialized fascia that is present only in the palm and in the sole of the foot, where its functional aspect is to give thickness and stability to the skin (Fig. 4–4). The palmar fascia starts from the heel of the hand and extends in various fiber arrangements up to the distal interphalangeal joint crease of the fingers and thumb. The attachments of the palmar fascia, the deep structures (including the bones), the skin along the various creases, and the skin of the palm restrict the skin of the hand from being freely mobile. The restriction of skin mobility is evident in the palmar triangle. The palmar fascia in the terminal phalangeal areas is replaced by strands of tough fibrous tissue called fibrous septae, which anchor the skin to the terminal phalanx and give stability to the tip of the digit (Fig. 4–5).

BONES

The skeleton of the hand consists of 29 bones that begin with the distal end of the radius and the head of the ulna at the wrist (Landsmeer, 1976; O'Brien and Eugene, 1988) (Figs. 4–6 and 4–7). The radius is the main forearm bone at the wrist joint, and the ulna is the main forearm bone at the elbow joint.

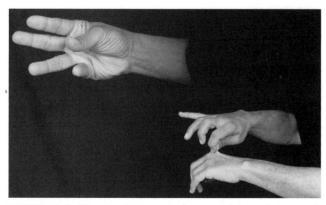

FIGURE 4–1. Note the difference between the thin loose skin on the dorsum and the thick, less-mobile skin on the palmar aspect.

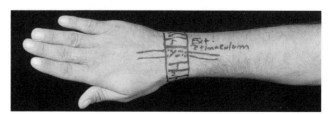

FIGURE 4–3. Extensor retinaculum.

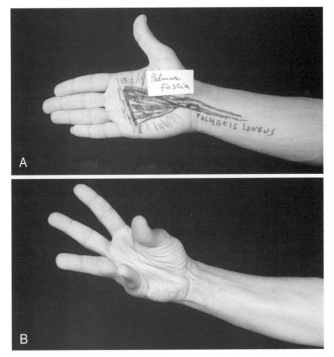

FIGURE 4–4. *A,* The palmaris longus inserts in the palmar fascia. *B,* The palmar fascia holds the skin of the volar aspect at the creases and in turn is attached to the bones and the deep intermuscular septae of the hand.

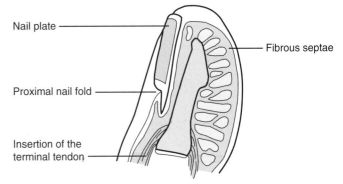

FIGURE 4–5. Anatomy of the terminal phalangeal area.

The carpus has eight carpal bones arranged transversely into the proximal and carpal rows and arranged longitudinally into the central and the two lateral columns. The scaphoid, lunate, triquetrum, and pisiform are in the proximal row. The trapezium, trapezoid, capitate, and hamate are in the distal row. The central longitudinal column consists of the lunate and the capitate, and the two lateral columns are made by the remaining carpal bones on each side of the central column (Fig. 4–8). Each carpal bone has a unique shape and size, which allows it to fit in its location. The carpal bones are arranged in such a way that they form the transverse carpal arch. This arch is concave toward the volar aspect and is the bony boundary of the carpal tunnel (Fig. 4–9). At its center, the deepest part of the transverse carpal arch forms the beginning of the center of the longitudinal arch and runs with the middle finger ray (Figs. 4–10 and 4–11). The distal carpal row articulates with the bases of the metacarpals. By itself, the thumb metacarpal only articulates with the trapezium. The remaining four metacarpals articulate with the other three distal row carpal bones.

The hand has five metacarpals. The thumb is the shortest and the widest, and the middle finger is the longest. All

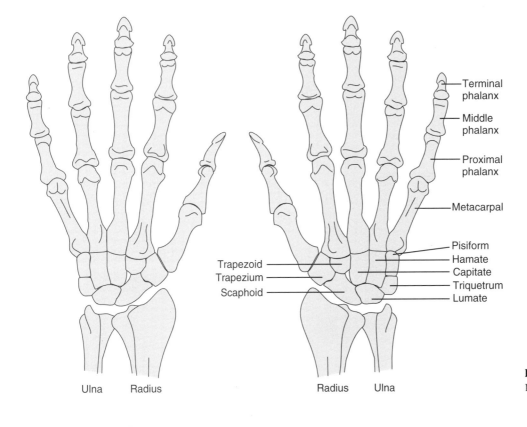

FIGURE 4–6 Bones of the hand, posterior aspect.

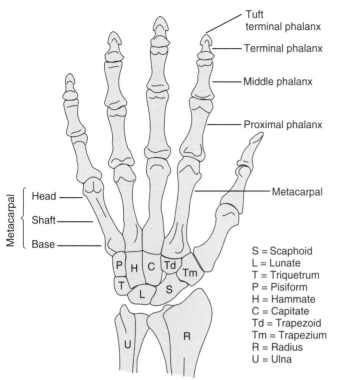

FIGURE 4–7. Bones of the hand, including parts of metacarpal.

S = Scaphoid
L = Lunate
T = Triquetrum
P = Pisiform
H = Hammate
C = Capitate
Td = Trapezoid
Tm = Trapezium
R = Radius
U = Ulna

metacarpals have a longitudinal gentle curve that is concave toward the palmar aspect, with the deepest part of the curve at the middle finger metacarpal. This is part of the longitudinal arch of the hand that extends from the wrist to the fingertips (Hollinshead, 1982; Milford, 1988) (see Fig. 4–7). Each metacarpal has a base, a shaft, and a head. The position of and the relationship between the metacarpal heads of the index, middle, ring, and little fingers make the base for the transverse metacarpal arch of the hand (Milford, 1988). The arch is concave toward the palm, with the deepest point of the arch at the metacarpal head of the middle finger. The middle finger is at the centermost, deepest part of the longitudinal arch. (see Fig. 4–7).

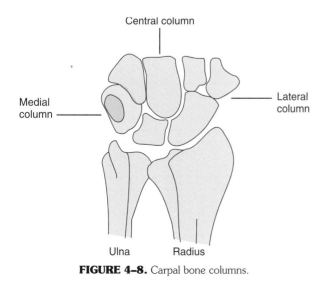

FIGURE 4–8. Carpal bone columns.

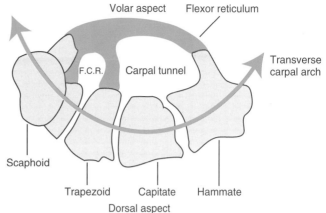

FIGURE 4–9. Cross-section of the carpal tunnel. F.C.R. = tunnel for the flexor carpi radialis.

Each finger has three phalanges (see Fig. 4 –7), and the thumb has two. Those of the thumb are the widest and the shortest. Those of the middle finger are the longest. Each phalanx has a concave wide base and a condylar head. They all have a gentle curve concave toward the palmar aspect to continue with the longitudinal arch of the hand. The terminal phalanx is the end of the hand skeleton and does not reach the tip of the digit but ends at a level around the junction of the proximal two thirds and the distal third of the nail bed. The end of the terminal phalanxes has an expanded round irregular shape, known as the tuft, that plays a major role in forming the shape of and contributing to the stability of the digit tip. The space between the skin of the tip at the distal end of the nail bed and the end of the terminal phalanx is occupied with fat and fibrous septae (see Fig. 4–5). It would be very painful if the end of the bone were to reach the skin because of the digit tip and the direct pressure of the bone on the skin. The terminal phalangeal area is supported partly by the terminal phalanx and partly by the nail plate, which compensate for the absence of the terminal phalanx in the distal third of the terminal phalangeal area.

JOINTS

Distal Radioulnar Joint. The distal radioulnar joint is located proximal to the radial carpal joint. The radial side of the head of the ulna articulates with a notch on the radial

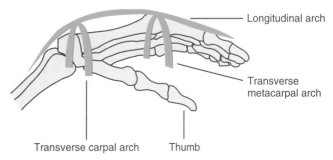

FIGURE 4–10. Arches of the hand, including transverse carpal arch.

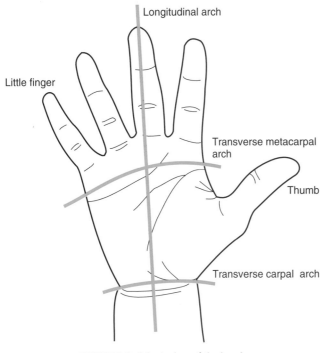

FIGURE 4-11. Arches of the hand.

side of the distal end of the radius and with the proximal surface of the triangular fibrocartilage. It is attached between the ulnar side of the end of the radius and the base of the styloid process of the ulna. No communication occurs between the distal radial ulnar joint and the radial carpal joint or the various components of the wrist joint itself. The distal radiulnar joint allows supination and pronation of movement to take place.

Radial Carpal Joint. The radial carpal joint is the main joint at the wrist. It only involves the scaphoid and part of the lunate to articulate with the radius and the triangular fibrocartilage, but the latter is only part of the joint in certain ranges of motion of the wrist.

Intercarpal Joints. Located between the various carpal bones, the intercarpal joints are a very complex set of joints that make the wrist area very unique and very well adapted to perform its function. These joints allow some of the carpal bones to be mobile in the very restricted space given, but it is the mobility of some of these bones that gives the intercarpal joints their uniqueness.

Carpometacarpal Joints. The carpometacarpal joints are formed by the distal carpal row and the basis of the five metacarpals. The basal joint, or the carpometacarpal joint, of the thumb between the trapezium and the first metacarpal is the most mobile. The carpometacarpal joint of the little finger between the base of the fifth metacarpal and the hamate bone is the second most mobile. The ring and index carpometacarpal joints have the least mobility. The middle finger carpometacarpal joint has no mobility at all, as it is the rigid, stable center of the longitudinal arch and is continuous with the central longitudinal rigid column of the carpal bones (see Fig. 4-11).

All these are important facts to remember, since fractures of the base of the metacarpal of the middle finger are to be treated quite differently from fractures of the base of the metacarpal of the thumb or the little finger. The difference in treatment is a result of the fact that the mobility varies from one digit to the other.

Metacarpophalangeal Joints. The metacarpophalangeal joints are located between the heads of the metacarpals and the base of the proximal phalanges, which are all primarily of the ball and socket variety. They allow flexion, extension, abduction, and adduction range of motion.

Interphalangeal Joints. The interphalangeal joints between the phalanges are of the bicondylar variety, that is, they have two convex condyles at the head with a groove, depression, and valley in between and allow flexion and extension range of motion.

LIGAMENTS

The stability of the joints depends on the bony structure of the joint, the shape of the articular surfaces, and the surrounding muscles and tendons, but more so on the integrity of the ligaments around the joints (Hollinshead 1982; Landsmeer, 1976; Taleisnik, 1976). Ligaments are specialized connective tissue structures, and their primary responsibility is to maintain stability while allowing mobility of the joints. At the wrist joint, numerous intricately arranged ligaments not only hold the carpal bones together but also hold the carpal bones to the metacarpals distally and the long bones of the forearm proximally. The ligaments are located in the volar, dorsal, radial, and ulnar sides between all the bony components, as shown in Figure 4-12. In the digits, however, the ligaments are in the volar and the lateral aspect. The dorsal aspect of the joints has no ligaments. On the volar aspect, ligaments are called the volar plates, but on the lateral aspect of the joints, they are called the collateral ligaments (Fig. 4-13) (*Kaplan's Functional and Surgical Anatomy of the Hand*, 1984; Landsmeer, 1976). The laxity or tightness of the ligaments depends on the position of the joints. When the joints are

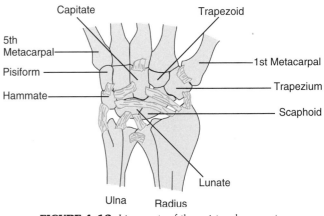

FIGURE 4-12. Ligaments of the wrist, volar aspect.

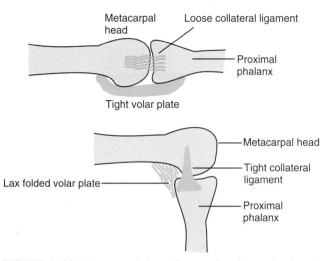

FIGURE 4–13. Metacarpophalangeal joint volar plate and collateral ligament in extension and in flexion.

flexed, the volar plates fold and become more lax and shorter. If they fibrose in this position, they shrink and become tight, which limits the extension of involved joints.

At the metacarpophalangeal joints, the collateral ligaments become tight with the metacarpophalangeal joints in 90 degrees flexion and become loose when the metacarpophalangeal joints are in the extended position and can allow abduction and adduction, as shown in Figure 4–14. At the interphalangeal joints, however, the collateral ligaments are tightest in the extended position and become loosest in the flexed position.

These are important facts because in positioning the joints during treatment, the conditions of these ligaments must be understood.

If the ligaments of the joints are disrupted, the joint becomes unstable. Consequently, the function of the hand is compromised. Some ligaments are much more vital than others. A good example is the ulnar collateral ligament of the metacarpophalangeal joint of the thumb, as compared

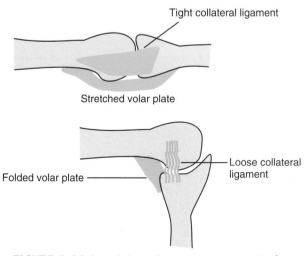

FIGURE 4–14. Interphalangeal joint in extension and in flexion.

with the radial collateral ligament of the same joint. A patient cannot use the thumb at all with an unstable ulnar collateral ligament. In the fingers, however, the radial collateral ligament of the proximal interphalangeal joint is more critical, as it takes the stress of the opposition between the thumb and the fingers. No deformities of the joints can develop without disruption to the ligaments, which renders joints unstable and sets the stage for deformities to occur in response to the various stress factors to which the joint is exposed.

MUSCLES

Muscles that play a direct role in hand function insert at various locations in the hand and are grouped into two divisions based on their location of origin. The first is the extrinsic group of muscles, which are located on the flexor and extensor aspects of the forearm. They originate in the forearm and are inserted in specific locations in the hand. The second is the intrinsic group of small muscles, which are located exclusively in the hand (i.e., they originate and insert inside the hand).

Extrinsic Muscles. Extrinsic muscles are located on the flexor and extensor aspects of the forearm. They are frequently referred to as the long flexors and long extensors. There are two flexor and two extensor surface muscles, which originate or insert away from the hand but indirectly affect the function of the hand. On the flexor surface, these two muscles are the pronator teres and the pronator quadratus. On the extensor aspect, the two muscles are the supinator and the brachioradialis.

Pronator Teres. This muscle has two origins: first, a humeral origin from the lower part of the medial supracondylar ridge and medial epicondyle and second, an ulnar origin from the coronoid process of the ulna. The pronator teres inserts into the middle of the lateral surface of the radius. Nerve supply is median nerve C6-7. To test the action of this muscle, the arm is held next to the body with the elbow in partial flexion, and the patient is asked to pronate the forearm (Fig. 4–15).

Pronator Quadratus. This muscle originates in the volar aspect of the distal ulna deep to the flexor tendons and is inserted in the volar aspect distal fourth of the radius. To test the action of this muscle, the arm is held next to the body with the elbow fully flexed, and the patient is asked to pronate the forearm. Nerve supply comes from median nerve C7-T1 (Fig. 4–16).

Brachioradialis. The brachioradialis originates from the upper third of the lateral supracondylar ridge of the humerus and inserts in the radial side of the lower end of the radius. Nerve supply is the radial C5-6. To test this muscle, the arm is held next to the body, elbow partially flexed, forearm in neutral position, and the patient is asked to flex the elbow (Fig. 4–17).

Supinator Muscle. This muscle originates in the lateral epicondyle of the humerus and inserts in the proximal third

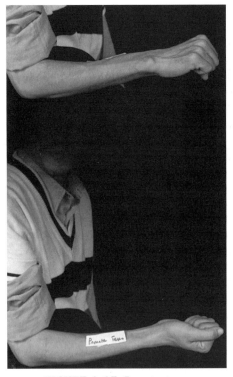

FIGURE 4–15. Pronator teres.

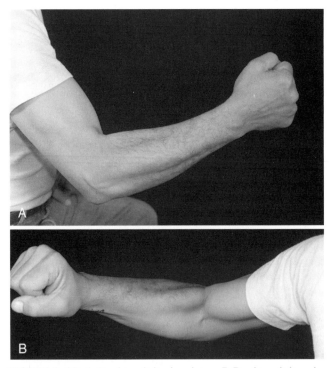

FIGURE 4–17. *A,* Brachioradialis, dorsal view. *B,* Brachioradialis, volar view.

of the lateral surface of the radius nerve supply. Nerve supply is radial nerve C5-6. To test the supinator, the forearm is held in neutral, with the elbow flexed fully. The muscle supinates the forearm (Fig. 4–18).

The long flexors that originate in the forearm and are inserted in the hand are the following:

1. Flexors of the wrist
   a. Flexor carpi radialis
   b. Flexor carpi ulnaris
   c. Palmaris longus, if present
2. Long flexors of the fingers
   a. Flexor digitorum superficialis "sublimis"
   b. Flexor digitorum profundus
3. Flexor pollicis longus (the long flexor to the thumb)

Flexor Carpi Radialis. This muscle's origin is in the common flexor origin in the medial epicondyle, and it inserts at the volar surface base of the second metacarpal. Nerve supply is the median nerve C7-8. To test this muscle, the

forearm is held in supination, and the elbow is partially flexed while this muscle flexes and radially deviates the wrist (Fig. 4–19).

Palmaris Longus. This muscle originates in the medial epicondyle and inserts into the flexor retinaculum and the palmar aponeurosis at the wrist and palm of the hand. This muscle is absent in 10 percent of the population. Nerve supply is median nerve C7-8. Its action is tested by holding the thumb and the little finger tip to tip and then flexing the wrist. If present, its tendon becomes the most prominent under the skin at the wrist area (Fig. 4–20).

Flexor Carpi Ulnaris. This muscle originates in the medial epicondyle, the medial border of the olecranon, and the upper part of the posterior border of the ulna. It is inserted in the pisiform bone. Nerve supply is the ulnar nerve

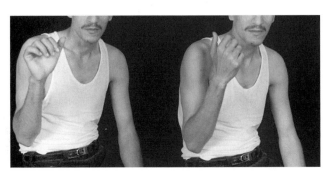

FIGURE 4–16. Pronator quadratus.

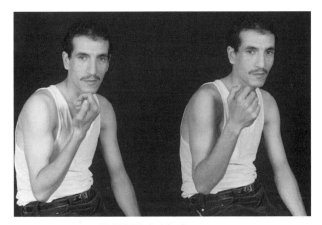

FIGURE 4–18. Supinator.

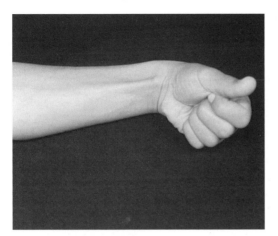

FIGURE 4–19. Flexor carpi radialis.

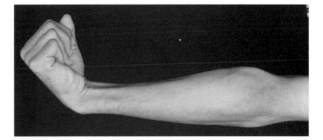

FIGURE 4–21. Flexor carpi ulnaris.

C8-T1. With the forearm supinated, it flexes and ulnarly deviates the wrist (Fig. 4–21).

Flexor Digitorum Superficialis "Sublimis." The origin of this muscle is in the medial epicondyle of the humerus, the medial border of the coronoid process of the upper two thirds of the anterior border of the radius, and from the ulnar collateral ligament. The superficialis tendons insert at the volar surface base of the middle phalanx. The superficialis to the little finger is absent in about 20 percent of hands and, if present, it is usually of a much smaller size than the superficialis tendon of the other fingers. Nerve supply is the median nerve C7-T1. To test for any of the sublimis units, the hand has to be held flat on the table with the forearm supinated and all the fingers blocked from movement, with the exception of the finger whose muscle unit is being tested. The patient is then asked to actively flex the proximal interphalangeal joint (Figs. 4–22 and 4–23).

Flexor Digitorum Profundus. The origin of this muscle is in the upper two thirds of the anterior and medial surfaces of the ulna and from the adjoining half of the interosseous membrane. It inserts at the base of the terminal phalanx of the index, middle, ring, and little fingers. Nerve supply to the muscle belly, which gives the profundus to the index and middle fingers, is from the median nerve through its anterior interosseous branch C7-T1. Nerve supply to the

muscle belly, which supplies the profundus to the ring and little fingers, is through the ulnar nerve C8-T1. The action of any unit of this muscle is tested by holding the hand in supination with the wrist and all the finger joints blocked from movement, except the distal interphalangeal joint to be tested (Figs. 4–24 and 4–25).

Flexor Pollicis Longus. This muscle originates in the forearm from the radius and interosseous membrane and, on occasion, partly from the coronoid process of the ulna.

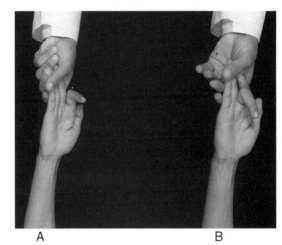

A   B

FIGURE 4–22. Isolating the sublimis flexor to the index finger (A) and to the middle finger (B).

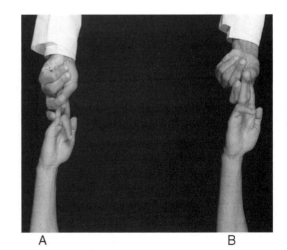

A   B

FIGURE 4–23. Isolating the sublimis flexor to the ring finger (A) and to the little finger (B).

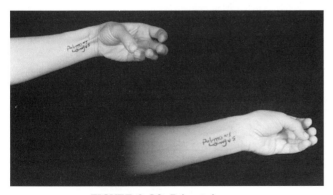

FIGURE 4–20. Palmaris longus.

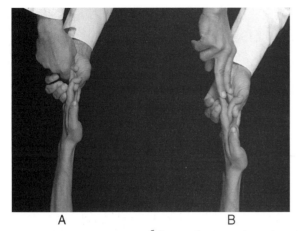

A   **B**

FIGURE 4–24. Isolating the action of the profundus tendon to the index finger *(A)* and to the middle finger *(B)*.

It is inserted into the base of the terminal phalanx of the thumb. Nerve supply is the median nerve through its anterior interosseus branch C7-T1. To test for its action, the hand is held in supination, the wrist and the metacarpophalangeal joint of the thumb are stabilized, and the patient is asked to flex the interphalangeal joint of the thumb (Fig. 4–26).

On the extensor side of the forearm, the following muscles are present:

1. Extensors to the wrist
   a. Extensor carpi radialis longus
   b. Extensor carpi radialis brevis
   c. Extensor carpi ulnaris
2. Extensors to the thumb
   a. Extensor pollicis longus
   b. Extensor pollicis brevis
3. Abductor pollicis longus
4. Extensor indicis proprius
5. Long common extensor proprius to the fingers (extensor digitorum communis)
6. Long independent extensor digiti minimi to the little finger

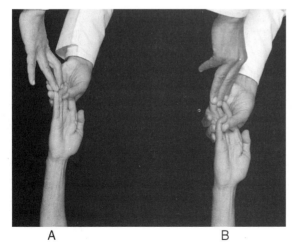

A   **B**

FIGURE 4–25. Isolating the action of the flexor digitorum to the ring finger *(A)* and to the little finger *(B)*.

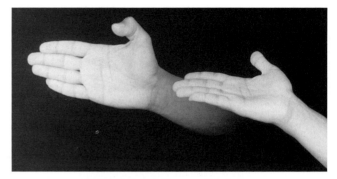

FIGURE 4–26. Flexor pollicis longus.

Extensor Carpi Radialis Longus. This muscle's origin is from the distal third of the lateral supracondylar ridge, and it inserts at the base of the second metacarpal on the extensor aspect. Nerve supply is the radial C6-7. This muscle is tested by holding the forearm in full pronation while the fingers are closed in a fist. The patient is then asked to extend the wrist with radial deviation. In testing, it is almost impossible to isolate this muscle from the extensor carpi radialis brevis (Fig. 4–27).

Extensor Carpi Radialis Brevis. This muscle originates in the lateral epicondyle of the humerus, which is called the common extensor tendon origin, and inserts at the extensor aspect of the base of the third metacarpal. Nerve supply and action are the same as for the extensor carpi radialis longus (see Fig. 4–27).

Extensor Carpi Ulnaris. This muscle originates in the lateral epicondyle of the common extensor tendon. It also has a partial origin in the middle part of the posterior border of the ulna. It inserts at the base of the fifth metacarpal on the extensor aspect. Nerve supply is the radial nerve C7-8. Its action is tested as other wrist extensors are tested but with the knowledge that this muscle extends the wrist with ulnar deviation (Fig. 4–28).

Extensor Digitorum Communis to the Fingers. This muscle originates in the anterior surface of the lateral humeral epicondyle from the fascia covering the muscle and from the intermuscular septum. The four tendons of this muscle insert partly in the base of the proximal phalanx of the fingers and partly in the extensor hood mechanism. Nerve supply is the radial nerve C7-8. To test this muscle, the forearm is held in pronation, the wrist is stabilized, the interphalangeal joints are fully flexed, and the

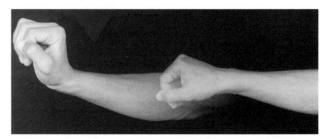

FIGURE 4–27. Extensor carpi radialis longus and brevis. They are very difficult to isolate clinically.

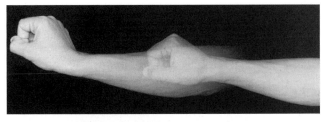

FIGURE 4–28. Extensor carpi ulnaris.

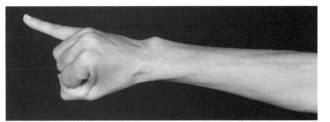

FIGURE 4–30. Extensor digiti minimi.

patient is asked to extend the metacarpophalangeal joints (Fig. 4–29).

Extensor Digiti Minimi. This muscle originates in the epicondyle and also from its own muscle fascia. The tendon inserts partly into the base of the terminal phalanx and partly into the extensor hood mechanism. Nerve supply is the radial nerve C7-8. To test this muscle, the forearm is held in pronation, the wrist is stabilized, all fingers are flexed, and the patient is asked to extend the little finger only (Fig. 4–30).

Extensor Indicis Proprius. This muscle originates deep in the forearm from the lower part of the ulna and the adjoining interosseous membrane. Its tendon inserts partly in the base of the proximal phalanx and partly in the extensor hood mechanism. Nerve supply is the radial C7-8. The muscle is tested in the same manner as the extensor digitiminimi, the only exception being that the patient is asked to extend the index finger (Fig. 4–31).

Extensor Pollicis Longus. This originates in the dorsal surface of the ulna and interosseous membrane. It inserts into the extensor hood mechanism of the thumb and through that into the base of the terminal phalanx of the thumb. Nerve supply is the radial nerve C7-8. The muscle is tested with the wrist and the metacarpophalangeal joint of the thumb stabilized in neutral and the forearm in pronation, supination, or neutral. The patient is asked to extend the thumb and, specifically, to hyperextend the interphalangeal joint (Fig. 4–32).

Extensor Pollicis Brevis. This originates in the radius and the interosseous membrane and inserts in the dorsal aspect of the base of the proximal phalanx and partly into the extensor mechanism of the thumb. Nerve supply is the radial nerve C6-7. To test this muscle, the wrist is stabilized in extension, and the patient is asked to extend the thumb independent of the position of the forearm (Fig. 4–33).

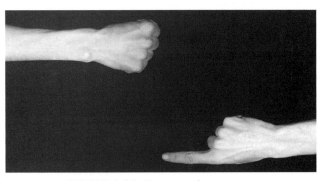

FIGURE 4–31. Extensor indicis proprius.

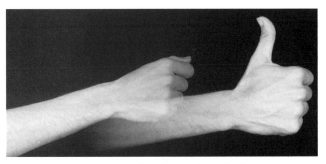

FIGURE 4–32. Extensor pollicis longus. Note the hyperextension at the interphalangeal joint of the thumb.

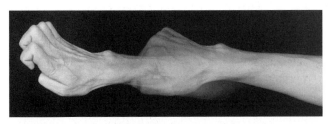

FIGURE 4–29. Extensor digitorum communis with isolated extension of metacarpophalangeal joints of the index, middle, ring, and little fingers.

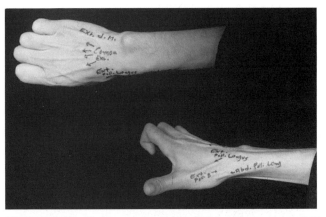

FIGURE 4–33. All of the extensors of the digits in action: extensor digiti minimi, common extensor "digitum extensor," extensor indicis proprius on the ulnar side of the common extensor part to the index, extensor pollicis longus, anatomic "snuff box," extensor pollicis longus.

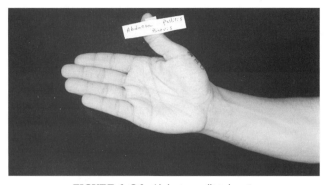

FIGURE 4–34. Abductor pollicis brevis.

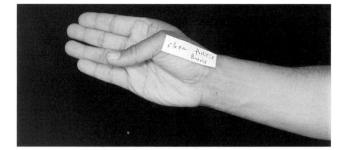

FIGURE 4–36. Flexor pollicis brevis.

Abductor Pollicis Longus. This muscle originates from the dorsal aspect of the radius, ulna, and the interosseous membrane between them. It is inserted sometimes through multiple slips into the lateral side of the base of the first metacarpal. Nerve supply is the radial nerve C6-7. With the forearm in neutral and the wrist stabilized, the patient is asked to abduct the carpometacarpal joint of the thumb. It is very difficult to isolate the function of this muscle from the interference of the other extensors of the thumb.

Intrinsic Muscles. These are the muscles that originate and insert inside the hand. The muscles are divided into four groups: 1) thenar muscles, 2) hypothenar muscles, 3) lumbrical muscles, and 4) interossei.

Thenar Muscle Group. The thenar muscles, also called the short muscles of the thumb, are located on the radial side of the hand. With the exception of the adductor pollicis and the deep head of the flexor pollicis brevis, they are supplied by the median nerve and act together as a group. It is very difficult to isolate the independent function of each muscle.

Abductor Pollicis Brevis. The abductor pollicis brevis is the most superficial of the group, is located on the radial side of the thenar eminence area, and originates from the flexor reticulum at the wrist, the scaphoid, the trapezium, and, more frequently, with a slip from the tendon of the abductor pollicis longus and occasionally with a slip from the tendon of the palmaris longus. That muscle is inserted into the base radial side of the proximal phalanx in the lateral tubercle and occasionally into the lateral sesamoid of the metacarpophalangeal joint and also partly into the extensor mechanism of the thumb (which will be discussed later), along with the extensor mechanism of the fingers (Fig. 4–34).

Opponens Pollicis. The opponens pollicis lies deeper than the abductor pollicis brevis and arises from the flexor retinaculum and the trapezium bone. It is inserted into the radial half of the shaft of the first metacarpal. Some parts might reach the palmar aspect of the metacarpophalangeal joint and the sesamoid bone (Fig. 4–35).

Flexor Pollicis Brevis. This muscle has both a superficial head and a deep head. The superficial head arises from the flexor retinaculum, trapezium, and the sheath of the flexor carpi radialis, and sometimes from the deep aspect of the palmar aponeurosis. The deep head arises from the capitate and the trapezoid, where it continues with the origin of the oblique head of the adductor pollicis. The two heads of the flexor pollicis brevis unite and are inserted into the lateral tubercle on the radial side of the base of the proximal phalanx. They also insert into the radial sesamoid of the metacarpophalangeal joint and into the extensor expansion of the thumb. The deep head is supplied by the ulnar nerve, and the superficial head, by the median nerve (Fig. 4–36).

Adductor Pollicis. The adductor pollicis arises by two heads: the oblique head from the sheath of the flexor carpi radialis; base of the second, third, and fourth metacarpal bones; trapezoid; and the capitate bones. The transverse head arises from the shaft of the third metacarpal. The adductor pollicis is inserted in the tubercle on the ulnar side of the base of the proximal phalanx into the ulnar sesamoid bone of the metacarpophalangeal joint and also into the extensor expansion of the thumb. It is supplied by the ulnar nerve. Its action is tested by stabilizing the wrist, regardless of the position of the forearm, and by asking the patient to adduct the thumb toward the index finger (Fig. 4–37). This is the basis for Froment's sign, which occurs when the patient is asked to hold a paper firmly between the thumb

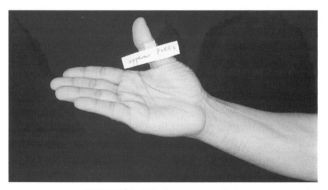

FIGURE 4–35. Opponens pollicis.

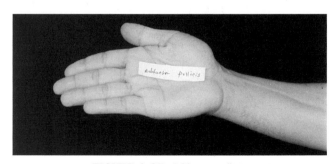

FIGURE 4–37. Adductor pollicis.

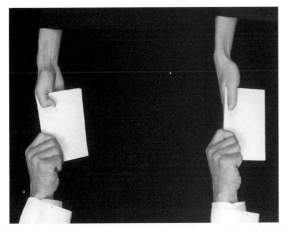

FIGURE 4–38. Froment's test—with paralysis of the first dorsal interosseous and the adductor pollicis "ulnar nerve injury," the patient has to use the flexor pollicis longus to flex the interphalangeal joints of the thumb to give power to thumb adduction.

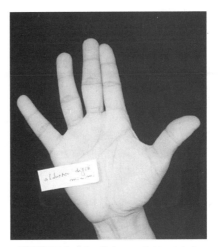

FIGURE 4–40. Abductor digiti minimi.

and the index finger; in case of paralysis of this muscle, the patient will not be able to hold the paper between the thumb and the index finger unless the thumb is flexed at the interphalangeal joint to hold the paper through the action of the flexor pollicis longus (Fig. 4–38).

Hypothenar Muscle Group. This group of muscles is located on the ulnar side of the hand. They are all supplied by the ulnar nerve and are easier to test independently than are the thenar muscles. With the wrist stabilized in neutral and the forearm supinated, the abductor digiti minimi abducts the little finger away from the ring finger. The flexor digiti minimi flexes the metacarpophalangeal and extends the interphalangeal joints of the little finger. The opponens digiti minimi brings the little finger toward the thumb (Fig. 4–39).

Abductor Digiti Minimi. The abductor digiti minimi arises from the tendon of the flexor carpi ulnaris at the wrist from the pisiform bone and also from the fibrous arch spanning or spreading over from the pisiform to the hook of the hamate. The hamate is the roof of the Guyon's canal. It is inserted into the medial side of the base of the proximal phalanx of the little finger and partly into the extensor

tendon. With the wrist in neutral position and resting on a flat surface with the palm up to cancel the action of the digit extensors, the little finger is abducted actively, and the rigid contracted muscle will be felt at the ulnar border of the hand (Fig. 4–40).

Opponens Digiti Minimi. The opponens digiti minimi arises from the hook of the hamate and the flexor retinaculum. It is inserted in the distal two thirds of the medial half of the palmar aspect of the fifth metacarpal. With the wrist in a neutral position, the little finger is twisted actively as if to meet the thumb. The muscle will be felt in the ulnar border of the hand (Fig. 4–41).

Flexor Digiti Minimi Brevis. This muscle is absent in about 20 to 30 percent of people, or in some cases it might just be joined as part of its neighboring small muscles in the hypothenar area. It originates from the flexor retinaculum, the hook of the hamate, and the fibrous arch, which unite the muscle to the origin of the abductor digiti minimi. It is inserted into the medial side of the base of the proximal phalanx of the little finger. With the wrist in neutral position, the little finger is actively flexed at the metacarpophalangeal joint, with the interphalangeal joints held in neutral (i.e., in full extension).

Palmaris Brevis. This is a very small subcutaneous muscle that arises from the medial border of the palmar aponeurosis and is inserted into the skin of the medial border of the

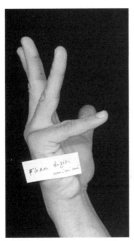

FIGURE 4–39. Flexor digiti minimi.

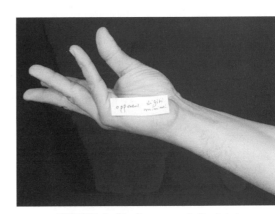

FIGURE 4–41. Opponens digiti minimi.

{

}

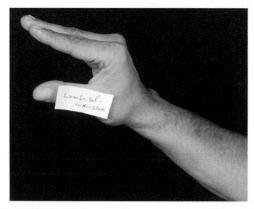

FIGURE 4–42. Lumbrical-interossei position "action."

hand. When present, its main function is to protect the ulnar nerve and the ulnar vessels.

Lumbrical Muscle Group. There are four lumbrical muscles. The medial two arise by two heads from the adjacent sides of the profundus tendon to the long, ring, and little fingers. The lateral two arise from the lateral side of the profundus tendon to the index and long fingers. These small muscles are inserted into the lateral edge of the extensor expansion to the fingers. The two lumbricals that originate from the profundus of the index and middle fingers are supplied by the median nerve. The two lumbricals that originate from the profundus of the ring and little fingers are supplied by the ulnar nerve. With the forearm pronated and the wrist stabilized, all the lumbricals extend the interphalangeal joints and simultaneously flex the metacarpophalangeal joints of all the fingers. They also extend the interphalangeal joints when the metacarpophalangeal joints are extended (Fig. 4–42).

Interossei Muscle Group. There are seven interossei muscles. The three palmar interossei arise from the metacarpals of the fingers on which they act. The first one arises from the ulnar side and adjoins the palmar aspect of the second metacarpal. The two remaining interossei arise from the radial side and adjoin the palmar surface of the

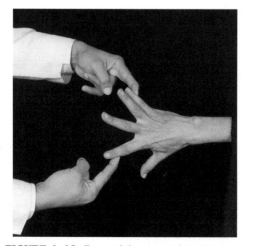

FIGURE 4–43. Finger abduction—palmar interossei.

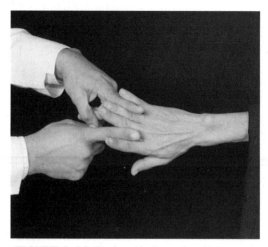

FIGURE 4–44. Finger adduction—dorsal interossei.

fourth and fifth metacarpals. The four dorsal interossei are much bigger than the palmar ones and arise from the adjacent metacarpals. The first dorsal interossei arise from the first and second metacarpal shafts by two heads, which form a kind of tunnel that transmits the radial artery into the palm. The three remaining dorsal interossei arise from the adjoining dorsal surfaces of the second, third, third and fourth, and fourth and fifth, respectively. They are inserted into the base of the proximal phalanx and the extensor expansion. All the interossei are supplied by the ulnar nerve. With the forearm pronated, the wrist stabilized, and the hand resting flat on a table to cancel the long tendons, the volar interossei adducts; the dorsal ones abduct the digits. The interossei also help the lumbricals with their action on the metacarpophalangeal and interphalangeal joints (Figs. 4–43 and 4–44).

TENDONS

Muscles are the contractile structure but tendons are specialized connective tissue that is designed to transmit contractions of the muscle into joint action through the process of gliding. Each muscle unit ends in single or multiple tendon units, which attach to the bone. All the tendons are primarily designed to perform a function that plays a major role in the harmony of the dynamics of the hand (Doyle and Blythe, 1975; Kleinert, 1975; Kleinert and Stormo, 1973; Verdan, 1964). Almost all the extrinsic muscles have long tendons, and the short muscles in the hand have short tendons. Tendons are always inserted distal to the joint on which they exert their function; consequently, the flexor profundus, which flexes the distal interphalangeal joint of the finger, is inserted in the base of the terminal phalanx just distal to that particular joint. Each tendon unit has to follow a certain path and is attached to the bone in a unique way that ultimately maximizes the actions of the muscle unit. Due to the uniqueness of the tendons, we will discuss each tendon separately.

In their journey from the end of the muscle to the insertion in the bone, some tendons curve, some go

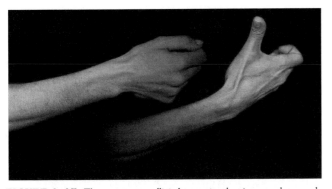

FIGURE 4–45. The extensor pollicis longus tendon is a good example of a tendon that partly goes straight, then around a curve, partly through a pulley on the dorsum of the wrist, and partly without a pulley on the more carpal; that is why the tendon pops out, as in bowstringing, and becomes obvious.

straight, and others go through tunnels (Fig.4–45). The tunnels are specialized compartments located at strategic locations in the hand. The function of these tunnels is to safeguard against bowstringing, and, consequently, they maximize the pulling forces of the muscle unit. One or more tendons might go through a specialized compartment. The compartments are located proximal or distal to joints, and if they have to cross in front of the joint, then structural changes in the pulley take place to allow the joint to move. The tendons have their own blood supply and are covered with a specialized tissue called the tenosynovium.

Flexor Carpi Radialis. The tendon of this muscle starts in the lower third of the forearm and travels in a separate deep compartment that is on the radial side of the wrist. The flexor carpi radialis tunnel is hidden behind the thenar muscle origin and is outside the carpal tunnel. It is such an active tendon and is squeezed in its tunnel so deep in the wrist area that it becomes vulnerable to an inflammatory condition known as flexor carpi radialis tendinitis.

Palmaris Longus. When the palmaris longus muscle is present, it has a very long tendon and short muscle belly. It is inserted in a widespread manner into the palmar aponeurosis of the hand. It is the length and size of this tendon that make it adequate to be used as a tendon graft to reconstruct another missing tendon in the hand. In addition, no specific functions are lost in its absence, making it an excellent donor tendon.

Flexor Pollicis Longus. The tendon of this muscle is fairly long and runs through the carpal tunnel deep to the flexor carpi radialis tunnel and then just distal to the carpal tunnel, it turns around superficial to it and then travels deep to the thenar muscles. It runs between the two sesamoids at the metacarpophalangeal joint of the thumb and then enters the fibrous flexor sheath or tunnel at the base of the proximal phalanx. It is inserted into the palmar aspect of the base of the distal phalanx. The tendon has a very well developed vinculum breve, which carries the blood supply to the tendon. Its synovial sheath, which extends proximally into the forearm, is significant because any infection in the thumb around the flexor pollicis longus can extend along the tendon and into the wrist area to the lower third of the forearm. The primary function of the flexor pollicis longus is flexion of the interphalangeal joint of the thumb and some flexion of the metacarpophalangeal joint.

Flexor Digitorum Superficialis "Sublimis." Usually four tendons (one for each finger) arise from the muscle belly around the middle of the forearm. The tendons for the long and ring fingers are almost always superficial to those for the index and little fingers. This position is maintained through the carpal tunnel but the tendons diverge (one to each finger) in the palmar triangle, and at the distal palmar crease, each tendon enters the fibrous flexor sheath along with the tendon of the profundus.

Around the level of the metacarpophalangeal joint, while still in the fibrous flexor sheath, each superficialis tendon splits into two segments, or slips. Each segment passes around and then posteriorly to the joining tendon of the profundus, where the segments partially join again. Each segment or slip continues distally to be inserted almost separately into the margins of the palmar surface of the middle phalanx. The tendons of the superficialis have the vincula breve and longus, which carry the blood vessels. The vinculum breve is a small triangular band in the interval between the terminal part of the tendon and the front of the proximal interphalangeal joint and the distal part of the proximal phalanx. The vinculum longus is a slender band extending from the tendon to the proximal part of the proximal phalanx. As previously mentioned, the superficialis tendon to the little finger is absent in about 20 percent of the population and is very small and less developed in the majority of the remaining population.

Flexor Digitorum Profundus. This tendon starts at the middle of the forearm. The most radial part of the muscle belly of the profundus forms the tendon to the index finger, and the most ulnar part forms the tendon to the little finger. The four tendons go through the carpal tunnel and lie deeply under the superficialis tendons. Each tendon of the profundus, after its exit from the carpal tunnel area, travels distally through the palmar triangle of the hand and then into the flexor fibrous sheath. As it enters the fibrous sheath, it runs behind the sublimis tendon to each digit and then goes through the decussation of the sublimis opposite the proximal phalanx. Each tendon has a vinculum breve, which is attached to the capsule on the volar aspect of the distal interphalangeal joint and is also supplied by the aforementioned long vincula. The tendon of the profundus is inserted in the volar aspect of the base of the terminal phalanx.

Abductor Pollicis Longus. The tendon of this muscle becomes superficial in the distal forearm. It travels on the radial side with the tendon of the extensor pollicis brevis, crosses the tendons of the two radial extensors of the wrist, and then travels through the first extensor compartment. The two tendons cross over the radial artery after they exit out of the first extensor compartment. The abductor pollicis longus splits into multiple tendon slips, and then it becomes attached to its point of insertion in the lateral side of the base of the thumb metacarpal. The abductor pollicis longus tendon acts as an abductor and stabilizer of the most dynamic part of the hand, which is the thumb metacarpal. Consequently, this makes it a very frequently used tendon, and because of its anatomic relationship as it travels through the first extensor compartment and as it lies on the distal border of the radius, it is vulnerable to irritation and inflammation. Inflammation of this tendon, along with its companion extensor pollicis brevis (located in the first extensor compartment), is what is known as tenosynovitis of the first extensor compartment (de Quervain's disease).

Extensor Pollicis Brevis. This tendon becomes superficial in the distal part of the forearm and travels along the tendon of the abductor pollicis longus through the first extensor compartment and continues distally as it inserts partly in the dorsal aspect of the base of the proximal phalanx and partly into the extensor expansion of the thumb. It extends and abducts the carpometacarpal joint and extends the metacarpophalangeal joint. It also plays a part in extension of the interphalangeal joint of the thumb, through its insertion in the extensor expansion.

Extensor Pollicis Longus. This tendon stays deep in the distal third of the forearm and in the wrist joint area until it gets out of its own third compartment, which is located on the ulnar side of the dorsal tubercle of the radius. At this point, it changes its direction to an oblique radial direction, crosses superficially to the tendons of the two radial extensors of the wrist, and continues distally until it becomes attached to the dorsal expansion of the extensor mechanism of the thumb and is inserted in a very wide flat tendon, which almost covers the whole width of the dorsal aspect of the base of the terminal phalanx. This muscle tendon unit extends all the joints of the thumb. Because of its oblique course and the side-to-side mobility on the dorsum of the first metacarpal, it can also abduct and adduct the thumb.

Extensor Digitorum Proprius "Communis." The tendons of the extensor digitorum proprius to the index, middle, ring, and little fingers start proximal to the wrist and travel through the fourth compartment of the extensor retinaculum over the center of the wrist. On the dorsum of the hand, the tendons are connected together by oblique bands, which allow these tendons to work together when the hand needs to function with the fingers extended in one unit. At the level of the metacarpophalangeal joints, these long extensors to the fingers divide into two parts. The deeper part of the tendon is inserted at the base of the proximal phalanx on the extensor aspect. The superficial part joins the extensor hood mechanism on the extensor aspect of the proximal phalangeal area of the fingers. This group of muscle tendons primarily extends the metacarpophalangeal joints. However, through the extensor hood expansion mechanism, these tendons play a role in the extension of the interphalangeal joints. In a hyperextended position of the metacarpophalangeal joints, these tendons have the tendency to abduct the fingers from the line of the long

finger bone. The same is true for extensor digiti minimi of the little finger.

Extensor Indicis Proprius. This tendon starts at the distal third of the forearm and then passes through the fourth compartment, along with the four common extensors. On the dorsum of the hand, it lies on the ulnar side of the extensor digitorum communis to the index finger and is inserted into the base of the terminal phalanx and the extensor hood mechanism. This muscle tendon unit, besides working along with the common extensors of the fingers, produces the independent extension of the index finger.

Extensor Digiti Minimi. This tendon starts at the lower third of the forearm and travels distally through a special fifth compartment in the extensor retinaculum. Either inside the compartment or just distal to it, it splits into two portions. This tendon, coupled with the extensor digitorum proprius to the little finger, is inserted in the extensor expansion on the dorsum of the proximal phalanx and partly in the base of proximal phalanx. The muscle tendon unit of the extensor digiti minimi extends the little finger in conjunction with the other extensors but also independently extends the little finger.

Lumbricals. From the muscle belly, the tendons travel distally through the lumbrical canal on the radial side of each digit and continue distally volar to the transverse axis of the metacarpophalangeal joint. The lumbrical tendons join the lateral edge of the extensor expansion of the extensor hood mechanism as they become the most distal part of what is known as the conjoint tendon of the small muscles of the hand. The other part of that conjoint tendon, which is proximal to the lumbrical, almost always belong to the interossei. As the lumbricals are volar to the axis of the metacarpophalangeal joints and are dorsal to the axis of the interphalangeal joints, they extend the latter, and with the fingers extended at these joints, they flex the first joints. Their attachment of origin to the flexor profundus and their attachment of insertion to the extensor system allow the lumbricals to play an important role in the balance between the flexor and extensor systems of the fingers.

Interossei. Like the other small muscles of the hand, the interossei tendons travel a very short distance dorsal to the deep transverse ligament of the palm but anterior to the axis of flexion at the metacarpophalangeal joint. They are inserted in the extensor expansion, forming the proximal part of the conjoint tendon of the small muscles of the hand into the digits. The action of the interossei depends on whether they are palmar or dorsal. The dorsal muscles abduct the other fingers away from the middle one. Those that act on the middle finger abduct the finger to the radial or the ulnar side. The first dorsal interosseus rotates the index finger radially at the metacarpophalangeal joint to allow for thumb-to-index pinching. The palmar interossei adduct the fingers toward the line of the long finger. Because of their line of pull and their relationship to the axis of the metacarpophalangeal and interphalangeal joints, the interossei, like the lumbricals, flex the metacarpopha-

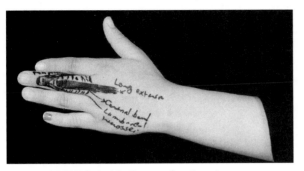

FIGURE 4–46. Extensor hood mechanism.

langeal joint and, through their insertion into the extensor expansion, extend the interphalangeal joints.

The Extensor Hood Mechanism. The extensor hood mechanism (Fig. 4–46), which starts at the level of the metacarpal head and extends to the middle of the middle phalanx, is a very complex area of tendon insertion and is a classic example of the uniqueness of tendon arrangement in the hand that allows it to perform its function in the most dynamic and harmonious way (Tubiana et al., 1984). In the fingers at the level of the metacarpophalangeal joint, the long extensor tendon, joined by the independent extensor to the index and little fingers, divides into a superficial and deep portion. The deep portion, as it crosses over the metacarpophalangeal joint, becomes adherent to the dorsal capsule and is inserted at the base of the proximal phalanx. The superficial portion passes into the extensor hood mechanism. The sagittal bands, which are the proximal part of the extensor hood mechanism, are joined and overlapped on each side toward the dorsal aspect by the interosseous tendon that passes from the hand to the fingers dorsal to the transverse metacarpal ligament but volar to the axis of the metacarpophalangeal joint. The superficial part of the interosseous tendon joins the lateral aspect of the sagittal bands. The deep portion of the interosseous tendon is attached to the base of the proximal phalanx on the side through which the tendon is passing. The lumbrical tendon, however, joins the extensor hood mechanism distal to the point of attachment of the interosseous tendon. From the description just given, it becomes quite obvious that overlying the extensor aspect of the proximal phalanx is the extensor hood mechanism, which is primarily a conjunction of the superficial part of the long extensor of the fingers, the conjoint tendon of the lumbrical, and the superficial part of the interossei tendon. At that particular location overlying the distal third of the proximal phalanx, the common extensor hood splits into two major groups: the central band and the lateral bands. The central band passes over the proximal interphalangeal joint capsule to be attached to the base of the middle phalanx. The lateral parts of the extensor hood mechanism pass on the lateral aspect of the proximal interphalangeal joint and then join together about halfway over the dorsal aspect of the middle phalanx. Together, they make the terminal tendon, which is inserted at the base of the

terminal phalanx. Overlying the proximal extensor aspect of the middle phalangeal area, just before the two lateral extensor bands become the terminal tendon, they are joined together with the triangular loose ligament, which maintains the lateral band's position dorsal to the proximal interphalangeal joints and in touch with the central slip at its insertion in the base of the middle phalanx. In the thumb, the extensor hood mechanism operates on the same principle as the other fingers but with some variation. None of the lumbricals or interossei in the hand contribute to the extensor mechanism of the thumb. There are the two extensor tendons that join the common extensor mechanism. On the radial side are the tendon of the abductor pollicis brevis and the flexor pollicis brevis. On the ulnar side is the tendon of the adductor pollicis.

NERVE SUPPLY

Three nerves are involved in the hand: the median nerve (C-5, C-6, C-7, C-8, and T-1), the radial nerve (C-5, C-6, C-7, C-8, and T-1), and the ulnar nerve (C-8 and T-1). In the forearm, the three nerves are mixed (motor and sensory). With the exception of the radial nerve, which becomes purely sensory in the hand area, the ulnar and median nerves continue to the hand as mixed sensory and motor. Knowledge of the course and the location of the nerve, its branches, and the muscles it supplies is absolutely crucial to properly evaluate and manage a neurologic problem. The accuracy of locating the site of an injury to the nerve becomes clear when considering as an example injury to the ulnar nerve at the elbow versus an injury to the same nerve at the wrist. In the first instance, a clinical picture of loss of sensation to the ring and little fingers, both in the volar and dorsal aspects, along with the ulnar half of the hand, is seen. Besides the sensory loss, paralysis of the flexor carpi ulnaris, the part of the flexor digitorum profundus to the ring and little fingers, and all the interossei, the hypothenar muscles, the two ulnar lumbricals, the adductor pollicis, and the deep head of the flexor pollicis brevis occurs. In the case of injury to the ulnar nerve at the wrist, however, the flexor carpi ulnaris, the flexor digitorum profundus to the ring and little fingers, along with the sensory function to the dorsum of the ring and little fingers and the ulnar side of the dorsum of the hand, will be spared from loss. The clinical presentation, the line of management, and the prognosis of an injury at any of these locations will be totally different.

The same principle does apply to all the nerves of the extremity. The only situation in which an injury to the ulnar nerve at the elbow will not result in intrinsic paralysis is the case of Martin-Gruder anastomosis (Fig. 4–47).

Ulnar Nerve. In the forearm, the ulnar nerve (Fig. 4–48) comes through the cubital canal behind the medial epicondyle of the elbow, enters through the flexor arch, and then gives its only motor branches in the forearm to the flexor carpi ulnaris (note "ulnar nerve distribution") and the part of the muscle belly of the flexor digitorum profundus,

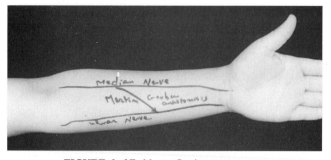

FIGURE 4–47. Martin-Gruder anastomosis.

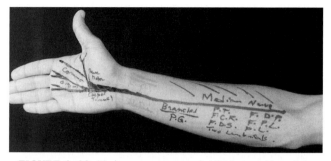

FIGURE 4–49. Median nerve course, distribution, and branches.

which inserts in the ring and little fingers (Lamb, 1970; Phalen, 1951.) The nerve continues distally in the forearm on the radial side of the flexor carpi ulnaris as it is joined by the ulnar artery until about 2 inches proximal to the wrist crease. At this point, the dorsal sensory nerve branches out and turns around to the ulnar side of the distal third of the ulna underneath the flexor carpi ulnaris musculotendinous junction to appear on the dorsal aspect of the lower end of the forearm. It then crosses over the wrist to the dorsum of the hand to supply sensory function to the ulnar dorsum overlying the fourth and fifth metacarpals and continues to the extensor side of the ring and little fingers.

The ulnar nerve continues to the wrist level and enters the hand through the Guyon's canal, distal to which it gives a palmar sensory branch for the hypothenar eminence area. It then divides into two branches: the deep ulnar nerve, which is primarily motor and goes through the hypothenar arch, and the superficial ulnar nerve, which is sensory. The latter remains superficial and then splits into the palmar digital nerves to supply both sides of the little finger and the ulnar side of the ring finger. The deep ulnar branch becomes purely motor and supplies all the small muscles of the hand, with the exception of the abductor pollicis brevis, the opponens pollicis brevis, the superficial head of the flexor pollicis brevis, and the two lumbricals that join the index and middle fingers.

Median Nerve. After the median nerve (Fig. 4–49) enters the forearm, it gives rise to the anterior interosseus (which is purely motor) that passes under the deep head of the pronator teres and continues moving toward the wrist Lamb and Kuczynski, 1981; Phalen, 1951). The median nerve itself continues distally between the two heads of the pronator teres and then under the flexor digitorum super-

ficialis, to which it remains attached until the lower third of the forearm, where it becomes superficial under the skin or under the palmaris longus, if the latter is present. About 2 inches proximal to the wrist, the median nerve gives its palmar cutaneous branch that travels distally under the skin on the ulnar side of the flexor carpi radialis and crosses over the base of the thenar eminence to end in the palmer triangle. It is because of the superficial location of this nerve that any surgical incisions on the radial side of the wrist are to be avoided. Injury to this nerve results in a very painful disabling neuroma. The median nerve continues its journey to enter the carpal tunnel, where it lies superficial to all the flexor tendons and is intimately attached to the undersurface of the flexor retinaculum. As it exits the tunnel, it gives its smallest branch, which is the motor to the thenar muscles that travel a very short distance before getting buried inside the thenar muscle's bulk. The motor branch, "the recurrent branch," is a very important nerve, and loss of its function severely compromises the workings of the hand. Distal to the carpal tunnel, the median nerve divides into an independent digital nerve to the radial side of the thumb and three common digital nerves. Each later divides into individual digital nerves that supply the adjoining sides of the thumb, index, middle, and ring fingers.

In the forearm, the median nerve supplies the flexor carpi radialis, the palmaris longus, the pronator teres, and the flexor digitorum sublimis. Through the anterior interosseous branch, it supplies the ulnar half of the flexor digitorum that inserts in the index and middle fingers, the flexor pollicis longus, and the pronator quadratus. In about 15 percent of the population, a branch from the anterior interosseus connects with the ulnar nerve in the forearm (Martin-Gruber anastomosis). In this case, an injury to the ulnar nerve proximal to the Martin-Gruber anastomosis results in prevention of the paralysis of the ulnar innervated intrinsic muscles (see Fig. 4–45). In the hand, the median nerve supplies the thenar muscles through its motor branch, with the exception of the deep head of the flexor pollicis brevis and the adductor pollicis. The two radial lumbricals are supplied by branches from the common digital nerves. Besides the motor supply, the median nerve is the sensory nerve to the radial half of the palm. It is also the sensory nerve of the palmar aspect of the thumb, index, and middle fingers and to the radial side of the ring finger.

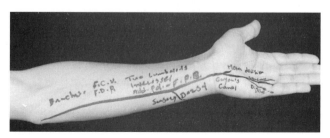

FIGURE 4–48. Ulnar course and distribution, including branches.

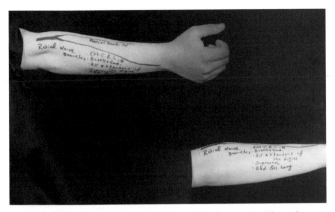

FIGURE 4–50. Radial nerve course, distribution, and branches.

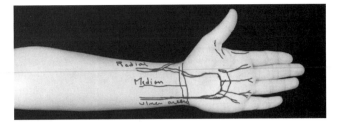

FIGURE 4–51. Diagrammatic representation of the arterial supply to the hand.

Radial Nerve. At the elbow, the radial nerve (Fig. 4–50) gives its first motor branches to the brachioradialis and the two radial extensors of the wrist. It then divides into a superficial and a deep branch. The deep branch, purely motor, is the posterior interosseous nerve. This nerve goes through the supinator tunnel and supplies all the remaining muscles of the extensor aspect of the forearm as it moves distally toward the wrist joint. The superficial branch that is purely sensory moves distally under the brachioradialis to the lower third of the forearm, where it becomes superficial, passing on the radial side of the forearm to the anatomic "snuff box" area. At this point, it divides into multiple branches that move distally to supply the extensor aspect of the radial half of the hand and the extensor aspect of the thumb, index, and middle fingers (Barton, 1973; Lister et al., 1979; Moss et al., 1983).

BLOOD SUPPLY TO THE HAND

The blood supply to the hand (Fig. 4–51 and 4–52) is primarily through the dominant radial artery the less dominant ulnar artery and partly through the anterior and posterior interosseous arteries (*Kaplan's Functional and Surgical Anatomy of the Hand,* 1984). The radial artery is a terminal branch of the brachial artery at the elbow. It travels distally on the radial side of the forearm, where, at the wrist level, it supplies a branch to the superficial palmar arch. Then it continues on, turning around the radial aspect of the distal end of the radius across the anatomic snuff box, deep to the abductor pollicis longus, the extensor pollicis brevis, and the extensor pollicis longus to enter in between the two heads of the first dorsal interossei muscle, through the first intermetacarpal space, to the palm between the two heads of the adductor pollicis. Finally, it ends up by anastomosing with the deep branch of the ulnar artery to form the deep palmar arch. Its branches include the two dorsal arteries to the thumb, the two dorsal arteries to the index, and a branch to the dorsal aspect of the carpus.

The ulnar artery, the second terminal branch of the brachial artery at the elbow, travels distally on the flexor surface of the forearm underneath the flexor carpi ulnaris, where it is joined by the ulnar nerve on its ulnar side, and then at the heel of the hand it enters Guyon's canal. As it comes out of Guyon's canal, it divides into the deep palmar and the superficial palmar branches. The deep palmar branch travels deep into the palm to join the deep palmar branch of the radial artery that makes the deep palmar arch. Its superficial branch makes the superficial arch, and that is what the superficial palmar branch of the radial artery joins.

The two vascular palmar arches (superficial and deep) are located in the palm. The superficial palmar arch is dominantly supplied by the ulnar artery and is located at the level of the midpalmar crease. Its branches are the three common palmar digital arteries that divide into the proper digital arteries for the adjacent sides of the four fingers and branch to the ulnar side of the little finger. The deep palmar arch is dominantly supplied by the radial artery and lies deeply under the flexor tendons. It gives two branches to the thumb and a branch to the radial side of the index finger

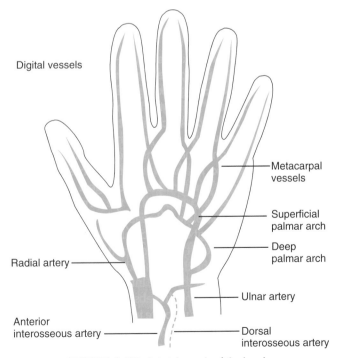

FIGURE 4–52. Arterial vessels of the hand.

BONES, JOINTS, AND LIGAMENTS

Along with the clinical evaluation, radiographs in the three basic standard positions of anteroposterior, lateral, and oblique are essential for the proper evaluation of the skeletal system of the hand. The alignment of the bones, integrity of the joint spaces, presence or absence of deformities, and type of bone structure are only a few of the elements to evaluate in the radiographs.

Based on the clinical condition and the history, special studies in addition to the basic radiographs might become necessary. Polytomography is a special radiographic technique that takes pictures of the part being imaged in slices; it is useful for a detailed evaluation of a bone area. A computed axial tomographic (CAT) scan uses much finer slices and can be more detailed and informative. Magnetic resonance imaging (MRI) is a special radiologic procedure that gives details about masses, tumors, bones, and ligaments. An arthrogram is done by injection of a special type of dye inside joint spaces; it allows the integrity of the joint spaces, the capsule, and the ligaments around it to be evaluated. Video fluoroscopy is a radiologic examination of the area of the hand with a television monitor. This last special test is very helpful in cases of suspected instability or in cases where reproduction of symptoms at filming could be done. A bone scan is a radiologic examination that follows the intravenous injection of a radioactive material. It is very useful in cases of pain with unknown origin, occult or difficult to see fractures, possible tumors, painful hand syndrome, and vascular lesions.

The presence of any signs of swelling, redness, deformity, or instability of an individual joint or multiple joints should be noted. Instability of the joints is checked by applying manual stress to any specific ligament. The stability of any joint is evaluated by holding the bone proximal to a joint and then by moving the bone distal to the joint to be examined in the desired position to evaluate the integrity of the various ligaments. The volar ligaments are to prevent unlimited hyperextension of the particular joint. The collateral ligaments, on the other hand, provide lateral stability to the joint. In the case of the metacarpalphalangeal joint, the joint has to be in 90 degrees flexion to check the stability of the collateral ligaments (Fig.

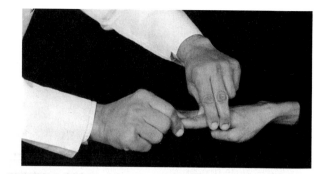

FIGURE 4–70. Checking the stability and the integrity of the collateral ligament on the radial side of the proximal interphalangeal joint of the left index finger. Note the neutral position of the joint to stretch the collateral ligament.

4–69). The interphalangeal joint must be held in a neutral position while the integrity and the stability of the collateral ligaments are checked at that joint (Fig. 4–70). The range of motion of any particular joint should be evaluated both actively and passively. The passive range of motion evaluates the integrity of the joint and all the structures related to it. The active range of motion evaluates not only the integrity of the joint and all the structures related to it but also the integrity of all the elements that allow the joint to work properly. Limitation of the passive range of motion alone is different in its significance from limitation of the active range of motion alone. Limitation of the passive and active range of motion has different significance. Measurements of both should be observed and recorded. The range of motion, active or passive, evaluates not only the bone and the joint structure of the hand but also all the other elements that contribute to the range of motion. The range of motion should be examined, not only from an individual joint aspect but also in conjunction with other joints (Figs. 4–71 to 4–78). It is very important to remember that the different parts of the hand work not only as individual units but also in conjunction with each other; therefore, the overall mode of function of the hand must be addressed.

MUSCULOTENDINOUS SYSTEM

When examining the muscles and tendons, each unit should be examined both individually and in conjunction with other units. It is very important that each muscle and tendon be isolated, evaluated, activated, and given an individual grade. When examining the muscles, look for the general appearance of tone, atrophy, and hypertrophy. A proper systematic muscle evaluation can enable the examiner identify any problems. Each examiner, through time and experience, will adopt a system of his or her own that will enable him or her to systematically evaluate the extremity.

Have the patient open the fingers and make a fist to show all the units together. Normally, in making a fist, the patient's fingertips should touch the distal palmar crease and the terminal phalangeal area of the thumb. The fingers

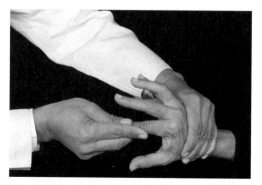

FIGURE 4–69. Checking the integrity of the collateral ligament on the radial-side metacarpophalangeal joint of the left index finger. Note the 90-degree flexion to stretch the collateral ligament.

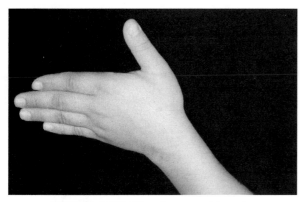

FIGURE 4–71. Ulnar deviation of the wrist.

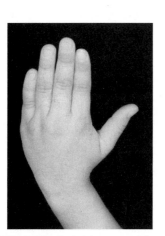

FIGURE 4–72. Radial deviation of the wrist.

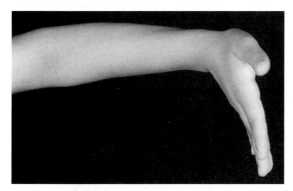

FIGURE 4–73. Extension of the wrist.

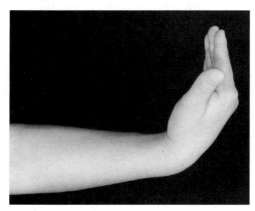

FIGURE 4–74. Volar flexion of the wrist.

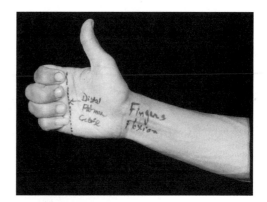

FIGURE 4–75. Full flexion of the interphalangeal joints with full extension of the metacarpophalangeal joints.

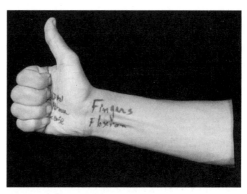

FIGURE 4–76. Full flexion of all the joints of the fingers.

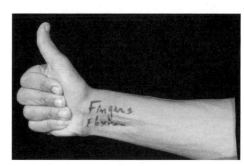

FIGURE 4–77. Full flexion of metacarpal and proximal interphalangeal joints but no flexion of the distal interphalangeal joints.

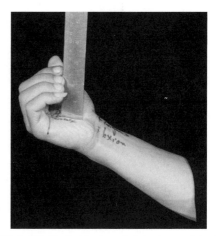

FIGURE 4–78. Limited flexion of all the joints of the fingers.

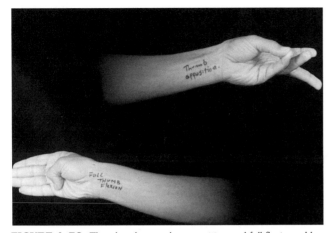

FIGURE 4–79. Thumb pulp-to-pulp opposition and full flexion adduction.

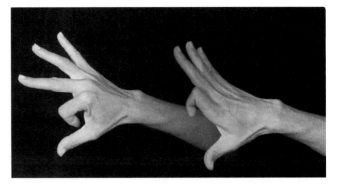

FIGURE 4–81. Relationship of joint flexion of the index finger and the other fingers.

should bend to cover the distal half of the middle phalangeal areas of the index and middle fingers. If, when the patient makes a fist, the patient reaches the tips of only distal to the distal palmar crease, then the problem is usually associated with the metacarpal phalangeal unit joints (see Fig. 4–75). If the fingertips touch proximal to the distal palmar crease, the problem is usually associated with the interphalangeal joint (see Fig. 4–77).

With the thumb fully adducted, full flexion at the metacarpal and interphalangeal joint should place the tip of the thumb at the palm at a point at the base of the little finger crease and the distal palmar crease at the ulnar side of the palm (Fig. 4–79). Any limitation in the patient's ability to bring the tip of the thumb to the desired point will be because of a limitation in thumb adduction or full flexion at the metacarpophalangeal or the interphalangeal joint. The pathologic reason for the limitation can be in the skin, tendons, muscles, bones, ligaments, or joints.

The hitchhiker position (Fig. 4–80) should be with the wrist in neutral between volar and dorsal flexion and forearm pronated or supinated fully, depending on which direction, east or west, north or south, or up or down, that the hitchhiker is going. The wrist will be in about 5 to 10 degrees ulnar deviation, and the thumb will be fully

abducted and extended at the basal and the metacarpophalangeal joints with hyperextension at the interphalangeal joint.

Pulp-to-pulp opposition (see Fig. 4–79) between the thumb and little finger is done with the wrist in about neutral or in dorsiflexion, the forearm pronated or supinated with full abduction at the basal joint of the thumb, full flexion at the metacarpophalangeal joint, and extension up to neutral only of the interphalangeal joint. The little finger on the other hand will have full flexion adduction opposition at the metacarpophalangeal joint and full extension at the interphalangeal joints. It is important to remember that full flexion at the metacarpophalangeal joint of the little finger with no adduction or opposition does not allow pulp-to-pulp opposition to be possible.

Full flexion of the interphalangeal joint of the index finger is possible with full extension of the remaining three fingers, but with full flexion of all the index finger joints, there will have to be flexion at the metacarpophalangeal joints of the remaining fingers (Fig. 4–81).

Independent full extension of the index or the little finger is possible (Fig. 4–82), as they each have an independent extensor, but the same is not possible for the middle and the ring fingers (Fig. 4–83).

All the flexors of the digits can flex their corresponding joints independently, with the exception of the profundus to the middle, ring, and little fingers, which work together in one unit. An obstruction of flexion at the distal interphalangeal joints of any of the three fingers blocks

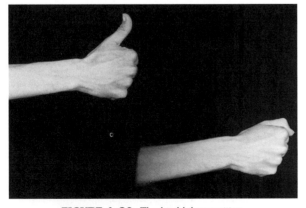

FIGURE 4–80. The hitchhiker position.

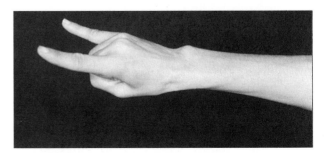

FIGURE 4–82. Independent full extension of index and little fingers.

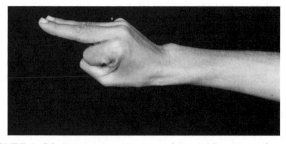

FIGURE 4–83. Independent extension of the middle and ring fingers is not possible, as these two digits do not have independent extensors.

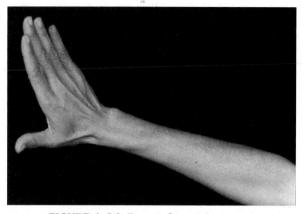

FIGURE 4–86. Extrinsic flexor tightness test.

flexion the profoundus action in the remaining two fingers (Fig. 4–84). This is an important fact that is utilized beneficially in surgical procedures and therapy when needed. In the same fingers, it is impossible to check the sublimis action without blocking the profundus of the remaining two fingers.

LENGTH-TENSION TESTS

Extrinsic Extensor Tightness Test: Composite Wrist Flexion Plus Finger Flexion (Fig. 4–85). Under normal circumstances, the patient should be able to fully close the digits with the wrist in full volar flexion (Brand et al., 1981). This position indicates no extensor tightness; if tightness were present, then the position mentioned would not be possible.

Extrinsic Flexor Tightness Test: Simultaneous Wrist Extension Plus Finger Extension (Fig. 4–86). Under normal circumstances, the patient should be able to fully extend the digits with the wrist fully extended. This posture is not possible if any long flexor tightness is present.

Intrinsic Tightness Test (Fig. 4–87). The examiner places the metacarpophalangeal in extension and flexes the interphalangeal joints. Passive and active flexion of the interphalangeal tests should be free; any limitations indicate a positive intrinsic tightness test.

Tenodesis (Fig. 4–88). This is a normal phenomena caused by the length-tension ratio of the extrinsic tendons (i.e., flex wrist–fingers extend and thumb is fully abducted and extended; extend wrist—fingers flex. Thumb is abducted and slightly flexed at the metacarpophalangeal and interphalangeal joints). For maximum function of the hand, this ratio must be preserved, as it is used in adjusting the length and tension of tendon transfers or tendon grafts in reconstruction procedures.

Extrinsic Finger Tightness Test. It should be possible with the wrist at least in neutral or preferably in full flexion to flex all of the joints of the fingers. This demonstrates gliding full length of the extensor mechanism.

Neurologic Examination

The median, ulnar, and radial nerves innervate the hand and possess a sensory and motor component. Various sensory tests are available and include evaluations of tactile sensation, e.g., Semmes-Weinstein Monofilaments, (Tubiana et al., 1984), deep sensation, temperature, pinwheel test, two-point discrimination, object identifica-

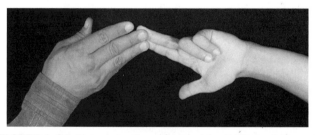

FIGURE 4–84. Note obstruction of flexion at the distal interphalangeal joint of the middle finger, which will interfere with the ability to flex the distal interphalangeal joints of the ring and little fingers.

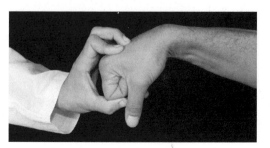

FIGURE 4–85. Extrinsic extensor tightness test.

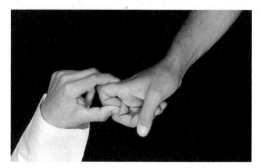

FIGURE 4–87. Intrinsic tightness test.

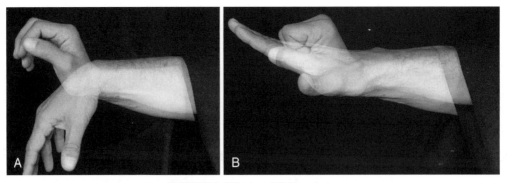

FIGURE 4–88. *A* and *B,* Tenodesis.

tion (stereognosis), texture identification, and Tinel's sign. The principle behind performing the last test is to irritate an already sensitive nerve. Assessment for Tinel's sign is done by gently tapping a sensory nerve with a blunt object that has the same circumference as the nerve. Unpleasant feelings (e.g., paraesthesia, hyperparasthesias) may occur in one of three locations or directions: at the site of tapping, at a direction going distal from the tapped area, or in a direction proximal from the tapped area. If the sensation travels proximally, it is not a positive Tinel's sign. The test is only positive when the unpleasant feelings are at the location of the tapping or in a direction distal to it.

Other useful tests are Phalen's and reverse Phalen's (Phalan, 1951). The principle behind performing these tests is to put the median nerve under maximum pressure by diminishing the size of the tunnel and by kinking or stretching the nerve in either test, which eventually causes irritation of the nerve. For Phalen's test, place the wrist in 90 degree palmar flexion, with the fingers relaxed, the elbow at 90 degrees of flexion, and the shoulder at 90 degrees abduction (Fig. 4–89).

For the reverse Phalen's test (Fig. 4–90), place the wrist in 90 degrees of dorsiflexion with the fingers relaxed, the elbow at 90 degrees of flexion, and the shoulder at 90 degrees abduction. Maintain the above positions for 0 to

60 seconds, and record if patient reports symptoms of tingling in median nerve–innervated sensory territory.

Special Tests

FINKELSTEIN'S TEST

When performing this test, you are assessing for the presence of tenosynovitis of the extensor pollicis longus

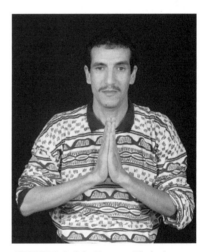

FIGURE 4–90. Reverse Phalen's test.

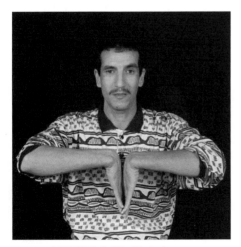

FIGURE 4–89. Phalen's test.

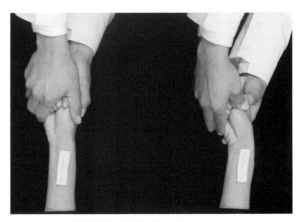

FIGURE 4–91. Finkelstein's test.

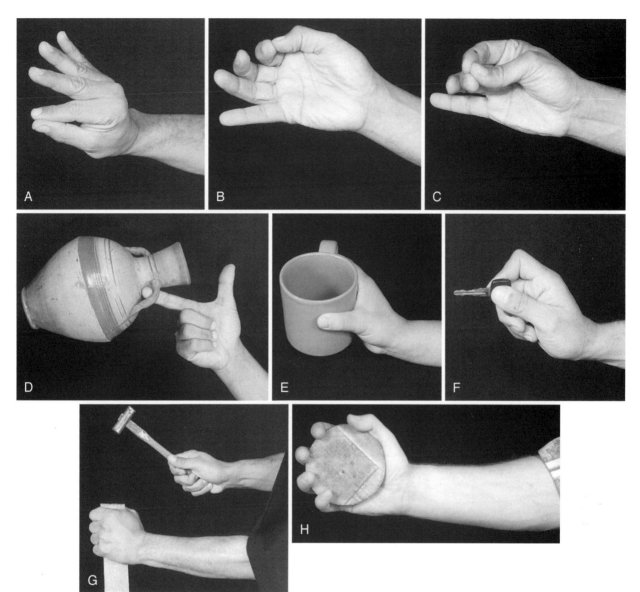

FIGURE 4–92. *A*, Tip-to-side grip. *B*, Tip-to-tip grip. *C*, Three-digit pinch. *D*, Hook grip. *E*, Special grip. *F*, Key grip. *G*, Power grip (hammer grip). *H*, Large object circular grip.

and abductor pollicis brevis tendons located in the first dorsal compartment. The pathology of de Quervain's disease includes swelling (inflammation), thickening (tendon sheath), tightness, and adhesions. Any attempt at distal gliding of the two tendons either passively or actively will be limited and very painful. (Positive Finkelstein's test results usually indicate de Quervain's disease). To perform the Finkelstein's test, place the patient's wrist in radial deviation and midway between pronation and supination with all the digits closed in a fist and the fingers covering the flexed thumb in the palm (Fig. 4–91). Ask the patient to relax. A gentle jerking motion in the direction of ulnar deviation is passively applied. A positive test result occurs when the movement causes pain; however, if the wrist is jerked too much, the patient may feel pain even if he or she does not have de Quervain's disease. The improper administration

of Finkelstein's test can lead to the patient developing de Quervain's.

WARTENBERG'S TEST

In this test, the little finger remains abducted if the patient has a weak palmar interossei and unbalanced action of the long extensor tendon, which indicates ulnar nerve weakness.

FROMENT'S TEST

This is a test of active thumb adduction, using a piece of paper between thumb and first finger (see Fig. 4–38). The patient is asked to hold paper without flexing the interphalangeal joint. An inability to hold without flexing indicates a positive test result and motor ulnar nerve palsy.

EVALUATION OF GRIP (FIG. 4–92)

The two types of grips are the precision grip, which is accomplished with the index, thumb, and middle fingers, and the power grip, which is accomplished with all digits. Examples of a power grip include grasp grip, spheric grip, and hook grip. Examples of precision grip include tip-to-tip grip, tip-to-side (lateral) grip, and three-jaw grip.

Using a dynamometer, power grip is evaluated at all five levels. Normal grip strength and appropriate patient participation produce a bell-shaped curve. Rapid alternating grip pattern at all levels or comfortable grip at level two or three assess "normal gripping" ability of the patient.

CIRCUMFERENCE MEASUREMENTS

Measures are made at specific levels of the forearm and arm for bulk to compare with those of future evaluations. A point is chosen at a fixed distance from an anatomic landmark, such as the elbow crease (Fig. 4–93). The circumference of the forearm is then measured at the chosen point. The measurement in one extremity is compared with the measurement at a similar point in the other extremity and with future measurements.

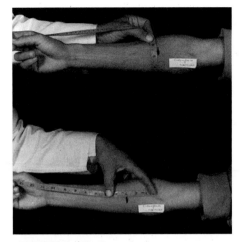

FIGURE 4–93. Circumference measurement.

VOLUMETRIC MEASUREMENTS

Measures for changes in size and for edema can also be taken. The circumference of the extremity at a chosen point is compared with measurements at a similar point in the other extremity. Swelling in one hand is measured by the amount of water spilled out from a marked container when the hand is immersed. The amount of water spilled out from one hand is compared with the amount spilled by immersing the other, uninvolved hand. Many other tests are designed to asses hand function; many of these are discussed in other chapters of this text.

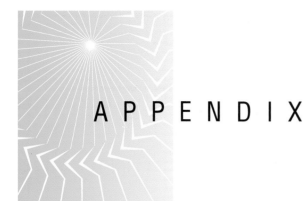

APPENDIX

Ramadan Hand Institute

850 E. Main Street Lake Butler, FL 32054 (904) 496-2323	6241 NW 23rd Street Gainesville, FL 32602 (904) 373-3130	407 N. Hernando Street Lake City, FL 32055 (904) 755-8688

HAND EVALUATION

NAME: _____ DATE: _____

Pt. NO: _____ AGE: _____

ADDRESS: _____

OCCUPATION: _____ HAND DOMINANCE: _____

INVOLVED HAND: _____ ATTENDING PHYSICIAN: _____

Present problem(s) to include functional limitations:

Past problems/injuries to the upper extremity:

Previous surgeries/treatments/medications/therapy:

Observations (posture of hand):

Illustration continued on following page

Soft Tissue Integrity: (Edema, Surface Irregularities, Moisture/Dryness, Wrinkling/Shininess, Tapering, Nodules, Scars—Location and Size) Diagram on last page

Joint Status: (Volar Plate, Collateral Ligaments, Grind Test, Stress Test)

Tendon Integrity: (Length, Glide, Excursion)

RIGHT			LEFT	
+	−	Middle Finger Extension	+	−
+	−	Finkelstein's	+	−
+	−	Adson's	+	−
+	−	Froment's	+	−
+	−	A of F	+	−

RIGHT		TINEL'S	LEFT	
+	−	Radial Nerve	+	−
+	−	Median Nerve	+	−
+	−	Ulnar Nerve	+	−

RIGHT		ALLEN'S	LEFT	
+	−	Radial Artery	+	−
+	−	Ulnar Artery	+	−

RIGHT			LEFT	
+	−	Phalen's	+	−
+	−	Reverse Phalen's	+	−

Strength:

Grip: (Level _____)	R _____ lbs.	L _____ lbs.
Lateral Pinch:	R _____ lbs.	L _____ lbs.
3 Jaw Pinch:	R _____ lbs.	L _____ lbs.
Tip Pinch:	R _____ lbs.	L _____ lbs.

Jamar Dynamometer—5 levels in lbs.

R 1_____   2_____   3_____   4_____   5_____
L 1_____   2_____   3_____   4_____   5_____

Forearm Circumference:

3 cm, 5 cm, 7 cm below volar elbow crease

R _____   3 cm   L _____
R _____   5 cm   L _____
R _____   7 cm   L _____

Comments: _____
_____
_____
_____

Motor Nerve Innervation: (Strength, Atrophy)

		RIGHT	LEFT
RADIAL	Wrist Ext.		
	Thumb Ext.		
	Finger Ext.		

		RIGHT	LEFT
MEDIAN	Wrist Flex.		
	Thumb Flex.		
	Thenars		

		RIGHT	LEFT
ULNAR	Wrist Flex.		
	Finger Flex.		
	Hypothenars		
	Intrinsics		

Illustration continued on following page

Range of Motion:

RIGHT

PASSIVE MOBILITY

	MP	PIP	DIP
I			
M			
R			
L			

ACTIVE MOBILITY

	MP	PIP	DIP
I			
M			
R			
L			

THUMB MOBILITY

MP		OPP	
IP		WB SP	
PMP		P OPP	
PIP		P WB SP	

WRIST MOBILITY

F		RD	
E		UD	
PF		PRD	
PE		PUD	

FOREARM   ELBOW

S		F		F	
P		E		E	
PS		PF		PF	
PP		PE		PE	

SHOULDER MOBILITY

AB		IP	
AD		EP	
PAB		PIR	
PAD		PER	

COMMENTS: _____
_____
_____
_____
_____

Range of Motion:

LEFT

PASSIVE MOBILITY

	MP	PIP	DIP
I			
M			
R			
L			

ACTIVE MOBILITY

	MP	PIP	DIP
I			
M			
R			
L			

THUMB MOBILITY

MP		OPP	
IP		WB SP	
PMP		P OPP	
PIP		P WB SP	

WRIST MOBILITY

F		RD	
E		UD	
PF		PRD	
PE		PUD	

FOREARM   ELBOW

S		F		F	
P		E		E	
PS		PF		PF	
PP		PE		PE	

SHOULDER MOBILITY

AB		IP	
AD		EP	
PAB		PIR	
PAD		PER	

COMMENTS: _____
_____
_____
_____
_____

Sensory Integrity: 2 Point Discrimination

	RIGHT				LEFT	
RADIAL SFC.	ULNAR SFC.			RADIAL SFC.	ULNAR SFC.	

RADIAL SFC.	ULNAR SFC.		RADIAL SFC.	ULNAR SFC.
		Thumb		
		Index		
		Middle		
		Ring		
		Small		

Illustration continued on following page

Other: (VIBRATION AT 30, 256 CPS, VONFREY)

_____
_____
_____

Sensory Testing: Semmes Weinstein

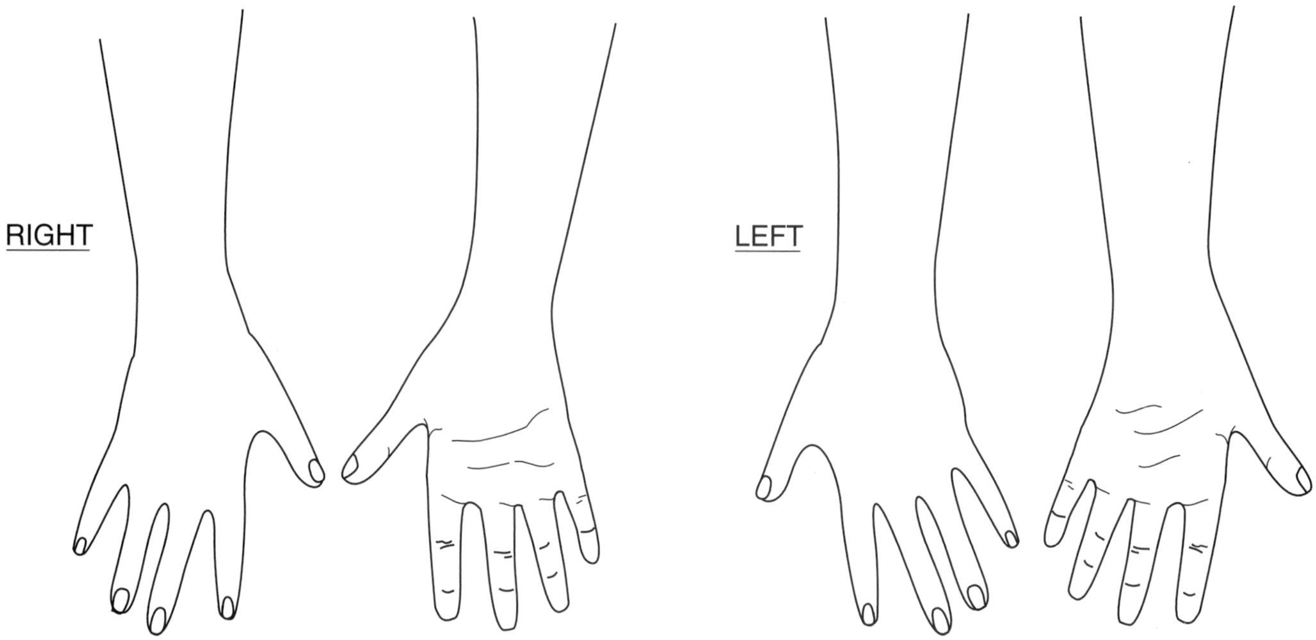

RIGHT   LEFT

   Volume of the Hands: Time of Day Administered: _____

   RIGHT _____ LEFT _____

Summary of Findings/Therapist's Impression _____

_____
_____
_____
_____
_____
_____
_____
_____

Patient's Hand: (Drawing to include scars, nodules, deformities, amputations)

Photo on file: _____ Yes _____ No

Plan: To forward a copy of this hand evaluation to the attending physician for use in determining the medical status of this patient.

_____	_____
Examiner	Date

The goals of this chapter are to 1) review basic physiology of pain, 2) identify the dimensions of pain, and 3) offer a full range of pain assessment scales available to the clinician for easy integration into the clinical setting.

THE PHYSIOLOGY OF PAIN

It is thought that pain is the result of tissue trauma or disease that initiates a complex set of chemical and electric events in the body. When a noxious mechanical, chemical, or thermal stimulus of sufficient intensity occurs, the body transforms this stimulus into electric activity in sensory nerve endings. Myelinated A-Δ and unmyelinated C fibers are first-order neurons that transmit this electrically coded nociceptive information from the periphery to the dorsal horn of the spinal cord (Fields, 1988). A-Δ and C fibers enter the dorsal horn where they synapse with second-order neurons.

The second-order, or relay, neurons ascend through the spinothalamic tract to the reticular formation of the brain stem, periaqueductal gray hypothalamus, and thalamus. In the thalamus, third-order neurons send axons to the somatosensory cortex and the limbic system, where the signal is interpreted as pain (Wallace, 1992).

During the transmission of nociceptive information from the spinal cord to these higher centers, the individual's perception of pain can be modified (Fields, 1988). The gate control theory (Melzack & Wall, 1965) explains the interaction of the peripheral afferents with a pain modulation system in the substantia gelatinosa within the gray matter of the spinal cord.

According to the gate control theory, pain modulation is the result of a balance of large-diameter A-β neurons transmitting nonnociceptive information, including touch, proprioception, and pressure, and small A-Δ and C sensory neurons transmitting nociceptive information.

A-beta, A-delta, and C neurons ascend into the substantia gelatinosa of the spinal cord. There, they synapse with both internuncial neurons in the substantia gelatinosa and second-order neurons called tract cells (T-cells). These T-cells are also termed wide-range dynamic neurons because they receive input from multiple sources, including A-beta, A-delta, and C fibers. The substantia gelatinosa acts as a "gate" or modulator to either inhibit or facilitate the transmission of noxious impulses to the T-cells.

The modulation of pain occurs when excessive large-diameter A-beta fiber activity stimulates the substantia gelatinosa. Excitation of the substantia gelatinosa "closes the gate" to nociceptive information transmitted by A-delta and C neurons to the T-cells and to higher centers. Excessive A-delta and C fiber activity can inhibit the substantia gelatinosa. When this occurs, the "gate opens," and increased nociceptive information is transmitted to the T-cells and higher centers, resulting in a more painful experience (Fig. 5–1). Pain can also be influenced by a

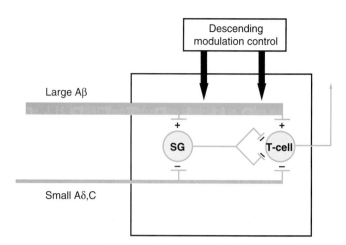

FIGURE 5–1. Diagram of the revised Melzack and Wall gate control theory. Aβ-Large A-β primary, first-order neuron; Aδ, C-small A-Δ, C primary, first-order neuron; SG-substantia gelatinosa; T-cell-second-order neuron.

descending modulation system that includes such structures as the corticospinal tract in the cortex and medulla (Wallace, 1992).

THE DIMENSIONS OF PAIN

Even with identifiable neuroanatomic pathways, it is still unclear why such great variability occurs in how people perceive pain. Clinically, we treat some patients with severe injuries who experience little pain and others with minor trauma who are totally debilitated by pain. These differences may be explained partially by the fact that pain is unique among all the senses. Pain involves two major components: the sensory component and the affective component.

The sensory component of pain has been described as discomfort that can often be identified and located to a particular part of the body and graded with respect to intensity (Fields, 1988). Clinically, we typically define pain intensity by *how much* a patient hurts (Jensen & Karoly, 1992).

The affective component of pain, however, is different. This component involves a complex series of behaviors that an individual may employ to minimize, escape, or terminate a noxious stimulus. It is this affective component of pain that may explain the uniquely different ways individuals perceive pain and the variability of their painful experience. For example, why do some patients require (or demand!) pain medication when their dentist fills a cavity, whereas others need none at all? Why do some women cope with the pain of childbirth by requesting medication whereas others use none?

Clinically, the most important difference between the sensory and affective aspects of pain is the distinction between pain detection and pain tolerance (Fields, 1988). Pain detection threshold relates to the sensory aspect and is highly repeatable in different people as well as in the same person at different times. Pain tolerance, on the other hand, is extremely variable as it is related to the affective component of pain. Due to its multidimensional nature, no two individuals tolerate pain in the same way (Turk & Kerns, 1983). To effectively assess pain in the clinical setting, therefore, the therapist must weigh and consider both the sensory and affective components of the pain experience.

ASSESSING THE SENSORY COMPONENT/PAIN INTENSITY

Three methods commonly used to assess pain intensity are the Verbal Rating Scale (VRS), the Visual Analogue Scale (VAS), and the Numerical Rating Scale (NRS).

Verbal Rating Scale

The VRS is a list of adjectives that describe different levels of pain intensity, ranging from no pain to extreme pain (Table 5–1). VRSs are effective tools for assessing pain because they are both valid and reliable. The VRSs are valid because they measure what they intend to measure—pain intensity. The VRSs are also reliable in that the results of a VRS for pain intensity are consistent and free from error (Downie et al., 1978; Jensen et al., 1986; Jensen et al.,

TABLE 5-1	
VERBAL RATING SCALES FOR PAIN INTENSITY	
5-Point Scale*	**15-Point Scale†**
None	Extremely weak
Mild	Very weak
Moderate	Weak
Severe	Very mild
Very severe	Mild
	Very moderate
	Slightly moderate
	Moderate
	Barely strong
	Slightly intense
	Strong
	Intense
	Very strong
	Very intense
	Extremely intense

* Reprinted from Gracely, R. H., McGrath, P., & Dubner, R. (1978). Ratio scales of sensory and affective verbal pain descriptors. *Pain, 5,* 5–18, with kind permission from Elsevier Science B. V., Amsterdam, The Netherlands.

† Reprinted from Gracely, R. H., McGrath, P., & Dubner, R. (1978). Validity and sensitivity of ratio scales of sensory and affective verbal pain descriptors: Manipulation of affect by diazepam. *Pain, 5,* 19–29, with kind permission from Elsevier Science B. V., Amsterdam, The Netherlands.

1989; Ohnhaus & Adler, 1975). One study evaluated four scales of pain intensity, including the NRS, VRS, and VAS, with 100 patients with a variety of rheumatic diseases. Correlation coefficients were high between pain scores derived from the different pain scales (Downie et al., 1978). In a second study, the effects of analgesics on pathologic pain in a double-blind study were assessed by the VRS and VAS. The comparison of the VRS and the VAS pain rating scales by a linear regression gave a highly significant correlation ($r = 0.81$, $P < 0.001$) (Ohnhaus & Adler, 1975).

The clinician must be aware of several important factors when evaluating VRS scores. First, VRSs are usually scored by assigning a number to each word, according to its rank on the order of pain intensity. For example, on the 5-point scale in Table 5–1, "none" would be given a score of 0; "mild," a score of 1; "moderate," a score of 2; "severe," a score of 3; and "very severe," a score of 4. The number associated with the adjective is then used for the patient's score of pain intensity. This information is ordinal data and must not be interpreted as interval data. That is, the difference between a score of 2 and 3 must not be viewed as the same as the difference between 3 and 4. For example, during an initial evaluation and subsequent treatment of a patient after total knee replacement, the patient is given four VRSs over a specific period of rehabilitation. The scores, using a 5-point VRS as described are "very severe" (4), "severe" (3), "moderate" (2), "mild" (1), and "none" (0). How should these scores be interpreted? The clinician can say objectively that the patient's pain intensity has decreased since the start of treatment. However, these rank scores do not allow for interpretation of the *magnitude* of the differences related by the patient.

Some limitations of VRSs are the inability of many patients to link the proper adjectives to their level of pain intensity and the inability of illiterate (of foreign language–speaking) patients to comprehend the adjectives used (Jensen & Karoly, 1992).

Numerical Rating Scale

An NRS asks patients to rate their perceived level of pain intensity on a numerical scale from 0 to 10 (an 11-point scale) or 0 to 100 (a 101-point scale). The 0 represents "no pain" and the 10 or 100, "pain as bad as it could be." Figure 5–2 outlines the NRS-101 and the 11-Point Box Scale.

With this scale, the clinician can obtain valuable baseline data and then use the scale at every subsequent treatment or on a weekly basis to monitor whether progress is occurring.

Numerical Rating Scales are valid measures of pain intensity and have demonstrated sensitivity to treatments expected to ameliorate pain intensity (Jensen et al., 1986; Jensen et al., 1989; Seymour, 1982). Furthermore, these

101-NUMERIC RATING SCALE

Please indicate on the line below the number between 0 and 100 that best describes your pain. A zero (0) would mean "no pain," and a one hundred (100) would mean "pain as bad as it could be." Please write only one response.

AN 11-POINT BOX SCALE

Zero (0) means "no pain," and a ten (10) means "the worst pain ever." On the 0 to 10 scale below, put an "X" through the number that best pinpoints your level of pain.

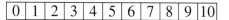

FIGURE 5–2. The 101-point Numerical Rating Scale and an 11-point box scale.

scales are extremely simple to administer and score, lending their application to a greater variety of patients than other scales (Jensen et al., 1986; Littman et al., 1985).

Visual Analogue Scale

The VAS is another measure used to assess pain intensity and typically consists of a 10- to 15-cm line, with each end anchored by one extreme of perceived pain intensity (Fig. 5–3). The VAS has one end of its line labeled "no pain" and the other, "pain as bad as it could be." The patient is asked to mark along the line what best approximates his or her level of perceived pain intensity. The distance measured from "no pain" to where the patient's marks the scale represents the score.

The visual analogue scale (VAS)

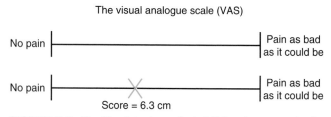

FIGURE 5–3. The Visual Analogue Scale (VAS) and an example of a completed VAS with a score of 6.3.

For example, during an initial evaluation, you choose the VAS as the scale to determine the patient's perceived pain intensity. After hearing a brief description of the scale, the patient makes a pencil slash through the 10-cm line at a measured distance of 6.3 cm. This becomes the patient's baseline score of pain intensity. Subsequently, you can administer and score a new VAS at regular intervals during the rehabilitation to chart the patient's progress.

Visual Analogue Scales provide a high number of response categories. As with the NRS-101 (with 101 responses), a VAS's 10-cm line can be measured in increments of millimeters, from 0 to 100 mm, allowing for 101 possible responses. This potentially makes the VAS (and the NRS-101) more sensitive to pain intensity than other measures with more limited responses such as the VRS 5-point scale. Also, the VAS may be more sensitive to changes in chronic pain rather than in acute pain (Carlsson, 1983; McGuire, 1984).

While the VAS is easy to administer, two potential sources of error exist. First, some patients, particularly older ones, may have difficulty working with graphic rather than verbal scales of their pain (Jensen et al., 1986; Kremer et al., 1981). Patients may find it difficult to rate their pain on the VAS because it is hard to understand. Therefore, proper supervision by the clinician may decrease the chance of error (Jensen et al., 1986). Inaccurate measurement of the patient's VAS is another source of error. If the clinician or researcher does choose the VAS, thoughtful patient explanation and thorough attention to scoring are vital (Jensen & Karoly, 1992).

Descriptor Differential Scale

Another method to assess pain intensity is the Descriptor Differential Scale (DDS) (Gracely & Kwilosz, 1988) (Table 5–2). Twelve descriptor items are presented in this scale. Each descriptor is centered over 21 horizontal dashes. At the extreme left dash is a minus sign, and at the extreme right dash is a plus sign. Patients are asked to rate the magnitude of their pain in terms of each descriptor. If their pain is equal to that of a specific descriptor, they place a check mark directly below the word. If their pain is greater than the descriptor, they place a check to the right, depending on how much more intense they rate their pain. If the pain is less than the specific descriptor, they place their check to the left, and so on. Each descriptor has a rating of intensity on a scale of 0 to 20. Thus, 21 responses are possible for each descriptor.

One advantage of the DDS is that it is a multiple-item measure, as compared with single-item measures. This may provide more reliable and valid assessments of pain than single-item scales (Jensen & Karoly, 1992). Since the DDS is of recent development, however, further research is needed to test its reliability among varying patient populations.

TABLE 5-2

DESCRIPTOR DIFFERENTIAL SCALE OF PAIN INTENSITY

Instructions: Each word represents an amount of sensation. Rate your sensation in relation to each word with a check mark.

Faint
(−) ————————————————— (+)

Moderate
(−) ————————————————— (+)

Barely strong
(−) ————————————————— (+)

Intense
(−) ————————————————— (+)

Weak
(−) ————————————————— (+)

Strong
(−) ————————————————— (+)

Very mild
(−) ————————————————— (+)

Extremely intense
(−) ————————————————— (+)

Very weak
(−) ————————————————— (+)

Slightly intense
(−) ————————————————— (+)

Very intense
(−) ————————————————— (+)

Mild
(−) ————————————————— (+)

Reprinted from Gracely, R. H., & Kwilosz, D. M. (1988). The descriptor differential scale: Applying psychophysical principles to clinical pain assessment. *Pain, 35,* 280, with kind permission from Elsevier Science B. V., Amsterdam, The Netherlands.

ASSESSING THE AFFECTIVE COMPONENT OF PAIN

Clinically, measurement of pain intensity alone is not sufficient to establish a complete picture of the patient's pain experience. It is necessary to measure the affective dimension as well. The following questions can be better understood by assessing the affective component of pain: How unpleasant or upsetting is the patient's pain? To what extent does the patient's pain disrupt his or her behavior? Can the patient cope with pain? Why do such differences exist among patients' abilities to cope with pain?

Verbal Rating Scale

Verbal Rating Scales for assessing pain affect consist of adjectives describing increasing levels of unpleasantness,

such as "distracting," "oppressive," "awful," or "agonizing." Patients are asked to select a word that best describes their affective pain (Table 5–3).

Verbal Rating Scales can be scored by a ranking method. With this method, the word representing the lowest level of pain is given a score of "0," the next a score of "1," and so on until each word has a rank score associated with it (Jensen et al., 1989). The patient's score equals the rank score of the word chosen. For example, in Table 5–3, if the patient selects the work "awful," his or her score would be an "8." As stated earlier, caution should be exercised when interpreting the VRS, as this method assumes equal intervals between each descriptor. This ranking method may not produce scores that are accurate numerical representations of pain.

Verbal Rating Scales for pain affect have two important drawbacks. The first is the question of validity. For a measure of pain affect to be valid, it must be distinct from measures of pain intensity. Recent research with postoperative patients (Jensen et al., 1989) indicates that VRSs designed to measure pain affect were not distinct from measures of pain intensity. It is recommended that further research be conducted into the validity of VRSs among different patient populations. Second, the patient must choose a descriptor even if none of the available descriptors adequately describe his or her affective response. This may result in a false representation of the pain.

Visual Analogue Scale

Visual Analogue Scales for pain affect are similar to those for pain intensity, except that the end points are different. The affective VAS scale (Fig. 5–4) typically uses a 10- to 15-cm line that is anchored at one end by "not bad

TABLE 5-3

VERBAL RATING SCALE OF PAIN AFFECT

15-Point Scale

Bearable
Distracting
Unpleasant
Uncomfortable
Distressing
Oppressive
Miserable
Awful
Frightful
Dreadful
Horrible
Agonizing
Unbearable
Intolerable
Excruciating

Reprinted from Gracely, R. H., McGrath, P., & Dubner, R. (1978). Ratio scales of sensory and affective verbal pain descriptors. *Pain, 5,* 11, with kind permission from Elsevier Science B. V., Amsterdam, The Netherlands.

Visual analogue scale (VAS) of pain affect

FIGURE 5–4. The Visual Analogue Scale (VAS) of pain affect.

at all'' and at the other end by "the most unpleasant feeling possible for me" (Price et al., 1987).

Visual Analogue Scales for pain affect are sensitive to changes in an individual's affective pain perception, making them valid measurements (Price et al., 1987). However, as with VASs for pain intensity, patients using the affective VAS may have difficulty with graphic representations of their pain. Therefore, therapists can easily measure the scale inaccurately if meticulous technique is not used.

Pain Discomfort Scale

A relatively new method of assessing pain affect is via the Pain Discomfort Scale (PDS) (Jensen et al., 1991) (Table 5–4). With the PDS, the patient is asked to indicate the level of agreement (from 0 = "This is very untrue for me" to 4 = "This is very true for me") for each of 10 items on the scale.

The PDS is a valid and reliable measure of pain affect for chronic pain patients. To assess test-retest stability of the PDS, subjects were administered the scale at discharge and at 1 month and at 4 months following discharge. The discharge/1-month follow-up correlation was 0.64 ($P < 0.001$, one-tailed test) and the 1-month/4-month follow-up correlation was 0.76 ($P < 0.001$, one tailed-test). The construct validity of the PDS was examined against two indices: depression, as assessed by Beck Depression Inventory (Beck, 1967), and the McGill Pain Questionnaire (MPQ) Affective Subscale (Melzack, 1975). The correlation coefficients were Beck Depression Inventory, 0.58 ($P < 0.001$, two-tailed test), and Affective Subscale, 0.38 ($P < 0.01$, two-tailed test) (Jensen et al., 1991).

The advantages of this measurement tool are that it can be quickly administered and it provides a broader range of response (10) than the VRS (choice of one descriptor) or the affective subscale of the MPQ (in which respondents choose from five categories). Also, the PDS is unique among affective measures since it is the only measure that directs patients to indicate their feelings of fear, helplessness, annoyance, and distress in response to pain.

The one drawback of the PDS is that the scale was developed and validated for chronic pain patients whose pain averaged 9 years' duration. Several of its items are inappropriate for acute and postoperative pain, such as item 4, "My pain does not stop me from enjoying life," or item 9, "I never let the pain in my body affect my outlook on life."

Descriptor Differential Scale

In addition to the scale for pain intensity, the DDS also has a separate scale for assessing pain affect (Gracely & Kwilosz, 1988). Table 5–5 outlines the DDS for pain affect. The patient has a choice of 12 descriptor items, each having a rating of "unpleasantness." Each descriptor is centered over 21 horizontal dashes. A minus sign is located to the extreme left, and a plus at the extreme right. The patient rates the unpleasantness of each descriptor. If the affective nature of the pain is equal to a specific descriptor, he or she places a check directly below the word. If the pain is less than the specific descriptor, a check is placed to the left, depending on how much less he or she rates the pain. If the pain is greater than the descriptor, a check is placed to the right, and so on. Each descriptor has 21 possible responses.

As previously explained, the DDS has recently been developed, and further research must be conducted on varying patient populations. However, its advantage lies in its potential ability to assess the sensory and affective components of pain.

McGill Pain Questionnaire

The most widely used and most thoroughly researched assessment tool for pain is the MPQ. The MPQ was developed from a two-part study (Melzack & Torgerson,

---

TABLE 5–4

THE PAIN DISCOMFORT SCALE

Instructions: Please indicate by circling the appropriate number whether each of the statements below is more true or false for you. Please answer every question and circle only one number per question. Answer by circling the appropriate number (0 through 4) according to the following scale:

    0 = This is very untrue for me.
    1 = This is somewhat untrue for me.
    2 = This is neither true nor untrue for me (or it does not apply to me).
    3 = This is somewhat true for me.
    4 = This is very true for me.

1. I am scared about the pain I feel.	0 1 2 3 4
2. The pain I experience is unbearable.	0 1 2 3 4
3. The pain I feel is torturing me.	0 1 2 3 4
4. My pain does not stop me from enjoying life.	0 1 2 3 4
5. I have learned to tolerate the pain I feel.	0 1 2 3 4
6. I feel helpless about my pain.	0 1 2 3 4
7. My pain is a minor annoyance to me.	0 1 2 3 4
8. When I feel pain I am hurting, but I am not distressed.	0 1 2 3 4
9. I never let the pain in my body affect my outlook on life.	0 1 2 3 4
10. When I am in pain, I become almost a different person.	0 1 2 3 4

Reprinted from Jensen, M. P., Karoly, P., & Harris, P. (1991). *Journal of Psychosomatic Research, 35* (2/3), 151, with kind permission from Elsevier Science Ltd., The Boulevard, Langford Lane, Kidlington OX5 1GB, UK.

TABLE 5–5

DESCRIPTOR DIFFERENTIAL SCALE OF PAIN AFFECT

Instructions: Each word represents an amount of sensation. Rate your sensation in relation to each word with a check mark.

Slightly unpleasant

(–) ———————————————— (+)

Slightly annoying

(–) ———————————————— (+)

Unpleasant

(–) ———————————————— (+)

Annoying

(–) ———————————————— (+)

Slightly distressing

(–) ———————————————— (+)

Very unpleasant

(–) ———————————————— (+)

Distressing

(–) ———————————————— (+)

Very annoying

(–) ———————————————— (+)

Slightly intolerable

(–) ———————————————— (+)

Very distressing

(–) ———————————————— (+)

Intolerable

(–) ———————————————— (+)

Very intolerable

(–) ———————————————— (+)

Reprinted from Gracely, R. H., & Kwilosz, D. M. (1988). The descriptor differential scale: Applying psychophysical principles to clinical pain assessment. *Pain, 35,* 283, with kind permission from Elsevier Science B. V., Amsterdam, The Netherlands.

1971). The first part categorized 102 words that describe different aspects of the pain experience. These words were classified into three major classes and 16 subclasses. These classes were 1) words that describe the *sensory* qualities of the experience in terms of time, space, pressure, heat, and related properties; 2) words that describe the *affective* qualities in terms of tension, fear, and autonomic properties that are part of the pain experience; and 3) *evaluative* words that describe the subjective overall intensity of the total pain experience. The second part of the study determines the pain intensities implied by words within each subclass.

The MPQ consists of a top sheet to record necessary patient medical information, line drawings of the body for the patient to indicate the pain location (part 1), words that describe temporal properties of pain (part 2), words that describe the pattern of pain (part 3), and a five-point rating scale for pain intensity (part 4) (Fig. 5–5).

The clinician should directly oversee the administration of the MPQ, rather than simply handing the MPQ to the patient along with a pencil. Initially, this test may take 15 to 20 minutes to administer; with experience administering the MPQ, the patient should be able to complete the MPQ in 5 minutes.

The line drawings of the body are anterior and posterior views, onto which the patient indicates the location of his or her pain. The patient marks an "E" for external pain, an "I" for internal pain, or an "EI" for both internal and external pain.

In part 2, the patient chooses one word from each of 20 categories that best describes his or her pain at that moment. If no single word is appropriate from any category, that category is left blank. In part 3, the patient describes the pattern of pain being experienced by choosing words from three, three-word columns with words such as "continuous," "intermittent," and "momentary." What activities the patient has found that relieve or exacerbate the pain are also written down. In part four, the patient rates the pain he or she is experiencing on a scale of 0 to 5, with 0 corresponding to "no pain," 1 to "mild," 2 to "discomforting," 3 to "distressing," 4 to "horrible," and 5 to "excruciating."

Three important scores are tabulated from the MPQ:
1. The descriptors in the first 20 categories are divided into four groups: 1 through 10, sensory; 11 through 15, affective; 16, evaluative; and 17 through 20, miscellaneous. Each descriptor is ranked according to its position in the category. For example, in column one, "flickering" would be given a rank of 1, and "quivering," a rank of 2. The sum of the rank values is assigned the Pain Rating Index (PRI).
2. The number of words chosen is determined.
3. The Present Pain Index (PPI) is tabulated from the patient's response to part 4.

Each MPQ score represents an index of pain quality and intensity at the time of administration. The clinician can administer the questionnaire before and after a series of treatment sessions. The difference can be expressed as a percentage change from the initial value.

For example, you might administer the MPQ to a patient who has just begun rehabilitation following spinal fusion surgery. Initial scores on the PRI and the PPI are 52 and 4 ("horrible"), respectively. You decide to administer the MPQ biweekly for 1 month. The scores of the PRI and PPI after the last MPQ are 21 and 2 ("discomforting"), respectively; this represents an objective change in the patient's pain experience.

The MPQ has been proven to be valid, reliable, and useful (Chapman et al., 1985; Graham et al., 1980; Reading 1989; Reading et al., 1982; Wilke et al., 1990). This assessment tool has also been used in over 100 studies of acute, chronic, and laboratory-induced pain. It has been modified and translated into several languages (Vanderlet et al., 1987; Melzack & Katz, 1992; Stein & Mendl, 1988).

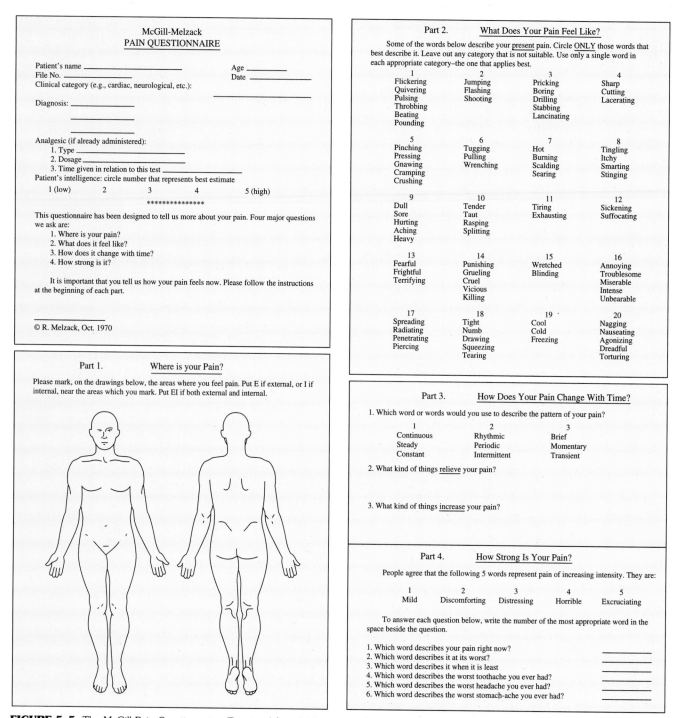

FIGURE 5–5. The McGill Pain Questionnaire. (Reprinted from Melzack, R. [1975]. The McGill Pain Questionnaire: Major properties and scoring methods. *Pain, 1,* 280, 281, with kind permission from Elsevier Science B. V., Amsterdam, The Netherlands.)

Perhaps one of the most interesting features of the MPQ is its potential for differentiating among pain syndromes. One study (Leavitt & Garron, 1980) found different descriptor patterns between two major types of low back pain. The authors found that patients with ''organic'' causes used different patterns of words from patients whose pain was ''functional''—having no physical causes. In a more recent study (Melzack et al., 1986), the MPQ was used to differentiate between trigeminal neuralgia and atypical facial pain. The results showed a correct prediction for 90 percent of the patients.

The MPQ is the most thorough clinical tool for assessing a patient's pain. However, the clinician must consider whether the MPQ is too complex and time consuming for the patient, since it involves answering 70 separate questions each time it is administered (Machin et al., 1988).

PAIN LOCATION, BODY DIAGRAMS, AND MAPPING

In addition to assessing pain intensity and pain affect, the location of the patient's pain is an important third dimension of the pain experience. Asking the patient, "Where is your pain?" may not be sufficient to pinpoint its location. The pain drawing is a reliable and valid instrument for assessing the location of pain (Margolis et al., 1988; Schwartz & DeGood, 1984). The pain drawing may be an appropriate assessment of pain location, particularly in the chronic pain population (Margolis et al., 1986; Ransford et al., 1976).

Figure 5–6 is a representative example. Patients are asked to color or shade areas on the line drawing of a human body that correspond to areas on their bodies that are painful. Additional symptoms such as "numbness" and "pins and needles," as well as more detailed descriptors of pain such as "deep," "superficial," "burning," "aching," and "throbbing," can be denoted by various symbols.

The pain drawing can be used to help establish treatment programs as well as a measure of treatment outcome. However, the clinician must consider how the pain drawing is interpreted. Recently, a scoring method has been

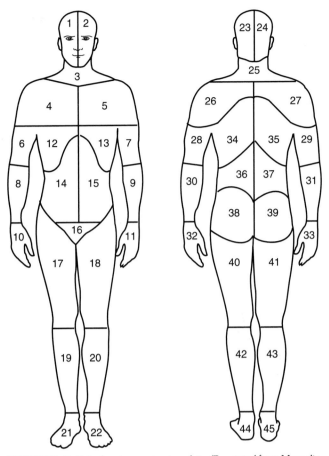

FIGURE 5–7. Pain drawing scoring template. (Reprinted from Margolis, R. B., Tait, R. C., & Krause, S. J. [1986]. A rating system for use with patient pain drawings. *Pain, 24,* 60, with kind permission from Elsevier Science B. V., Amsterdam, The Netherlands.)

developed, based on the presence or absence of pain in each of 45 body areas (Margolis et al., 1986) (Fig. 5–7). For each of the 45 areas, a score of 1 was assigned if a patient's shadings indicated that pain was present and a score of 0 if pain shadings were absent. To score the drawings, weights were assigned to body areas equal to the percentage of body surface they covered. This scoring system is similar to the system used for assessing burn victims (Feller & Jones, 1973).

CONCLUSIONS

This chapter has reviewed the physiology of pain, explored the dimensions of the pain experience, and provided a variety of scales to assess pain intensity, pain affect, and pain location in the clinical setting. Although every patient's pain experience is unique and influenced by numerous factors, a thorough pain evaluation should include an assessment of pain intensity, pain affect, and pain location.

Many of the measures presented are clinically reliable

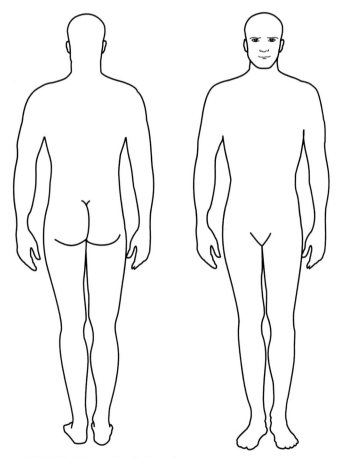

FIGURE 5–6. Example of a body diagram.

and valid, whereas others have not yet been thoroughly tested. Ironically, these scales have been used in research endeavors rather than by physical therapists and occupational therapists in the clinical setting. Without question, more clinical research is needed to further detail the effectiveness of these assessment tools with a variety of patient populations. Even so, these pain assessment scales are simple and effective tools that can and should be used clinically.

GLOSSARY

Affective dimension of pain—The complex series of behaviors a person uses to escape a painful stimulus. Pain tolerance is a principal aspect of the affective dimension.

First-order neurons—Myelinated and unmyelinated nerve fibers that transmit electronically coded information from the periphery to the dorsal horn of the spinal cord.

Internuncial neurons—Cells located in the substantia gelatinosa of the spinal cord that can either facilitate or inhibit the transmission of noxious stimuli.

Second-order neurons—Cells that transmit information from the spinal cord to the higher centers in the brain.

Sensory dimension of pain—Pain that can be identified and located to a specific part of the body and graded by intensity.

Somatosensory cortex—A region in the posterior section of the central sulcus (in the parietal lobe) that is important in the localization of pain.

Verbal rating scale—A list of adjectives to describe either pain intensity or pain effect. The patient is asked to choose a word from the list that best describes the intensity or unpleasantness, respectively, of his or her pain.

Visual analogue scale—A line, usually 10 to 15 centimeters long with each end achored by extremes of either pain intensity or pain effect. A patient is asked to place a mark on the line that best describes his or her pain.

Wide-range-dynamic neurons—Cells located in the spinal cord that respond to a broad spectrum of noxious and nonnoxious stimuli.

REFERENCES

Beck, A. T. (1967). *Depression: Clinical, experimental and theoretical aspects.* New York: Hoeber.

Bonica, J. J., & Benedetti, C. (1980). Post-operative pain. In R. E. Condon & J. J. Decosse (Eds.), *A physiological approach to clinical management.* Philadelphia: Lea & Febiger.

Carlsson, A. M. (1983). Assessment of chronic pain, Part I. Aspects of the reliability and validity of the visual analogue scale. *Pain, 16,* 87–101.

Cole, B., Finch, E., Gowland, C., & Mayo, N. (1992). In B. Cole, E. Finch, C. Gowland, & N. Mayo (Eds.): *Physical rehabilitation outcome measures* (1st ed.). The Canadian Physical Therapy Association.

Chapman, C. R., Casey, K. L., Dubner, R., Foley, K. M., Gracely, R. H., & Reading A. E. (1985). Pain measurement: An overview. *Pain, 22,* 1–31.

Downie, W. W., Leatham, P. A., Rhind, V. M., Wright, V., Branco, J. A., & Anderson, J. A. (1978). Studies with pain rating scales. *Annals of the Rheumatic Diseases, 37,* 378–381.

Fields, H. L. (1988). *Pain* (2nd ed.). New York: McGraw-Hill.

Feller, I., & Jones, C. A. (1973). *Nursing the burned patient.* Ann Arbor, MI: Braun-Bromfield.

Gracely, R. H., & Kwilosz, D. M. (1988). The Descriptor Differential Scale: Applying psychophysical principles to clinical pain assessment. *Pain, 35,* 279–288.

Gracely, R. H., McGrath, P., & Dubner, R. (1978). Validity and sensitivity of ratio scales of sensory and affective verbal pain descriptors: Manipulation of affect by diazepam. *Pain, 5,* 19–29.

Graham, C., Bond, S. S., Gerkousch, M. M., & Cook, M. R. (1980). Use of the McGill Pain Questionnaire in the assessment of pain: Replicability and consistency. *Pain, 8,* 377–387.

Jensen, M. P., & Karoly, P. (1992). Self-report scales and procedures for assessing pain in adults. In D. C. Turk & R. Melzack (Eds.), *Handbook of pain assessment* (pp. 135–151) (1st ed.). New York: Guilford Press.

Jensen M. P., Karoly P., & Braver, S. (1986). The measurement of clinical pain intensity: A comparison of six methods. *Pain, 27,* 117–126.

Jensen, M. P., Karoly, P., & Harris, P. (1991). Assessing the affective component of chronic pain: Development of the pain discomfort scale. *Journal of Psychosomatic Research, 35*(2/3), 149–154.

Jensen, M. P., Karoly, P., O'Riordan, E. F., Bland, F., & Burns, R. S. (1989). The subjective experience of acute pain: An assessment of the utility of 10 indices. *The Clinical Journal of Pain, 5*(2), 153–159.

Knapp, D. A., & Koch, H. (1984). The management of new pain in office ambulatory care. *National ambulatory medical care survey.* Hyattsville, MD: National Center for Health Statistics, 1980 and 1981. Advance data from vital and health statistics, No. 97 (DHHS Publication No. PHS 84-1250).

Koch, H. (1986). The management of new pain in office ambulatory care. *National ambulatory medical care survey.* Hyattsville, MD: National Center for Health Statistics. Advance data from vital and health statistics, No 123 (DHHS Publication No. PHS 86-1250).

Kremer, E., Atkinson, J. H., & Igneli, R. J. (1981). Measurement of pain: Patient preference does not confound measurement. *Pain, 10,* 241–248.

Leavitt, F., & Garron, D. C. (1980). Validity of a back pain classification for detecting psychological disturbances as measured by the MMPI. *Journal of Clinical Psychology, 36,* 186–189.

Littman, G. S., Walker, B. R., & Schneider, B. E. (1985). Reassessment of verbal and visual analog ratings in analgesic studies. *Clinical Pharmacology Therapy, 1*(3), 16–23.

Machin, D., Lewith, G. T., & Wylson, S., (1988). Pain measurement in randomized clinical trials. *The Clinical Journal of Pain, 4,* 161–168.

Margolis, R. B., Chibnall, J. T., & Tait, R. C. (1988). Test-retest reliability of the pain drawing instrument. *Pain, 3,* 49–51.

Margolis, R. B., Tait, R. C., & Krause, S. J. (1986). A rating system for use with patient pain drawings. *Pain, 24,* 57–65.

Melzack, R., & Casey, K. L. (1968). Sensory, motivational and central control determinants of pain: A new conceptual model. In D. Kenshal (Ed.), *The skin senses* (pp. 423–439). Springfield, Il: Charles C. Thomas.

Melzack, R. (1975). The McGill Pain Questionnaire: Major properties and scoring methods. *Pain, 1,* 277–299.

Melzack, R., & Katz, J. (1992). The McGill Pain Questionnaire: Appraisal and status. In D. C. Turk & R. Melzack (Eds.), *Handbook of pain assessment* (pp. 152–168) (1st ed.). New York: Guilford Press.

Melzack, R., Terrance, C., Fromm, G., & Amsel, R. (1986). Trigeminal neuralgia and atypical facial pain: Use of the McGill Pain Questionnaire for discrimination and diagnosis. *Pain, 27,* 297–302.

Melzack, R., & Torgerson, W. S. (1971). On the language of pain. *Anesthesiology, 34,* 50–59.

Melzack, R., & Wall, P. D. (1965). Pain mechanisms: A new theory. *Science, 150,* 971–979.

McGuire, D. B. (1984). The measurement of clinical pain. *Nursing Research, 33*(3), 152–156.

Ohnhaus, E. E., & Adler, R. (1975). Methodological problems in the measurement of pain: A comparison between verbal rating scale and the visual analogue scale. *Pain, 1,* 379–384.

Price, D. D., Harkins, S. W., & Baker C. (1987). Sensory-affective relationships among different types of clinical and experimental pain. *Pain, 28,* 297–307.

Ransford, A. O., Cairns, & Mooney, V. (1976). The pain drawing as an aid to the psychologic evaluation of patients with low-back pain. *Spine, 1,* 127–134.

Reading, A. E., Everitt, B. S., & Sledmere, C. M. (1982). The McGill Pain Questionnaire: A replication of its construction. *British Journal of Clinical Psychology, 21,* 339–349.

Reading, A. E. (1989): Testing pain mechanisms in persons in pain. In P. D. Wall & R. Melzack (Eds.), *The textbook of pain* (2nd ed.) (pp. 269–280). Edinburgh: Churchill Livingstone.

Schwartz, D. P., & DeGood, D. E. (1984). Global appropriateness of pain drawings: Blind ratings predict patterns of psychological distress and litigation status. *Pain, 19,* 383–388.

Seymour, R. A. (1982). The use of pain scales in assessing the efficacy of analgesics in post-operative dental pain. *European Journal of Clinical Pharmacology, 23,* 441–444.

Stein, C., & Mendl, G. (1988). The German counterpart to the McGill Pain Questionnaire, *Pain, 32,* 251–255.

Turk, D. C., & Kerns, R. D. (1983). Conceptual issues in the assessment of clinical pain. *International Journal of Psychiatry in Medicine, 13,* 57–68.

Turk, D. C., & Melzack, R. (1992). The measurement of pain and the assessment of people experiencing pain. In D. C. Turk & R. Melzack (Eds.), *Handbook of pain assessment* (pp. 3–12) (1st ed.). New York: Guilford Press.

Vanderlet K., Andriaensen, H., Carton, H., & Vertommen, H. (1987). The McGill Pain Questionnaire constructed for the Dutch language (MPQ-DV). Preliminary data concerning reliability and validity. *Pain, 30,* 395–408.

Wallace, K. G. (1992). The pathophysiology of pain. *Critical Care Nursing, 15*(2), 1–13.

Wilke, D. J., Savedras, M. C., Hozemer, W. L., Esler, M. D., & Paul, S. M. (1990). Use of the McGill Pain Questionnaire to measure pain: A meta-analysis. *Nursing Research, 39,* 36–41.

CHAPTER 6

Cardiovascular and Pulmonary Function

Elizabeth T. Protas, PT, PhD, FACSM

SUMMARY The measurement of cardiovascular and pulmonary function is crucial to assessing the patient's status, planning an exercise program, and establishing the outcomes of an intervention. The clinician needs to be familiar with a number of standard tests for assessing these functions. In this chapter the discussion is focused on the evaluation of exercise capacity and endurance using standard exercise testing protocols, clinical measures of exercise capacity, and other measures of exertion. Another means for measuring the difficulty of a task is to monitor heart rate responses. The clinician must be able to accurately record the heart rate and interpret the results. Blood pressure is an easily accessible measure of cardiovascular and autonomic responses. Standardizing the methods of measuring blood pressure will greatly increase the reliability of these values. Another aspect of the ability to perform functional activity or to exercise is the ability of the lungs to deliver oxygen to the working muscles and to eliminate carbon dioxide. Observation of breathing patterns may be the simplest way for the clinician to detect the stress of an activity, but there are instruments available for recording pulmonary responses to activities. Finally, monitoring blood oxygenation is important, especially in an individual who has pulmonary disease. Current methods available to the clinician are discussed.

Functional activities require that an individual be able to draw on the cardiovascular and pulmonary systems to respond to a wide variety of demands. The reserves in these systems provide a range from resting to maximal ability. Physical and occupational therapists are interested in the patient's ability to respond to activities of daily living. Endurance from this perspective is often submaximal. Most persons would rarely need to draw on maximal capacities. On the other hand, clinicians frequently encounter individuals whose reserves have been severely restricted through disease, deconditioning, or both. In this instance, a patient may become short of breath when transferring from the bed to a wheelchair. Physical and occupational therapists need to assess a patient's endurance and use these assessments to plan treatment programs.

Improved endurance is one of the most common clinical goals for occupational and physical therapists; however, there are no widely accepted standards for measuring and evaluating endurance in patient populations. This is true despite the fact that there are a number of good measures or tests that can be used. These methods range from very simple to more complex tests requiring considerable instrumentation. In this chapter the focus is on measuring cardiovascular, autonomic, and pulmonary responses to activities; on the clinical applications of these tests; and on test interpretation.

Cardiovascular responses include the ability of the heart to pump an adequate amount of blood, the distribution of the blood through changing blood pressure, and the delivery of the blood through the blood vessels. The pulmonary system responds to exercise by increasing the rate and depth of ventilation to provide adequate gas exchange. By matching ventilation with the blood perfused in the lung, the blood will be adequately oxygenated and carbon dioxide eliminated. Under normal circumstances, the cardiovascular and musculoskeletal systems or both limit exercise capacity and endurance. The pulmonary system's capacity is much greater and is not thought to normally limit exercise capacity.

An additional consideration for the clinician is that cardiovascular disease is the most common chronic disease in American adults (Hahn et al., 1990). Many patients referred for physical or occupational therapy have overt or latent cardiovascular disease. A number of therapists are also involved in cardiac and pulmonary rehabilitation programs. These programs require that the therapist recognize the normal as well as the abnormal responses of the systems.

Both cardiovascular and pulmonary measures are discussed in this chapter. Measures of heart rate, blood pressure, and exercise capacity are presented, in addition to measures of ventilation and oxygen saturation.

HEART RATE

The heart rate is probably the easiest means for the clinician to monitor cardiovascular responses to activity. The validity of the heart rate as a cardiovascular measure is based on the linear relationship between heart rate, the intensity of aerobic exercise, and the oxygen consumption (Montoye et al., 1996). (Fig. 6–1). Resting heart rate is 70 to 75 beats per minute and increases incrementally with gradually increasing aerobic activity until maximal exercise capacity is reached. Variability in heart rate responses between persons is created by age, level of fitness, and presence or absence of disease. A 65-year-old individual who is not fit will have higher submaximal heart rates and lower maximal heart rates than a fit 65-year-old.

Determining the heart rate by palpating either the radial or the carotid pulse is the most common means used in rehabilitation settings. Heart rates are palpated either for a fixed period of time (i.e., 10, 15, or 60 seconds) and extrapolated to establish the beats per minute or a given number of beats are counted (i.e., 30 beats). The latter method is much easier to use during exercise activities. The

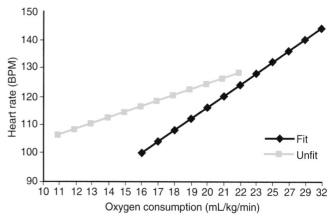

FIGURE 6–1. Heart rate compared with increasing oxygen consumption during exercise for fit and unfit individuals.

heart rate is determined using a conversion table (Sinacore & Ehsani, 1985) (Table 6–1). Standardizing the procedures as much as possible should increase the accuracy of heart rate assessments. Procedural considerations include noting the position of the measure (e.g., either supine or sitting for resting heart rates), using a similar time period, avoiding using the thumb, and using the same artery. Excessive pressure on the carotid artery can cause a reflex slowing of the heart rate (White, 1977). Palpated radial and carotid heart rates are not significantly different from heart rates recorded with an electrocardiogram (ECG) during exercise in healthy subjects (Sedlock et al., 1983).

TABLE 6–1

HEART RATE CONVERSION DETERMINED BY TIMING 30 CARDIAC CYCLES

Time*	Rate†
22.0	82
21.0	86
20.0	90
19.0	95
18.0	100
17.5	103
17.0	106
16.5	109
16.0	113
15.5	116
15.0	120
14.5	124
14.0	129
13.5	133
13.0	138
12.5	144
12.0	150
11.5	157
11.0	164
10.5	171
10.0	180
9.5	189
9.0	200

*Time for 30 beats.
†Heart rate per minute.

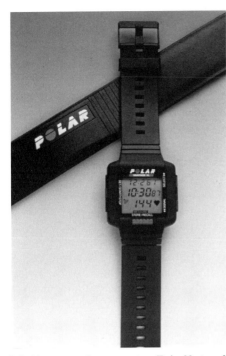

FIGURE 6–2. Heart rate telemetry system (Polar Vantage XL) showing heart rate wrist monitor and chest belt transmitter. (Courtesy of Polar CIC, Inc., Port Washington, NY.)

Many clinical situations do not allow the therapist to palpate the pulse rate during an activity. For example, when doing gait training with a patient who requires contact guarding, the pulse rate may need to be taken immediately after the exercise stops. Generally, the pulse should be palpated within 15 seconds of exercise cessation because the pulse begins to decrease rapidly after the activity is stopped (Pollock et al., 1972). The number of beats should be counted for 10 seconds and extrapolated to the minute value. Although postexercise heart rates are significantly lower, the difference is only about 4 percent lower than the heart rate recorded during exercise (Cotton & Dill, 1935: McCardle et al., 1969; Sedlock et al., 1983). Accuracy is improved if the pulse is located rapidly and the measure taken as quickly as possible. My colleagues and I have found intertherapist reliability of palpated carotid pulses in elderly postoperative patients performing assisted ambulation to be poor (Protas et al., 1988).

Portable heart rate telemetry systems can also be used to record exercise heart rates. These devices are composed of a chest band with a sensor and a telemetry receiver that can be worn on the patient's wrist or on the therapist (Fig. 6–2). The heart rate can be displayed on the receiver and stored so that heart rate trends over time can be recorded. The rate is derived by averaging four beats over a period of time. The higher the heart rate, the shorter the measurement time. Many devices can also be programmed to record the rate at different intervals (e.g., every 15 seconds for 4 hours). Some devices have computer interfaces so that a record of heart rates over several hours or days can be determined. Some of these devices corre-

spond well with simultaneous ECG recordings whereas others are less accurate (Leger & Thivierge, 1988; Treiber et al., 1989). Gretebeck and colleagues (1991) reported that a portable heart rate monitor they tested missed few beats but that its operation was influenced by proximity to a computer or microwave oven, traffic signals, and car driving, among other things. The chest sensor must be snugly attached to the subject and located on a rib or bony prominence to decrease the possibility of muscle interference. These devices have been found to be reliable during assisted ambulation with elderly nursing home residents (Engelhard et al., 1993); however, there is little information on the use of these devices in clinical settings with various patient populations. Clinicians should monitor the accuracy of these devices for their own application and setting.

A more detailed record of heart rate, rhythm, and the analysis of the ECG can be obtained by using standard ECG monitoring. This is more frequently used in intensive care, cardiac, or pulmonary rehabilitation. Lead placement is either a bipolar, single-lead system or 10 leads, which provides a standard 12-lead ECG (Gamble et al., 1984) (Fig. 6–3). A bipolar system is less sensitive in detecting ischemic ECG changes during exercise than a 12-lead system. (Froelicher, 1983; Hanson, 1988); however, a bipolar lead is recommended for exercise testing in pulmonary patients unless ischemic heart disease is suspected (American Association of Cardiovascular and Pulmonary Rehabilitation, 1993). Rate determination from the recording is possible because of the standard paper speed of the ECG. An ECG heart rate ruler or other methods using the interval between two R waves provides the rate (Schaman, 1988) (Fig. 6–4). ECG rate determination is accurate as long as interference from motion artifact is minimized during exercise by proper skin preparation and the use of adequate, gelled electrodes with secure placement.

ECG rhythm is the determination of the interval between

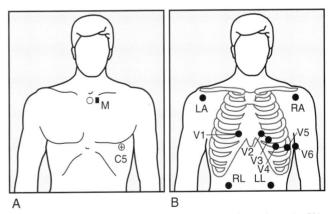

FIGURE 6–3. *A,* Bipolar lead CM5 has a positive electrode on the fifth rib interspace (C5) and the other on the manubrium (M). *B,* The 10-lead placements for a standard 12-lead electrocardiogram. (*A* from Froelicher, V. F., et al. [1976]. A comparison of two-bipolar electrocardiographic leads to lead V5. *Chest, 70,* 611–616. *B* from Gamble, P., McManus, H., Jensen, D., Froelicher, V. [1984]. A comparison of the standard 12-lead electrocardiogram to exercise electrode placements. *Chest, 85,* 616–622.)

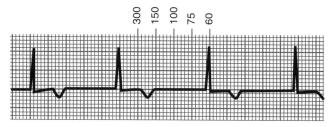

FIGURE 6–4. Heart rate determination from an electrocardiogram can be performed by using a rate scale for each heavy line on the tracing.

each R wave. Normally, the rhythm should be regular with equal intervals between each R wave. Irregular intervals between R waves are referred to as arrhythmias. Variations in rhythm can occur sporadically or at a fairly predictable interval, for example, every third or fourth beat. Although some arrhythmias can be detected while palpating a pulse as an uneven pulse rate, identification of the arrhythmia can only be done with an ECG.

The value of ECG monitoring during activity or exercise is one of safety. If a therapist is working with a patient whose condition is unstable, who is at high risk for arrhythmias or coronary artery disease, or who has a recent history of cardiovascular disease, detecting abnormal responses may indicate the need for a different exercise intensity or pace to lessen the cardiovascular stress. Evidence from supervised cardiac rehabilitation programs indicates that the rate of myocardial infarction is 1 per 300,000 patient-hours, with a mortality rate between 1 in 790,000 patient-hours of exercise (Van Camp & Peterson, 1986) and 1 in 60,000 participant hours (Haskell, 1994). There are no published accounts of myocardial infarctions or sudden death during physical or occupational therapy exercise. This may suggest that medically supervised exercise programs are relatively safe with or without ECG monitoring even though the risk of a serious event cannot be eliminated. Clinicians should be aware of a number of risk classification systems available for detecting individuals at risk for a cardiac event during exercise (American College of Sports Medicine, 1995).

BLOOD PRESSURE

Resting and exercise measurements of blood pressure, just as heart rate, are easily monitored by most clinicians. The procedure is a bit more complicated but, if precise, is accurate. Resting blood pressure values are used to determine hypertension. Table 6–2 provides a classification system for blood pressure.

The methods for taking resting blood pressure are straightforward (Altug et al., 1993; American College of Sports Medicine, 1995; American Heart Association, 1987). The patient should be seated for at least 5 minutes. The arm should be bare, slightly flexed with the forearm supinated, and supported by a table or the clinician's hand.

The arm should be positioned at the level of the heart and the cuff wrapped firmly around the arm about 2.5 cm above the antecubital fossa with the arrows on the cuff aligned with the brachial artery. Three cuff sizes are available—child (13 to 20 cm), adult (17 to 26 cm), and large adult (32 to 42 cm)—and should be used for different body sizes. The stethoscope should be placed about 1 cm below the antecubital fossa over the brachial artery. Palpating the artery before placing the stethoscope will enhance accuracy. The cuff should be inflated quickly to about 200 mm Hg, or 20 mm Hg above the expected blood pressure. The air in the cuff should be released slowly at 2 to 3 mm Hg per heartbeat. Systolic pressure is the pressure when the first Korotkoff's sound is heard. The Korotkoff's sounds are created by turbulence when the cuff pressure goes below the pressure in the brachial artery. Diastolic pressure can be read at two points as the pressure in the cuff is released. The first is the pressure when the sounds become muffled, called the fourth phase diastolic blood pressure, or when the sound disappears completely, known as the fifth phase diastolic blood pressure. I prefer the fourth phase measure for accuracy. Because there may be differences between the pressure readings for the right and left arms, the pressure should consistently be taken from either right or left. At least two readings should be averaged, especially if the reading differs by more than 5 mm Hg (National Heart Lung and Blood Institute, 1988).

Exercise blood pressures require additional considerations. First, since the patient is probably moving with the exercise, the arm on which the blood pressure is being taken should be as relaxed as possible. A standing mercury sphygmomanometer is preferred during exercise to reduce motion artifact. An aneroid manometer (the most common available clinically) must be regularly calibrated according to the manufacturer's instructions and is more difficult to read

TABLE 6–2

CLASSIFICATION OF BLOOD PRESSURE FOR ADULTS*

Systolic (mm Hg)	Diastolic (mm Hg)	Category
<130	<85	Normal
130–139	85–90	High normal
140–159	90–99	Mild (stage 1) hypertension
160–179	100–109	Moderate (stage 2) hypertension
180–209	110–119	Severe (stage 3) hypertension
≥210	≥120	Very severe (stage 4) hypertension

*Not taking antihypertensive medication and not acutely ill. When systolic and diastolic pressures fall into different categories, the higher category should be selected.

Reprinted with permission from National Heart, Lung, and Blood Institute. (1993). The fifth report of the Joint Committee on Detection, Evaluation, and Treatment of High Blood Pressure. *Archives of Internal Medicine, 153,* 154–183.

Reprinted with permission from American College of Sports Medicine. (1995). *ACSM's Guidelines for Exercise Testing and Prescription* (5th ed.) Baltimore: Williams & Wilkins.

TABLE 6-3
POTENTIAL SOURCES OF ERROR IN BLOOD PRESSURE ASSESSMENT
Inaccurate sphygmomanometer Improper cuff size Auditory acuity of clinician Rate of inflation or deflation of cuff pressure Experience of clinician Reaction time of clinician Improper stethoscope placement or pressure Background noise Arm not relaxed Certain physiologic abnormalities (e.g., damaged brachial artery)

with motion. A mercury manometer should be at approximately eye level of the clinician. The systolic pressure should increase with increasing intensity of exercise activity. Abnormal responses include a systolic pressure that does not increase with increasing exercise or a systolic pressure that falls with increasing exercise. Blood pressure should be taken again immediately if the systolic pressure seems to be decreasing with increasing exercise (Dubach et al., 1989). Table 6–3 summarizes potential sources of error in blood pressure measurement. The time of day in which the measurements are made does not impact exercise blood pressure responses in some clinical populations. For example, there appear to be no significant differences between morning and afternoon blood pressure during walking in frail elderly persons (Engelhard et al., 1993).

EXERCISE TESTS

Many standardized exercise or stress testing protocols have been developed (Balke & Ware, 1959; Bruce et al., 1973; Naughton et al., 1964; Taylor et al., 1955). The most common applications of exercise tests in physical and occupational therapy are (1) exercise prescription, (2) assessment of exercise endurance, (3) treatment evaluation, and (4) to ensure patient safety. These applications are considerably different from the more usual application of exercise tests in relation to the detection, diagnosis, and prognosis of coronary artery disease (Bruce et al., 1973). Reviews of the most common protocols are available elsewhere (Altug et al., 1993; American College of Sports Medicine, 1995). The test selected may depend on the purpose of the test, the test environment, the availability of special equipment, and the characteristics of the patient. For example, different tests may be needed for home care than in a hospital setting.

The most common method of distinguishing exercise tests is by the endpoint of the test. Tests can be classified as maximal versus submaximal. A number of criteria are used to determine if a test is considered maximal. The most widely accepted are volitional fatigue, a respiratory exchange ratio (RER = volume of carbon dioxide exhaled/volume of oxygen consumed) over 1.15, reaching age-predicted maximal heart rate, and a plateau in the oxygen consumption (an increase of less than 150 ml/min with increasing exercise) (Froelicher, 1994). These criteria are often difficult to obtain with elderly persons and individuals with various disabilities (Shephard, 1987). Repeated measures derived from maximal exercise tests tend to be reliable regardless of the population being tested. Coefficients of variation for maximal oxygen consumption have been reported of between 2.2 and 6 percent (Shephard, 1987; Wright & Sidney, 1978). Submaximal tests can be ended when a predetermined heart rate or workload is reached, signs of myocardial ischemia occur, or symptoms cause the test to be terminated (Altug, 1993; American College of Sports Medicine, 1995; Astrand & Rhyming, 1954; Sinacore & Ehsani, 1985). Submaximal tests are used (1) to determine the relationship between heart rate response and oxygen consumption during exercise to predict maximal oxygen consumption, (2) to screen for safety during an activity, and (3) to estimate cardiovascular endurance during functional activities. Submaximal tests are of more value to most physical and occupational therapists because these tests can determine the patient's current status, be used to establish a treatment plan, and assess the outcomes of the treatment. The clinician should be aware that submaximal tests when used to predict maximal capacity introduce considerable inaccuracy into the estimate. Maximal oxygen consumption can be underestimated by between 5 to 25 percent for any one individual (Ward et al., 1995). If you look at Figure 6–1, you can see that an extrapolation from several of the measures of submaximal heart rate and oxygen consumption for a fit versus an unfit individual can result in significantly different predictions of the maximal values. Also in some populations, such as the elderly and individuals with chronic disabilities, a linear relation between heart rate and oxygen consumption may not exist. Prediction of maximal values based on submaximal responses assumes a linear relationship between heart rate and oxygen consumption (Skinner, 1993).

Exercise tests can also be distinguished by the mode and protocol of the test. The mode refers to the method or type of equipment used. Treadmills, cycle ergometers, arm-crank ergometers, and wheelchair ergometers are the most common equipment used for exercise tests. There are advantages and disadvantages for all of these devices. Individuals can achieve the highest maximal oxygen consumption when tested on treadmills; therefore, the highest estimates of exercise capacity are determined with treadmills (McKiran & Froelicher, 1993). Treadmills have the additional advantages of having normative values based on thousands of tests, requiring the familiar activity of walking or running, having many potential workloads, and being the least limited of the testing devices by local muscle fatigue. Cycle ergometers are useful for testing individuals who have gait or balance disturbances such as in Parkinson's disease or cerebral palsy, whereas arm-crank or wheelchair ergometers are used in testing individuals who have limited use of the lower extremities, such as patients with spinal cord injuries (Pitetti et al., 1987). Maximal oxygen consumption and maximal heart rate are 20 to 30 percent lower during arm-cranking than treadmill or cycle ergometry (Pollock & Wilmore, 1990; Protas et al., 1996). As a result, there is a poor correlation between maximal values achieved during upper extremity and lower extremity testing (McCardle et al., 1991). This makes it difficult to predict responses to upper extremity exercise from lower extremity tests (Protas et al., 1996). Exercise programs for enhancing cardiovascular endurance of the upper extremities should be based on upper extremity exercise tests. Arm-crank activities, however, are less familiar to most persons and are more difficult to perform.

The test-retest reliability of exercise tests is quite high. This is true for treadmills, bicycle ergometers, and arm-crank ergometers (Bobbert, 1960; Ellestad et al., 1979; Fabian et al., 1975; Pollock et al., 1976; Protas et al., 1996). Several factors influence the outcomes of exercise tests. In elderly persons, higher maximal oxygen consumptions are reached with a repeated test; therefore, an elderly person may require more than one exercise test session to become familiar with the test (Thomas et al., 1987). The work increments used in the test changes the maximal oxygen consumption reached. If the increment is too large or too small, a lower maximal oxygen consumption occurs (Buchfuhrer et al., 1983). For example, the increment between stage 3 (3.4 mph, 14 percent grade treadmill elevation) and stage 4 (4.2 mph, 16 percent grade) of a Bruce protocol is the difference between fast walking up a slight hill and running up a moderate hill. This may be an accurate increment for a healthy young person but too challenging for a frail elderly person. On the other hand, if the increment is too small, it makes the test excessively long (Lipkin et al., 1986). It is recommended that exercise test increments be individualized so that the test length is 8 to 12 minutes (Froelicher, 1994).

CLINICAL TESTS AND OTHER MEASURES OF EXERCISE INTENSITY

An increase in the physical and occupational therapy care administered in the home or in sites such as nursing homes and community health centers has enhanced the need for measures of exercise tolerance that do not require much equipment. Several tests that are based on walking or running for a specific time or distance have been developed (Balke, 1963; Cooper, 1968; Guyatt et al., 1985; Kline et al., 1987). The timed tests measure the distance covered when walking or running as fast as possible for 15, 12, 9, 6, or 5 minutes. Higher distances and faster walking are associated with a greater estimate of exercise capacity.

Distances covered in the 6-minute walk test can differentiate between healthy elderly persons and individuals with New York Heart Association Class II and III heart disease. My colleagues and I have found the 5-minute distance to be moderately correlated with peak oxygen consumption in elderly women (Stanley & Protas, 1991) and that timed walking distances are reliable in elderly postoperative patients (Protas et al., 1988). Nursing home patients walked significantly farther in the late afternoon than in the morning with a walk test (Englehard et al., 1993). These observations suggest that distance walked during short walking tests in several patient populations are valid and reliable if readministered during the same time of day. Table 6–4 presents some of the distances and the potential clinical meaning of these values.

A more useful approach to a walk test for clinicians may be looking at what a clinically significant improvement might be after an exercise intervention. Price and associates (1988) reported an increase from 1598 feet to 1774 feet (176 feet) during a 5-minute walk after a 3-month exercise program consisting of flexibility and strengthening exercises and walking to improve endurance in 5 patients with either osteoarthritis or rheumatoid arthritis. A similar absolute increase in walking distance of 161 feet was reported for 47 individuals with osteoarthritis after an 8-week exercise intervention compared with a control group not participating in the exercise program (Peterson et al., 1993). A change in 5-minute walk distance after elective total hip replacement was reported from 631 to 894 feet at 3 months after surgery and 1115 feet with 2 years of recovery (Laupacis et al., 1993). Test-retest reliability of a 5-minute walk test with elderly persons yields a standard error of the measurement of 135 feet, suggesting that a clinical improvement should be at least 135 feet to be meaningful and greater than the variability of the test.

A continuous, progressive chair step test has been developed for exercise-testing frail elderly individuals (Smith & Gilligan, 1983). Subjects sit comfortably in a chair and kick up to a target that is 6, 12, or 18 inches high. The kicking rate should be controlled at 1/second, alternating right and left legs so that there are 30 kicks/second. Each target is used for a 3-minute period. For the fourth and final stage, the subject continues to kick to the 18-inch target while simultaneously raising the ipsilateral upper extremity. Heart rate is observed for each stage of exercise. The test

TABLE 6–4

PERFORMANCE ON A 5-MINUTE WALK TEST FOR MIDDLE-AGED OR OLDER SUBJECTS

Classification	Distance (feet)
Average or above	>1500
Fair (moderate impairment)	1000–1300
Poor (severe impairment)	<1000

TABLE 6–5

RATINGS OF PERCEIVED EXERTION

Original Scale		Revised Scale	
6		0	Nothing at all
7	Very, very light	0.5	Very, very weak
8		1	Very weak
9	Very light	2	Weak
10		3	Moderate
11	Fairly light	4	Somewhat strong
12		5	Strong
13	Somewhat hard	6	
14		7	Very strong
15	Hard	8	
16		9	
17	Very hard	10	Very, very strong
18		•	Maximal
19	Very, very hard		
20			

From Noble, B. J., Borg, G. A. V., Jacobs, I., Ceci, R., & Kaiser, P. (1983). A category ratio perceived exertion scale: Relationship to blood and muscle lactates and heart rate. *Medicine and Science of Sports Exercise, 15,* 523–528.

lasts between 6 and 12 minutes. The endpoints are volitional fatigue (particularly hip muscle fatigue), inability to maintain the pace, knee pain, or 70 percent of age-predicted heart rate is reached. I have found that many frail nursing home residents can perform this test safely.

Ratings of perceived exertion have been devised for use in reflecting individual exercise intensity (Borg, 1982; Noble et al., 1983). Table 6–5 shows the rating scales used, either a 6 to 20 or a 0 to 10 point scale. An explanation of the scales must be given before the exercise. The patient is told that a 6 on the 6 to 20 scale is comparable to walking at a comfortable pace without noticeable strain, whereas a 20 is the most difficult exercise the patient has experienced comparable to exercise that cannot be continued without stopping. The ratings can be differentially used to indicate central exertion from the heart and lungs, local muscle fatigue, or a combination of both. The scale values are strongly correlated with exercise intensity, oxygen consumption, heart rate, and, for the 0 to 10 scale, blood lactate levels and ventilation. An intensity necessary for a cardiorespiratory training effect and a threshold for blood lactate accumulation can be achieved at a rating of "somewhat hard" or "hard" or between 13 and 16 on the 6 to 20 scale or 4 or 5 on the 0 to 10 scale (American College of Sports Medicine, 1995). This may be an easier method to use than to teach a patient to take his or her pulse as a means of monitoring exercise intensity. Much of the application of ratings of perceived exertion have been with healthy normal subjects and individuals with cardiovascular disease.

One method of nonexercise estimation of maximal oxygen consumption has been suggested (Jackson et al., 1990). The estimate is based on regression equations that use age, physical activity status, and percent body fat or body mass index to derive maximal oxygen consumption.

The equations were developed on individuals representing a wide age range (20 to 59) and fitness levels. Physical activity status (PA-R) is grossly classified according to the subject's usual activity pattern. The percent body fat model is slightly more accurate (r = .81, SEE = 5.35 ml/Kg/min) than the model based on body mass index (r = .78, SEE = 5.70 ml/kg/min). The equations are as follows:

Percent Body Fat Model:

$$Vo_2peak = 50.513 + 1.589 (PA\text{-}R) - 0.289 (age) - 0.552 (\% \ fat) + 5.863 (F = 0, M = 1)$$

Body Mass Index (BMI):

$$Vo_2peak = 56.363 + 1.921 (PA\text{-}R) - 0.381 (age) - 0.754 (BMI) + 10.987 (F = 0, M = 1)$$

These equations have not been validated with populations with chronic disabilities seen by physical and occupational therapists, nor with an aging population, but the simplicity may make this an option for estimates of exercise capacity by the therapist. The clinician should keep in mind that considerable error may occur with these estimates.

RESPIRATORY RATE

Observing respiratory rate can be easily done by most clinicians. The resting rate in adults is generally 12 to 16 breaths per minute. A full breath occurs from the beginning of inspiration to the end of expiration. The accuracy of the observation of resting ventilation is enhanced if the patient is unaware that the therapist is noting breathing frequency (Wetzel et al., 1985). Breathing frequency increases up to 36 to 46 breaths per minute during maximal exercise (Astrand 1960; Wasserman & Whipp, 1975). Lower maximal breathing rates occur in older individuals (Astrand, 1960). Exercise breathing frequencies that exceed 55 breaths per minute are associated with ventilatory limitation (Wasserman et al., 1994). Breathing frequencies during exercise are most reliably measured with open circuit methods. Normal maximal ventilatory breathing values during exercise are shown in Table 6–6.

TABLE 6–6

NORMAL MAXIMAL BREATHING VALUES DURING EXERCISE

Value	Rate
Respiratory frequency	< 50 breaths per minute
Tidal volume (V_T)	< Inspiratory capacity
Minute ventilation/maximal voluntary ventilation ($\dot{V}_E$/MVV)	72% ± 15
Breathing reserve (MVV – $\dot{V}_E$ max)	38 ± 22 L/min

TIDAL VOLUME AND MINUTE VENTILATION

Tidal volume is the volume of air breathed in one inhalation or exhalation. The resting tidal volume is 0.50 ml ± 0.10 ml. Tidal volume can increase to an average of 1.9 to 2.0 L during maximal exercise (Astrand, 1960). The absolute value of the maximal tidal volume is related to an individual's height, age, and gender. The highest values are seen in tall, 20-year-old men. The maximal tidal volume is between 50 and 55 percent of the vital capacity for men and between 45 and 50 percent for women (Cotes, 1975; Spiro et al., 1974). The maximal tidal volume is generally 70 percent of the inspiratory capacity (Wasserman & Whipp, 1975). Exercise, even at a maximal value, does not use all of the lung capacity but only uses up to 70 percent of the available capacity. This is another way of looking at the fact that, under normal circumstances, exercise is limited by the cardiovascular and musculoskeletal systems, not the lungs. In individuals with restrictive lung disease the maximal exercise tidal volume approaches 100 percent of the inspiratory capacity, suggesting that lung capacity is implicated in limited exercise when restrictive lung disease is present.

The minute ventilation is the product of the tidal volume times the breathing frequency. Minute ventilation increases linearly with increasing exercise until the ventilation threshold is reached, where ventilation increases faster than the oxygen consumption. During mild to moderate exercise, the minute ventilation is increased primarily by increasing the tidal volume (the depth of breathing.) With harder exercise, increased minute ventilation is accomplished by increased breathing frequency (Spiro et al., 1974). The maximal minute ventilation is between 50 and 80 percent of the maximal voluntary ventilation (Hansen et al., 1984). The maximal voluntary ventilation is the volume of air that can be breathed in 12 to 15 seconds. The difference between the maximal voluntary ventilation and the maximal exercise minute ventilation reflects the breathing reserve, or the functional difference between respiratory capacity and what is used during exercise. The breathing reserve tends to be reduced in individuals with chronic obstructive lung disease (Bye et al., 1983; Pierce et al., 1968).

DYSPNEA SCALES

Dyspnea is a primary symptom that limits exercise in individuals with pulmonary or cardiovascular disease. Dyspnea is the subjective sensation of difficulty with breathing. The patient often reports being "short of breath" or not being able to "catch" his or her breath. Dyspnea occurs when the demand for ventilation outstrips the patient's

TABLE 6–7
RATING OF DYSPNEA

DYSPNEA INTENSITY*
1—Mild, noticeable to patient but not to observer
2—Some difficulty, noticeable to observer
3—Moderate difficulty, but can continue
4—Severe difficulty, patient cannot continue

DYSPNEA LEVELS†
0—Able to count to 15 easily (no additional breaths necessary)
1—Able to count to 15 but must take one additional breath
2—Must take two additional breaths to count to 15
3—Must take three additional breaths to count to 15
4—Unable to count
The patient is asked to inhale normally and then to count out loud to 15 over a 7.5- to 8.0-second period. Any shortness of breath can be graded by levels.

*From Hansen, P. (1988). Clinical exercise testing. In S. N. Blair, P. Painter, R. R. Pate et al. (Eds.). Resource manual for guidelines for exercise testing and prescription (p. 215). Philadelphia: Lea & Febiger.
†From Physical therapy management of patients with pulmonary disease. Downey, CA: Ranchos Los Amigos Medical Center, Physical Therapy Department.

ability to respond to the demand and is distinct from tachypnea (rapid breathing) or hyperpnea (increased ventilation) (West, 1982). Several methods have been described for rating the intensity of the dyspnea. These methods are based on ordinal scales and operational definitions of dyspnea intensity (Table 6–7). These scales have not been well validated; however, the clinician should keep in mind that it is difficult to measure a subjective sensation.

PULMONARY FUNCTION TESTS

Pulmonary function tests provide information on the functional characteristics of the lung. These tests measure air flow and air flow resistance, lung volumes, and gas exchange. For a review of individual tests and measurement issues related to pulmonary function tests the reader is referred elsewhere (Protas, 1985).

Pulmonary function tests have limited applications in many rehabilitation settings. For instance, rehabilitative interventions for individuals with chronic lung disease often do not change pulmonary function values of diseased lungs, even though the patient may demonstrate improved function. The relationship between pulmonary function measures, walking ability, and submaximal exercise performance has been shown to be poor in individuals with chronic bronchitis (Mungall & Hainesworth, 1979). Likewise, there is no correlation between regional lung secretion clearance as measured by a radiolabeled technique, the maximal expiratory flow during either a cough or a forced expiratory technique (e.g., "huffing"), viscoscity or elasticity of the sputum, and the amount of sputum expectorated during the maneuvers (Hasani et al., 1994). This suggests that maximal expiratory flow during a cough or forced expiratory technique and the sputum production provide no guide to the efficacy of secretion clearance in the lung. On the other hand, pulmonary function values do improve in individuals with cystic fibrosis who were hospitalized for an acute exacerbation of the disease and who underwent either cycle ergometer exercise and one bronchial hygiene treatment or three bronchial hygiene treatments alone each day during the hospital stay (Cerny, 1989). Likewise, pulmonary function tests have been used to assess treatment outcomes after either inspiratory resistive muscle training or abdominal weight training in a group of individuals with cervical spinal cord lesions. A 7-week period of training produced significant increases in pulmonary function values for both treatment interventions, but there were no differences between the two interventions (Derrickson et al., 1992). The value of pulmonary function measures to the clinician may depend on the type of patients seen, as well as on the interventions used. The clinician may need to monitor the pulmonary function of the individual with a high cervical spinal cord lesion more closely than the individual with stable, chronic obstructive pulmonary disease.

EXERCISE TESTS

Although exercise tests have been previously discussed in this chapter, several additional comments are appropri-ate in relation to the assessment of pulmonary function. Exercise tests with the observation of pulmonary gas exchange provide important information about the functional status of an individual patient that cannot be provided by pulmonary function tests. In essence, what the clinician wants to know is whether a patient's ability to function or to exercise is limited. Using a standard, incremental, progressive exercise testing protocol offers the chance to observe cardiopulmonary responses under controlled exercise conditions.

Several pulmonary measures provide information on the ventilation, gas exchange, and metabolism. The respiratory exchange ratio (RER) is the ratio between exhaled carbon dioxide and oxygen consumed (Vco_2/Vo_2). The RER is normally 0.70 at rest (less carbon dioxide produced per unit of oxygen) and increases to greater than $1:1$ with maximal exercise. As exercise increases, the metabolic demands increase and the pulmonary system begins to buffer the blood pH by eliminating more carbon dioxide (Wasserman & Whipp, 1975). Observing the ventilatory equivalents for carbon dioxide and oxygen (minute ventilation/carbon dioxide exhaled, $\dot{V}_E/\dot{V}co_2$, and minute ventilation/oxygen consumed, $\dot{V}_E/\dot{V}o_2$) gives a noninvasive, indirect measure of ventilation-perfusion ($\dot{V}_A/\dot{Q}$) matching or the physiologic dead space to tidal volume ratio (V_D/V_T).

The ventilatory equivalents normally decrease until the ventilatory threshold for $\dot{V}_E/\dot{V}co_2$ or lactate threshold for $\dot{V}_E/\dot{V}o_2$ (Fig. 6–5). The $\dot{V}_E/\dot{V}co_2$ value is normally between 26 and 30, while the $\dot{V}_E/\dot{V}o_2$ is between 22 and 27 (Wasserman et al., 1994). Elevated ventilatory equivalents

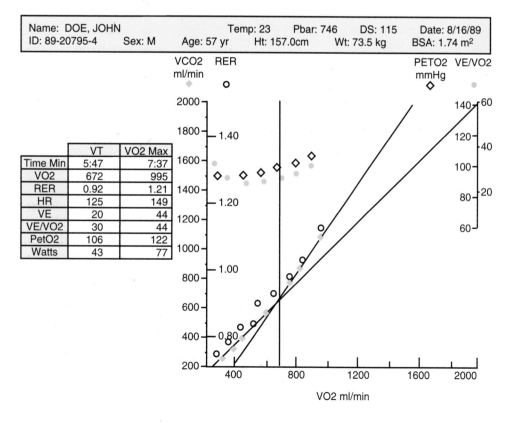

	VT	VO2 Max
Time Min	5:47	7:37
VO2	672	995
RER	0.92	1.21
HR	125	149
VE	20	44
VE/VO2	30	44
PetO2	106	122
Watts	43	77

FIGURE 6–5. A comparison of the ventilatory equivalent for carbon dioxide ($\dot{V}_E/\dot{V}co_2$) and the ventilatory equivalent for oxygen ($\dot{V}_E/\dot{V}o_2$) during increasing exercise. The ventilation threshold is the point at which $\dot{V}_E/\dot{V}co_2$ begins to increase. (Courtesy of Medical Graphics Corp., St. Paul, MN.)

indicate either hyperventilation or uneven $\dot{V}_A/\dot{Q}$ (increased $\dot{V}_D/\dot{V}_T$). Individuals with obstructive lung disease often have $\dot{V}_A/\dot{Q}$ mismatching and have increased ventilatory equivalent values.

OXYHEMOGLOBIN SATURATION

The degree to which arterial blood is oxygenated (partial pressure of arterial oxygen, Pa_{O_2}) is reflected by the oxyhemoglobin saturation of arterial blood (Sa_{O_2}). Arterial oxygenation at rest decreases with age from approximately 100 mm Hg for a 20-year-old to 80 mm Hg for an 80-year-old (Marini, 1987). During heavy exercise in individuals without cardiopulmonary disease, the Pa_{O_2} values may increase slightly. Hypoxemia is decreased Pa_{O_2} and is a condition that can be harmful to a patient. The Sa_{O_2} values at rest are 95% or higher and do not normally decrease with exercise (Wasserman, 1994).

The Sa_{O_2} can be monitored using an indwelling catheter to draw blood samples; however, outside the intensive care unit the use of catheters in most clinical situations is impractical. Pulse oximeters are a noninvasive method of monitoring Sa_{O_2} under a variety of circumstances. In one review it was suggested that the accuracy of pulse oximeters is variable, even within the same model; however, versions that use finger-probe sensors may be more accurate than devices that use earlobe sensors (Mengelkoch et al., 1994). Accuracy is improved when Sa_{O_2} is greater than or equal to 85 percent in nonsmokers. Because these devices are most useful during exercise, the clinician should carefully secure the probe to the finger and should select activities that will reduce motion artifact (cycle ergometer vs. treadmill). The estimates of Sa_{O_2} when saturation is below 78 percent tend to be inaccurate and can miss undetected hypoxemia. Thus, the value of these devices is limited in individuals with severe pulmonary disease.

GLOSSARY

Body mass index—Weight in kilograms per height in meters squared.

Breathing reserve—Difference between maximum voluntary ventilation and the maximum exercise minute ventilation.

Chair step test—A progressive test with four levels or stages conducted sitting by kicking to increasingly higher targets. The last stage adds reciprocal arm movements with kicking.

Dyspnea—The subjective sensation of breathing difficulty.

Dyspnea scales—Numeric ratings of dyspnea intensity.

Electrocardiogram rhythm—Determination of the interval between each R wave on the ECG.

Exercise test mode—Type of equipment used for test.

Exercise test protocol—Standard combination of intensities, stage progressions, and stage durations.

Fifth phase diastolic blood pressure—Blood pressure when the Korotkoff's sounds disappear completely.

Fourth phase diastolic blood pressure—Blood pressure when the Korotkoff's sounds become muffled.

Hypoxemia—Decreased partial pressure of arterial oxygen.

Korotkoff's sounds—Created by turbulence when the blood pressure cuff goes below the blood pressure in the brachial artery.

Maximal exercise test—Maximal ability to perform exercise with large muscle groups. The individual is not able to continue the exercise and reaches several other criteria indicating maximum exercise.

Maximum voluntary ventilation—Volume of air that can be breathed in 12 to 15 seconds.

Minute ventilation—Volume of air breathed in 1 minute. Measured in liters per minute.

Oxyhemoglobin saturation (Sa_{O_2})—Oxygen saturation of hemoglobin in arterial blood. The resting normal value is generally 95% of higher.

Partial pressure of arterial oxygen (Pa_{O_2})—Degree of arterial blood oxygenation.

Percent body fat—Measured by skin calipers or impedance devices, which determine the percent of body weight that is attributed to fat.

Pulse oximeters—Noninvasive measure of oxyhemoglobin saturation.

Respiratory exchange ratio (RER)—Ratio of volume of exhaled carbon dioxide to volume of oxygen consumption.

Respiratory frequency—Number of breaths per minute.

Submaximal exercise test—A test which ends at a predetermined endpoint, such as a heart rate of 150 bpm or with the appearance of significant symptoms.

Tidal volume—Volume of air breathed in one inhalation or exhalation.

Ventilation perfusion matching ($\dot{V}_A/\dot{Q}$)—Ratio of alveolar ventilation to pulmonary circulation.

Ventilation threshold—Ventilation increases faster than oxygen consumption. Approximately the point with increasing exercise intensity where more carbon dioxide needs to be exhaled.

Ventilatory equivalent for oxygen or carbon dioxide—Ratio of minute ventilation to oxygen or carbon dioxide consumed.

Walk test—An indirect means to measure cardiovascular endurance in the clinical setting by noting the distance walked in a fixed period of time such as 5, 6, or 12 minutes with the patient walking as far and as fast as possible.

REFERENCES

Altug, Z., Hoffman, J. L., & Martin, J. L. (1993). *Manual of clinical exercise testing, prescription, and rehabilitation* (pp. 49–51). Norwalk, CT: Appleton & Lange.

American Association of Cardiovascular and Pulmonary Rehabilitation. (1993). In G. Connors, & L. Hilling (Eds.), *Guidelines for pulmonary rehabilitation programs* (p. 42). Champaign, IL: Human Kinetics Publishers.

American College of Sports Medicine. (1995). *ACSM's guidelines for exercise testing and prescription* (5th ed., pp. 13–25, 53–69, 94–96). Baltimore: Williams & Wilkins.

American Heart Association. (1987). *Recommendations for human blood pressure determination by sphygmomanometers.* Dallas: American Heart Association.

Astrand, I. (1960). Aerobic work capacity in men and women with special reference to age. *Acta Physiology Scandinavia, 49,* 1–89.

Astrand, P. O., & Rhyming, I. A. (1954). A nomogram for calculation of aerobic capacity (physical fitness) from pulse rate during submaximal work. *Journal of Applied Physiology, 7,* 218–221.

Balke, B. (1963). A simple field test for the assessment of physical fitness. *Civil Aeromedical Research Institute Report, 63,* 1–8.

Balke, B., & Ware, R. (1959). An experimental study of physical fitness of Air Force personnel. *United States Armed Forces Medical Journal, 10,* 675–688.

Bobbert, A. C. (1960). Physiological comparison of three types of ergometry. *Journal of Applied Physiology, 15,* 1007–1012.

Borg, G. (1982). Psychophysical bases of perceived exertion. *Medicine and Science of Sports and Exercise, 14,* 377–387.

Bruce, R. A., Kusami, F., & Hosmer, D. (1973). Maximal oxygen intake and nomographic assessment of functional aerobic impairment in cardiovascular disease. *American Heart Journal, 85,* 546–562.

Buchfuhrer, M. J., et al. (1983). Optimizing the exercise protocol for cardiopulmonary assessment. *Journal of Applied Physiology, 55,* 1558–1564.

Bye, P. T. P., Farkas, G. A., & Roussos, C. H. (1983). Respiratory factors limiting exercise. *American Review of Physiology, 45,* 439–451.

Cerny, F. (1989). Relative effects of bronchial drainage and exercise for in-hospital care of patients with cystic fibrosis. *Physical Therapy, 69,* 633–639.

Cooper, K. (1968). A means of assessing maximal oxygen intake. *Journal of the American Medical Association, 203,* 201–204.

Cotes, J. E. (1975). *Lung function: Assessment and application in medicine* (3rd ed., p. 394). Oxford: Blackwell Scientific Publications.

Cotton, F. S., & Dill, D. B. (1935). On the relation between heart rate during exercise and the immediate post-exercise period. *American Journal Physiology, 111,* 554.

Derrickson, J., Ciesla, N., Simpson, N., & Imle, P. C. (1992). A comparison of two breathing exercise programs for patients with quadriplegia. *Physical Therapy, 72,* 763–769.

Dubach, P., Froelicher, V. F., Klein, J., Oakes, D., Grover-McKay, M., & Friis, R. (1989). Exercise induced hypotension in a male population: Criteria, causes and prognosis. *Circulation, 78,* 1380–1387.

Ellestad, M. H., Allen, W., Wan, M. C. K., & Kemp, G. L. (1979). Maximal treadmill stress testing for cardiovascular evaluation. *Circulation, 39,* 517–524.

Englehard, C., Protas, E. J., Stanley, R. (1993). Diurnal variations in blood pressure and walking distance in elderly nursing home residents. *Physical Therapy, 73,* S60.

Fabian, J., Stolz, I., Janota, M., & Rohac, J. (1975). Reproducibility of exercise tests in patients with symptomatic ischaemic heart disease. *British Heart Journal, 37,* 785–793.

Froelicher, V. R. (1983). *Exercise testing and training* (pp. 15–17). Chicago: Year Book Medical Publishers.

Froelicher, V. F. (1994). *Manual of exercise testing.* (2nd ed., pp. 12–13, 41–44). St. Louis: C. V. Mosby.

Froelicher, V. F., et al. (1976). A comparison of two-bipolar electrocardiographic leads to lead V5. *Chest, 70,* 611–616.

Gamble, P., McManus, H., Jensen, D., Froelicher, V. (1984). A comparison of the standard 12-lead electrocardiogram to exercise electrode placements. *Chest, 85,* 616–622.

Gretebeck, R. J., Montoye, H. J., Baylor, D., & Montoye, A. P. (1991). Comment on heart rate recording in field studies. *Journal of Sports Medicine and Physical Fitness, 31,* 629–631.

Guyatt, G. H., Sullivan, M. J., Thompson, P. J., Fallen, E. L., Pugsley, S. O., Taylor, D. W., Berman, L. B. (1985). The six-minute walk: A new measure of exercise capacity in patients with chronic heart failure. *Canadian Medical Association Journal, 132,* 919–923.

Hahn, R. A., Teutsch, S. M., Paffenbarger, R. S., Marks, J. S. (1990). Excess deaths from nine chronic diseases in the United States, 1986. *Journal of the American Medical Association, 264,* 2654–2659.

Hansen, J. E., Sue, D. Y., & Wasserman, K. (1984). Predicted values for clinical exercise testing. *American Review of Respiratory Disease, 129*(Suppl.), S49–S55.

Hanson, P. (1988). Clinical exercise testing. In S. N. Blair, P. Painter, R. R. Pate, L. K. Smith, & C. B. Taylor (Eds.). *Resource manual for guidelines for exercise testing and prescription* (pp. 205–222). Philadelphia: Lea & Febiger.

Hasani, A., Pavia, D., Agnew, J. E., & Clarke, S. W. (1994). Regional lung clearance during cough and forced expiratory technique (FET): Effects of flow and viscoelasticity. *Thorax, 49,* 557–561.

Haskell, W. L. (1994). The efficacy and safety of exercise programs in cardiac rehabilitation. *Medicine and Science of Sports and Exercise, 26,* 815–823.

Jackson, A. S., Blair, S. N., Mahar, M. T., Wier, L. T., Ross, R. M., & Stuteville, J. E. (1990). Prediction of functional aerobic capacity without exercise testing. *Medicine and Science of Sports and Exercise, 22,* 863–870.

Kline, G. M., Porcari, J. P., Hintermeister, R., Freedson, P. S., Ward, A., McCarron, R. F., Ross, J., & Rippe, J. M. (1987). Estimation of VO$_2$ max from a one-mile track walk, gender, age and body weight. *Medicine and Science of Sports and Exercise, 19,* 253–259.

Laupacis, A., Bourne, R., Rorabeck, C., Feeny, D., Wong, C., Tugwell, P., Leslie, K., & Ballas, R. (1993). The effect of elective total hip replacement on health-related quality of life. *Journal of Bone and Joint Surgery, 75,* 1619–1626.

Leger, L., & Thivierge, M. (1988). Heart rate monitors: Validity, stability, and functionality. *Physician and Sports Medicine, 16,* 143–151.

Lipkin, D. P., Canepa-Anson, R., Stephens, M. R., & Poole-Wilson, P. A. (1986). Factors determining symptoms in heart failure: Comparison of fast and slow exercise tests. *British Heart Journal, 55,* 439–445.

Marini, J. J. (1987). *Respiratory medicine for the house officer* (2nd ed.). Baltimore: Williams & Wilkins.

McCardle, W. D., Katch, F. I., Katch, V. L. (1991). *Exercise physiology: Energy, nutrition and human performance* (3rd ed). Philadelphia: Lea & Febiger.

McCardle, W. D., Zwiren, L., & Magel, J. R. (1969). Validity of the post exercise heart rate as a means of estimating heart rate during work of varying intensities. *Research Quarterly of American Association of Health and Physical Education, 40,* 523–530.

McKiran, M. D., and Froelicher, V. F. (1993). General principles of exercise testing. In J. Skinner (Ed.), *Exercise testing and exercise prescription for special cases* (pp. 3–27). Philadelphia: Lea & Febiger.

Mengelkoch, L. J., Martin, D., & Lawler, J. (1994). A review of the principles of pulse oximetry and accuracy of pulse oximeter estimates during exercise. *Physical Therapy, 74,* 40–49.

Montoye, H. J., Kemper, H. C. G., Saris, W. H. M., & Washburn, R. A. (1996). *Measuring physical activity and energy expenditure* (pp. 98–99). Champaign, IL: Human Kinetics.

Mungall, I. P., Hainesworth, B. (1979). Assessment of respiratory function in patients with chronic obstructive airway disease. *Thorax, 34,* 254–261.

National Heart, Lung and Blood Institute (National High Blood Pressure Education Program). (1993). The fifth report of the Joint Committee on Detection, Evaluation and Treatment of High Blood Pressure. *Archives of Internal Medicine, 153,* 154–183.

Naughton, J., Balke, B., & Nagle, F. (1964). Refinement in methods of evaluation and physical conditioning before and after myocardial infarction. *American Journal Cardiology, 14,* 837–843.

Noble, B. J., Borg, G., Jacobs, I., Ceci, R., & Kaiser, P. (1983). A category-ratio perceived exertion scale: Relationship to blood and muscle lactates and heart rate. *Medicine and Science of Sports Exercise, 15,* 523–528.

Peterson, M. G. E., Kovar-Toledano, J. C., Allegrande, J. P., Mackenzie, C. R., Gutlin, S., & Kroll, M. A. (1993). Effect of a walking program on gait characteristics in patients with osteoarthritis. *Arthritis Care and Research, 6,* 11–16.

Pierce, A. K., Luterman, D., Loundermilk, J., et al. (1968). Exercise ventilatory patterns in normal subjects and patients with airway obstruction. *Journal of Applied Physiology, 25,* 249–254.

Pitetti, K. H., Snell, P. G., Stray-Gunderson, J. (1987). Maximal response of wheelchair-confined subjects to four types of arm exercise. *Archives of Physical Medicine and Rehabilitation, 68,* 10–13.

Pollock, M. L., Bohannon, R. L., Cooper, K. H., Ayres, J. J., Ward, A., White, S. R., & Linnerud, A. C. (1976). A comparative analysis of four protocols for maximal treadmill stress testing. *American Heart Journal, 92,* 39–45.

Pollock, M. L., Broida, J., & Kendrick, Z. (1972). Validity of palpation technique of heart rate determination and its estimation of training heart rate. *Research Quarterly, 43,* 77–81.

Pollock, M. L., & Wilmore, J. H. (1990). *Exercise in health and disease: Evaluation and prescription for prevention and rehabilitation* (2nd ed.). Philadelphia: W. B. Saunders.

Price, L. G., Hewett, H. J., Kay, D. R., & Minor, M. M. (1988). Five-minute walking test of aerobic fitness for people with arthritis. *Arthritis Care and Research, 1,* 33–37.

Protas, E. J. (1985). Pulmonary function testing. In J. M. Rothstein (Ed.). *Measurement in physical therapy* (pp. 229–254). New York: Churchill-Livingstone.

Protas, E. J., Cole, J., & Haney, K. (1988). Reliability of the three-minute walk test in elderly post-operative patients. *Journal of Cardiopulmonary Rehabilitation, 3,* 36.

Protas, E. J., Stanley, R. K., Jankovic, J., & MacNeill, B. (1996). Cardiovascular and metabolic responses to upper and lower extremity exercise in men with idiopathic Parkinson's disease. *Physical Therapy, 76,* 34–40.

Schaman, J. P. (1988). Basic electrocardiographic analysis. In S. N. Blair, P. Painter, R. R. Pate, L. K. Smith, & C. B. Taylor (Eds.), *Resource manual for guidelines for exercise testing and prescription* (p. 183). Philadelphia: Lea & Febiger.

Sedlock, D. A., Knowlton, R. G., Fitzgerald, P. I., Tahamont, M. V., & Schneider, D. A. (1983). Accuracy of subject-palpated carotid pulse after exercise. *Physician and Sports Medicine, 11,* 106–116.

Shephard, R. J. (1987). *Physical activity and aging.* (2nd ed., pp. 81–86). Rockville, MD: Aspen Publishers.

Sinacore, D. R., & Ehsani, A. A. (1985). Measurements of cardiovascular function. In J. Rothstein (Ed.), *Measurement in physical therapy* (pp. 255–280). New York: Churchill-Livingstone.

Skinner, J. S. (1993). Importance of aging for exercise testing and exercise prescription. In J. S. Skinner (Ed.), *Exercise testing and exercise prescription for special cases: Theoretical basis and clinical application* (pp. 75–86). Philadelphia: Lea & Febiger.

Smith, E. L., Gilligan, C. (1983). Physical activity prescription for the older adult. *Physician and Sports Medicine, 11,* 91–101.

Spiro, S. C., Juniper, E., Bowman, P., & Edwards, R. H. T. (1974). An increasing work rate test for assessing the physiological strain of submaximal exercise. *Clinical Science and Molecular Medicine, 46,* 191–206.

Stanley, R. K., & Protas, E. J. (1991). Validity of a walk test in elderly women. *Physical Therapy, 71,* S73.

Taylor, S. A., Buskirk, E., & Henschel, A. (1955). Maximal oxygen intake as an objective measure of cardiorespiratory performance. *Journal of Applied Physiology, 8,* 73–80.

Temes, W. C. (1994). Cardiac rehabilitation. In E. Hillegass, & S. Sadowsky (Eds.), *Essentials of cardiopulmonary physical therapy* (pp. 633–675). Philadelphia: W. B. Saunders.

Thomas, S., Cunningham, D. A., Rechnitzer, P. A., Donner, A. P., & Howard, J. H. (1987). Protocols and reliability of maximum oxygen uptake in the elderly. *Canadian Journal of Sport Science, 12,* 144–150.

Treiber, F. A., Musante, L., Hartdagan, S., Davis, H., et al. (1989). Validation of a heart rate monitor with children in laboratory and field settings. *Medicine and Science of Sports and Exercise, 21,* 338–342.

Van Camp, S. P., & Peterson, R. A. (1986). Cardiovascular complications of outpatient cardiac rehabilitation programs. *Journal of American Medical Association, 256,* 1160–1163.

Ward, A., Ebbeling, C. B., & Ahlquist, L. E. (1995). Indirect methods for estimation of aerobic power. In Maud, P. J. & Foster, C. (Eds.). *Physiological assessment of human fitness* (pp. 47–56) Champaign, IL: Human Kinetics.

Wasserman, K., Hansen, J. E., Sue, D. S., Sue, D. Y., Whipp, B. J., & Casaburi, R. (1994). *Principles of exercise testing* (pp. 123–127). Philadelphia: Lea & Febiger.

Wasserman, K., & Whipp, B. J. (1975). Exercise physiology in health and disease. *American Review of Respiratory Diseases, 112,* 219–249.

West, J. B. (1982). *Pulmonary pathophysiology* (2nd ed., pp. 52–53). Baltimore: Williams & Wilkins.

Wetzel, J., Lunsford, B. R., Peterson, M. J., & Alvarez, S. E. (1985). Respiratory rehabilitation of the patient with a spinal cord injury. In S. Irwin & J. S. Tecklin (Eds.), *Cardiopulmonary physical therapy* (pp. 395–420). St. Louis: C. V. Mosby.

White, J. R. (1977). EKG changes using carotid artery for heart monitoring. *Medicine and Science of Sports and Exercise, 9,* 88–94.

Wright, G. R., Sidney, K. H., & Shephard, R. J. (1978). Variance of direct and indirect measurements of aerobic power. *Journal of Sports Medicine and Physical Fitness, 18,* 33–42.

CHAPTER 7

Psychosocial Function

Melba J. Arnold, MS, OTR/L

Elizabeth B. Devereaux, MSW, ACSW/L, OTR/L, FAOTA

SUMMARY   Since the early 1800s, the assessment of psychosocial functional performance has existed as a philosophical foundation for occupational therapy in support of "holistic" therapy. Occupational therapy promotes the concept of holism in treatment, operating under the belief that full recovery from illness requires both physical and psychological treatment. Implementation of the holistic approach involves the use of a variety of occupational therapy theories and assessment techniques. Assessment of psychosocial dysfunction may be performed independently or as a component of a major functional performance evaluation. Psychosocial assessment addresses the loss of functional performance in areas of work, play or leisure, and interpersonal and emotional behavior. Psychosocial dysfunction can be a result of physical illness or a psychological condition. Treatment approach is determined by results from the psychosocial functional evaluation.

HISTORIC PERSPECTIVE

Ocupational therapy for psychosocial dysfunction dates back to the era in which "moral treatment" was advocated. Moral treatment evolved in the early 1800s in response to unbearable and inhumane conditions that existed for people who were mentally ill. Those identified as mentally ill were thought to be demonic and a danger to society and, as such, were totally isolated from their environment of origin. The emphasis of moral treatment was humanitarianism. The moral movement occurred during a time of political change and was based on the belief that "man could control his environment and improve his life on earth" (Hopkins & Smith, 1993, p. 27).

Numerous people were major promoters of the moral treatment movement, the first of whom was Philippe Pinel, who promoted reform throughout Europe and America. A strong influence in England was the Tuke family, who provided mentally ill individuals with clothes, educated them in self-control, and engaged them in employment situations for self-reliance. Other supporters included Benjamin Rush, a physician considered to be the father of American psychiatry and the first to use moral treatment in the United States, and Dr. Thomas S. Kirkbride, who organized what is now known as the American Psychiatric Association (APA).

The "arts and crafts" movement followed the moral treatment period. Later, the movement was viewed as both educational and therapeutic with a vocational and a diversional approach, respectively. The diversional approach became synonymous with the therapeutic practice of occupational therapy in psychiatry, and the vocational approach became the basis for occupational therapy in people with physical disabilities. Promoters of the arts and crafts movement engaged mentally and physically ill individuals in the production of various useful goods and services, which encouraged self-reliance.

Guided by changes in thought by the APA on the etiology of mental illness, the occupational therapy approach progressed from moral treatment, promoted by Adolph Meyer, psychiatrist and founder of the occupational therapy profession, to that of "habit training." Habit training was introduced by Eleanor Clarke Slagle, co-founder of the occupational therapy profession. Slagle's concept of healthy habits included behavior that was "industrious, hard working, neat, clean, polite, self controlled, and emotionally restrained." Slagle's treatment approach consisted of training in socially acceptable conduct (Hopkins & Smith, 1993). Because habit training and moral treatment neglected the affective and interpersonal experiences of clients, both perspectives were eventually abandoned (Mosey, 1986).

By the mid-1900s, the occupational therapy approach had progressed from a symptomatology perspective promoted by William Rush Dunton, also a cofounder of the profession, to that of a psychoanalytic and sociological orientation. Major proponents of this new perspective were Gail S. Fidler and Jay W. Fidler, coauthors of *Introduction to psychiatric occupational therapy* (1954) and *Occupational therapy: A communication process in psychiatry* (1963). The writings and clinical contributions made by the Fidlers provided a stable treatment foundation in psychiatric occupational therapy that continues to exist as a component of present-day approaches (Mosey, 1986).

The remainder of this chapter presents three major psychosocial theories and examples of assessments used in occupational therapy: the analytic perspective of the Fidlers, the cognitive disability perspective by Claudia Allen, and the model of human occupation by Gary Kielhofner. Finally, occupational therapy assessment of interpersonal skills and emotional behavior is specifically addressed.

PSYCHOSOCIAL FUNCTION–DYSFUNCTION

Successful psychosocial functioning requires harmony between one's psychological capability and the skills required to perform routine daily tasks. It is the ability to be able to take care of one's daily needs in a responsible and safe manner. An individual may experience the loss of this harmony for various reasons. Specifically, the effects of a psychiatric illness, a physical illness or accident, or a neurologic impairment that affects the function of the brain can result in a range of performance difficulties or psychosocial dysfunction.

Literature from a variety of sources indicates that successful psychosocial functioning involves both emotional and cognitive components (Allen, 1985; Levy,

1993; Mosey, 1986; Perry & Bussey, 1984). How we perform daily routine tasks and the manner in which we socially interact with others and exhibit psychological behavior depend on emotional, as well as cognitive, abilities. Recovering from a mental illness or a psychological condition is considered by some theorists to be a result of an analytic process that addresses ego functioning and unconscious actions leading to need fulfillment. A return to cognitive functioning is thought to be a result of the natural healing process of the neurologic structures of the brain combined with environmental adjustments. These neurologic structures are responsible for functions of the brain referred to as occupational performance components (American Occupational Therapy Association [AOTA], 1994). Occupational performance components include three main categories: sensory motor components, cognitive integration components, and psychosocial or psychological components (AOTA, 1994).

According to "Uniform terminology for occupational therapy" (AOTA, 1994), human function occurs in three performance areas: activities of daily living (ADL), work, and play or leisure activities. The lowest level of functional independence in humans is the ability to perform basic self-care needs. If the primary self-care skills of feeding, hygiene, grooming, toileting, and dressing are lost due to illness or disease, a loss of independent functioning can occur (AOTA, 1994). Additional performance skills that can be affected by functional impairment are known as instrumental activities of daily living (IADL). These IADL are tasks that are vital to total functional independence and involve greater complexity in skill and cognitive capability. Examples of IADL include following a medication routine, shopping, preparing a meal, doing housework, using a telephone, managing money and time, and traveling (Hopkins & Smith, 1993).

When effective psychosocial function is interrupted by psychiatric or physical illness or by an injury to the brain, some aspects of the occupational performance components and occupational performance areas may become affected. Those areas affected can be revealed through psychosocial assessment processes as a part of the total evaluation. Assessment of performance may be required for one or several performance components or areas. The type of psychosocial assessment performed should be supported by a frame of reference. The chosen frame of reference would support the underlying purpose of the assessment process being utilized and would guide the overall treatment approach.

ACTIVITIES THERAPY AND ANALYTIC FRAMES OF REFERENCE

In occupational therapy, the use of activities as a therapeutic process was first based on the psychoanalytic and psychodynamic theoretical perspectives of Sigmund

Freud and followers such as Sullivan, Jung, Erikson, Mahler, and others (Bootzin et al., 1993; Gallatin, 1982; Mears & Gratchel, 1979). The psychoanalytic theorists postulate that abnormal behavior is a result of unconscious intrapsychic motivational conflict of a sexual or aggressive nature, a result of an inferiority complex, or problems with object relations involving strong emotional ties. These intrapsychic conflicts are believed to be established during childhood and are thought to be a result of interpersonal interactions that at some point involve one or both parents. The intrapsychic conflicts are thought to be the impetus for how one thinks, feels, or behaves (Bootzin et al., 1993).

According to the psychoanalytic theory, a return to normal function is accomplished by exploring the origin and symbolism of the unconscious conflicts and bringing them into conscious awareness, thus developing greater insight on the part of the individual about the nature of the behavior. The establishment of insight is thought to occur through an analytic process that also includes what Freud termed "loose association," in which the patient is able to freely express thoughts without judgment from the therapist to allow repressed content to surface and to achieve need fulfillment. The patient's ability to return to the community at a productive level is thought to occur only after successfully working through the intrapsychic conflict (Fidler, 1982).

From the psychoanalytic perspective, dysfunctional behavior among patients varies significantly and does not present in any particular order because dysfunction is considered to be any form of behavior that is unexplainable. Mosey (1986) identified categories that could serve as individual function-dysfunction continuums: (1) intrapsychic conflict that is developmental in nature according to Freud; (2) nondevelopmental types of intrapsychic conflict such as conflicts concerning love, hate, autonomy, trust, aggression, and others; and (3) intrapsychic conflict areas involving maladaptive ideas about self or others.

In occupational therapy, Fidler and Fidler (1963), Fidler (1982), and Mosey (1970, 1973, 1986) have made significant therapeutic contributions using the analytic frames of reference that reflect the treatment of intrapsychic conflict through the use of activities and objects. They believe that effective treatment in the psychoanalytic process must go beyond logistical dialogue that reveals the origin of intrapsychic conflict to include symbolic activities that provide further confirmation of conflict and engage the patient in attempts to alter maladaptive behavior. According to Mosey (1970, 1973, 1986), therapeutic intervention based on the analytic frames of reference is most effective with patients who possess a high degree of cognitive ability. Average intelligence is required for the thinking, problem-solving, and psychological finesse that is necessary for insight that leads to the resolution of intrapsychic conflict and need gratification.

Using the analytic frames of reference, occupational therapy intervention is based on the disease and medical model focusing mainly on the pathology and nature of the mental illness. The pioneers in occupational therapy treatment using the analytic frames of reference were the Fidlers. Although their work occurred during a time when the medical model defined most health professions, their theoretical approach included emphasis on rehabilitation and the resumption of responsibilities within the environment (Fidler & Fidler, 1963).

The Fidlers' theoretical base and function-dysfunction continuum were similar in focus to that of other psychoanalytic theorists, e.g., unconscious conflict, interpersonal relations, communication, object relations, and symbolic activity. Identification of specific behavior is not possible under this frame of reference, since dysfunction is defined as any unexplainable form of conduct (Bootzin et al., 1993; Gallatin, 1982; Mosey, 1986). Three evaluation categories are offered: the patient's relationship to the therapist, group, and activity. The clinician is required to interpret the individual's behavior according to the theoretical base or function-dysfunction continuum. Consistent with the absence of specific behavior identification, the process for change is also unclear and relegated to examples of how occupational therapy as a modality could be included in the overall treatment process (Mosey, 1986).

Object relations analysis as a part of the analytic frames of reference is a process based primarily on the contributions of theorists such as Freud, Jung, Azima, Maslow, Mahler, Fidler and Fidler, Mosey, Naumberg, and others. For this reason, the object relations analysis is considered to be an eclectic process involving the synthesis of several theories. In the object relations analysis, the individuals' relationship and interaction with objects for need gratification and self-actualization are explored. Objects are defined as people, things, and ideas (Bruce & Borg, 1987; Mosey, 1970, 1986). Because this framework is eclectic, the theoretical base involves several concepts: "needs, drives and objects, affect, will, attending and the formation of complexes, cognition, and symbolism" (Mosey, 1970, pp. 37–62).

Mosey (1970, p. 232) defines a complex as "a gestalt of repressed affect, energy and intrapsychic content associated with some type of conflict." Almost any experience can form the nucleus of a complex. The complexes carry great significance, as they serve as indices for the function-dysfunction continuum. Examples of the complexes include feelings related to inferiority, trust, gratification of needs for safety, and love and self esteem.

Assessment Instruments. Projective techniques have been the primary evaluation approach utilized in occupational therapy with the psychoanalytic treatment concept (Fidler & Fidler, 1954, 1963; Fidler, 1982; Hemphill, 1982; Mosey, 1986). The distinguishing feature of projective techniques exists in the assignment of a relatively unstructured task, i.e., one that permits an almost unlimited variety of possible responses. To encourage the unlimited variety of possible responses, only brief, general instructions are provided to the examinee. Projective testing is based on the hypothesis that "the way in which the individual perceives and interprets the test material, or structures the situation, will reflect fundamental aspects of psychological functioning" (Anastasi, 1971, p. 464). In projective testing, the procedures are disguised in that the individual is usually unaware of the type of psychological interpretation that will be made of the responses (Anastasi). Projective testing involves an interview and discussion process followed by interpretation of the examinee's performance by the examiner.

The following are examples of psychoanalytic projective techniques used in occupational therapy (Hemphill, 1982; Hopkins & Smith, 1993; Moyer, 1981).

1. *The Fidler Diagnostic Battery*: Projective testing that consists of presenting the examinee with three sequential tasks; drawing, finger painting, and clay. The examinee is required to discuss each task production. The examiner makes interpretations of the examinee's performance and discussions. (Developed by Fidler and Fidler; from Hopkins & Smith, 1993.)
2. *Azima Occupational Therapy Battery*: Projective battery using pencil drawing, figure drawing, finger-painting, and clay modeling. (Developed by Azima and Azima; from Hemphill, 1982.)
3. *B. H. Battery*: Projective test with finger-painting and tile. (Developed by Hemphill; from Hemphill, 1982.)
4. *Draw-A-Person*: Projective drawings of people. (Developed by Urban; from Western Psychological Services, Los Angeles, CA.)
5. *House-Tree-Person*: Freehand drawing by examinee of a house, a tree, and a person. (Developed by Buck, revised manual; from Western Psychological Services, Los Angeles, CA.)
6. *Magazine Picture Collage*: Pictures are cut out of available magazines and glued on a sheet of paper. (Unstructured reporting format by Buck and Lerner, 1972 and by Ross, 1977.)
7. *Object History*: The examinee is asked to remember something that was important or valued at earlier periods of life and also to explain why. (From Hopkins & Smith, 1993.)
8. *Shoemyen Battery*: Contains four tasks: mosaic tile, finger painting, plaster sculpture, and clay modeling with an interview-discussion to gain information about attitudes, mood, cognitive and social skills, dexterity, attention, suggestibility, independence, and creativity. (Developed by Chemin; from Shoemyen, 1970.)
9. *Goodman Battery*: Consists of tasks of decreasing structure. Purpose is to assess cognitive and affective ego assets and deficits affecting function. (Developed by Evaskus; from Hemphill, 1982.)

COGNITIVE DISABILITY

Mosey (1986, p. 45) defines cognitive function as "a cortical process that involves the use of information for the purpose of thinking and problem solving." Cognitive function involves the following occupational performance components: arousal, orientation, recognition, concentration, attention span, memory, intellect, problem solving, and learning (AOTA, 1994; Abreu & Toglia, 1987). The integrative effects of the cognitive components result in the ability to problem-solve and make decisions. These abilities result in the capacity to exhibit independent functioning in the occupational performance areas, enabling the individual to carry out his or her daily living skills. In situations in which this integrative effect is absent, cognitive dysfunction exists.

The cognitive disability model (CDM) developed by Claudia Allen was initially designed as an evaluation and treatment format for clients with psychiatric illnesses. Further refinement of the model led to its use in the treatment of a variety of clients whose cognitive disability had physical disability origins.

Based on her research and on accounts published by Piaget, other theorists, and Soviet psychologists, Allen learned that the manifestations of psychiatric illnesses revealed strong similarities to those of medical illnesses (Allen, 1985; AOTA, 1988). Allen ruled out theories that involved learning and normal memory based on her presumption that with cognitive impairment, these abilities would be permanently impaired. To this end, the pursuit of evaluation and treatment methods that would provide measurable results of cognitive performance for clients with psychiatric illnesses led to the development of the CDM.

According to Allen (AOTA, 1988), the theoretic foundation of the CDM is a neuroscience approach that is based on the belief that cognitive disabilities are due to illness or injury to the brain, resulting in limitations in functional capability. Although the nature of the illness or injury results in a variety of effects on cognitive ability, the diagnostic category may be any condition that can have an effect on the brain. Diagnostic categories may include cerebrovascular accidents, acquired immunodeficiency syndrome, schizophrenic disorders, acute and chronic organic brain syndromes, traumatic brain injury, primary affective disorders, personality disorders, eating disorders, substance abuse, and developmental disabilities. With each condition, cognitive ability that influences normal performance of human activities may be temporarily or permanently affected. The CDM places emphasis on the functional consequences of cognitive impairments.

Use of the CDM requires an understanding of normal human function, disability impairment, and functional independence. Allen presents the CDM in the form of six cognitive levels that are graded from normal functioning to severe functional disability. The cognitive levels measure performance competence by providing explanations of how information is processed during task performance. To use the CDM, the clinician must acknowledge that improvements in cognitive levels of performance are due to natural healing or the use of medication. Evaluation and treatment are directed toward making necessary adjustments to the remaining cognitive abilities a client may possess.

Cognitive Levels. The CDM describes six levels of cognitive dysfunction. The following is a summary description of function-dysfunction for each level (Allen, 1985, 1987; Allen et al., 1992; Allen and Reyner, 1991).

1. *Level one:* Patient does not respond to the environment, including primary aspects such as eating and toileting. Change is gradual, but food and water intake remains a primary concern. Arousal level is very low; thus, training is usually impossible.
2. *Level two:* Patient often exhibits unusual postures, gestures, or repetitive motions. Gross motor activity for proprioceptive experiences may be exhibited when the patient is guided.
3. *Level three:* Actions are directed toward physical objects in the environment. Patient lacks awareness of the connection between his or her actions and goal achievement. Actions are guided, repetitive, and may have a destructive nature.
4. *Level four:* Patient exhibits actual attempt at task completion, usually an exact match of a sample provided. Attention is concrete, so objects in peripheral field cause confusion. Patient is compliant, so routines can be followed and situational training can occur.
5. *Level five:* Patient demonstrates more flexibility in attending to elements of the physical environment, but the deficit is still present. He or she learns by exploration and trial and error, as he or she is unable to preplan or anticipate the consequences of his or her actions.
6. *Level six:* Patient is able to calculate a plan of action and to use symbolic cues, images, and words to guide own behavior. Motor behavior is spontaneous and based on ability to associate with symbolic cues.

Cognitive Disability Model Assessment Process. The CDM involves three phases of assessment that are used in determining functional level of performance: the routine task inventory, the Allen Cognitive Level (ACL), and the lower cognitive level (LCL) test (Allen, 1985).

The *routine task inventory (RTI)* is an interview process that is administered to either the patient or the caregiver or by observation of the patient's performance. It includes 14 routine tasks in two subscales, the physical scale and the instrumental scale. The physical scale contains six tasks: grooming, bathing, toileting, dressing, feeding, and walking. The instrumental scale has eight tasks: housekeeping, preparing food, spending money, taking medication, doing laundry, traveling, shopping, and telephoning. Each of the

14 tasks is supplemented with behavioral descriptions that reflect each of the cognitive levels. The behavioral descriptions may also serve as potential observations of performance. By matching the patient's reported or observed performance to the descriptions under each task, the therapist is able to determine the patient's level of cognitive functioning, as well as make discharge recommendations (Allen, 1985).

The ACL test is a screening tool designed to provide a quick assessment of a person's ability to function. The ACL involves the use of a leather lacing activity to identify a patient's cognitive level of functioning. The leather activity is graded according to complexity, ranging from a simple running stitch (levels two and three) to a whip stitch (level four) to a more complicated single cordovan stitch. Although each stitch involves repetitive manual activity, the running stitch is thought to be more universal in terms of familiarity and the absence of biases. The administration and scoring of the ACL have been standardized. A larger version of the ACL is also available for individuals with visual impairments (Allen, 1985).

The LCL test was designed to assess the performance of patients functioning at levels one, two, and three, e.g., patients who are diagnosed as having senile dementia. The LCL uses the imitation of motor action to assess the patient's cognitive level of function. The patient is instructed to imitate hand-clapping actions. Lack of patient response reveals level one function; one or two inaudible responses or other imitated movements reveal level two function; three consecutive audible responses reveal level three function (Allen, 1985).

To assist the clinician with the assessment and treatment process, Earhart and coworkers (1993) developed the *Allen Diagnostic Module (ADM)*, which is a set of 24 standardized craft activities that have been rated according to their cognitive complexity. Use of the ADM provides the clinician with the opportunity to observe general functional performance as well as the ways in which the individual may process new information. The ADM is intended to be used following the ACL but prior to the RTI.

Task analysis is also a viable part of the CDM. With the CDM, task analysis is a systematic process of identifying the complexity of task procedures step by step, with an emphasis on those steps that the patient is unable to perform. By performing task analysis, the therapist can guide the patient in accomplishing routine daily tasks. Through task analysis, any activity can be adapted to eliminate procedures that patients cannot do while permitting them to use remaining abilities.

Research. Allen (1985) cited several research findings in support of the effectiveness of the CDM in determining cognitive deficits. Research done on the CDM involved a study of four patient populations.

In a study of hospitalized patients diagnosed with schizophrenia, the ACL was found to have an interrater reliability of $r = 0.99$ with the Pearson product-moment correlation. Validity of the ACL was determined by rating the patient's performance for appropriateness of group placement. Before establishing validity, the interrater reliability for group performances was determined where $r = 0.69$. The validity for group placement was $r = 0.76$ (Allen, 1985). Group placement categories were limited to cognitive levels three and four versus five and six.

A study of schizophrenic subjects from a work rehabilitation unit of a psychiatric hospital investigated the relationship between cognitive levels at the time of discharge and social adjustment in the community. While results revealed a significant but low correlation between cognitive function and pay earnings at the time of discharge ($r = 0.33$, $P < 0.05$), no comparative information was available following discharge. Additionally, a very low correlation between cognitive function and social adjustment ($r = -0.2$ to $r = +0.3$) was evident by the end of 3 months following discharge. Similar studies involving schizophrenic subjects, cognitive levels, and community adjustment revealed no conclusive results (Allen, 1985).

A criterion-related validity study of the ACL was done with patients diagnosed with major depression to investigate cognitive impairment and its relation to ability to function. The results revealed Pearson r correlation between all test scores for admission ranging from 0.01 to 0.42 when compared with the ACL ($n = 32$). The Pearson r between all test scores and the ACL at discharge ranged from 0.05 to 0.24 ($n = 32$). Other results supported the ACL as a sensitive measure of cognitive levels based on the significant increase of the mean score from admission to discharge; 75% rating at levels four to six and 91% rating at levels five to six, respectively, with $n = 32$ (Allen, 1985).

Comparisons were made between the studies for both schizophrenia and depression, which supported the construct validity of the ACL. Results revealed significant differences, which indicated that the ACL was able to differentiate between the two patient populations, identifying the schizophrenic patients as being more severely impaired in cognitive ability.

A study between disabled and nondisabled adult populations investigated their similarities and differences in performance on the ACL. Results also supported construct validity, revealing the disabled adults to be functioning at a lower cognitive level than the nondisabled group. Another important finding that is difficult to interpret was that demographic data such as social class, level of education, and others were greater indicators of cognitive ability than was the ACL (AOTA, 1988).

Lastly, a study involving subjects with senile dementia was designed to investigate the relationship between cognitive disability and the performance of ADL. Results of the study revealed that cognitive impairment produces observable limitations in routine task behavior. Results further supported validity, revealing a significant relationship between the ACL scores and the scores on the Physical Self-Maintenance Scale and the Instrumental Activities of Daily Living Scale in patients with senile dementia.

The aforementioned studies primarily involved observation of performance. Findings by Ottenbacher revealed that cognitive assessment was mainly a result of subjective determination based on clinical observations and, as such, it is difficult to verify treatment success (Abreu & Toglia, 1987).

Backman (1994) concluded that because of its novelty, the RTI has yet to undergo the intense standardization process necessary to legitimize its claim as a valid and reliable tool in assessing change in behavior. Backman asserts that without standardization, the RTI's greatest use is to provide an explanation of a client's ability (or disability) to perform self-care tasks. Thus, although some studies have provided data in support of the validity and reliability of the Allen tests, much work is still needed before they can be accepted by rehabilitation professionals as valid and reliable assessment tools. Because of the precise description inherent in the Allen tests and the favorable attitude their author holds toward research, investigations of these assessment instruments are continually in progress.

HUMAN OCCUPATION

Early formal work that identified occupational behavior as a core philosophy in occupational therapy was first presented by Mary Reilly in her 1961 Eleanor Clarke Slagle lecture (Reilly, 1962). Other occupational therapy contributors to the philosophy of occupational behavior include Matsutsuyu, Florey, Shannon, Burke, and Barris (AOTA, 1986). Over the years, Reilly's development of the occupational behavior model has provided a foundation for other perspectives in identifying the relationship between human occupational behavior and occupational therapy.

"A model of human occupation," originally published by Kielhofner and Burke in 1980, was based on Reilly's work. This earlier model was based on the postulate that human behavior is innate, spontaneous, and occurs because of an urge to explore and master the environment (AOTA, 1988; Kielhofner, 1985; Miller, 1993). In his most recent edition of *A model of human occupation: Theory and application*, Kielhofner (1995) revised his theoretical perspective of the human being, basing it on the general, dynamical, and open systems theories. This revised model continues to view the human as a system but as one that is complex and dynamic. The dynamical concept is based on the dynamical systems theory relative to the physical sciences. According to Kielhofner, the complexity and dynamical aspects of the human system are inherent in the system's ability to readily adjust to varying situations. The human system's ability to readily adjust is accomplished by creating a form of new energy to establish new order to one's life situation. Kielhofner (1995) refers to this process as self-organization through behavior. The model continues to incorporate the holistic approach to occupational dysfunction and involves synthesizing other theoretical approaches to address dysfunction and conceptual clinical reasoning.

The revised model maintains the view of the human system consisting of three subsystems that interact with the environment. These three subsystems make it possible for the human system to choose based on motivation, to organize, and to produce occupational behavior. Volition is the subsystem responsible for motivation, choices, and will. Habituation is the subsystem responsible for organizing behavior into patterns and routines. The mind-body-brain performance subsystem is responsible for the skills that produce behavior for interacting with the environment (Kielhofner, 1985). These three subsystems interact in a collaborative manner to influence occupational behavior.

The revised model's view of dysfunction is based on the inability of an individual to organize, choose, or perform what David Nelson refers to as occupational forms (Kielhofner, 1995). Occupational forms are the inherent aspects of a task that guide how an individual should perform. Occupational forms are *"rule-bound sequences of action which are at once coherent, oriented to a purpose, sustained in collective knowledge, culturally recognizable and named"* (Kielhofner, 1995, p. 102). Occupational dysfunction exists when an individual is unable to demonstrate behavior that would meet his or her own needs or the demands of the environment. A number of factors may influence occupational dysfunction, which can result in a negative effect on the structures of the human system, i.e., the volition, habituation, and mind-body-brain subsystems. Clinicians attempting to understand occupational dysfunction must determine the restrictions placed on each subsystem and the environment as a result of dysfunction and understand the collaborative effect on the human system.

Change in occupational behavior is the result of the interaction of the three subsystems with the environment. Change is initiated through the volition subsystem based on the client's motivation, sense of efficacy, interests, and values. Treatment is directed toward organizing occupational behavior so that adaptive functioning is restored, resulting in a balance between the individual's inner needs and the environmental requirements. Use of the model is not limited to a specific patient population (Kielhofner, 1995).

Assessment Instruments. Assessment of occupational status involves an interactive analysis of the three subsystems as well as environmental constraints. The assessment process involves the use of a collection of instruments to gather information on the patient's current occupational status, including occupational performance history data. Evaluation results are interpreted and synthesized to determine the client's current occupational status. Because of the constant interaction between the human system and the environment, collection and synthesis of assessment data are ongoing (Kielhofner, 1995).

Numerous psychosocial assessment tools are applicable to the model. Because of the assessment diversity, each performance component of occupational therapy uniform terminology can be addressed as indicated by the client's performance dysfunction (See Table 7–1). Additionally, observation of behavior during the assessment process provides necessary information about social interaction and self-management skills. Table 7–1 is based on Kielhofner's (1985) assessment "instrument library," which provides descriptive information on 64 instruments. In his instrument library, Kielhofner identifies the contents of each assessment tool, standardization information, applicable patient populations, and reference sources. Each assessment tool is matched to the components of the model of human occupation to assist the examiner in effective application of each instrument to the model. In the revised edition (1995), Kielhofner provides more recent and expanded assessment information for greater reinforcement and support of the model.

Assessment Tools and Research Data. The following is a partial collection of data on assessment tools commonly used under this model.

1. *Bay Area Functional Performance Evaluation (BaFPE)*: A task performance and observation rating scale used to evaluate daily living skills in areas of cognition, affect, and performance (Task-Oriented Assessment [TOA] Scale and Social Interaction Skills [SIS] Scale). The SIS is a rating scale used to assess patients' social behavior based on observation or self-report.

   Interrater reliability was determined through four pairs of occupational therapists, each of whom studied an individual group of 25 patients. The four patient groups were titled county inpatient mental health center, longer term; Veteran's Hospital, acute inpatient; private, for-profit acute psychiatric; and university-affiliated psychiatric, acute inpatient.

   Interrater reliability was determined for the TOA and the SIS. Correlations for the TOA are in excess of 0.90, with 80 percent of the correlations equaling or exceeding 0.80 in three of four test groups.

   Another reliability study investigated comparison of the correlations for items changed in the revised TOA with those in the original version. Findings revealed improvement in 10 of the original 16 scales on the TOA. Results also showed high correlations for the items added to the revised TOA. Finally, internal consistency among certain subscales within the TOA was studied. Findings revealed an average correlation of 0.60, with a range of 0.29 to 0.84.

   Interrater reliability correlations for the SIS are lower than those for the TOA, with a range of 0.76 to 0.79. To improve the validity of the SIS, five observation situations were substituted for those in the original version. With these substitutions, results revealed an increase in all correlations, including reliability (Asher, 1989; Kielhofner, 1985; Williams & Bloomer, 1987).

TABLE 7–1

PSYCHOSOCIAL ASSESSMENT INSTRUMENTS

Performance Components	Values	Interests	Self-concept	Role performance	Social conduct	Interpersonal skills	Self-expression	Coping skills	Time management	Self-control	Chronological	Developmental	Life cycle	Disability status	Physical	Social	Cultural
	1. PSYCHOLOGICAL			*2. SOCIAL*				*3. SELF-MANAGEMENT*			*A. TEMPORAL ASPECTS*				*B. ENVIRONMENT*		
Activity Questionnaire	X	X	X						X		X			X			
Adolescent Role Assessment	X			X					X		X	X				X	X
Bay Area Functional Performance Evaluation						X	X	X	X	X	X						
Behavior Setting Observations													X		X	X	X
Environmental Questionnaire								X							X	X	X
Expectancy Questionnaire	X																
Group Interaction Skills					X	X	X	X		X	X						
Hopelessness Scale			X					X			X						
Interest Checklist			X					X			X						
Internal-External Scale		X						X			X						
Leisure History Interview	X	X	X	X					X		X	X					
Leisure Satisfaction Scale	X							X			X						
Occupational Case Analysis Interview	X	X	X	X	X	X	X	X	X	X	X						
Occupational Functioning Tool	X	X	X	X	X	X	X	X	X	X	X						
Occupational Role History	X	X	X	X	X	X	X	X	X	X	X		X		X	X	
Paracheck Geriatric Rating Scale					X	X	X										
Pleasant Events Schedule		X						X									
Role Checklist	X			X				X			X						
Role Performance Scale				X	X	X	X	X	X		X		X				
Self-Attitude Questionnaire	X		X					X			X						
Self-Directed Search		X	X														
Self-Esteem Scale			X					X			X						
Social Climate Scale	X							X			X				X		
Time Reference Inventory	X							X			X	X					

Based on information from American Occupational Therapy Association. (1994). *Uniform terminology for occupational therapy. American Journal of Occupational Therapy, 48*(11), 1047–1059; In Kielhofner, G. (ed.) (1985) model of human occupation. Baltimore, MD; Williams & Wilkins.

In two separate studies by Mann and colleagues (1989) and Mann and Klyczek (1991), use of the BaFPE was effective in identifying deficits in the three component areas of cognition, performance, and affect. In the 1989 study, the authors presented normative data for the total TOA in the form of actual scores and "z" scores on 144 psychiatric inpatients. A significant difference was identified between patients evaluated within the first 14 days of admission and those evaluated after more than 14 days of hospitalization. A table of standard scores that resulted from the study allows the clinician to compare information acquired on recently tested patients with the normative data provided by Mann and associates (1989). Data comparison may reveal a need for or a lack of treatment in a certain component area.

In the study by Mann and Klyczek (1991), results from the 1989 study were used to determine normative data for 266 psychiatric inpatients. Study results revealed standard scores for cognitive, performance, and affective components for each task; each parameter of the cognitive, performance, and affective components; and each total task summary score. Standard scores were presented in table form for comparing and reporting results of testing patients. Data comparison may reveal a need for treatment in either a component area or in a specific parameter. In summary, Mann and coworkers (1989) and Mann and Klyczek (1991) concluded that the BaFPE is a valid tool to be used in identifying performance difficulties of psychiatric inpatients. They further suggest that for best results, clinicians should establish local norms and standard scores for comparison based on test results from their own inpatient environment.

The BaFPE is available through Maddak, Inc., Pequannock, NJ.

2. *Occupational Case Analysis Interview and Rating Scale (OCAIRS)*: A semistructured interview and rating scale designed for data gathering, analysis, and reporting a client's occupational adaptation. Results of the interrater reliability study revealed 57 percent of the components with correlation coefficients ranging between 0.50 and 0.80; 36 percent had lower than 0.50, and 7 percent had in excess of 0.80 (Kaplan & Kielhofner, 1989).

Investigation of content validity revealed 81.8 percent to 100 percent correct matches between the interview questions and 9 of the 11 model components (Kielhofner, 1985).

The OCAIRS is available through the Model of Human Occupation Clearinghouse, Department of Occupational Therapy, M/C 811, University of Illinois at Chicago.

3. *Role Checklist*: A self-report checklist for adult psychiatric patients designed to assess productive roles in life by indicating their perception of their past, present, and future roles. Reliability is based on percent agreement and kappa measure of agreement on categorical responses between the test and retest. Findings were based on 124 nondisabled adults ranging from 18 to 79 years of age. Results were as follows (Asher, 1989; Kielhofner, 1985, 1995; Oakley et al., 1986):

a. Individual roles for a given time category—kappa estimates ranged from slight to near perfect agreement. Percent agreement was 73 to 97, with an average of 88 percent.

b. Each role over three time categories—kappa estimates ranged from moderate to substantial. Percent agreement was 77 to 93, with an average of 87 percent.

c. Each time category for the 10 roles assessed— kappa estimates were substantial for present time and moderate for past and future. Percent agreement averaged 87 across time categories.

d. Age of subjects (two age groups) and time between test administration—kappa estimates were moderate to substantial. Percent agreement was 73 to 95.

e. Valuation of each role—kappa estimates were moderate. Percent agreement was 79.

f. Reportedly has content validity founded on literature review.

The Role Checklist is available through the Model of Human Occupation Clearinghouse.

4. *Self-Esteem Scale*: A self-report scale that measures feelings about oneself, abilities, and accomplishments. Primarily used with adolescents but has also had a history of use with elderly clients. Reliability based on Guttman scale, with correlations of 0.92 for reproducibility and 0.72 for scalability. Test-retest reliability was 0.85 (Asher, 1989; Kielhofner, 1985).

The Self-Esteem Scale is available through Princeton University Press, Princeton, NJ.

5. *Occupational Functioning Tool (renamed Assessment of Occupational Functioning, 1995)*: An interview and observation screening tool for assessing the three subsystems; volition, habituation, and performance. Primary use is with institutionalized clients. Standardization results were based on 49 institutionalized older adults. Reliability measures revealed interrater correlation coefficients of 0.48 to 0.65, with 0.78 as a total score. Test-retest coefficients ranged from 0.70 to 0.90 based on Pearson product-moment correlations (Kielhofner, 1985, 1995).

Criterion-related validity moderately supported by significant correlations of -0.42 to -0.84 when related to similar screening tools (Kielhofner, 1985, 1995).

The Assessment of Occupational Functioning is available through the Model of Human Occupation Clearing House.

6. *Assessment of Communication and Interaction Skills (ACIS)*: an observation assessment tool designed to measure social performance in personal communication and group interactions. Studies revealed (Kielhofner, 1995) modest interrater reliability, indicating a need for further refinement of the tool. Subsequent studies for construct validity, based on revision of the tool, revealed that the assessment items do form a single unidimensional scale (Kielhofner).

The ACIS is available through the Model of Human Occupation Clearinghouse.

7. *Fisher's Assessment of Motor and Process Skills (AMPS)*: An observation assessment tool designed to evaluate quality and effectiveness (not impairment) of motor and process performance skills while the individual performs IADL, e.g., meal preparation, driving (Kielhofner, 1995).

Studies support the reliability and validity of the AMPS. Construct validity, test internal consistency, score stability over time, and interrater reliability have all been supported (Kielhofner, 1995). A major advantage of the AMPS is that test task choice is available to the patients.

Administration of the AMPS requires formal training. Training is available through the AMPS Project, Occupational Therapy Building, Colorado State University, Fort Collins, CO.

INTERPERSONAL SKILLS AND EMOTIONAL BEHAVIOR

Interpersonal skills are defined as the ability to use verbal and nonverbal communication to interact with others in casual and formally sustained relationships in individual and group settings (AOTA, 1994; Mosey, 1986). Interpersonal skills involve both social interaction and emotional behavior. The ability to successfully interact in society and process emotions is perhaps the greatest challenge for humans. Social interaction and emotional control are psychosocial daily life tasks that are interwoven into major daily life tasks of work, school, leisure, and family relations, as well as numerous other routine activities (AOTA, 1994).

Interpersonal skill dysfunction results in an inability to effectively communicate and interact with others in various settings. Mosey (1986) describes the communication and interaction as processes that involve skills and abilities in initiating and responding to sustained verbal exchanges, assertiveness, expression of ideas and feelings, awareness of others' needs and feelings, compromise and negotiation, and the ability to take part in cooperative and competitive events. Assessment of interpersonal skill dysfunction should reflect the appropriate life task area(s) affected. Mosey (1986) identified two methods of assessing

social interaction: the Interpersonal Skill Survey and the Group Interaction Skill Survey. Both are used to collect data while observing clients in an evaluation group setting.

The *Interpersonal Skill Survey* is a six-item format of interaction and affective behaviors that are rated on a scale of 1 to 4. The rating results are followed by an interview process involving a discussion between the client and the therapist to review and clarify any discrepancies between the therapist's and the client's observations.

The *Group Interaction Skill Survey* is a format arranged according to group types: parallel, project, egocentric-cooperative, cooperative, and mature groups. The survey is used as a guide to determine the client's level of social interaction development. Scoring involves checking off behaviors exhibited by the client in the evaluation setting. The completion of the survey is followed by an interview process to highlight the client's successes and to discuss social interaction behaviors that may not have been mastered.

Mosey (1986) also provides the clinician with evaluation tools and guidelines to assess social interaction in life tasks for work, school, family relations, and play or leisure. Each survey lists behaviors typical to the life task area and can be utilized as a preassessment tool to record responses based on an interview with the client, family member, or caregiver, or the survey may be used as a guide in scoring observed behavior during evaluation or in simulated treatment situations.

Fidler addresses the evaluation of interpersonal skills in the context of a *Life-style Performance Profile* (AOTA, 1988). The profile identifies and organizes performance skills and deficits according to the client's sociocultural environment. The profile can also provide information on potential resources for improving skills and can identify factors that may interfere with skill development or progression. By creating a profile about the client's history of performance including all components and life task areas, a distinct pattern of behavior is revealed regarding social interaction in work, school, play or leisure, and family relationships.

Emotional behavior as defined by the AOTA's "Uniform terminology for occupational therapy" (1994) is self-management and includes coping skills and self-control. The ability to maintain emotional control when faced with stressful events depends on coping skills developed during childhood and carried forward into adulthood.

Theorists on emotional development agree that childhood is the point of origin; however, they disagree on the primary source of emotional behavior (Bee, 1985; Perry & Bussey, 1984). Bee (1985) identified three theoretical viewpoints on the development of emotional behavior: the *temperament theory* operates on the belief that emotional behavior is of a biologic origin and that individuals are born with certain characteristics that influence how they interact with the environment and how others may respond. The *psychoanalytic theorists* hypothesized that emotional behavior is influenced by the three personality structures:

the id, ego, and superego, or that emotional behavior is influenced by social demands that occurred throughout life in stages of development. Lastly, *social theorists* postulate that one's emotional behavior is learned through observation of modeled behaviors.

The occupational therapy evaluation and treatment process strongly supports the social theorist's position on learned behavior. Occupational therapy assessment of emotional behavior is typically performed as a component of an overall functional evaluation, i.e., observation of social interaction, frustration tolerance, problem solving, judgment, and overall coping relative to the productive use of defense mechanisms. The following are examples of assessment tools commonly used in determining an individual's emotional capability:

1. *AAMD Adaptive Behavior Scale*: Evaluation of the subject's effectiveness in coping with environmental demands through behavioral adaptation. Twenty-four areas of social and personal behavior are addressed. Reliability measures revealed interrater reliability correlations of 0.86 for part one (psychosocial, sensory-motor, and daily living skills) and 0.57 for part two (maladaptive behaviors, behavior disorders, and medication). (Developed by the American Association on Mental Deficiency, Washington DC; from Asher, 1989; Moyer, 1981.)

2. *Bay Area Functional Performance Evaluation (BaFPE)*: Includes the SIS, which rates behavior in seven parameters. Behavioral information can be acquired through an interview process with a caregiver or by actual observation of performance. Although the greatest emphasis is on social interaction, the seven-item scale also addresses related emotional aspects of behavior. Refer to the section on model of human occupation for research data related to the SIS. (Developed by Bloomer & Williams; from Maddak Inc., Pequannock, NJ.)

3. *Emotions Profile Index*: A brief, standardized personality test for adolescents and adults. The profile index provides information about various basic traits and conflicts. Literature search did not reveal research data on this index. (Developed by unknown source; from Moyer, 1981.)

4. *Functional Independence Measure (FIM)*: A seven-level scale assessment tool ranging from independent to dependent behavior that is designed to measure disability regardless of the actual diagnosis. The FIM measures self-care, sphincter control, mobility, locomotion, communication, and social cognition. Although the FIM is primarily designed to measure physical dysfunction, the psychosocial aspects related to patient treatment are also addressed by assessing social interaction skills relative to patient progress. Standardization measures were based on the use of the FIM by clinicians. Measures revealed an ANOVA correlation of 0.86 on patients admitted to rehabilitation services and 0.88 for those discharged from the service. Face validity was based on three areas: 88 percent did not have difficulty understanding the FIM, 97 percent believed there were no unnecessary items in the FIM, and 83 percent believed there was not a need for additional items. (Developed by The Center for Functional Assessment Research, State University of New York at Buffalo; from The Center for Functional Assessment Research, 1990.)

SUMMARY

This chapter is by no means conclusive regarding the psychosocial assessment tools available in occupational therapy. What has been provided is a manner in which the assessment process can be approached based on a chosen theoretical frame of reference. Interpersonal skills and emotional behavior have been addressed to identify their manifestation in the psychosocial assessment process in occupational therapy and to provide examples of instruments commonly used to determine the degree of dysfunction.

GLOSSARY

Cooperative group—A homogeneous non–task-oriented group whose aim is to promote sharing of thoughts and feelings and acceptance among its members.

Egocentric cooperative group—A task-oriented group whose aim is to promote self-esteem through activities that emphasize cooperation, competition, leadership, and other group roles.

Holistic—Relates to the "whole" and assumes the whole is greater than the sum of its parts. In occupational therapy, treating the whole of the patient, both the physical condition and the associated psychosocial situations.

Loose association—A type of thinking that is typical of schizophrenic patients in which they may ramble or freely express their thoughts during therapy.

Medical model—Patient treatment that is based on the nature of the disease and considers the disease to be a separate entity from the patient. Treatment does not consider the patient's functional capabilities.

Parallel group—An activity group in which interaction is not required.

Projective technique—A method of studying personality in which the individual is given an unstructured task that allows for a range of characteristic responses. The responses are interpreted or analyzed by the examiner.

Task analysis—A systematic process of identifying the complexity of task procedures step by step. Emphasis is placed on steps that the patient is unable to perform.

REFERENCES

Abreu, B. C., & Toglia, J. P. (1987). Cognitive rehabilitation: A model for occupational therapy. *American Journal of Occupational Therapy, 41*(7), 439–448.

Allen, C. K. (1987). Activity: Occupational therapy's treatment method, Eleanor Clarke Slagle lecture. *American Journal of Occupational Therapy, 41*(9), 563–575.

Allen, C. K. (1985). *Occupational therapy for psychiatric diseases: Measurement and management of cognitive disabilities.* Boston, MA: Little, Brown & Co.

Allen, C. K., & Allen, R. (1987). Cognitive disabilities: Measuring the social consequences of mental disorders. *Journal of Clinical Psychiatry, 48*(5), 185–190.

Allen, C. K., Earhart, C., & Blue, T. (1992). *Occupational therapy treatment goals for the physically and cognitively disabled.* Bethesda, MD: The American Occupational Therapy Association.

Allen, C. K., & Reyner, A. (1991). *How to start using the cognitive levels.* Colchester, CT: S & S Worldwide.

American Occupational Therapy Association. (1988). *FOCUS: Skills for assessment and treatment in mental health.* Rockville, MD: American Occupational Therapy Association.

American Occupational Therapy Association. (1986). *SCOPE: Strategies, concept, and opportunities for program development and evaluation in mental health.* Rockville, MD: American Occupational Therapy Association.

American Occupational Therapy Association. (1994). Uniform terminology for occupational therapy. *American Journal of Occupational Therapy, 48*(11), 1047–1059.

Anastasi, A. (1971). *Psychological assessment.* New York: Macmillan.

Asher, I. E. (1989). *The annotated index of occupational therapy evaluation tools.* Bethesda, MD: American Occupational Therapy Association.

Backman, C. (1994). Assessment of self-care skills. In C. Christiansen (Ed.), *Ways of living* (1st ed.) (pp. 51–75). Bethesda, MD: American Occupational Therapy Association.

Bee, H. (1985). *The developing child* (4th ed.). New York: Harper & Row.

Bootzin, R., Accoella, J., & Alloy, L. (1993). *Abnormal psychology: Current perspectives.* New York: McGraw-Hill.

Bruce, M. A., & Borg, B. (1987). *Frames of reference in psychosocial occupational therapy.* Thorofare, NJ: Slack, Inc.

Buck, R., & Provancher, M. A. . (1972). Magazine picture collages as an evaluative technique. *American Journal of Occupational Therapy, 26*(1), 36–39.

Center for Functional Assessment Research. (1990). *Guide for use of the uniform data set for medical rehabilitation including the functional independence measure (FIM).* Buffalo, NY: State University of New York at Buffalo.

Earhart, C., Allen, C. K., & Blue, T. (1993). *Allen diagnostic module.* Colchester, CT: S & S Worldwide.

Fidler, G. (1982). The lifestyle performance profile: An organizing frame. In B. Hemphill (Ed.), *The evaluation process in psychiatric occupational therapy.* Thorofare, NJ: Slack, Inc.

Fidler, G., & Fidler, J. (1954). *Introduction to psychiatric occupational therapy.* New York: Macmillan.

Fidler, G., & Fidler, J. (1963). *Occupational therapy: A communication process in psychiatry.* New York: Macmillan.

Gallatin, J. (1982). *Abnormal psychology: Concepts, issues, trends.* New York: Macmillan.

Hemphill, B. J. (1982). *The evaluative process in psychiatric occupational therapy.* Thorofare, NJ: Slack, Inc.

Hopkins, H., & Smith, H. (1993). *Willard and Spackman's occupational therapy.* Philadelphia, PA: J. B. Lippincott.

Kaplan, K., & Kielhofner, G. (Eds.). (1989). *Occupational case analysis interview and rating scale.* Thorofare, NJ: Slack, Inc.

Kielhofner, G. (Ed.). (1985). *A model of human occupation.* Baltimore, MD: Williams & Wilkins.

Kielhofner, G. (Ed.). (1995). *A model of human occupation* (2nd ed.). Baltimore, MD: Williams & Wilkins.

Kielhofner, G., & Burke, J. (1980). A model of human occupation, part one. Conceptual framework and content. *American Journal of Occupational Therapy, 34*(9), 572–581.

Lerner, C., & Ross, G. (1977). The magazine picture collage: Development of an objective scoring system. *American Journal of Occupational Therapy, 31*(3), 156–161.

Levy, L. (1993). Cognitive disability frame of reference. In H. Hopkins & H. Smith (Eds.), *Willard and Spackman's occupational therapy* (8th ed.) (pp. 67–71). Philadelphia, PA: J. B. Lippincott.

Mann, W. C., & Klyczek, J. P. (1991). Standard scores for the Bay Area Functional Performance Evaluation Task Oriented Assessment. *Occupational Therapy in Mental Health, 11*(1), 13–24.

Mann, W. C., Klyczek, J. P., & Fiedler, R. C. (1989). Bay Area Functional Performance Evaluation (BaFPE): Standard scores. *Occupational Therapy in Mental Health, 9*(3), 1–7.

Mears, F., & Gratchel, R. J. (1979). *Fundamentals of abnormal psychology.* Chicago, IL: Rand McNally.

Miller, R. (1993). Gary Kielhofner. In R. Miller & K. Walker (Eds.), *Perspectives on theory for the practice of occupational therapy* (pp. 179–218). Gaithersburg, MD: Aspen Publications.

Mosey, A. C. (1973). *Activities therapy.* New York, NY: Raven Press.

Mosey, A. C. (1986). *Psychosocial components of occupational therapy.* New York, NY: Raven Press.

Mosey, A. C. (1970). *Three frames of reference for mental health.* Thorofare, NJ: Slack, Inc.

Moyer, E. (1981). *Index of assessments used by occupational therapists in mental health.* Birmingham, AL: University of Alabama.

Oakley, F., Kielhofner, G., Barris, R., & Reichler, R. K. (1986). The role checklist: Development and empirical assess of reliability. *The Occupational Therapy Journal of Research, 6*(3), 157–170.

Perry, D. G., & Bussey, K. (1984). *Social development.* Englewood, CA: Prentice-Hall.

Reilly, M. (1962). Occupational therapy can be one of the great ideas of twentieth century medicine. The Eleanor Clarke Slagle lecture. *The American Journal of Occupational Therapy 16,* 1–9.

Shoemyen, C. W. (1970). Occupational therapy orientation and evaluation: A study of procedure and media. *American Journal of Occupational Therapy, 24*(4), 276–279.

Smith, H. D. (1993). Assessment and evaluation: Overview. In H. Hopkins & H. Smith (Eds.), *Willard & Spackman's occupational therapy* (pp. 169–191). Philadelphia, PA: J. B. Lippincott.

Williams, S. L., & Bloomer, J. (1987). *Bay Area Functional Performance Evaluation (BaFPE).* Pequannock, NJ: Maddak, Inc.

CHAPTER 8

Body Image

Julia Van Deusen, PhD, OTR/L, FAOTA

SUMMARY In this chapter, I discuss assessment of body image disturbance of adult patients likely to be evaluated by occupational or physical therapists in a rehabilitation setting. Three models related to assessments are described. Body image assessment is pertinent to intervention for patients with neurologic disorders, acute dismemberment, other kinds of physical impairment, and some psychiatric diagnoses. Two illustrative case reports are given. I discuss the instrumentation for body image disturbances in which neural scheme disturbance is primary and for body image disturbances in which the psychological representation is the dominant disturbance. The validity and reliability of the various instruments are documented.

The construct of body image is a complex one (Cash & Pruzinsky, 1990; Tiemersma, 1989). It incorporates both the neural body scheme, which is subject to disturbance from lesions, and its psychological representation formed through cultural and environmental input, also subject to disturbance. This latter aspect of body image includes a perceptual component involving estimation of the real body shape and size, as well as its attitudinal aspect pertaining to knowledge of and feelings about the body. Of particular importance to occupational therapy and to physical therapy is the notion that our body image incorporates images of the function of the body and its parts necessary for skilled performance, images dependent on both its psychological and physical components (Cash & Pruzinsky, 1990; Keeton et al., 1990). A social aspect to the body image also exists and is researched by addressing subjects' ideal body image (Fallon & Rozin, 1985; Keeton et al., 1990). It is assumed that the ideal body image is based on cultural influences.

Since body image is complex and many faceted, it logically follows that disturbances are diverse. Body image disturbance refers to problems in the integration of the neural body scheme and its psychosocial representation.

Problems can result from neural lesions, which result in bodily inattention, or in misperception of body shape, size, or relationships. They can result from actual physical bodily impairments such as loss of a limb, or from psychosocial influences affecting the mental representation of some aspect of the body. Body image is a holistic construct and seldom is encountered without psychological and physical manifestations. Consequently, assessment of body image has been addressed by both neurology and psychology. Because of their relation to these disciplines, applied fields such as occupational therapy have also been concerned with body image instrumentation. Typically, several instruments addressing the many aspects of body image are needed for adequate assessment (Butters & Cash, 1987; Lacey & Birtchnell, 1986; Thompson, 1990; Van Deusen, 1993).

HISTORY

According to Tiemersma (1989), body image is a very old construct. The notion of body image extends back to

159

ancient and medieval times, and actual medical records of body image phenomena date from the 16th century. In clinical neurology during the first part of the 20th century, the notion was elaborated and popularized through the works of Head and Schilder (cited in Tiemersma, 1989). Head defined the neural body scheme as a dynamic schema resulting from past postures and movements. Schilder emphasized the mental image from psychosocial and psychoanalytic perspectives.

Following the period of classical definition of body scheme in clinical neurology, interest in this area declined until the introduction of assessment tools by psychologists in the 1950s. This was the time of development of body image projective tests and attitude scales and the refinement of neurologic evaluation.

Although body image concepts were compatible early in the century with those of Gestalt psychology, the midcentury work of Fisher and Cleveland (cited in Tiemersma, 1989) was the first major body image research from the field of psychology. Their primary work, in which body boundary relationships were focal, was strongly influenced by the psychoanalytic theorists. Assessment was through projective technique (Fisher, 1990). However, Fisher recently advocated the multidimensional complexity of the body image construct, necessitating a diversity of measuring tools. His explanation of the vast amount of body image research in psychology over the decades was that "Human identity cannot be separated from its somatic headquarters in the world. How persons feel about their somatic base takes on mediating significance in most situations" (p. 18).

During the 1970s, interest in body image research temporarily declined for a number of reasons, such as the nebulousness of its definition and incompatibility with popular theoretical positions. The widespread concern about anorexia nervosa brought a resurgence of body image research by the late 1970s and 1980s. This was a period in which body image test development flourished (Thompson, 1990).

In the current era, deliberate attempts have been made to integrate approaches from neurology and psychology (Lautenbacher et al., 1993; Tiemersma, 1989). Body image authority, Thompson, writing in 1990, predicted ". . . an expanding role into the 1990s for the researcher and clinician interested in the assessment . . . of body image disturbance" (p. xiv). Appropriately, at the present time, the creation of new tests has declined, but refinement of old tests has not.

BODY IMAGE MODELS

Many theories concerning body image exist (Tiemersma, 1989; Thompson, 1990). Several theoretical positions are of particular relevance to assessment in occupational therapy and physical therapy. The neurophysiologic explanation of body scheme is fundamental to assessment for body image disturbances associated with neural lesions. The sociocultural model and the schema model in cognitive psychology can be useful guides to assessment procedures for body image disturbance related to problems with mental representation.

Neurophysiologic Theory

Tiemersma (1989) described a neurophysiologic explanation for body scheme. The Finger Localization Test (Benton et al., 1994) and the Behavioural Inattention Test (BIT) (Wilson et al., 1987a) are sample assessments related to neurophysiologic theory. According to Tiemersma (1989), the muscle spindles, tendon organs, joint, and cutaneous receptors are the sensory receptors of particular importance to the body scheme. Information from these receptors is transmitted by means of afferent tracts to the somatic sensory association area of the parietal cortex, a primary site for body scheme function. The brain has many somatosensory maps, each specialized for a specific modality, such as joint position. Somatosensory processing is by means of a complex network within the central nervous system, which is considered very plastic since damage to the nervous system results in much cortical reorganization. From this perspective, body scheme can be viewed as the function of patterns of excitation in the brain. The limbic system is associated with affective aspects of body image, and the motor system with images of bodily performance. Although he has described body scheme in terms of neuroscience, Tiemersma's position on body image is by no means limited to this domain.

The position of Lautenbacher and colleagues (1993) is not inconsistent with that of Tiemersma (1989). These authors believe there is strong agreement that the mental representative of the body is dependent on the integration of sensory stimuli. The first stage of central nervous system processing (in sensory cortical areas) results in many body schemes, schemes that can be affected by disturbances in sensory input. If the discrepancy among these multischemes is not too great, they become integrated (in the temporal lobes) into one "body self." Like Tiemersma, Lautenbacher and associates consider the body self plastic and integration subject to cognitive and affective influences. Final integration of the body self is dependent on the activity of widespread cortical and subcortical areas.

Sociocultural Model

Many authors, including Cash and Pruzinsky (1990), Lacey and Birtchnell (1986), and Van Deusen (1993), have recognized the influence of culture on body image. However, Thompson (1990) emphasized the importance of the sociocultural body image model. Inherent in the sociocultural model is the assumption that current societal standards are the major factor relating to body image disturbance. Propositions of this model include the following for our society:

1. Physical attractiveness is highly valued
2. Thinness equals beauty, and obesity is negatively valued
3. Beauty equals goodness so that thinness is also equated with goodness
4. Society encourages women's preoccupation with the pursuit of beauty
5. Society reinforces the bodily alteration of women to enhance society's notion of beauty
6. A build emphasizing upper extremity musculature is the ideal masculine body
7. Men show less body image disturbance than do women

Assessments relating to this sociocultural model include those dealing with ideal size and shape relative to the personally known or felt body image. An example of this kind of instrument is the Body Image Assessment developed by Williamson (1990).

Model From Psychology

Another model of theoretical interest for assessment of body image disturbance is the schema organization in cognitive psychology, especially when integrated with the ecologic perspective. In general, it is agreed that schemata are cognitive structures that organize prior, guide new, and retrieve stored information (Safran & Greenberg, 1986). Paradoxically, with the advent of cognitive psychology in the 1970s, body image research decreased (Tiemersma, 1989). Probable contributing factors were the close ties of body image research with the gestalt and psychoanalytic views of psychology.

However, the schema model in cognitive psychology derives quite basically from the body image writings of Sir Henry Head, which influenced the ideas about schema elaborated by Bartlett, by Piaget, and by Neisser (Safran & Greenberg, 1986; Tiemersma, 1989). Furthermore, it has at least a limited theoretical link with cognitive behavioral therapy, a major current treatment approach for body image disturbances (Butters & Cash, 1987; Freedman, 1990; Van Deusen, 1993).

Safran and Greenberg (1986) believe that the work of Neisser in particular integrates the two positions in cognitive psychology with value for therapy. According to their perspective, Neisser combined the best of the information processing position, the idea of schemata, with the ecologic position, which emphasizes environmental interaction. Neisser maintained that we both act on and are acted on by the environment. Because of this action, internal schemata experience ongoing revision. The Feelings of Fatness Questionnaire (FOFQ) (Roth & Armstrong, 1993) is a particularly good example of an assessment tool congruent with this theoretical perspective.

KINDS OF BODY IMAGE DISTURBANCES

Lacey and Birtchnell (1986) have categorized body image disturbances into four groups: 1) those due to neurologic disorder, 2) those following acute dismemberment, 3) those associated with actual physical problems, and 4) those accompanying psychiatric diagnosis and without physical disability. Van Deusen (1993) used these groups to organize body image disturbances likely to be encountered in patients treated by rehabilitation specialists. Although assessment tools may be useful for more than one type of disturbance, often instruments have data related to only one category.

Neurologic Disorder

Lesions of the central nervous system leading to impaired neurologic function can disturb the body scheme. Under these conditions, psychosocial factors may add to the body image disturbance beyond that from the neurologically impaired scheme. Cumming (1988) described the various body scheme disturbances from neurologic disorders. Many problems have been observed, including 1) denial of paralysis or paresis of the involved limbs, 2) inability to identify body parts or relationships, 3) a special condition of inability to identify parts, namely finger agnosia, 4) inability to distinguish right from left on one's own body or on a confronting body, 5) disturbed use of body parts, particularly in writing, 6) perception of body parts as abnormally large or small, 7) inability to identify the area of body part touched, 8) inattention to the stimulated body side contralateral to the brain lesion, 9) extinction of stimuli to the involved side when simultaneously administered to the uninvolved side, and 10) inability to use body parts to address the hemispace contralateral to the side of brain lesion.

Patients treated in rehabilitation facilities who may have one or more of these neurologic body scheme disorders are those challenged by stroke, by traumatic head injury, by substance abuse, by brain tumor, or by other pathologic conditions affecting the central nervous system. Both psychologists and neurologists have developed many instruments for assessment of body image disturbances in this category (Van Deusen, 1993).

Acute Dismemberment

This category of body scheme disorders includes those patients who experience the phantom phenomena following amputation of a body part. The temporary phantom sensation of the missing part is almost universal after adult limb loss. Phantom sensation is attributable to continued existence of the neurologic scheme after loss of the actual physical part. Because of interactions of central nervous system mechanisms and loss of the sensory receptors of the missing part, phantom pain may occur but, as yet, is not fully understood. A logical estimate is that more than 60% of adults experience phantom pain following limb amputation. Although phantom sensation may actually aid rehabilitation by providing the trainee with a complete body perception, phantom pain must be considered a disturbance of body image that can greatly interfere with performance. Phantom pain can also occur after breast surgery or spinal cord injury but has not been as extensively studied as for limbs. Phantom pain can be assessed in rehabilitation settings by use of instruments designed to evaluate chronic pain in relation to functional activity (Van Deusen, 1993).

Actual Physical Problem

Adults who are challenged by physical disabilities such as burns or rheumatoid arthritis may be susceptible to body image disturbances. Persons in this category may be basically well adjusted, but because of unfavorable societal input can suffer body image disturbances in the process of adjusting their image to their new physical reality. The body image disturbance in this category is secondary to the physical problem (Lacey & Birtchnell, 1986). Attitudinal body image assessment is necessary for this category of disturbances since disturbances would be in the psychological representative aspect of the body image.

Psychiatric Diagnosis

Body image disturbances are a condition of many psychiatric diagnoses and problems. Persons with disturbances in this category have no visible physical problem to account for the body image disturbance.

Disturbances vary widely from that of the person with a normal nose insisting on surgery to correct the deformity to the major body image distortions of the person challenged by schizophrenia (Lacey & Birtchnell, 1986). Although many disturbances in this category are seldom encountered by occupational and physical therapists, some, such as the attitudinal body image problem of the youth with bulimia nervosa, may be seen. Others may be encountered by occupational therapists in psychiatric settings where assessment would involve projective techniques or psychiatric interviews, making it beyond the scope of this chapter. Assessment for this category involves instrumentation addressing the psychological representation of the body image.

Illustrative Cases

Occupational therapists and physical therapists seldom address intervention only for body image disturbances. Rather, enhanced or improved body image is one of a complex of rehabilitation goals. The illustrative case reports presented here are hypothetical, particularly in that they address only one facet of the total assessment process in the rehabilitation setting. An example is given for a patient requiring body image assessment for neural scheme disturbance and for a patient requiring body image assessment for disturbance of psychological representation.

Neurologic Disorder: Neural Scheme Disturbance. Mrs. B. is a 52-year-old African-American homemanager married to an executive in Pasadena, California. She is a right hemisphere stroke survivor with mild hemiparesis of her left upper and lower extremities. Mrs. B. is in the rehabilitation unit being assessed by the occupational therapist, the physical therapist, and the language pathologist. The language pathologist has found no speech impairment. While evaluating Mrs. B.'s status in activities of daily living (ADL), the therapists found her unable to respond to stimuli presented to her left. The BIT (described in the Instrumentation section) was administered, and scores confirmed the presence of severe left side neglect. Major objectives incorporated into Mrs. B.'s rehabilitation programming were for enhanced left body side awareness and for improved function with objects to her left. Although Mrs. B. anticipates being able to afford weekly assistance with her home chores when discharged, improved body scheme is vital for her return to her full role as a homemanager in a conservative residential setting.

Physical Problem: Disturbance of Psychological Representation. J. T. is a 23-year-old white man severely burned in a camping accident. The involved areas include most of the shoulder and neck area and lower face. He has undergone two surgeries as well as rehabilitation at a well-known institution. His girlfriend of 2 years became involved with another man a month after J. T.'s accident. His parents are divorced. He lives with his mother, who is a waitress at a local chain restaurant, and J. T. has essentially no contact with his father. He was enrolled in general education courses at the community college at the time of his accident. Since his discharge from the rehabilitation center, J. T. has been unwilling to resume college work. He applied for two retail sales positions and was rejected. He has recently been admitted to a work hardening program for assessment by occupational therapy and physical therapy. The initial impression of the therapists was that J. T. has the physical capacity for many kinds of employment. Several sarcastic comments by J. T. about his appearance led to administration of an attitudinal body image self-report questionnaire. Results indicated severe body image disturbance. The therapists recommended a psychological consultation since J. T.'s body image problem was apparently a major hindrance to employment.

INSTRUMENTATION

Because of its many facets, innumerable instruments for assessing body image are described in the literature. Many of these tools are appropriate for use by rehabilitation personnel for assessing body image dysfunction. Others are better used as research instruments. Furthermore, the various instruments can be categorized as to whether they are primarily used to assess disturbances of the neural scheme or to assess disturbances in the psychological representation component of the body image. I have necessarily had to limit the number of instruments discussed and have categorized those selected under their function relative to the neural scheme or psychological representation. My selections were based on the desire to 1) provide examples of the different kinds of tools available (e.g., self-report questionnaires, size estimation techniques), 2) include instruments suitable for clinical intervention and for research purposes, 3) include samples of instruments for assessment of all four categories of body image disturbance, and 4) provide information on those tools that my literature review showed to be best researched. In addition, I have provided some examples of the more recent, innovative instruments that hold promise for future development.

From a practical point of view, it must be understood that much overlap in assessment occurs. Clear-cut categorization by function is not always possible. A tool or technique may be designed to ascertain presence of a neural body scheme deficit but ultimately be more useful for assessment of a psychological disturbance. An example is the size estimation technique widely used for perceptual body image research in anorexia nervosa studies. Directions requesting responses of how subjects feel about their bodies or comparison of actual image with their ideal have differentiated subjects with eating disorders from those without, although both groups have been found to overestimate their size (Keeton et al., 1990; Van Deusen, 1993).

Neural Scheme Disturbances

Disturbances of the neural body scheme were traditionally evaluated by neurologists and psychiatrists by means of interviews or clinical observations. This tradition was incorporated into occupational therapy assessment procedures (Zoltan et al., 1986) and is widely in use today, despite the availability of standardized instruments. Some clinicians prefer the flexibility of patient assessment allowed by nonstandardized tools and appreciate such practical advantages as low cost.

From those standardized or semistandardized instruments discussed in the literature and appropriately used by occupational therapists and physical therapists, I have

selected four to represent those available for assessment of body image disturbances associated with disruption of the central nervous system scheme. Assessments are for the categories of neurologic disorder and acute dismemberment. I have also included a computerized tool that deserves further research. These instruments are

1. Right-Left Orientation Test (Benton et al., 1994)
2. Finger Localization Test (Benton et al., 1994)
3. BIT (Wilson et al., 1987a)
4. Pain Disability Index (Pollard, 1984).
5. Computerized Test of Visual Neglect and Extinction (Anton et al., 1988)

Right-Left Orientation Test. Among the tests for neuropsychological assessment developed by Arthur Benton and his colleagues is the Right-Left Orientation Test (Benton et al., 1994). There are four forms of this test, the original form (A), a "mirror image" version (B) for use as an alternate form, and forms R and L, designed for use with patients unable to use their right or left hands. Form R is shown in Figure 8–1. Performance on this 5-minute test requires verbal comprehension and slight motor skill as well as the spatial-symbolic aspects of right-left discrimination it is designed to evaluate. Items included to assess the hierarchical skills in right-left orientation are orientation toward one's own body (lowest on hierarchy), orientation toward a confronting person, and orientation toward one's own body combined with a confronting person.

Normative data are available from 126 men and 108 women without brain disease and from 94 adults with brain disease (Benton et al., 1994). Various problems in right-left disorientation can thus be identified from the standard administration of this test. Data are provided that define a generalized defect, a confronting person defect, and an own body defect. If systematic reversal occurs (all left when it should be right), it is assumed that right-left orientation is intact but the person is confused with verbal labels, as might be the case with patients challenged by aphasia.

I found no reliability data on this specific measure of right-left orientation. However, Baum obtained an interrater reliability coefficient of $r = 0.94$ for a similar instrument used with adults having had head injury (cited by Zoltan et al., 1986). Also, some evidence of construct validity was found. An early version of Benton's Right-Left Orientation Test (Sauguet et al., 1971) as well as the current test (Benton et al., 1994) discriminated aphasic from nonaphasic persons in respect to orientation to one's own body. Benton and collaborators believe that right-left orientation has symbolic as well as spatial determinants. A case study of Gerstmann syndrome (Mazzoni et al., 1990) also supported the construct validity of this test. This complex of dyscalculia, dysgraphia, right-left disorientation, and finger agnosia was shown to be present in a patient with a very proscribed area of cerebral trauma. Although the specific items of Benton's test for right-left orientation were apparently not used, the instrument

RIGHT-LEFT ORIENTATION, FORM R

(For use with patients who cannot execute commands with the right hand)

Name _____ No. _____ Date _____

Age _____ Sex _____ Education _____ Handedness _____ Examiner _____

Own Body	Response	Score
1. Show me your <u>left</u> hand.	_____	+ – R
2. Show me your <u>right</u> eye.	_____	+ – R
3. Show me your <u>left</u> ear.	_____	+ – R
4. Show me your <u>right</u> hand.	_____	+ – R
5. Touch your <u>left</u> ear with your <u>left</u> hand.	_____	+ – R
6. Touch your <u>right</u> eye with your <u>left</u> hand.	_____	+ – R
7. Touch your <u>right</u> knee with your <u>left</u> hand.	_____	+ – R
8. Touch your <u>left</u> eye with your <u>left</u> hand.	_____	+ – R
9. Touch your <u>right</u> ear with your <u>left</u> hand.	_____	+ – R
10. Touch your <u>left</u> knee with your <u>left</u> hand.	_____	+ – R
11. Touch your <u>right</u> ear with your <u>left</u> hand.	_____	+ – R
12. Touch your <u>left</u> eye with your <u>left</u> hand.	_____	+ – R
	SUM _____	

Examiner's Body	Response	Score
13. Point to my <u>right</u> eye.	_____	+ – R
14. Point to my <u>left</u> leg.	_____	+ – R
15. Point to my <u>left</u> ear.	_____	+ – R
16. Point to my <u>right</u> hand.	_____	+ – R
17. Put your <u>left</u> hand on my <u>left</u> ear.	_____	+ – R
18. Put your <u>left</u> hand on my <u>left</u> eye.	_____	+ – R
19. Put your <u>left</u> hand on my <u>right</u> shoulder.	_____	+ – R
20. Put your <u>left</u> hand on my <u>right</u> eye.	_____	+ – R
	SUM _____	

Performance Pattern

A. Normal   _____   Total Score _____
B. Generalized Defect   _____   Reversal Score _____
C. "Confronting Person" Defect   _____   Comments: _____
D. Specific "Own Body" Defect   _____   _____
E. Systematic Reversal   _____

FIGURE 8–1. Right-left orientation test, Form R for persons unable to use their right hand. (From Benton, A. L., deS. Hamsher, K., Varney, N. R., & Spreen, O. CONTRIBUTIONS TO NEUROPSYCHOLOGICAL ASSESSMENT. Copyright ©1983 by Oxford University Press, Inc.)

defining this construct in the reported case followed Benton's hierarchy and used similar items. Benton and associates (1994) cited a study showing small but significant relationships between right-left orientation scores and the pertinent variables of brain atrophy, EEG slowing, and educational background. Finally, construct validity was further supported by Fischer and colleagues (1990). These researchers showed that the "confronting" items on the Right-Left Orientation Test discriminated persons with dementia of the Alzheimer type at all stages not only from control subjects but also from persons with multiinfarct dementia. Scores for visuospatial dysfunction and aphasia did not differentiate these groups. An abbreviated version of the Right-Left Orientation Test was used because of the age of the subjects. Further research is needed for documentation of the reliability and validity of Benton's test of right-left orientation. Particularly, the relationship between right-left orientation and task performance must be determined to support the use of the Right-Left Orientation Test in rehabilitation assessment.

Finger Localization Test. A second test designed by Benton and colleagues (Benton & Sivan, 1993; Benton et al., 1994) pertinent to an aspect of the body scheme is that for the localization of fingers to assess finger agnosia. Again, verbal comprehension and a slight amount of motor skill are required to perform. This test is in three parts graded as to ease of localization. Tasks require localization of single fingers with vision and then without vision, followed by localization of pairs. Depending on the patient's choice, responses can be made by verbal name or finger number or by pointing to a finger on a drawing. Normative data were collected from 104 hospitalized patients aged 16 to 65 years with no history of psychiatric or brain disease. Data also were obtained from 61 patients with brain disease (Benton et al., 1994). From the normative data, several problems in finger localization were defined from those scores outside the total score limits, outside single hand score limits, and outside the difference score between hands. Borderline scores were also recorded.

I could not locate any report of reliability studies with Benton's Finger Localization Test. However, evidence of its construct validity suggests that it must measure in a consistent manner. On an early version of this test, controls made no errors and response mode was only nonverbal. This test discriminated between persons with and without aphasia (Sauguet et al., 1971).

When vision was not used, Benton's Finger Localization Test discriminated between subjects with brain disease and control subjects (Benton et al., 1994). The case reported by Mazzoni and coworkers (1990), which I discussed in relation to right-left orientation, also supported the construct validity of the Benton test of finger localization.

I found no study relating scores on Benton's Finger Localization Test with those from tests of ADL or occupational performance, although occupational therapists have suggested that finger agnosia is related to poor dexterity for activities requiring finger movements in relation to each other (Zoltan et al., 1986). It would be of interest to research the Finger Localization Test in this respect and to obtain other data to further verify its reliability and validity.

Behavioural Inattention Test. The BIT (Wilson et al., 1987a, 1987b) was designed in England as a measure of unilateral visual neglect (UN). According to Heilman and collaborators (1985), the neglect syndrome includes both lack of intention to act in the space contralateral to the site of the brain lesion and inattention to sensory input to the body side contralateral to the site of the lesion. The BIT addresses the former aspect of the neglect syndrome and is concerned with the body function aspect of body image rather than identification of the body parts. Tests such as that by MacDonald (1960) have long been used by occupational therapists to identify patient problems with body part recognition, including those resulting from inattention to sensory input to a body side.

The BIT has changed through the usual developmental process involved in test construction, and the current version (Wilson et al., 1987a) is distributed in the United States. The unique feature of the BIT is that it includes ADL tasks. The intent of these ADL behavioral subtests is to increase the tester's understanding of the specific daily living problems of a patient with unilateral neglect toward more effective rehabilitation procedures. Content validity was sought by having these behavioral tasks selected by occupational therapists and psychologists who understood the daily living problems of patients challenged by unilateral neglect (Stone et al., 1987; Wilson et al., 1987a). Initially, the criterion-related validity of these ADL subtests as measures of neglect was estimated by correlation with scores from six conventional tests of UN. Except for a line bisection test, coefficients ranged from $r = 0.59$ to 0.87. The current test manual (Wilson et al., 1987a) gives a coefficient of $r = 0.67$ for the relation between questionnaire responses by patient therapists and the scores of patients on the ADL subtests. Estimates of reliability were also acceptable for these ADL subtests, with alternate form reported as $r = 0.83$ and 100% agreement between two raters (Wilson et al., 1987b). The current version of this test (Wilson et al., 1987a) has the following nine behavioral (ADL) subtests:

Picture scanning, in which subjects identify daily living items in three color photographs, and omissions are scored

Telephone dialing, in which the task is to dial a disconnected telephone

Menu reading, in which a menu is opened and items are read (or pointed to) and omissions scored

Article reading, in which a short newspaper article is read aloud and errors scored; this subtest is not given to language-impaired persons

Telling and setting time, in which the time is read from a digital and an analogue clock, and the time is set on the analogue clock

Coin sorting, in which 18 coins are prearranged and must be pointed out when named by the tester

Address and sentence copying, in which an address and a sentence are copied

Map navigation, in which three sets of sequential directions are traced with a finger on a maplike item

Card sorting, in which the person points to a selection of playing cards as named by the tester

Test materials are presented opposite the subject's midline, and, although other errors may be noted for further investigation, only errors of omission are scored.

In addition to the ADL behavioral subtests, the BIT has six simple pencil and paper conventional subtests of UN: line crossing, letter cancellation, star cancellation, figure and shape copying, line bisection, and representational drawing. According to the test authors (Wilson et al., 1987a), these subtests may be used to diagnose the presence or absence of unilateral neglect. Small and Ellis (1994) found these six subtests of the BIT discriminated between their control subjects and a patient group with dual diagnoses of anosognosia and visuospatial neglect. A principal components analysis clearly showed that these six conventional subtests were contributing to the same construct, defined as visual neglect. The star cancellation was the most sensitive measure of the six subtests (Halligan et al., 1989). In a New Zealand study (Marsh & Kersel, 1993), 13 subjects were found to have visual neglect when assessed with the line crossing and star cancellation subtests and two other tests of neglect. The star cancellation was the most sensitive of these four measures and the only one found to correlate significantly with scores from a measure of ADL, the Modified Barthel Index ($r = 0.55$). The test manual gives a correlation coefficient of $r = 0.92$ between scores from the ADL behavioral subtests and those from the six conventional subtests for 80 rehabilitation patients with unilateral cerebral lesions.

The BIT is being used in research because of its functional relevance. One group (Robertson et al., 1990) considered it as their principal measure in a controlled study of the effects of computerized treatment for UN patients after stroke. Although the BIT did not discriminate between groups, neither did five of their other six measures of UN. In another intervention study using single system design, the researchers found that with two subjects, the BIT did discriminate between pretest and six-month performances (Cermak et al., 1991). The suggestion of Cermak and Hausser (1989) that the behavioral subtest items be validated against real-life ADL performance makes sense in view of the use of the BIT for its functional properties.

The current test manual (Wilson et al., 1987a) shows excellent reliability data for the Behavioural Inattention Test in its entirety. The 15-day interval test-retest coefficient for 10 subjects with brain damage was $r = 0.99$; the interrater coefficient was $r = 0.99$; and the parallel form coefficient was $r = 0.91$. Small and Ellis (1994) observed two control subjects, testing them each week with the six

conventional BIT subtests for a 1-month period. Their scores did not vary by more than one point over time. Considering the evidence for test stability of the BIT, it is of interest that Small and Ellis (1994) found inconsistent scores from a long-term follow-up study of neglect patients. These authors attributed this inconsistency to brief periods of remission in the unilateral neglect of their sample.

The BIT (Wilson et al., 1987a) was standardized on 80 rehabilitation patients averaging 2 months post stroke. The manual provides normative data from only 50 persons without cerebral lesion. Cermak and Hausser (1989) have justifiably criticized these normative data. On the positive side, the cutoff score from these data defined as having neglect the expected greater proportion of subjects who had right hemisphere, as opposed to left hemisphere, strokes. Research should address improved normative data for the BIT. Although there is little reason to expect data from the United States to differ from the British data, a study confirming this expectation would also be of interest to the American therapist.

Stone and colleagues (1991) successfully shortened the BIT for use with short-term acute stroke patients. This shortened version was validated by comparing the test scores with occupational therapists' assessments of unilateral neglect from ADL evaluations. Further research on this shortened BIT is needed.

Pain Disability Index. No instrument was found specifically designed to assess the phantom pain associated with dismemberment. The Pain Disability Index (PDI) developed by Pollard (1984) is an easily administered scale assessing chronic pain in relation to activity and, consequently, applicable to phantom limb pain. The PDI, consisting of self-report ratings of the extent that chronic pain interferes with seven categories of life activity (family and home responsibilities, recreation, social activity, occupation, sexual behavior, self-care, and life support activity), is a well-researched tool (Gronblad et al., 1993; Gronblad et al., 1994; Jerome & Gross, 1991; Tait et al., 1987; Tait et al., 1990). Originally, ratings of the seven categories were summed, but factor analyses by the Tait research group (1987, 1990) showed the instrument to have a two-factor structure, discretionary (voluntary) versus obligatory activities, so that an overall score has little meaning. The PDI results should be interpreted in terms of ratings of discretionary activities (home, recreation, social, occupation, and sexual) and of ratings of the obligatory activities essential for living (self-care, such as dressing, and life support, such as eating). Reasonable internal consistency was obtained for each factor (alpha = 0.85, discretionary; 0.70, obligatory). The test-retest reliability coefficient was low for the Tait research group (1990), but a 2-month time span can explain the coefficient of $r = 0.44$ (n = 46). The Gronblad group (1993) obtained 1-week, test-retest intraclass correlation coefficients of 0.91 (total PDI), 0.87 (discretionary factor), and 0.73 (obligatory factor) for 20 subjects randomly selected from their total of 94 patients with chronic back pain.

A number of studies have been completed that support the construct validity of the PDI. Initially, Pollard (1984) showed that this scale discriminated between nine persons with lower back pain with a current work history from nine who had just received surgery. The Tait research group (1987, 1990) showed that the PDI discretionary and obligatory factors discriminated outpatients with pain from inpatients with pain, the former, as expected, being less disabled by their pain. In a major study, 197 PDI high scorers (greater disability) were compared with 204 low scorers. The high scorers reported more psychological distress, pain, and disability, stopped activity more, were in bed more during the day, and spent more total time in bed than did low scorers. Two other studies also supported the construct validity of this instrument. Multiple regression procedure showed that time in bed, stopping of activity, psychological distress, and work status predicted PDI scores. Patients who were employed had lower PDI scores than did those unemployed. Finally, it was found that high PDI scorers had higher rates of pain behaviors such as verbal complaints and grimaces than did low scorers. Gronblad and collaborators (1993, 1994) provided still further support for the construct validity of the PDI, since the PDI total values correlated $r = 0.83$ with those from the extensively used and researched Oswestry Disability Questionnaire. The coefficient for the discretionary factor was $r = 0.84$ but only $r = 0.41$ for the obligatory factor, showing less support for the validity of this part of the PDI. The PDI was also related to a measure of pain intensity at $r = 0.69$. Further work showed the PDI to discriminate persons with chronic pain who were working from those on sick leave. Since the PDI is a self-report measure, Gronblad and associates (1994) studied its relation to objective physical therapist observations of activities requiring back and leg muscle use. Subjects were 45 outpatients with chronic back pain. Activities included a sit-up test emphasizing abdominal muscles, an arch-up test for back muscles, and a squatting test for lower extremity muscles. Although correlation coefficients were low (0.30s and 0.40s), these researchers did find significant relationships between PDI results and observed activity scores, even after adjustment for age and gender. Jerome and Gross (1991) were concerned that the PDI scores might not provide any useful information beyond that of a pain intensity scale. For 74 subjects from a university pain clinic, they correlated PDI results to several variables used to assess functional status in chronic pain. Although pain intensity was highly related to PDI, when intensity was partialled out, discretionary PDI scores were still related to level of depression, lack of employment, and use of pain medication. Thus, the PDI does provide information on disability beyond that provided by a pain intensity scale.

In summary, an impressive body of research supports the construct validity of the PDI with chronic pain patients. I concur with the researchers who consider the PDI a feasible clinical instrument if used as part of a battery to assess the relation of chronic pain and activity level. The PDI should be a valid tool for use with patients suffering from phantom pain, but specific research in this area would be valuable. The PDI would be an instrument of choice for assessment in longitudinal studies of rehabilitation in which chronic pain is a factor.

Computerized Tests. In this information age, computer aided testing is a given. However, because of time and cost constraints, use of a well-developed paper and pencil test often may be of more practical value in the clinic than the use of elaborate electronic measuring devices. Computerized tests that are useful to the clinician are obviously desirable. Anton and colleagues (1988) reported such a test designed to assess visual neglect and extinction. In this test situation, the subject, with gaze fixed centrally, responded to randomly appearing lights (Fig. 8–2). Lights appeared to the subject's right side, to the left, or simultaneously to right and left sides. Testing with 30 "normal" volunteers showed that, although errors were made, no difference was made in the number on the right and left sides. When used with patients after right cerebrovascular accident (CVA), greater response to right than to left lights would indicate neglect. Response only to right with simultaneous lights would show extinction. Relative to clinical evaluation by a physician and identification by occupational therapists from paper and pencil testing, the computerized test was found to be highly sensitive, identifying visual neglect in 16 and extinction in 13 of 24 subjects with right CVA. In every instance, when neglect and extinction were identified by the physician or occupational therapist, they were also identified by the computerized testing, but the computerized test identified five more cases of extinction than did the physician and six more cases of neglect than did the occupational therapist.

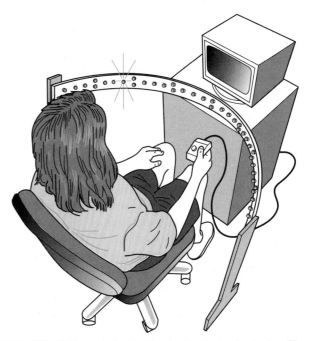

FIGURE 8–2. Computerized test for visual neglect and extinction. (From Anton, H., Hershler, C., Lloyd, P., & Murray, D. [1988]. Visual neglect and extinction: A new test. *Archives of Physical Medicine and Rehabilitation, 69,* 1013–1016.)

Anton and coworkers (1988) reported limited information on reliability, merely stating that three each of control and experimental subjects were retested within 2 to 3 weeks, with no change in test results. Construct validity was supported. The data from this computerized test supported the position of neurologists that neglect is a severe manifestation of extinction since neglect never occurred in the absence of extinction.

Because this computerized test of Anton and colleagues (1988) appears to be well worth the effort of those researching this type of testing, I was surprised to locate only one later study. Beis and collaborators (1994) described a modification of the Anton test, which was designed to detect visual field deficits as well as visual neglect. From 63 subjects with brain injury, 17 were identified as having visual field defects and 12 as having neglect. Identifications of visual field defects by the computer test did not differ significantly from those by ophthalmologist tests. The array of 64 light emitting diodes (LEDs) for this study (in a somewhat tighter semicircular arrangement than that for the Anton test) allowed for well-defined control data. All errors by the 31 control subjects were limited to the final five lights to the right or left sides. Further research is needed on this type of testing for unilateral neglect.

To summarize, one aspect of body image that needs assessment in rehabilitation is neural scheme disturbance. Persons with conditions such as phantom limb pain or unilateral neglect are examples of patients needing such assessment. Five examples of instruments of research and clinical interest were discussed.

Disturbances of Psychological Representation

Many instruments were reviewed that purport to assess body image disturbances associated strongly with psychological or social conditions. These tools have been used for assessment of body image disturbances of persons with actual physical disabilities or with psychiatric diagnoses but with no known neural lesion to distort the neural scheme.

Thompson (1990) was among those who recognized that, even with the neural body scheme disturbance excluded, body image disturbance remained a multidimensional construct. Thus, he discussed measures designed to assess the perceptual and the subjective components of disturbances. Keeton and associates (1990) also categorized assessment tools for the psychological representation aspect of the body image into these same categories (perceptual and attitudinal). Measures of body size estimation (width of body parts) and whole-image distortion procedures have been termed perceptual, but this term can cause them to be confused with measures used to assess neural body scheme disturbances often classified as perceptual (Zoltan et al., 1986), so I prefer the term used by Meermann (1983), *psychophysical methods.*

These psychophysical methods are of two types: body-size estimation procedures and the whole-image distortion methods. In the former, using lights, calipers, or other instruments, subjects estimate the width of their various body sites (such as hips or chest), and distortion scores are computed by comparing estimates to actual measures, typically taking variables such as height and weight into consideration. The whole-image distortion procedures use photographic or video methods for subjects to estimate their bodies as a whole (Van Deusen, 1993). I selected a body size procedure, the Body Image Detection Device (BIDD) (Ruff & Barrios, 1986) to illustrate this kind of body image assessment instrument.

The attitudinal measures have been subdivided in various ways (Ben-Tovin & Walker, 1991; Thompson, 1990; Van Deusen, 1993). I believe that three categories incorporate instruments of major use to occupational therapists and physical therapists: 1) self-report tools requiring responses to figures or silhouettes; 2) self-report tools requiring responses to verbal statements about size, shape, or other aspects of body image; and 3) the semantic differential technique (Van Deusen, 1993).

The instruments I selected to illustrate the wide array of measures of the psychological representation aspect of body image include examples from each category:

1. Body Image Detection Device (BIDD) (Ruff & Barrios, 1986)—psychophysical measure
2. Body Image Assessment (Williamson, 1990)—self-report, silhouette measure
3. Multidimensional Body-Self Relations Questionnaire (MBSRQ) (Cash & Pruzinsky, 1990)—self-report, verbal statements measure
4. Body Shape Questionnaire (BSQ) (Cooper et al., 1987)—self-report, verbal statements measure
5. Body Image Assessments Using the Semantic Differential Technique (Isaac & Michael, 1981)—bipolar adjective attitude scales

I also included two recently developed instruments with minimal research work, the FOFQ (Roth & Armstrong, 1993) and the Color-a-Person Body Dissatisfaction Test (CAPT) (Wooley & Roll, 1991). These tests provide varied scores as body image changes within situational context, and both instruments deserve further research attention.

Body Image Detection Device. Of those devices and techniques developed for research investigating body size estimation accuracy, particularly for subjects challenged by anorexia or bulimia nervosa, one tool receiving research attention was the BIDD originated by Ruff and Barrios (1986). The BIDD projects light onto a wall for the subjects to adjust to their estimated body site widths by manipulating the templates of the apparatus. The subjects' site sizes (face, chest, waist, hips, thighs), estimated one at a time, are compared with their actual widths measured by the investigator, so that a ratio can be computed for over- or underestimation of size (estimated/actual discrepancy index). By requesting subjects to show estimates of their ideal sizes, a self/ideal discrepancy index can also be computed.

Data from college students, 20 with bulimia and 20 without, in the Ruff and Barrios study (1986) showed internal consistency coefficients (Cronbach's alpha) of 0.79 to 0.93. Interrater reliability coefficients were $r = 0.98$ or better. All 3-week test-retest reliability coefficients were in the 0.70s and 0.80s for bulimic and control subjects, except for the waist estimate of bulimic subjects (0.44). The authors' second study (cited by Thompson, 1990) showed much lower coefficients among college women. Keeton and associates (1990) in their use of the BIDD found a coefficient (alpha = 0.93) indicating high interrater reliability of the measurement of the actual body site sizes.

Considerable evidence exists for the construct validity of the data obtained from the BIDD. The estimated/actual index discriminated between three weight groups, 12 each of normal, over-, and underweight nonclinical subjects (Cash & Green, 1986), between 20 each of bulimic subjects and controls (Ruff & Barrios, 1986), and between 47 male and 78 female college students (Keeton et al., 1990). The self-estimate scores and self/ideal discrepancy index showed moderate correlations (0.42 to 0.67) with those from a silhouette tool. For women, the self/ideal discrepancy index was also significantly related to scores on a test for bulimia, but the coefficient was low at $r = 0.38$. Evidence indicated that BIDD results were independent from those of attitudinal measures (Keeton et al., 1990).

A modification of the BIDD, the Adjustable Light Beam Apparatus, allows the projected light to be simultaneously adjusted for the three body sites (waist, hips, and thighs) after practice with the face (Thompson & Spana, 1988). The authors provided detailed directions for construction of this device. It has also received research attention showing acceptable reliability coefficients and evidence that size estimation data are independent from those of attitudinal measures (Altabe & Thompson, 1992; Coovert et al., 1988; Thompson & Spana, 1988).

Body Image Assessment. A number of researchers have used figures or silhouettes graded from very thin to very obese as stimuli for response by subjects in their body image studies (Bell et al., 1986; Fallon & Rozin, 1985). A computer program version has also been evaluated (Dickson-Parnell et al., 1987).

One such silhouette assessment procedure for body image was designed and researched by Williamson and colleagues (Williamson, 1990; Williamson et al., 1989; Williamson et al., 1993). Nine silhouettes (Fig. 8–3) graded from thin to obese are presented to subjects on cards. Cards are presented in a fixed order since no difference was found from the random display originally used. Standard instructions are used to request first accurate and then preferred body size choices from the cards. Administration time is less than 1 minute. Normative data of subjects' height and weight were established by cluster analysis (Williamson et al., 1989). These data may be used to determine if testees show body images outside of normal limits.

Data estimating the reliability and validity of the Body Image Assessment were obtained (Keeton et al., 1990; Williamson, 1990; Williamson et al., 1989; Williamson, et al., 1993). Test-retest reliability data were gathered from 1-week, 2-week, and 3- to 8-week intervals between administrations. All reliability estimates were in the 0.70s, 0.80s, or 0.90s.

Williamson and colleagues provided evidence for the construct validity of the Body Image Assessment (Williamson, 1990; Williamson et al., 1989; Williamson et al., 1993). In two separate studies, as hypothesized, it discriminated between persons with bulimia nervosa and control subjects and between persons with anorexia nervosa and control subjects. No score differences were found between eating-disordered subjects. As hypothesized, relationships were found between scores on tests of eating attitudes and bulimia and those of the Body Image Assessment. Furthermore, another research team, Keeton and coworkers

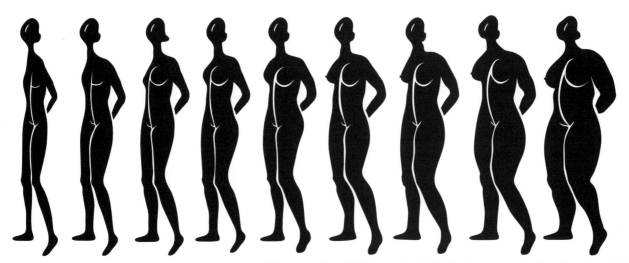

FIGURE 8–3. Silhouettes for the Body Image Assessment by Williamson. (From Williamson, D. A. [1990]. *Assessment of eating disorders: Obesity, anorexia, and bulimia nervosa.* Needham Hights, MA: Allyn & Bacon.)

(1990), also supported the construct validity of a modified version of the Body Image Assessment in their study examining a number of body image measurements.

Body-Self Relations Questionnaire. Many self-report scales of the Likert type using verbal statements have been used by body image researchers for investigation of disturbances of persons challenged by anorexia nervosa, mastectomy, severe burns, and other problems (Van Deusen, 1993). The self-report questionnaire devised and researched by Winstead, Cash, and collaborators (Cash & Pruzinsky, 1990) is an outstanding example of this type of assessment procedure. Their conceptual framework was a multidimensional, psychosocial one in which body image was originally assessed by the nine subscales of the Body-Self Relations Questionnaire (BSRQ), which addressed the cognitive, affective (evaluative), and behavioral dimensions of three somatic domains: physical appearance, fitness, and health. For the various subscales, internal consistency coefficients were reported from alpha = 0.68 to 0.91 (Winstead & Cash, cited in Cash & Pruzinsky, 1990), alpha = 0.91 (Noles et al., 1985), 0.83 to 0.92 (Cash & Green, 1986), and the 0.80s (Butters & Cash, 1987). Test-retest scores from the physical appearance domain over 1 month were 0.85 to 0.91 (Cash & Green, 1986).

Evidence exists of the construct validity of the physical appearance domain items from the BSRQ. Noles and associates (1985) found the affective dimension to discriminate depressed from nondepressed subjects. Cash and Green (1986) showed these items to discriminate among nonclinical subjects by weight group. Pasman and Thompson (1988) found these items to differentiate between male and female runners, the latter being less satisfied with their physical appearance. Keeton and collaborators (1990) found scores from the affective/appearance domain to be related to several other attitudinal body image measures, as well as to a measure of eating disorders. Thompson and Psaltis (1988) found BSRQ scores related to those from a figure rating scale. Of particular importance was the evidence provided by Butters and Cash (1987) that the BSRQ (all domains) showed significantly improved body image following cognitive-behavioral treatment of experimental relative to control subjects. Although these experimental subjects had shown dissatisfaction with their body images, they were functioning college students, not patients.

From a magazine survey (Cash, 1990; Cash et al., 1986), data were obtained on the BSRQ from 30,000 persons. Norms were established (N = 2000) from a random sample of these data stratified for age and gender. Since this sample contained 91% white, 84% college-educated subjects and 37% never-married persons, it is not representative of the general population. These BSRQ data clearly differentiated persons who did poorly from those who did not on a psychosocial adjustment scale included with the survey. The BSRQ also showed women as having less positive body images than men, although not to the extent anticipated. Adolescents showed less positive body images than did other age groups.

From their survey data, Cash and collaborators (Brown et al., 1990) refined the BSRQ. The current instrument, the Multidimensional Body-Self Relations Questionnaire (MBSRQ), was reduced to 69 items from the original 140 and to six subscales from the original nine. Because of the correlation of data, the cognitive and behavioral dimensions were combined to one orientation dimension, with the affective (evaluation) dimension maintaining independence. The revised BSRQ part of the MBSRQ has 54 items, and the other items make up a body areas satisfaction and a weight attitude scale. Sample items are "Most people would consider me good-looking" and "I am very well coordinated" (Cash & Pruzinsky, 1990). To validate their conceptual frame of reference, Brown and colleagues (1990) analyzed the factor structure of the BSRQ with separate split-sample factor analyses for each gender. The survey data from 1064 women and 988 men were used. It was expected that the analyses would reveal factors that could be defined by the six subscales: appearance, fitness, and health evaluation; and appearance, fitness, and health orientation. The six predicted factors were generated by each of the four analyses plus a seventh, an illness orientation factor. Items loading on the illness orientation factor pertained to alertness to symptoms of illness, as distinguished from items about motivation toward bodily wellness, which loaded on the health orientation factor. Further study showed marked stability of the factor structure between and within genders. The construct validity of the MBSRQ as a measure of the psychological representation aspect of body image has continued to be demonstrated through research results obtained with the use of this instrument (Cash et al., 1991; Denniston et al., 1992). Unquestionably, the MBSRQ is a body image tool with very acceptable reliability and validity data. Computer software is available to facilitate the use of this instrument (Cash & Pruzinsky, 1990).

Body Shape Questionnaire. British researchers Cooper, Taylor, Cooper, and Fairburn (1987) perceived the lack of a body image tool dealing specifically with body shape concerns. They developed a measure directing subjects to respond in terms of how they felt about their appearance over the past four weeks. Sample items from their BSQ follow:

Have you felt so bad about your shape that you have cried? (p. 491)
Have you felt excessively large and rounded? (p. 492)
Have you felt ashamed of your body? (p. 492)
Have you pinched areas of your body to see how much fat there is? (p. 493)

Items were obtained through interviews with women having eating disorders and with nonclinical university women. From statistical analyses of data from nonclinical and clinical female samples, 51 items were reduced to 34. A single score is obtained by adding items (Cooper et al., 1987). That the BSQ has a unitary structure has been supported by several factor analytic studies (Mumford et al., 1991; Mumford et al., 1992). Internal consistency reliability was excellent (alpha = 0.93).

Concurrent validity of the BSQ was supported by significant relationships with well-known eating disorder and attitude tests (Cooper et al., 1987). Concurrent validity was substantiated by other researchers (Rosen et al., 1990) with a correlation of $r = 0.78$ between eating disorder scales and the BSQ in a sample of 106 female subjects.

Research with the BSQ showed it to discriminate between patients with bulimia nervosa and comparable nonclinical women, between women rated as concerned and not concerned about their shape, and between probable bulimics and other women in a community sample (Cooper et al., 1987). In a discriminant analysis (Rosen et al., 1990), eating disorder scales contributed nothing beyond the BSQ to group placement (control vs. eating-disordered subjects).

Cross-cultural validity of the BSQ was shown in several studies, including one on subjects from New Zealand and Asia. According to these authors, evidence was strong because of similar factor structures across cultures (Mumford et al., 1991, 1992). By modifying items slightly for male subjects, Kearney-Cooke and Steichen-Asch (1990) used the BSQ to divide 112 male college students into those at risk for eating disorders and those not at risk. These authors then found the expected differences between these groups on eating attitudes and body satisfaction; even greater differences were found with their clinically diagnosed anorexic/bulimic subjects. To summarize, considerable evidence supports the construct validity of the BSQ.

Because the BSQ is measuring only one construct (Mumford et al., 1991, 1992) and because of the current need for efficient measures, Evans and Dolan (1993) investigated short forms of the BSQ. Their analysis and replication showed internal consistency coefficients in the 0.90s for the short, 16-item alternate forms. These authors supported construct validity of these short forms by obtaining results consistent with their hypotheses in several instances. For example, moderately high correlations were found with eating attitude scores, and the short form BSQ could separate subjects reporting eating problems from those not reporting them. Certainly, more efficient measurement tools are necessary in view of current health care trends.

The Semantic Differential Technique. Citing the work of Osgood and collaborators, Isaac and Michael (1981) described the use of the semantic differential method for measuring the meaning of concepts. It consists of a five- to nine-step scale anchored by bipolar adjectives. On a form with items randomly arranged, the subject marks the step best describing his or her attitude toward the concept being considered (Fig. 8–4). The semantic differential has been a very useful tool, and literally thousands of references verify its value. This technique is well suited to the assessment of body image. For this purpose, its use with clinical samples challenged by anorexia nervosa, burns, and rheumatoid arthritis is next described.

I chose the semantic differential technique for assessment of body image in our studies with adults diagnosed

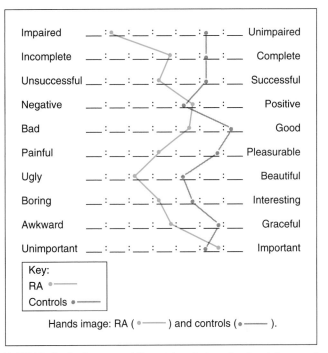

FIGURE 8–4. Semantic differential technique for hand image of persons with rheumatoid arthritis. (From Van Deusen, J. [1993]. *Body image and perceptual dysfunction in adults.* Philadelphia: W. B. Saunders.)

with rheumatoid arthritis (Van Deusen, 1993). It was used simply as an attitude scale consisting of scales for self-reports on trunk, arms, hands, and legs (see Fig. 8–4). Harlowe, my coinvestigator, and I found this semantic differential to discriminate subjects with rheumatoid arthritis from nonclinical control subjects. The scale for hands also discriminated between subjects with arthritis who had traditional programming from those subjects participating in an experimental dance experience.

The semantic differential also was found to be an effective method to assess body image of persons with severe burns. Orr and colleagues (1989) used this tool to show that perceived social support (especially by peers) was the variable most highly associated with body image adjustment of young adults with burns.

A study reported from Germany (Steinhausen & Vollrath, 1992) used the semantic differential approach to assess body image of adolescents with anorexia nervosa. Bipolar adjectives used were beautiful-ugly, desirable-undesirable, dirty-clean, soft-hard, proportional-unproportional, light-heavy, powerful-weak, pleasant-unpleasant, fragile-massive, attractive-repulsive, large-small, inactive-active, firm-flabby, bad-good, and uncomfortable-comfortable. This scale differentiated 46 subjects with anorexia from 109 control subjects. Two analyses showed a similar factor structure (attractiveness and body mass dimensions) for the subjects with and without anorexia nervosa. This semantic differential also showed sensitivity to the therapeutic body image changes of anorexic subjects.

To summarize, the semantic differential technique has

been found from my personal experience, as well as from reports in the literature, to be a valuable method for assessing, from an attitudinal perspective, the body image of clinical subjects.

I am not aware of any study in which this technique has been used to assess body image in changing environments. Because of a recent interest in measuring a "dynamic" body image in varying environments, research of this type is desirable.

Contextual Body Image Tools. It is likely that two newer instruments will be receiving increased research attention: the CAPT and the FOFQ. These body image assessment instruments apparently measure a dynamic body image, so that scores can be expected to vary with context. Research has shown CAPT score fluctuation with environmental change, and the FOFQ was designed as a dynamic measure.

The CAPT (Wooley & Roll, 1991) consists of a figure of the same sex as the subject. Five color markers are used by subjects to indicate their level of satisfaction with various body parts. With nonclinical and clinical subjects, internal consistency and test-retest reliability coefficients were in the 0.70s and 0.80s. CAPT scores were significantly greater ($P < 0.0001$) after bulimic subjects received therapy. Moderate correlations with traditional tests (0.50s) were obtained. Haimovitz and collaborators (1993) showed that the CAPT scores varied under different environmental situations. Face, hair, and hands were the only aspects of body image unaffected by beach, lunch, private, and dressing room situations for a sample of 144 undergraduate women. Furthermore, the CAPT appeared to measure body image when subjects were especially self-critical rather than body image in general.

Unlike the CAPT, the FOFQ was designed specifically as an affective measure of body image across contexts. The authors of FOFQ (Roth & Armstrong, 1993) proposed to measure the subjective experience of fatness across a variety of situations. Content validity was established by contributions of items from experienced mental health professionals expressing feelings of fatness in achievement, affective, social, somatic, and self-focused situations. Internal consistency reliability was 0.98. Analysis showed two factors defined as troubles and satisfactions. Test scores were related to eating attitude scales but not with a psychophysical size estimation measure. Through statistical procedures, considerable variability of test scores was found across situations in a sample of 132 undergraduate women. A need exists for thorough investigation of body image tests that can be used to assess body image changes within varied contexts.

To summarize, instrumentation for assessment of body image has received much attention across disciplines. Because the construct of body image is so complex, assessment must deal with both neurologic and psychosocial aspects. Because body image is not stable, assessment also must consider context.

GLOSSARY

Body image disturbance—Problems in the integration of the neural body scheme and its psychosocial representation.

Body scheme disturbance—Interference with the patterns of excitation in the brain that are basic to posture and movement.

Cognitive behavioral therapy—Psychological intervention that emphasizes restructuring of attitudes in the area of the patient's dysfunction.

Concurrent validity—Favorable comparison of test scores to other variables, considered to provide a direct measure of the characteristic under consideration.

Construct validity—Definition of explanatory concepts reflected in test performance by supporting logical hypotheses related to test scores. Demonstration of concurrent validity may be part of the construct validation process.

Factor analysis—A statistical process in which a large number of variables can be reduced to a small number of concepts through the interrelationship of these variables.

Finger agnosia—Confusion in identification of one's fingers.

Internal consistency reliability—Consistency of performance on the items of a test.

Phantom pain—Painful sensations referred to a lost body part.

Phantom sensation—The feeling that an amputated part is still present.

Psychophysical method—Procedures developed by researchers of eating disorders that allow subjects to estimate their body size by such means as adjusting lights, calipers, or video images.

REFERENCES

Altabe, M., & Thompson, J. K. (1992). Size estimation versus figural ratings of body image disturbance: Relation to body dissatisfaction and eating dysfunction. *International Journal of Eating Disorders, 11,* 397–402.

Anton, H., Hershler, C., Lloyd, P., & Murray, D. (1988). Visual neglect and extinction: A new test. *Archives of Physical Medicine and Rehabilitation, 69,* 1013–1016.

Beis, J., Andre, J., & Saguez, A. (1994). Detection of visual field deficit and visual neglect with computerized light emitting diodes. *Archives of Physical Medicine and Rehabilitation, 75,* 711–714.

Bell, C., Kirkpatrick, S., & Rinn, R. (1986). Body image of anorexic, obese, and normal females. *Journal of Clinical Psychology, 42,* 431–439.

Benton, A., & Sivan, A. (1993). Disturbances of the body schema. In K. Heilman & E. Valenstein (Eds.), *Clinical neuropsychology* (3rd ed.) (pp. 123–140). New York: Oxford University Press.

Benton, A., Sivan, A., deS. Hamsher, K., Varney, N., & Spreen, O. (1994). Contributions to neuropsychological assessment (2nd ed.) New York: Oxford Press.

Ben-Tovin, D., & Walker, M. K. (1991). Women's body attitudes: A review of measurement techniques. *International Journal of Eating Disorders, 10,* 155–167.

Brown, T., Cash, T., & Mikulka, P. (1990). Attitudinal body-image assessment: Factor analysis of the Body-Self Relations Questionnaire. *Journal of Personality Assessment, 55,* 135–144.

Butters, J., & Cash, T. (1987). Cognitive-behavioral treatment of women's body-image dissatisfaction. *Journal of Consulting and Clinical Psychology, 55,* 889–897.

Cash, T. (1990). The psychology of physical appearance: Aesthetics, attributes, and images. In T. Cash & T. Pruzinsky (Eds.), *Body images, development, deviance, and change* (pp. 51–79). New York: Guilford Press.

Cash, T., & Green, G. (1986). Body weight and body image among college women: Perception, cognition, and affect. *Journal of Personality Assessment, 50,* 290–301.

Cash, T., & Pruzinsky, T. (Eds.). (1990). *Body images, development, deviance, and change.* New York: Guilford Press.

Cash, T., Winstead, B., & Janda, L. (1986). The great American shape-up. *Psychology Today, 20,* 30–37.

Cash, T., Wood, K., Phelps, K., & Boyd, K. (1991). New assessments of weight-related body image derived from extant instruments. *Perceptual and Motor Skills, 73,* 235–241.

Cermak, S., & Hausser, J. (1989). The Behavioral Inattention Test for unilateral visual neglect: A critical review. *Physical and Occupational Therapy in Geriatrics, 7,* 43–53.

Cermak, S., Trombly, C., Hausser, J, & Tiernan, A. (1991). Effects of lateralized tasks on unilateral neglect after right cerebral vascular accident. *Occupational Therapy Journal of Research, 11,* 271–291.

Cooper, P., Taylor, M., Cooper, Z., & Fairburn, C. (1987). The development and validation of the Body Shape Questionnaire. *International Journal of Eating Disorders, 6,* 485–494.

Coovert, D., Thompson, J., & Kinder, B. (1988). Interrelationships among multiple aspects of body image and eating disturbance. *International Journal of Eating Disorders, 7,* 495–502.

Cumming, W. (1988). The neurobiology of the body schema. *British Journal of Psychiatry, 153*(suppl 2), 7–11.

Denniston, C., Roth, D., & Gilroy, F. (1992). Dysphoria and body image among college women. *International Journal of Eating Disorders, 12,* 449–452.

Dickson-Parnell, B., Jones, M., & Braddy, D. (1987). Assessment of body image perceptions using a computer program. *Behavior Research Methods, Instruments, & Computers, 19,* 353–354.

Evans, C., & Dolan, B. (1993). Body Shape Questionnaire: Derivation of shortened "alternate forms." *International Journal of Eating Disorders, 13,* 315–321.

Fallon, A., & Rozin, P. (1985). Sex differences in perceptions of desirable body shape. *Journal of Abnormal Psychology, 94,* 102–105.

Fischer, P., Marterer, A., & Danielczyk, W. (1990). Right-left disorientation in dementia of the Alzheimer type. *Neurology, 40,* 1619–1620.

Fisher, S. (1990). The evolution of psychological concepts about the body. In T. Cash & T. Pruzinsky (Eds.), *Body images, development, deviance, and change* (pp. 3–20). New York: Guilford Press.

Freedman, R. (1990). Cognitive-behavioral perspectives on body-image change. In T. Cash & T. Pruzinsky (Eds.), *Body images, development, deviance, and change* (pp. 272–295). New York: Guilford Press.

Gronblad, M., Hupli, M., Wennergrand, P., Jarvinen, E., Lukinmaa, A., Kouri, J., & Karaharju, E. (1993). Intercorrelation and test-retest reliability of the Pain Disability Index (PDI) and the Oswestry Disability Questionnaire (ODQ) and their correlation with pain intensity in low back pain patients. *The Clinical Journal of Pain, 9,* 189–195.

Gronblad, M., Jarvinen, E., Hurri, H., Hupli, M., & Karaharju, E. (1994). Relationship of the Pain Disability Index (PDI) and the Oswestry Disability Questionnaire (ODQ) with three dynamic physical tests in a group of patients with chronic low-back and leg pain. *The Clinical Journal of Pain, 10,* 197–203.

Haimovitz, D., Lansky, L., & O'Reilly, P. (1993). Fluctuations in body satisfaction across situations. *International Journal of Eating Disorders, 13,* 77–84.

Halligan, P., Marshall, J., & Wade, D. (1989). Visuospatial neglect: Underlying factors and test sensitivity. *Lancet, ii,* 908–911.

Heilman, K., Valenstein, E., & Watson, R. (1985). The neglect syndrome. In J. Fredericks (Ed.), *Handbook of clinical neurology. Vol 45–1: Clinical neuropsychology* (pp. 153-183). New York: Elsevier Science.

Isaac, S., & Michael, W. (1981). *Handbook in research and evaluation* (2nd ed). San Diego, CA: EDITS.

Jerome, A., & Gross, R. (1991). Pain Disability Index: Construct and discriminant validity. *Archives of Physical Medicine and Rehabilitation, 72,* 920–922.

Kearney-Cooke, A., & Steichen-Asch, P. (1990). Men, body image, and eating disorders. In A. E. Andersen (Ed.), *Males with eating disorders. Eating Disorders Monograph* (Series NO. 4) (pp. 54–74). New York: Brunner/Mazel.

Keeton, W., Cash, T., & Brown, T. (1990). Body image or body images?: Comparative, multidimensional assessment among college students. *Journal of Personality Assessment, 54,* 213–230.

Lacey, J., & Birtchnell, S. (1986). Review article—Body image and its disturbances. *Journal of Psychosomatic Research, 30,* 623–631.

Lautenbacher, S., Roscher, S., Strian, F., Pirke, K., & Krieg, J. (1993). Theoretical and empirical considerations on the relation between body image, body scheme and somatosensation. *Journal of Psychosomatic Research, 37,* 447–454.

Macdonald, J. (1960). An investigation of body scheme in adults with cerebral vascular accident. *American Journal of Occupational Therapy, 14,* 72–79.

Marsh, N., & Kersel, D. (1993). Screening tests for visual neglect following stroke. *Neuropsychological Rehabilitation, 3,* 245–257.

Mazzoni, M., Pardossi, L., Cantini, R., Giorgetti, V., & Arena, R. (1990). Gerstmann syndrome: A case report. *Cortex, 26,* 459–467.

Meermann, R. (1983). Experimental investigation of disturbances in body image estimation in anorexia nervosa patients and ballet and gymnastics pupils. *International Journal of Eating Disorders, 2,* 91–99.

Mumford, D., Whitehouse, A., & Choudry, I. (1992). Survey of eating disorders in English-medium schools in Lahore, Pakistan. *International Journal of Eating Disorders, 11,* 173–184.

Mumford, D., Whitehouse, A., & Platts, M. (1991). Sociocultural correlates of eating disorders among Asian schoolgirls in Bradford. *British Journal of Psychiatry, 158,* 222–228.

Noles, S., Cash, T., & Winstead, B. (1985). Body image, physical attractiveness, and depression. *Journal of Consulting and Clinical Psychology, 53,* 88–94.

Orr, D., Reznikoff, M., & Smith, G. (1989). Body image, self-esteem, and depression in burn-injured adolescents and young adults. *Journal of Burn Care Rehabilitation, 10,* 454–461.

Pasman, J., & Thompson, J. K. (1988). Body image and eating disturbance in obligatory runners, obligatory weight lifters and sedentary individuals. *International Journal of Eating Disorders, 7,* 759–770.

Pollard, C. (1984). Preliminary validity study of pain disability index. *Perceptual and Motor Skills, 59,* 974.

Robertson, I., Gray, J., Pentland, B., & Waite, L. (1990). Microcomputer-based rehabilitation for unilateral left visual neglect: A randomized controlled trial. *Archives of Physical Medicine and Rehabilitation, 71,* 663–668.

Rosen, J., Vara, L., Wendt, S., & Leitenberg, H. (1990). Validity studies of the eating disorder examination. *International Journal of Eating Disorders, 9,* 519–528.

Roth, D., & Armstrong, J. (1993). Feelings of Fatness Questionnaire: A measure of the cross-situational variability of body experience. *International Journal of Eating Disorders, 14,* 349–358.

Ruff, G., & Barrios, B. (1986). Realistic assessment of body image. *Behavioral Assessment, 8,* 237–252.

Safran, J., & Greenberg, L. (1986). Hot cognition and psychotherapy process: An information-processing/ecological approach. In P. Kendall (Ed.), *Advances in Cognitive-Behavioral Research and Therapy* (pp. 143–177). Vol. 5. Orlando: Academic Press.

Sauguet, J., Benton, A., & Hecaen, H. (1971). Disturbances of the body scheme in relation to language impairment and hemispheric locus of lesion. *Journal of Neurology, Neurosurgery, and Psychiatry, 34,* 496–501.

Small, M., & Ellis, S. (1994). Brief remission periods in visuospatial neglect: Evidence from long-term follow-up. *European Neurology, 34,* 147–154.

Steinhausen, H., & Vollrath, M. (1992). Semantic differentials for the assessment of body-image and perception of personality in eating-disordered patients. *International Journal of Eating Disorders, 12,* 83–91.

Stone, S., Wilson, B., & Clifford-Rose, F. (1987). The development of a standard test battery to detect, measure and monitor visuo-spatial neglect in patients with acute stroke. *International Journal of Rehabilitation Research, 10,* 110.

Stone, S., Wilson, B., Wroot, A., Halligan, P., Lange, L., Marshall, J., & Greenwood, R. (1991). The assessment of visuo-spatial neglect after acute stroke. *Journal of Neurology, Neurosurgery, Psychiatry, 54,* 345–350.

Tait, R., Chibnall, J., & Krause, S. (1990). The Pain Disability Index: Psychometric properties. *Pain, 40*, 171–182.

Tait, R., Pollard, A., Margolis, R., Duckro, P., & Krause, S. (1987). The Pain Disability Index: Psychometric and validity data. *Archives of Physical Medicine and Rehabilitation, 68*, 438–441.

Thompson, J. K. (1990). *Body image disturbance assessment and treatment.* New York: Pergamon Press.

Thompson, J. K., & Psaltis, K. (1988). Multiple aspects of body figure ratings: A replication and extension of Fallon and Rozin (1985). *International Journal of Eating Disorders, 7*, 813–817.

Thompson, J. K., & Spana, R. (1988). The adjustable light beam method for the assessment of size estimation accuracy: Description, psychometrics, and normative data. *International Journal of Eating Disorders, 7*, 521–526.

Tiemersma, D. (1989). *Body schema and body image: An interdisciplinary and philosophical study.* Amsterdam: Swets & Zeitlinger.

Van Deusen, J. (1993). *Body image and perceptual dysfunction in adults.* Philadelphia: W. B. Saunders.

Williamson, D. (1990). *Assessment of eating disorders: Obesity, anorexia, and bulimia nervosa.* New York: Pergamon Press.

Williamson, D., Cubic, B., & Gleaves, D. (1993). Equivalence of body image disturbances in anorexia and bulimia nervosa. *Journal of Abnormal Psychology, 102*, 177–180.

Williamson, D., Davis, C., Bennet, S., Goreczny, A., & Gleaves, D. (1989). Development of a simple procedure for assessing body image disturbances. *Behavioral Assessment, 11*, 433–446.

Wilson, B., Cockburn, J., & Halligan, P. (1987a). *Behavioural Inattention Test.* Tichfield, Hampshire: Thames Valley Test Company. (Distributed in the United States by Western Psychological Services, Los Angeles, CA.)

Wilson, B., Cockburn, J., & Halligan, P. (1987b). Development of a behavioral test of visuospatial neglect. *Archives of Physical Medicine and Rehabilitation, 68*, 98–102.

Wooley, O., & Roll, S. (1991). The Color-A-Person Body Dissatisfaction Test: Stability, internal consistency, validity, and factor structure. *Journal of Personality Assessment, 56*, 395–413.

Zoltan, B., Siev, E., & Freishtat, B. (1986). *The adult stroke patient, a manual for evaluation and treatment of perceptual and cognitive dysfunction* (revised 2nd ed.). Thorofare, NJ: Slack Inc.

CHAPTER 9

Electrodiagnosis of the Neuromuscular System

Edward J. Hammond, PhD

SUMMARY   In this chapter, traditional electrodiagnostic studies including nerve conduction velocity studies, the electromyogram, and somatosensory evoked potential are surveyed. Newer techniques, the motor evoked potential, the surface EMG, and dermatomal evoked potentials, are also considered. Detailed technical considerations and interpretations are not discussed, but emphasis is placed on assisting the nonelectrophysiologist in understanding basic principles of, and indications for, commonly used diagnostic tests. Limitations and benefits of each technique are clearly stated, and areas for future improvement and research are discussed.

The anatomic system of interest in clinical electrodiagnosis consists of the peripheral nerves, the neuromuscular junction, the skeletal muscles, and the somatosensory and motor pathways in the spinal cord and brain. During normal movements, these components interact with each other to bring about the contraction and relaxation of muscle. Various types of electrodiagnostic tests discussed in this chapter can be used to determine physiologic abnormalities occurring in one of these anatomic subdivisions. Historically, specific electrodiagnostic tests were developed because careful clinical examination is sometimes not enough for accurate diagnosis (and, therefore, treatment). The degree to which electrodiagnostic tests are pertinent to diagnosis and treatment depends on the extent to which we can integrate this "subclinical neurology" with clinical neurology. This chapter discusses basic principles, limitations, and benefits of currently used electrodiagnostic tests. Tests of peripheral nerves and muscles are discussed first, then central nervous system testing. The chapter necessarily contains many technical and specialized terms, and the reader unfamiliar with electrophysiologic terminology is urged to consult the glossary at the end of the chapter.

NERVE CONDUCTION STUDIES

Classification of Peripheral Nerves. The peripheral nerve contains sensory and motor fibers of various diameters and conduction speeds. Peripheral nerve fibers can be classified into different types known as the A, B, and C fibers. The largest fibers transmit nerve impulses the fastest. The A fibers are large myelinated fibers that innervate skeletal muscle (efferent or motor fibers) and also conduct impulses from proprioceptive receptors in skeletal muscles and other receptors in the skin (afferent or sensory fibers). The B nerves are small myelinated, efferent, preganglionic autonomic nerves. The C fibers are unmyelinated autonomic nerve fibers. Some C fibers serve as sensory afferents that mediate various types of sensation, mostly deep pain. A typical peripheral nerve contains A and C fibers. Within a peripheral nerve, all nerve fibers are not of equal size but actually cover a wide range of diameters. Another classification is frequently used to describe sensory nerve fibers. In this classification, the fibers are also grouped according to diameter, but a Roman numeral classification is used: Group I contains the largest afferent fibers; Group II, the next largest; Group III, the third largest; and then Group IV, which corresponds to the small unmyelinated C fibers. Within these main groups are further subdivisions—labeled a, b, c. One often sees a nerve classified as Ia; this means that the nerve is of the largest diameter and fastest conduction.

Classification of Peripheral Nerve Injuries. Peripheral nerve injuries are often classified as neuropractic, axonotmetic, or neurotmetic. Neuropraxia is a reversible injury in which some loss of distal function occurs, with no associated structural change of the nerve axon. Causes of neuropraxia can include neural ischemia or local electrolyte imbalance or trauma (e.g., as in the transient alteration in sensation sometimes associated with leg crossing or in a nerve block caused by a local injection of an anesthetic).

Acute compression neuropathies such as Saturday night palsy or crutch palsy of the ulnar nerve, as well as chronic entrapments such as carpal tunnel syndrome or tardy ulnar palsy, are considered neuropraxic (although the latter two can later be associated with focal demyelination). In neuropraxia, nerve action potentials can be generated above and below the injury site but are not recorded across the site of injury; therefore, the lesion can be precisely delineated electrophysiologically. Axonotmesis is of more increased severity and is characterized by a loss of axons and myelin, with preservation of the surrounding connective tissue. A more severe type of peripheral nerve trauma is neurotmesis. In this case, the axons and myelin are destroyed, with additional disruption of the surrounding connective tissue. An example of this would be a complete nerve transection.

Pathophysiology of Peripheral Nerves. Neuropraxia, axonotmesis, and neurotmesis produce certain electrophysiologic alterations, which can be classified into disorders

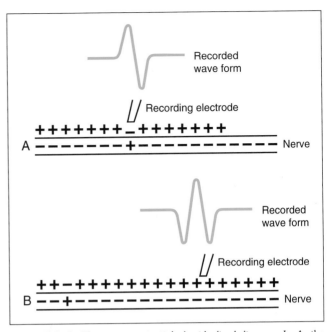

FIGURE 9–1. The action potential. An idealized diagram. In *A*, the potential arises underneath the electrode and propagates away from it. The *plus* and *minus signs* represent ions situated outside and inside the nerve. This is recorded as a biphasic negative-positive wave. The waveform (as seen on an oscilloscope screen) of the potential recorded by the electrode is drawn above the electrode; negativity is drawn upward. Another situation common in clinical practice is shown in *B*; the potential (i.e., ion exchange) approaches the electrode and passes underneath it. In this case, a positive-negative-positive triphasic wave is recorded.

characterized by the much more usable terms *conduction slowing* and *disorders with conduction block*. Disorders with slowing of conduction can occur with demyelination of the axons; a conduction block occurs with a metabolic alteration in the membrane, as with anesthetic block or a structural alteration in the axon. Reduced or absent responses are the result of nerve degeneration after axonal interruption.

Electrophysiology of Peripheral Nerves. Current electrophysiologic techniques and concepts are the result of continual refinements made over 300 years. The nerve "impulse" or "discharge" is a wave of changing electric charge that passes down the axon from the neuron's cell body (Fig. 9–1).

A resting or unstimulated neuron has an active mechanism that maintains the interior of the cell in a state of negative charge while the area immediately outside the cell membrane is positively charged. When a neuron is stimulated, the permeability of the membrane alters, which lets in positively charged sodium ions. This momentarily reverses the charge on both sides of the nerve membrane. This area of reversed charge is the nerve impulse, which is recorded by electrophysiologic recording equipment. The nerve impulse induces an identical change in the area of the axon adjacent to it, and the impulse then travels down the nerve axon. Once the nerve impulse has passed, sodium ions are pumped back out of the cell, and after a brief recovery period, the original charged (polarized) state is restored. When a nerve impulse arrives at the end of the axon (the synapse), it causes release of a chemical neurotransmitter, which travels across the narrow gap between one neuron and the next, triggering an impulse in the second.

TECHNIQUE AND WAVEFORM NOMENCLATURE

Nerve conduction studies (NCSs) assess peripheral sensory and motor function by recording the response evoked by stimulation of selected peripheral nerves. Sensory NCSs are performed by electrically stimulating a peripheral nerve and making a recording at a measured distance, either proximally or distally from the stimulation site. Motor NCSs are performed by stimulating a peripheral nerve and recording from a muscle innervated by that nerve (Figs. 9–2 through 9–5). These studies have been used clinically since the 1950s to localize peripheral nerve disease and to differentiate it from disorders of the muscle or neuromuscular junction. Comprehensive reviews are found in references (Aminoff, 1992; Ball, 1993; Buchthal et al., 1975; Daube, 1985, 1986; Gilliatt, 1982; Johnson, 1988; Kimura, 1983, 1984; Oh, 1984).

Motor Nerve Conduction Studies. The clinical utility for motor NCSs was first described by Hodes and associates (1948). The functional integrity of motor fibers in any peripheral nerve can be evaluated by motor conduction studies if this nerve can be adequately stimulated and the response of one or more of the muscles that it innervates can be recorded. Typically, the more accessible nerves—the median, ulnar, tibial and peroneal nerves—are more readily studied. The musculocutaneous, radial, facial, femoral, phrenic, suprascapular, intercostal, and others can also be studied. The electric response of the muscle is called the compound muscle action potential (CMAP). This CMAP is the summated electric activity of the muscle fibers

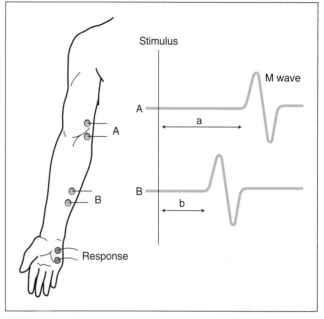

FIGURE 9–3. General scheme for motor nerve conduction studies. The general idea in conducting peripheral nerve conduction studies is to stimulate the peripheral nerve with a bipolar electrode and then to calculate the so-called conduction velocity of the nerve. The electrode is applied to the skin over the nerve, which is stimulated. This produces an activation of the nerve fiber. The response to stimulation is recorded from the muscle. The muscle response is usually measured with surface electrodes. The earliest muscle response is termed the M wave. The interval between the time of stimulation and the onset of the M wave is the latency of the response. To calculate a pure nerve conduction velocity, the nerve is stimulated at two separate points (A and B), and two latency measurements are then obtained (a and b). The distance between points A and B is measured in millimeters. The conduction velocity in meters per second is equal to

$$\frac{\text{distance between A and B in mm}}{\text{conduction time between A and B (in msec)}}$$

The conduction time between A and B is equal to the latency (msec) from point A minus the latency at point B.

in the region of the recording electrode that are innervated by the nerve that is stimulated.

The CMAP recorded after stimulation of a peripheral nerve is called the *M wave*. With supramaximal stimulation, all of the fibers in a muscle innervated by the stimulated nerve contribute to the potential. The earliest part of the M wave is elicited by the fastest-conducting motor axons. The M wave is described by its latency, amplitude, and configuration. The *latency* is the time in milliseconds from the application of the stimulus to the initial recorded deflection from baseline, and this is the time required for the action potentials in the fastest-conducting fibers to reach the nerve terminals in the muscle and activate the muscle fibers (see Fig. 9–2). As mentioned before, the latency varies directly with the distance of the stimulating electrode to the muscle.

Typically, the peripheral nerve is studied at more than one site along its course to obtain two or more CMAPs. The latencies, amplitudes, and configuration of these evoked responses are then compared (see Figs. 9–3 through 9–5).

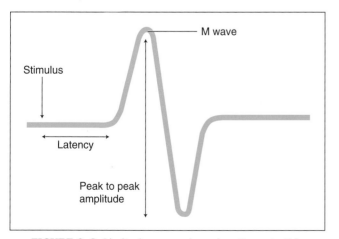

FIGURE 9–2. Idealized compound muscle action potential.

Normal conduction velocities in the upper extremities range from 50 to 70 meters per second and in the lower extremities, from 40 to 55 meters per second.

Sensory Nerve Conduction Studies. Sensory nerve action potential studies were first demonstrated in humans by Dawson and Scott in 1949. Evaluation of sensory axons in peripheral nerves may be directly evaluated by electrically stimulating the nerve and recording sensory nerve action potentials (SNAPs). Recording of SNAPs is technically more difficult than recording M waves because of much smaller amplitudes; nevertheless, potentials can readily be recorded from the median, ulnar, radial, plantar, and sural nerves, and, with some difficulty, from the musculocutaneous, peroneal, lateral femoral cutaneous, and saphenous nerves, as well as others. Gilliatt and Sears (1958) demonstrated the clinical utility of such responses, and since that time these tests have been widely used and an immense literature has emerged. By 1960, performing motor and sensory NCSs was considered the standard of care by most physical medicine specialists.

The latency of the evoked response is directly related to the speed of conduction of the nerve and the distance

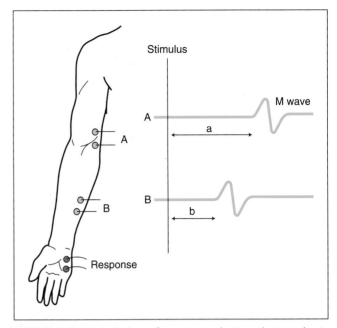

FIGURE 9–5. General scheme for motor conduction velocity studies in axonal neuropathies (axonotmesis). If axons are damaged in addition to myelin, then nerve conduction studies will show only 1) a diminished amplitude CMAP, 2) normal or only slightly slowed conduction velocity, and, paradoxically, 3) no evidence of conduction block. The CMAP would look the same regardless of whether one has stimulated above or below the lesion. This is because wallerian degeneration (which takes only 3 to 5 days to complete) would make it impossible to stimulate damaged fibers below the site of the lesion. For example, if some process destroyed 80 percent of the axons, stimulating above the lesion would excite all of the fibers, but only 20 percent would conduct past the lesion, while stimulating below the lesion would excite only the same 20 percent of the fibers since the other 80 percent have degenerated. To localize the site of the injury, the physician has to rely on clinical information and electromyography.

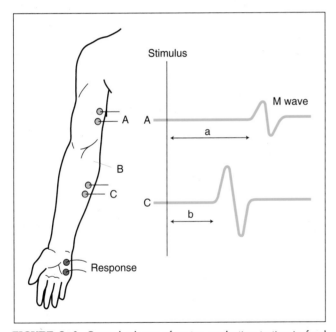

FIGURE 9–4. General scheme of motor conduction testing in focal injury. This type of lesion is seen with mild to moderate degrees of nerve compression or other neuropractic local change, such as neural ischemia or local electrolyte imbalance. The nerve is normal except for a localized area of partial injury indicated at point B. The axons are intact and therefore are conductive. This means that as many normal nerve axons are below the lesion as above. If 20 percent of the fibers in the region of the lesion can still conduct impulses, then stimulating at point A only 20 percent of the fibers will conduct through the lesion (the other 80 percent being "blocked" by their dysfunction). The resulting CMAP will be small. Stimulating below the lesion at point C, the recorded CMAP will be of normal amplitude since all of the fibers under this stimulating electrode will conduct normally. Therefore, by merely recording the amplitude of the CMAP, a focal conduction block of the nerve can be readily demonstrated. In addition, if the conduction velocity is measured at various points along the nerve (see discussion in legend for Fig. 9–3), a local slowing of conduction can also usually be found across the area of the lesion.

between the stimulating and recording electrodes. The differences in latency and distance at different sites allow for calculations of conduction velocity.

Late Responses (F Waves and H Reflexes). From the foregoing discussion and from Figures 9–3 through 9–5, it might be apparent that these techniques for assessing peripheral nerves are not applicable to studying the proximal segments of nerves. However, techniques have been developed for studying these proximal segments, including the anterior and posterior roots and the intraspinal segments, which are inaccessible using traditional sensory and motor nerve conduction stimulation. These responses are generally called long latency responses or late responses. The so-called F wave is a late response that can be recorded from numerous muscles (Fig. 9–6). In the initial studies, potentials were studied in the foot muscles, hence, the designation F wave. To elicit an F wave from a muscle, a supramaximal stimulus is delivered to a motor nerve and potentials ascend up to the spinal cord and then descend from the spinal cord out to the muscle. The latency of the F wave then includes the time required for the action potential to ascend (antidromically) to the anterior horn cell and then descend (orthodromically) from the anterior horn cell to the muscle fibers. F waves, then, provide an

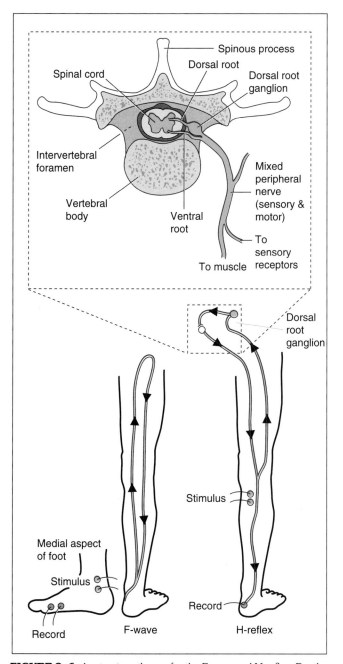

FIGURE 9–6. Anatomic pathways for the F wave and H reflex. For the F wave, the motor fiber is the afferent as well as the efferent pathway, and for the H reflex, the Ia peripheral nerve fiber is the afferent pathway and the motor fiber is the efferent pathway. There is a monosynaptic reflex arc in the H reflex pathway but no synapse involved for the F wave. The *insert* shows an axial view showing anatomic relationships of dorsal and ventral nerve roots, spinal cord, and intervertebral foramen.

the site of stimulation. F waves can be recorded from muscles in the upper and lower extremities.

The H reflex is another type of late response (see Fig. 9–6). Its name derives from its discoverer, Paul Hoffman. In adults, it is generally only studied in the gastrocnemius-soleus muscle after stimulation of the tibial nerve at the popliteal fossa. It is thought that this electric response is analogous to the monosynaptic ankle jerk. The afferent arc of this reflex is mediated by the large afferent nerves that synapse in the spinal cord on the efferent alpha motor fibers of the nerve root.

If the soleus muscle is studied, then the H reflex is thought to reflect activity of the proximal segments of the peripheral nerve as well as the S1 nerve root. In clinical reports, one sees reference to the "predicted latency," which is the time that the H reflex should occur. (The electromyographer knows how fast the nerves should conduct and also has measured the length of the patient's leg.) The electromyographer then reports on the observed latency and then also makes a left/right comparison. From this, inferences often can be made about the functional integrity of the S1 nerve root.

Like all other electrophysiologic tests, F waves and H reflexes have their proponents (Shahani & Young, 1980), who find them extremely useful, and those who find them diagnostically disappointing (Wilbourn, 1985). A main benefit of these responses is that abnormalities in these responses can be detected long before nerve degeneration occurs. F waves and H reflexes have been shown to reliably document slowed proximal conduction in hereditary and acquired demyelinating neuropathies and neurogenic thoracic outlet syndrome but are somewhat limited in the diagnosis of radiculopathy. The F wave is rarely abnormal without abnormal EMG changes (discussed later). Similarly, the H reflex is rarely abnormal without significant alteration of the ankle jerk.

Long Latency (Long Loop) Reflexes. As has always been the case in clinical electrophysiology, whenever a potential is termed a short latency response or a long latency response, inevitably an even shorter latency or longer latency response is soon discovered; the H reflex and F waves are no exception. Although these are called long latency responses, even longer latency responses are known and have interesting properties.

Long latency reflexes of human hand and forearm muscles have been described in voluntarily contracted muscles. These long latency reflexes can be elicited by various stimuli, including muscle stretch, electric stimulation of pure muscle afferents, mixed nerves, or pure cutaneous afferent nerves. At least for the muscles acting at the wrist and fingers, evidence exists that indicates these responses are mediated pathways ascending the spinal cord up to the brain and then down from the brain through the spinal cord out through the motor neurons. A large, and somewhat difficult to read, literature concerns various reflexes in this category. In a review, Deuschl and Lucking (1990) summarize the different terminologies for various

opportunity to measure conduction along the most proximal segment of motor axons, including the nerve root. Usually the F wave does not occur at a constant fixed latency from trial to trial but varies slightly; therefore, the electromyographer generally records 10 or more F wave potentials and reports on the best (shortest) latency. The latency of this "late response" is between 20 and 50 meters per second, depending on the nerve stimulated and components of these responses. Another readable and thorough review was presented by Marsden and colleagues (1983).

Although no special equipment (other than normal NCS equipment) is required for analysis of these responses, they are typically not studied in the neurology/physical medicine clinic, partly because clinical correlations are not as well established for these potentials. These responses obviously reflect integrated activity in ascending and descending pathways involved in neuromuscular control, but the functional significance of these responses is a matter of much discussion.

CLINICAL UTILITY OF NERVE CONDUCTION STUDIES

Peripheral Neuropathies. Peripheral neuropathy can affect peripheral nerve axons, their myelin sheaths, or both. Various types of pathologic changes in peripheral neuropathy can result in different patterns of electrophysiologic abnormality. Peripheral neuropathies are manifested by sensory, motor, and autonomic signs and symptoms. NCSs are sensitive tests for evaluating polyneuropathies, and such studies can define the presence of a polyneuropathy, the location of the nerve injury, and usually the pathophysiology (demyelination vs. focal axonal block).

Common types of peripheral neuropathy are a mononeuropathy of the median nerve at the wrist (carpal tunnel syndrome), ulnar neuropathy at the elbow, and peroneal nerve at the knee with localized slowing of conduction or conduction block in these regions. Jablecki and colleagues (1993, p. 1392) reviewed 165 articles on the use of NCSs in carpal tunnel syndrome and concluded that "NCSs are valid and reproducible clinical laboratory studies that confirm a clinical diagnosis of CTS with a high degree of sensitivity and specificity." In diabetes, a wide variety of abnormalities can be seen in NCSs (Kimura, 1983). In the Guillain-Barré syndrome, or inflammatory polyradiculopathy, a wide range of electrophysiologic abnormalities also exists (Kimura, 1983). Often, electrophysiologic studies can provide longitudinal information concerning the course of a polyneuropathy and can usually be used for prognosis, as in the Guillain-Barré Syndrome.

Axonal neuropathies can often be found in toxic and metabolic disorders. The major abnormality found by nerve conduction studies is a reduction in amplitude of the CMAP or SNAP, simply because fewer nerve fibers are present. Some axonal neuropathies, such as vitamin B_{12} deficiency, carcinomatous neuropathy, and Friedreich's ataxia, predominantly affect sensory fibers, while others such as the lead neuropathies seem to affect motor nerve fibers more.

Radiculopathies. Electrophysiologic studies can identify the specific level of root injury and also differentiate between root injury and other peripheral nerve problems that might cause similar symptomatology. Evaluation of functional integrity of nerve roots can be important for patient management with regard to further diagnostic evaluation and surgical intervention.

Usually in radiculopathies the most common clinical presentation is with sensory symptoms. In nerve root dysfunction, the locus of the injury is at or proximal to the foraminal opening (see Fig. 9–6, *insert*). Normal studies of sensory nerves in the distribution of the sensory complaints or abnormal clinical sensory examination would be consistent with a radiculopathy, while abnormalities of sensory conduction would indicate a more distal site of injury. Similarly, slowing of motor conduction velocity would argue for peripheral nerve dysfunction rather than nerve root dysfunction.

The H reflex can be effectively used to assess the S1 dorsal root, but somatosensory evoked potentials (discussed later) are needed to adequately study nerve roots at other levels. Abnormal H reflexes or F waves by themselves do not establish a diagnosis of a radiculopathy but can complement other electrophysiologic information. Conventional nerve conduction studies are usually normal in cervical and lumbosacral radiculopathies (Eisen, 1987). In radiculopathy, most lesions can occur proximal to the dorsal root ganglion; therefore, the sensory nerve fibers are intact, and, consequently, distal sensory nerve potentials are normal, even if the patient has a sensory deficit. However, in radiculopathy, damage to motor nerve fibers may occur, and, consequently, a slowing of motor conduction can often be detected.

Plexopathies. Diagnosis of nerve root damage localized to nerve plexi often poses a clinical challenge. NCS techniques that can localize lesions to the plexi are available. Such studies can also provide evidence against peripheral nerve abnormalities, which could produce similar symptoms. Serial studies can follow the course of plexus injuries and aid in management and prognosis.

System Degenerations. Some system degenerations of the central nervous system involve either the dorsal root ganglia or the anterior horn cells. Motor neuron diseases such as amyotrophic lateral sclerosis, spinal muscular atrophy, Charcot-Marie-Tooth disease, Kugelberg-Welander disease, and others are characterized by degeneration of anterior horn cells and, therefore, loss of peripheral motor axons. This is reflected by a reduction in amplitude of the CMAP, which is proportional to the loss of axons innervating the muscle. Sensory system degenerations are found in spinal cerebellar degeneration, vitamin B_{12} deficiency, and carcinomatous sensory neuropathy. The degeneration seen in sensory pathways in the spinal cord is due to degeneration of the cells of origin in the dorsal root ganglia; these cells are the source of the large sensory fibers in the peripheral nerves and therefore show abnormalities with sensory nerve testing. A moderate number of sensory axons must be involved before SNAP amplitudes become noticeably lower, and even more motor axons must be affected to result in an abnormally low amplitude CMAP.

Disorders of the Neuromuscular Junction. The myasthenic syndrome and botulus poisoning are likely to show changes in nerve conduction studies. Both of these conditions result in a low rate of release of acetylcholine from nerve terminals and, therefore, a block of neuromuscular transmission to a large portion of the muscle fibers. The CMAPs are usually of low amplitude.

Disorders of Involuntary Activity. Some disorders are manifested as stiffness of muscles, myokymia, and cramping. These are due to excessive discharges in peripheral motor axons. Numerous clinical patterns and a wide variation in electric abnormalities have been seen. Each has different findings on clinical needle electromyography (discussed below), but abnormalities can also be seen on nerve conduction studies.

In these cases, motor nerve stimulation produces a repetitive discharge of the muscle. Instead of a single CMAP after a single stimulus, a group of two to six potentials can be seen.

ELECTROMYOGRAPHY

In 1938, Denny-Brown and Pennybacker pointed out the clinical utility of analyzing the electric activity of muscle, and electromyography has been in clinical use since that time. The term *electromyography* (EMG) has sometimes been used to refer to the entire array of electrodiagnostic tests for nerve and muscle diseases, but strictly speaking, it refers only to the examination of the bioelectric activity of muscles with a needle or surface electrode. The EMG examination, then, unlike NCSs, assesses only muscle fibers and, indirectly, motor nerve fibers but not sensory nerves.

Some Anatomy

Discussion of much of the scientific basis for these tests is relegated to the figures and legends in this chapter, and the reader is urged to consult these frequently. The motor nerve fibers that innervate voluntary muscles (except those in the head) are axons of cells in the anterior gray matter of the spinal cord (Fig. 9–7). The junction between the terminal branch of the motor nerve fiber and the muscle fiber is located at the midpoint of the muscle fiber and is called the motor end-plate (see Fig. 9–7). Each axon generally contributes to the formation of a single end-plate innervating one muscle fiber. Where the motor nerve enters the muscle is termed the motor point.

Each mammalian skeletal muscle fiber is innervated by only one motor neuron, but a motor neuron innervates more than one muscle fiber (see Fig. 9–7). In the 1920s, Sir

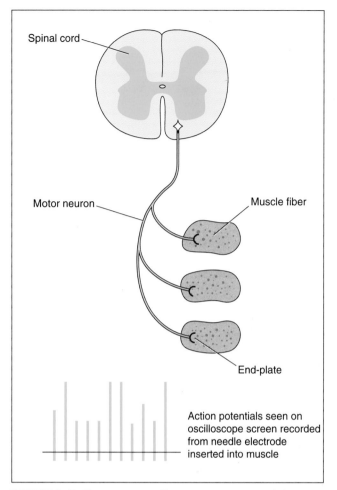

FIGURE 9–7. The motor unit. The motor unit consists of the motor neuron and the population of muscle fibers that it innervates; three motor neurons and their population of muscle fibers are shown. The muscle fibers innervated by a single motor neuron generally are not adjacent to one another. However, a needle electrode inserted into the muscle will record a motor unit potential when the unit is activated, because synaptic transmission at the neuromuscular junction ensures that each action potential in the nerve produces a contraction in every muscle fiber innervated by that motor neuron. The size of the motor unit potentials varies as a function of the number of muscle fibers that contribute. (Adapted, with permission, from Kandel, E., & Schwarz, J. H. [1981]. *Principles of Neural Science.* Stamford, CT: Appleton & Lange.)

Charles Sherrington introduced the term *motor unit* to refer to the motor neuron in the spinal cord and the population of muscle fibers that it innervates. The motor unit, then, is composed of three components: 1) the cell body of the motor neuron, 2) its axon, which runs in the peripheral nerve, and 3) muscle fibers innervated by that neuron (see Fig. 9–7). The number of muscle fibers innervated by a single motor neuron varies according to its function: Motor units involved in fine movements (e.g., in the small muscles of the hand) consist of only three to six muscle fibers, but motor units of the gastrocnemius muscle of the leg can contain as many as 2000 muscle fibers. Good reviews on the anatomy and physiology of motor units can be found in Buchthal (1961) and in Burke (1981).

Most diseases of the motor unit cause weakness and atrophy of skeletal muscles. Various types of motor unit diseases were characterized by pathologists in the 19th century. Some patients showed pronounced pathologic changes in the cell bodies of the motor neuron but no or minor changes in the muscle (motor neuron diseases). Other patients had a degeneration of muscle with little or no change in motor neurons (myopathies). Other patients had pathologic changes that affected only the axons of peripheral nerves (peripheral neuropathy). Diseases of the motor unit can be divided into two classes: 1) *neurogenic* diseases, which affect the cell body or peripheral axon; and 2) *myopathic* diseases, which affect the muscle (Figs. 9–8 and 9–9).

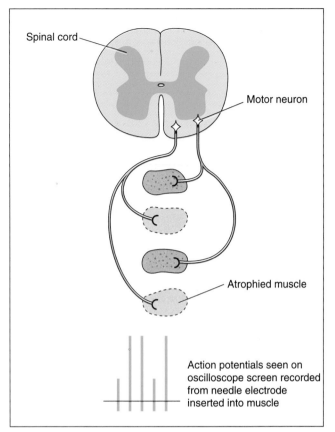

FIGURE 9–9. Diagram of motor unit in muscle disease (myopathy). Some muscles innervated by the motor neuron have become diseased. The motor unit potential is reduced in amplitude. (Adapted, with permission, from Kandel, E., & Schwarz, J. H. [1981]. *Principles of Neural Science.* Stamford, CT: Appleton & Lange.)

Technique and Waveform Nomenclature

The clinical utility of EMG lies in its ability to detect abnormalities in muscle activity resultant to injury to the nerve innervating that muscle. The EMG examination includes four phases: the evaluation of spontaneous (resting) muscle activity, insertional activity, activity during minimal muscle contraction, and activity during maximal muscle contraction. During these four phases, the electromyographer looks for abnormal electric activity of the muscle. The activity from the needle electrode is led into powerful amplifiers, and the activity is displayed on an oscilloscope screen. The electromyographer often leads the output of the amplifier to a loudspeaker; various abnormal patterns produce distinctive sounds, which can often facilitate recognition. These needle EMG changes are discussed under "Abnormal EMG Activity."

The waveforms of various types of normal EMG activity are shown in Figure 9–10.

Spontaneous Activity. A very important point is that normal muscle fibers, with normal nerve supply, show no spontaneous (i.e., at rest) electric activity.

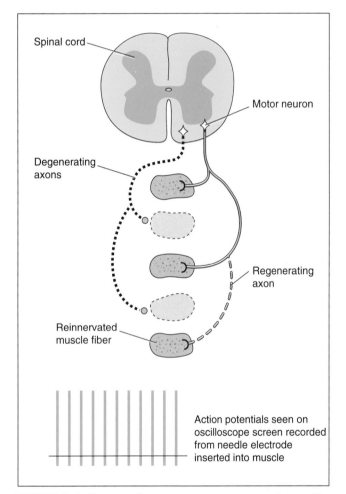

FIGURE 9–8. Diagram of motor unit in motor neuron disease. The motor neuron on the left is degenerating. Its muscle fibers have become atrophic (symbolized by dotted lines), and units innervated by the degenerated nerve no longer produce motor unit potentials. This is apparent on the oscillograph screen by decreased rate of action potentials (compared with Fig. 9–7). However, the neuron on the right has sprouted additional axonal branches that reinnervate some of the denervated muscle fibers. These muscle fibers produce a larger than normal motor unit potential (compared with Fig. 9–7), and they also fire spontaneously at rest (fasciculations). (Adapted, with permission, from Kandel, E., & Schwarz, J. H. [1981]. *Principles of Neural Science.* Stamford, CT: Appleton & Lange.)

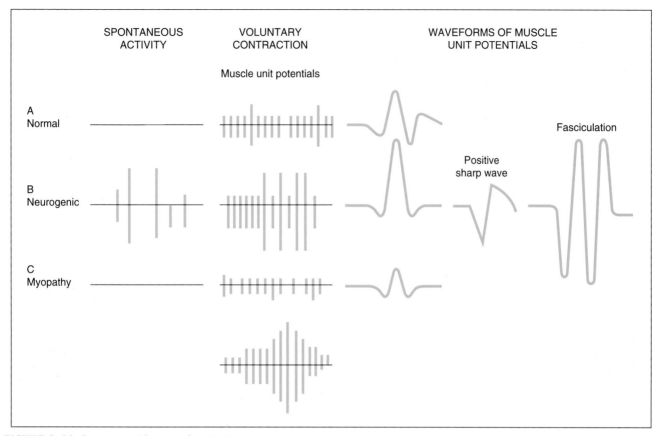

FIGURE 9–10. Some general features of the EMG in normal subjects *(A)*, in patients with neurogenic diseases *(B)*, and in myogenic diseases *(C)*. The rising and falling pattern of action potentials *(bottom trace)* seen on the oscilloscope is referred to as "myotonic discharge." (Adapted, with permission, from Kandel, E., & Schwarz, J. H. [1981]. *Principles of Neural Science*. Stamford, CT: Appleton & Lange.)

Voluntary Activity. The motor unit potential (MUP) is the sum of the potentials of muscle fibers innervated by a single anterior horn cell. Motor unit potentials are characterized by their firing pattern and their morphology. Recruitment is the initiation of firing of additional motor units as the active motor unit potentials increase their rate of discharge, as when a patient is asked to contract a muscle.

Abnormal EMG patterns are diagrammed in Figure 9–10*B* and *C*.

Neuromuscular diseases can show abnormal spontaneous discharges or abnormal voluntary MUPs. Abnormal spontaneous activity includes *fibrillation potentials, fasciculation potentials, myotonic discharges, neuromyotonic discharges, complex repetitive discharges, myokymic discharges, and cramps*. Only the first two are encountered frequently in the EMG laboratory.

Motor unit potentials are characterized by their morphology—they can have abnormal duration, be polyphasic, or can vary in size. The recruitment pattern of MUPs can be altered; all of these are noted by the electromyographer. Early on, Adrian and Bronk (1929, p. 10) noted that recognition of abnormal EMG patterns was made easier if the amplified electric activity was run into a loudspeaker, " . . . for the ear can pick out each new series

of slight differences in intensity and quality which are hard to detect in the complex electrometer record." For readers who might visit an EMG laboratory, these various "sounds" are described.

Fibrillation Potentials. Fibrillation potentials are action potentials of single muscle fibers that are twitching spontaneously in the absence of innervation. Fibrillation potentials can have two different forms: a brief spike or a positive wave. Spikes are considered to be muscle fiber action potentials recorded extracellularly, and positive waves are muscle fiber action potentials recorded from an injured part of the muscle fiber. When run into a loudspeaker, fibrillation potentials sound like the "ticking of a clock," i.e., they occur at regular intervals. Any muscle fiber that is denervated can produce fibrillation potentials, and because of this, a wide variety of both neurogenic and myopathic processes can show fibrillation potentials. Fibrillation potentials can therefore be seen in lower motor neuron diseases, neuromuscular junction diseases, and muscle diseases. Fibrillation potentials do not appear immediately after motor axon loss but have an onset 14 to 35 days after injury. They persist until the injured muscle fiber either gets reinnervated or degenerates due to lack of nerve supply (generally about 1.5 to 2 years after denervation).

Fasciculation Potentials. Fasciculation potentials are the action potentials of a group of muscle fibers innervated by an anterior horn cell, i.e., action potentials of an entire motor unit. When run into a speaker, fasciculation potentials sound (to some) like "raindrops on a roof." As opposed to fibrillation potentials, fasciculation potentials require an intact motor unit; their appearance indicates motor unit "irritation." Fasciculation potentials can occur in normal subjects and in a wide variety of neuromuscular disorders.

Myotonic Discharges. These discharges consist of high-frequency trains of action potentials that are provoked by electrode movement or percussion or contraction of the muscle. The frequency and amplitude of these potentials wax and wane and, consequently, if the signal is run into a speaker, it produces a sound like that of a "dive bomber." The pathogenesis of the myotonic discharge is uncertain but it is thought to be related to a disorder of the muscle fiber membrane.

Neuromyotonic Discharges (Neurotonic Discharges). These are motor unit potentials associated with continuous muscle fiber activity. The activity is rapid—100 to 300 per second. Such activity can be seen in chronic spinal muscular atrophy, tetany, and anticholinesterase poisoning.

Complex Repetitive Discharges (Bizarre High-Frequency Potentials). Complex repetitive discharges are the action potentials of groups of muscle fibers discharging at high rates (3 to 40 per second.). The sound of the signal run into a speaker has been described as a "motorboat that misfires occasionally." Complex repetitive discharges are seen in a variety of myopathic and neurogenic disorders, such as poliomyositis, amyotrophic lateral sclerosis, spinal muscular atrophy, chronic radiculopathies, chronic neuropathies, poliomyositis, and other myopathies. An experienced electromyographer can distinguish complex repetitive discharges from other trains of high-frequency discharges such as neuromyotonic discharges, myokymic discharges, cramps, tremor, and others.

Myokymic Discharges. Myokymic discharges are spontaneous muscle potentials associated with fine quivering of muscles, usually in the face. Myokymic discharges rise in the lower motor neuron or axon. They are differentiated from fasciculation potentials by their distinct pattern (fluttering and bursts), and the discharges have been described as the sound of "marching soldiers." Myokymic discharges have a distinct clinical significance. They are seen in patients with multiple sclerosis, brain stem neoplasm, polyradiculopathy, facial palsy, radiation plexopathy, and chronic nerve compression.

Cramp Potentials. Cramp potentials resemble MUPs. They fire at a rate of 30 to 60 per second. They fire when a muscle is cramping, i.e., when it is activated strongly in a shortened position. Cramps are a normal phenomenon but can also be indicative of some disorders, including salt depletion, chronic neurogenic atrophy, and uremia.

A common "complaint" about conventional NCS and EMG testing is that very little has changed over the last 40 years. The founder of modern EMG, Adrian, would feel right at home in a modern EMG laboratory, as would the developers of sensory and motor NCSs. This is in marked contrast to the almost yearly advances in imaging techniques such as computed tomography (CT) and magnetic resonance imaging (MRI). However, several new EMG techniques to study the fine points of motor unit physiology have been developed over the last decade or so. These are *single fiber EMG, macro EMG, and scanning EMG*. Despite the enthusiasm of "early adopters" of these techniques, they are, for the most part restricted to research laboratories or at least very large academic centers. These techniques are concerned with measuring activity in individual muscle fibers, or displaying the spatiotemporal activity of an entire motor unit. The interested reader should consult the article by Stalberg and Dioszeghy (1991), which discusses normal and clinical examples and has a good reference list. For purposes here, discussion of these emerging techniques is relegated to the glossary.

Clinical Utility

The reader is referred to some of the numerous comprehensive references on clinical correlations of EMG (Aminoff, 1992; Ball, 1993; Brown and Bolton, 1987; Daube, 1985, 1986; Johnson, 1988; Kimura, 1983, 1984; Oh, 1984; Shahani 1984; Willison, 1964). Only a brief summary is presented here.

Myopathy. Disorders of muscle can be often defined by examining the characteristics of motor units. Such characteristics include the morphology of individual motor units, as well as recruitment and interference patterns. The physiologic abnormality in myopathies is lessened tension generated by muscle fibers. This is accompanied by decreased size, increased duration, and increased complexity of motor unit potentials. In many muscle diseases, electromyographic abnormalities of resting muscle due to disruption of the normal connections between the nerve and muscle are present. By evaluating these changes, a myopathic process can be ruled in or ruled out. Electroneurophysiologic studies are important for patient management, as they can establish the presence of a myopathy and can also be helpful prior to muscle biopsies in identifying exactly which muscles are clinically involved. Serial studies can be used to follow the course of a myopathy and monitor the effect of therapy.

Nerve conduction should be normal in patients with pure myopathy. However, in many myopathies, including myotonic dystrophy, hypothyroidism, sarcoidosis, polymyositis, and carcinomatous neuromyopathy, peripheral neuropathy is usually present. Regarding electromyographic abnormalities, an increased amount of insertion activity (i.e., electric activity recorded immediately on insertion of the needle electrode) may be found in myopathic disorders, and abnormal spontaneous activity is often present. Abnormalities are seen in the recruitment pattern of motor unit potentials during a strong voluntary contraction. A full interference pattern is recorded, but the potentials are lower in amplitude and have altered wave forms.

Neuromuscular Junction Disorder. Electrophysiologic examinations can accurately localize clinical disorders of neuromuscular transmission to the neuromuscular junction. These disorders include myasthenia gravis, Lambert-Eaton syndrome, botulism, and the congenital myasthenic syndromes. Disturbances of the neuromuscular junction can also be seen in certain peripheral neuropathies, neuronopathies, myopathy, and myotonic disorders. These can be distinguished from primary disturbance of the neuromuscular junction by clinical examination and by peripheral NCSs. Individual motor unit potentials show a marked variation in morphology because of blocking of impulse transmission to individual fibers within the motor unit.

Radiculopathy. Abnormalities in a myotomal distribution can define a root injury. Needle EMG in radiculopathies is abnormal only when the injury is of sufficient degree to produce axonal transection or a conduction block.

SURFACE ELECTROMYOGRAPHY

In traditional needle EMG, action potentials are recorded intramuscularly through thin needles. In contrast, the frequency and amplitude of single motor unit firing measured with surface EMG muscle activity is recorded from the surface of the skin via a disk electrode. What is measured is a summation of muscle action potentials, providing a general measure of muscle contraction. Thus, needle EMG cannot provide general information concerning whole muscle contraction, and surface EMG cannot give specific information regarding individual motor units.

The use of surface EMG has been in two main areas: 1) as biofeedback in pain management; and 2) to try to quantify low back pain due to muscular dysfunction.

The use of surface EMG as a biofeedback modality has been extensively reviewed by Headley (1993). Since the 1960s, biofeedback has been used as a technique to promote muscle relaxation. The basic premise of the relaxation model of pain management is that pain causes stress, and this stress in turn increases anxiety of the patient, thereby further increasing the pain. The use of biofeedback for relaxation was based on the assumption that muscle activity is at a higher level because of anxiety or stress and that muscles are overreactive to stressful activity. In 1985, Bush and colleagues demonstrated that many patients with chronic low back pain do not have elevated paraspinal EMG activity, and they raised the question of whether relaxation training of chronic low back patients was a desired protocol. Most research papers, at least early ones, on surface EMG and low back pain are hampered by lack of control subjects and unclear relationship between the experience of pain and surface EMG measurements.

The elucidation of the role of trigger points in myofascial pain syndromes has explained many patients' complaints (Travell and Simons 1983, 1992), and Headley (1993) has described a role for surface EMG in various phenomena, which could be attributable to trigger points. One is the concept of referred reflex muscle spasm caused by activation of a trigger point in another, sometimes distant, muscle. Another phenomenon described by Headley is reflex inhibition of muscle activity by a trigger point in a distant muscle. This inhibition may be movement specific; i.e., a given muscle might work normally during one movement but not during another movement. Headley has provided intriguing examples of how surface EMG can be used to study such phenomena, and she uses this technique as part of a treatment protocol.

The relationship between paraspinal surface electromyography and low back pain is controversial. Pertinent studies can be found in DeLuca (1993), Roy and associates (1989, 1990), and Sihvonen and colleagues (1991).

A problem with selecting patients with low back pain for scientific studies is picking patients with similar pathophysiology. Aside from disk disease, a number of musculoskeletal disorders need to be considered, including muscle tension, lumbosacral sprain, strain, and mechanical pain. Clearly, many more studies with large numbers of patients are needed to clarify the role of surface EMG in electrodiagnosis.

It should be emphasized that surface EMG is currently considered to be a technique that is not diagnostically useful, and its performance is generally not reimbursed by third-party payers. Traditional electromyographers generally tend to totally discount surface EMG as being of very limited usefulness. One reason is that the technique seems to be technically unsophisticated, but a more important reason is that consistent descriptions of surface EMG characteristics in back pain patients have not been presented. Every possible result has been reported in the literature. For example, some studies have shown patients to have an elevated EMG activity, some have shown them to have a similar EMG pattern to normals, and some report lowered EMG activity. In some studies, patients with low back pain have been found to have asymmetries between left and right paraspinal muscles. Asymmetries in EMG activity are thought to be the result of excessive and chronic bracing and guarding. For patients with elevated EMG activity, high muscle tension is proposed in a muscle spasm model, and in patients with lowered amounts of EMG activity, low muscle tension is proposed by a muscle deficiency model.

EVOKED POTENTIALS

Evoked potentials are electric potentials that are generated in the central nervous system in response to sensory (auditory, visual, somatosensory) stimuli. The existence of

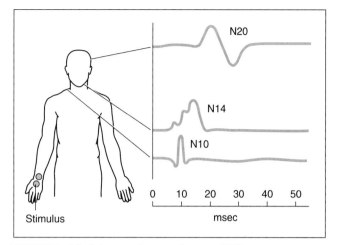

FIGURE 9–12. Schematic diagram of a normal SEP in response to arm stimulation. Recordings from top to bottom show the scalp recorded N20; the cervical SEP, N13; and the clavicular (Erb's point), N10.

can be recorded from the peripheral nerve over the popliteal fossa, lumbar region of the spinal cord, and over the foot sensory area of the cortex (Fig. 9–13).

In 1994, the International Federation for Clinical Neurophysiology published recommended standards for SEP recordings (Nuwer et al., 1994). Recording montages differ slightly from the protocol described here. In the author's opinion, this new guideline introduces arguably unnecessary complications into what should be a simple test, and, as with Chiappa's (1983) recommendations, there are published objections (Zeyers de Beyl, 1995).

Waveform Nomenclature and Neural Generators

The scalp-recorded SEP is thought to be mediated solely through activation of the large Ia peripheral nerves (Burke et al., 1981). Various components of the SEP are often described in clinical reports and in the literature, so these are briefly summarized here. By convention, an evoked potential component is designated by its electric polarity (by a P or N, for positive or negative) and by its latency in milliseconds. Thus, an N10 potential is a negative potential with a peak latency of 10 milliseconds. For several of the SEP components, the polarity depends on the choice of reference electrode, so several authors designate the polarity as P/N. Consult Figure 9–11 for pertinent anatomic pathways.

Upper Extremity Stimulation (see Fig. 9–12). In the clinical setting, SEPs in response to stimulation of nerves in the upper extremity are usually recorded from the following three levels:

a) *Clavicle (N10)*. Potentials at this level are best recorded from Erb's point in the supraclavicular fossa or from just above the midpoint of the clavicle. Under these conditions, a triphasic wave (positive-negative-

positive) with a very prominent negativity is recorded. The negativity occurs with a peak latency of around 10 milliseconds for median nerve stimulation and is generally referred to as the N10 potential (sometimes called the Erb's point potential, or N9). This is a near-field potential generated in the nerve fibers in the brachial plexus underlying the electrode.

b) *Posterior neck (N12, N14)*. The N12 is thought to be generated at the level of the cervical dorsal root, and the N14 generated either in the dorsal column pathway or at the cuneate nucleus in the medulla or possibly in the caudal portion of the medial lemniscus.

c) *Sensory cortex (N20)*. This potential, a negative potential with a peak latency of around 20 milliseconds, is recorded from a scalp electrode overlying the sensory cortex, which is in the contralateral cerebral hemisphere (i.e., for right upper extremity stimulation, the potential is recorded from left brain).

Lower Extremity Stimulation (see Fig. 9–13). SEPs in response to stimulation of nerves in the lower extremity can be recorded at the following levels:

a) *Lumbothoracic spine (N20)*. This potential is recorded best by placing an active skin electrode over the spinous process of L1 or T12 and using a distant lateral reference (e.g., over the iliac crest). With this recording set-up, a negative deflection with a latency of around 20 milliseconds is recorded (N20). Most investigators agree that this potential reflects activity in the dorsal spinal cord.

b) *Neck (N27)*. Here, the main potential consists of a negative deflection of around 27 milliseconds. It is probably generated at the level of the foramen magnum, either in the dorsal columns themselves or in the dorsal column nucleus (nucleus gracilis), or perhaps in the caudal part of the medial lemniscus. (For routine clinical use, potentials recorded over the

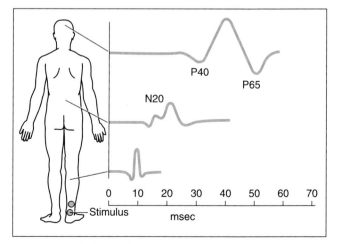

FIGURE 9–13. Schematic diagram of a normal SEP in response to stimulation of the posterior tibial nerve at the ankle. The recordings from top to bottom show the scalp recorded P40 and P65, low thoracic and lumbar spinal SEPs, and peripheral nerve potential recorded at the popliteal fossa.

lower thoracic spine and also the neck are usually somewhat difficult to record, mainly due to myogenic contamination by paraspinal muscles. They are best recorded in very thin people and cannot be recorded in overweight people with any reliability. Because of poor reproducibility and excessive false positives, these potentials are often not used in routine clinical screening exams.)

c) *Cortex (P40)*. This potential is best recorded from a scalp electrode overlying the foot area of the brain, which lies midline just posterior to the middle of the top of the head. A well-formed positive wave peaking at 40 to 45 milliseconds is recorded in response to posterior tibial nerve stimulation at the ankle. Obviously, patient height and limb length are some determinants of the latency of this potential. Potentials evoked by sural nerve stimulation at the same level have a slightly longer latency because of slightly smaller (and therefore slower conducting) peripheral nerve fiber diameters.

Clinical Utility

In evaluation of the central nervous system, the main role for SEPs is for the detection of lesions. A primary use for neurologists has been for confirmation of this diagnosis in a patient with a presumptive diagnosis on the basis of clinical and imaging studies. The presence of somatosensory abnormalities has often been useful in detecting subclinical lesions in multiple sclerosis and thus in establishing the presence of multiple lesions in the central nervous system. As with NCS or EMG, evoked potential abnormalities never provide a diagnosis by themselves. They must be interpreted within the clinical context of the case.

Somatosensory evoked potentials can also be abnormal in a wide variety of other disorders affecting the brain and spinal cord such as tumors and strokes, depending on whether these lesions affect the afferent pathways. With regard to a hemispheric stroke or in the evaluation of patients following anoxic-ischemic events, SEP findings are often useful in providing a guide to the prognosis of such patients. For example, Hume and coworkers (1979) correctly predicted the outcome in 38 of 49 comatose patients; basically, the principle is that the worse the morphology of the somatosensory evoked potentials, the worse the prognosis.

An important use for SEPs is in the operating room to monitor spinal cord and brain functioning during surgery. Discussion of this widespread but somewhat controversial topic is beyond the scope of this chapter. The interested reader can consult several textbooks on this subject or the chapter by Owen (1991).

For routine clinical testing, Eisen and associates (1983) popularized a technique of analyzing "segmentally specific" evoked potentials in an attempt to increase specificity of SEPs when trying to isolate a radiculopathy. Basically,

the technique involves stimulation of several different nerves in the extremity being studied in an effort to localize slowing at one particular nerve root. Unfortunately, most peripheral cutaneous nerves contain fibers from two or more roots. Therefore, an abnormality restricted to one root might be masked by activity in the normal roots. Another problem in using SEPs for the diagnosis of radiculopathies is that one is attempting to detect a small segment of conduction slowing, usually only a few millimeters long, and this small area can easily be masked or diluted along the long length of the normally conducting nerve distal to the root. This is true for stimulation of both upper and lower extremities. Despite these practical and theoretic difficulties, the author has found this technique to be quite sensitive and easy to perform and interpret.

Peripheral Neuropathy. There are several indications for using SEPs to evaluate the integrity of peripheral nerves:

1. Some peripheral nerves, such as the lateral femoral cutaneous or pudendal nerve, are not easily accessible for stimulation or recording using standard EMG methods, and SEPs can be used to measure conduction along such nerves.

2. In processes such as Charcot-Marie-Tooth disease, the peripheral neuropathy makes NCSs difficult to quantify.

3. For the evaluation of radiculopathies, especially when sensory signs and symptoms are present. As discussed previously, often peripheral nerve testing is inadequate because in such problems the actual conduction deficit lies proximal to the dorsal root ganglion.

4. SEPs can be used to evaluate plexopathies.

Usually, however, it is considered good practice to use more routine techniques such as peripheral nerve conduction and EMG, and if these are shown to be of little value, then SEP testing might then be employed.

Radiculopathy. In SEP testing, a bilateral segmental analysis (described earlier) is often useful for pinpointing a radiculopathy. Eisen and colleagues (1983) studied 28 patients with either cervical or lumbosacral pathology and found that 16 (57%) had abnormal SEPs. Using the technique of segmental stimulation, Perlik and colleagues (1986) studied 27 patients with low back pain; 21 patients had SEP abnormalities that correlated with symptomatology and CT scanning. The authors also described 15 cases in which no associated clinical deficit or peripheral nerve or EMG, electrophysiologic abnormality was present and believed that the SEP was often useful for detecting subclinical nerve root pathology. These authors found the most common abnormality to be a prolongation in the evoked potential latency. Walk and colleagues (1992) studied SEPs in 59 patients with signs or symptoms suggestive of lumbosacral radiculopathy and compared them with CT myelography, MRI, and other electrophysiologic studies. Thirty-eight patients had abnormal CT myelograms, and 32 of these had abnormal SEPs, but only 11 demonstrated EMG abnormalities. Interestingly, all 21 patients with normal

Fasciculation—The random, spontaneous twitching of a group of muscle fibers that may be visible through the skin. The electric activity associated with the spontaneous contraction is called the *fasciculation potential.*

Fibrillation—The spontaneous contractions of individual muscle fibers that are ordinarily not visible through the skin.

Frequency analysis—Determination of the range of frequencies composing a potential waveform, with a measurement of the absolute or relative amplitude of each component frequency. It is similar to the mathematic technique of Fourier analysis.

F wave—A long latency compound action potential evoked from a muscle by supramaximal electric stimulus to a peripheral nerve. Compared with the maximal amplitude M wave of the same muscle, the F wave has a reduced amplitude and variable morphology and a longer and more variable latency. It can be found in many muscles of the upper and lower extremities, and the latency is longer with more distal sites of stimulation (see Fig. 9–6).

H wave reflex—A long latency compound muscle action potential having a consistent latency evoked from a muscle by an electric stimulus to a peripheral nerve. It is regularly found only in a limited group of physiologic extensors, particularly the calf muscles. A stimulus intensity sufficient to elicit a maximal amplitude M wave reduces or abolishes the H wave. The H wave is thought to be due to a spinal reflex, the Hoffman reflex, with electric stimulation of afferent fibers in the mixed nerve to the muscle and activation of motor neurons to the muscle through a monosynaptic connection in the spinal cord (see Fig. 9–6).

Insertional activity—Electric activity caused by insertion or movement of a needle electrode.

Interference pattern—Electric activity recorded from a muscle with a needle electrode during maximal voluntary effort, in which identification of each of the contributing action potentials is not possible because of the overlap or interference of one potential with another. When no individual potentials can be identified, this is known as a *full interference pattern.* A *reduced interference pattern* is one in which some of the individual potentials may be identified, while other individual potentials cannot be identified because of overlapping.

Jitter—In single-fiber EMG, the jitter is characterized by the mean difference between consecutive interpotential intervals (MCD). The MCD is 10 to 50 μsec in normal subjects; when neuromuscular transmission is disturbed, the jitter (i.e., MCD) is increased.

Latency—Interval between the onset of a stimulus and the onset of a response unless otherwise specified. Latency always refers to the onset unless specified, as in *peak latency.* Generally, in cerebral evoked potential studies, peak latency is measured (see Fig. 9–2).

Macroelectromyography—In this technique, electric activity within a muscle is recorded by a modified electrode that is used for single-fiber EMG. During a voluntary muscle activity, an averaging computer is triggered from activity arising in a single muscle fiber. It is thought that the resultant wave form measures the contribution from one entire motor unit. As such, macro motor unit action potentials reflect abnormalities seen in myopathies and can show when reinervation has occurred in peripheral neuropathies.

Membrane instability—Tendency of a cell membrane to depolarize spontaneously or after mechanical irritation or voluntary activation.

Monopolar needle electrode—A solid wire, usually of stainless steel, coated (except at its tip) with an insulating material. Variations in voltage between the tip of the needle in a muscle and a conductive plate on the skin surface (reference electrode) are measured. This recording setup is referred to as a monopolar needle electrode recording.

Motor unit potential (MUP)—Action potential reflecting the electric activity of that part of a motor unit that is within the recording range of an electrode.

M wave—A *compound action potential* evoked from a muscle by a single electric stimulus to its motor nerve. By convention, the M wave elicited by supramaximal stimulation is used for motor nerve conduction studies.

Myokymia—Involuntary, continuous quivering of muscle fibers that may be visible through the skin as a vermiform movement. It is associated with spontaneous, rhythmic discharge of *motor unit potentials.*

Myotonic discharge—Repetitive discharge of 20 to 80 Hz recorded after needle insertion into muscle.

Needle electrode—An electrode for recording or stimulating, shaped like a needle.

Nerve conduction studies—Refers to all aspects of electrodiagnostic studies of peripheral nerves. However, the term is generally used to refer to the recording and measurement of *compound nerve* and *compound muscle action potentials* elicited in response to a single supramaximal electrical *stimulus.*

Neuromyotonic discharges—Bursts of *motor unit potentials* firing at more than 150 Hz for 0.5 to 2 seconds. The amplitude of the response typically wanes. Discharges may occur spontaneously or be initiated by needle movement.

Orthodromic—Refers to *action potentials* or stimuli eliciting action potentials propagated in the same direction as physiologic conduction, e.g., motor nerve conduction away from the spinal cord and sensory nerve conduction toward the spinal cord. Contrast with *antidromic.*

Polarization—The presence of an electric potential difference across an excitable cell membrane. The potential across the membrane of a cell when it is not excited by input or spontaneously active is termed the *resting poten-*

tial; it is at a steady state with regard to the electric potential difference across the membrane. *Depolarization* describes a decrease in polarization. *Hyperpolarization* describes an increase in polarization (see Fig. 9–1).

Positive sharp wave—Strictly defined, one form of electric activity associated with fibrillating muscle fibers (see Fig. 9–10B).

Recording electrode—Device used to monitor electric current or potential. All electric recordings require two *electrodes*. The electrode close to the source of the activity to be recorded is called the *active electrode*, and the other electrode is called the *reference electrode*. The commonly used term *monopolar recording* is, strictly speaking, not correct because all recording requires two electrodes; however, it is commonly used to describe the use of an intramuscular needle active electrode in combination with a surface disk or subcutaneous needle reference electrode.

Recruitment—The orderly activation of motor units with increasing strength of voluntary muscle contraction.

Repetitive stimulation—The technique of utilizing repeated supramaximal stimulation of a nerve while analyzing *M waves* from muscles innervated by the nerve.

Resting membrane potential—Voltage across the membrane of an excitable cell (nerve or muscle fiber) at rest.

Scanning electromyography—In this technique, an electrode used for single-fiber EMG is inserted into a slightly contracted muscle and advanced in small steps (on the order of 50 μm). What is displayed is a spatiotemporal analysis of firing of the motor units. This term is also used in surface EMG to describe the recording from several muscles.

Single-fiber electromyography (SF-EMG)—A relatively new technique that allows for recording activity in individual muscle fibers with a very small needle electrode. The muscle is under slight voluntary activation, and the electrode is positioned so activity is recorded from one or two individual muscle fibers. A temporal variability, *the jitter*, is analyzed. This is the time between two consecutive discharges (see *jitter*). Measurement of jitter is a sensitive means of evaluating neuromuscular transmission. This technique can be used for analysis of myopathic and neurogenic disorders. The technique has also been used to estimate the number of motor units in a muscle.

Somatosensory evoked potential (SEP or SSEP)—Electric waves recorded from the head or trunk in response to stimulation of peripheral sensory fibers. Recordings over the spine may be referred to as *spinal evoked potentials* (see Figs. 9–12 and 9–13).

Spike—Transient wave with a pointed peak and a short duration (a few milliseconds or less). See *end-plate spike* and *fibrillation potentials*.

Spinal evoked potential—Electric waves recorded from the head or trunk in response to stimulation of peripheral sensory fibers. Recordings over the spine may be referred to as *spinal evoked potentials* (see Fig. 9–13).

Spontaneous activity—Action potentials recorded from muscle or nerve at rest after insertional activity has subsided and when no voluntary contraction or external stimulus occurs.

Stimulating electrode—Device used to apply electric current. All electric stimulation requires two electrodes; the negative terminal is termed the *cathode,* and the positive terminal, the *anode.* By convention, the stimulating electrodes are called bipolar if they are roughly equal in size and separated by less than 5 cm. Electric stimulation for *nerve conduction studies* generally requires application of the cathode to produce depolarization of the nerve trunk fibers.

Stimulus—In clinical nerve conduction studies, an electric stimulus is generally applied to a nerve or muscle. With respect to the evoked potential, the stimulus may be graded as subthreshold, threshold, submaximal, maximal, or supramaximal. Ordinarily, supramaximal stimuli are used for nerve conduction studies, and submaximal stimuli are used for SEPs.

Surface EMG—Recording of electromyographic activity with recording electrodes attached to the surface of the skin. Contrasted with *needle electromyography*.

Visual evoked potential—Electric waveforms of biologic origin recorded over the cerebrum and elicited by light stimuli.

Volume conduction—Spread of current from a potential source through a conducting medium, such as the body tissues.

Voluntary action—In electromyography, the electric activity recorded from a muscle with consciously controlled muscle contraction (see Fig. 9–10).

Waveform—The shape of an electric potential (wave).

REFERENCES

Adrian, A. D., & Bronk, D. W. (1929). The discharge of impulses motor nerve fibers. Part II. The frequency of discharge in reflex and voluntary contractions. *Journal of Physiology (London), 67,* 119–151.

American Association of Electrodiagnostic Medicine. (1992). Guidelines in electrodiagnostic medicine. *Muscle and Nerve, 15,* 229-253.

American EEG Society. (1994). Guidelines for evoked potentials. *Journal of Clinical Neurophysiology, 11,* 40–77.

Aminoff, M. J. (Ed.). (1992). *Electrodiagnosis in clinical neurology* (3rd ed.) (p. 822). New York: Churchill Livingstone.

Aminoff, M. J. (1978). *Electromyography in clinical practice.* Menlo Park, CA: Addison-Wesley.

Aminoff, M. J., & Goodin, D. S. (1988). Dermatomal somatosensory evoked potentials in lumbosacral root compression. *Journal of Neurology, Neurosurgery and Psychiatry, 51,* 740.

Ball, R. D. (1993). Electrodiagnostic evaluation of the peripheral nervous system. In J. A. DeLisa (Ed.). *Rehabilitation Medicine: Principles and practice* (pp. 269–306). Philadelphia: J. B. Lippincott..

Boden, S. D., Davis, D. O., Dina, T. S., Patronas, N. J., & Wiesel, S. W. (1990). Abnormal magnetic-resonance scans of the lumbar spine in asymptomatic subjects. *Journal of Bone and Joint Surgery, 72A,* 403–408.

TABLE 10-3				
TRANSTIBIAL AMPUTEE METABOLIC COST OF AMBULATION				
Author	**Type**	**Rate of Oxygen Uptake (ml/kg/min [±])**	**Net Oxygen Cost (ml/kg/m [±])**	**Heart Rate (beats/min [±])**
Waters et al. (1976)	D	11.7 (1.6)	0.26 (0.05)	105 (17)
Waters et al. (1976)	T	15.5 (2.9)	0.20 (0.05)	106 (11)
Pagliarulo et al. (1979)	T	15.5 (2.8)	0.22 (0.4)	106 (10)
Huang et al. (1979)	T	10.0	0.20	
Waters et al. (1988)	N	12.1	0.15	99

D = Dysvascular; N = nonamputee; T = traumatic.

Waters et al., 1976). In an attempt to reduce oxygen uptake and heart rate, amputees may adopt a slower walking speed (Table 10–3).

Other influencing factors such as age, self-selected walking speed, prosthetic weight (Gailey et al., 1994), and the type of prosthetic foot, such as the "energy storing" prosthetic feet or dynamic feet versus the use of conventional prosthetic feet such as the SACH foot, do not reduce the metabolic cost of amputee walking (Lehmann et al., 1993; Perry & Shanfield, 1993). The length of the residual limb (Gailey et al., 1994; Gonzalez et al., 1974) and the cause of amputation (Waters et al., 1976) appear to have the most significant effect on the metabolic energy cost of walking for transtibial amputees.

TRANSFEMORAL AMPUTEES— VARIATIONS FROM NORMAL GAIT

- Transfemoral amputees have been described as having an increase in stride width during ambulation, increasing the displacement of the COM laterally (James & Oberg, 1973; Murray et al., 1964; Zuniga et al., 1972). One suggested reason for the increase in walking width is prosthetic side hip abductor weakness, which would require greater lateral stability (Jaegers et al., 1995; James & Oberg, 1973). Another possible explanation expands on the lateral stability concept. As with transtibial amputees, the COM of the transfemoral amputees may have a tendency to shift over the nonprosthetic limb, providing greater stability; therefore, the sound limb adducts. If the prosthetic limb were to follow the natural forward progression, the width of walking base would be more narrow, resulting in the prosthetic limb's having to exert greater muscular stability as the COM moves laterally during prosthetic stance. If the prosthetic limb is slightly more abducted, a strut effect occurs during stance, requiring less muscular effort and greater lateral stability.
- Increased lateral bending of the trunk over the

prosthetic limb is a common gait deviation (Jaegers et al., 1995; James, 1973c; Klopsteg et al., 1968). James (1973c) noted that with a decrease in the width of the walking base, there is decreased lateral trunk bending. The assumption is that decreasing step width decreases the lateral displacement in COM; consequently, less contractile effort would be necessary to control trunk movement. Another reason for lateral trunk bending over the prosthetic side is that the amputee is attempting to reduce weight-bearing directly over the prosthetic limb because of pain, instability, poor balance, or lack of trust in the prosthesis.

- The inability of the prosthetic knee to flex during early stance results in an upward acceleration of the trunk as the body progresses over the prosthetic limb toward mid-stance (Klopsteg et al., 1968). The most significant consequence is the loss of smooth progression of the vertical displacement of COM and, as a result, an increase in the metabolic cost of walking (Peizer et al., 1969).
- Because of the loss of musculoskeletal tissue, there is a loss of muscle strength and a greater difficulty in balancing over the prosthesis. Balance problems and loss of strength are directly related to the length of the residual limb: amputees with shorter limbs experience greater difficulties than those with longer limbs (Jaegers et al., 1995; James, 1973a; James, 1973c; Ryser et al., 1988). Consequently, transfemoral amputees compensate for the decreased ability to maintain single-limb balance over the prosthesis by taking a shorter stride length with the sound limb, a faster prosthetic step, or a lateral lean of the trunk over the prosthetic limb in an attempt to reduce weight bearing and maintain balance.
- Lack of ankle plantar flexion in the prosthetic limb results in the amputee relying on the hip flexors to flex the hip and prosthetic knee during terminal stance. To flex the knee, a contraction of the hip greater than normal is required, and in addition, flexion must be initiated considerably earlier than normal (Hale, 1991; Klopsteg et al., 1968). However, most transfemoral amputees tend to flex the

prosthetic knee about 20 percent later than non-amputees, just prior to entering the swing phase (Jaegers et al., 1995). Additionally, medium- to short-limbed transfemoral amputees demonstrate faster transition from hip extension to hip flexion to assist in flexing the prosthetic knee (Jaegers et al., 1995). Restoration of rotation of the pelvis in the transverse plane assists in passively flexing the knee (Inman et al., 1981; Peizer et al., 1969; Stokes et al., 1989) and may eliminate the need to over-compensate with the hip flexors. Unfortunately, many amputees lose pelvic rotation because they use their hip flexors to "kick" the prosthetic leg forward.

■ More time is spent on the anatomic heel-midfoot and midfoot-toe and less at midfoot than on the prosthetic side (Zuniga et al., 1972). The loss of smooth transition and normal timing of weight transfer over the sound stance limb may be attributed to altered pelvic and hip mechanics of the prosthetic limb. Because the amputee typically attempts to generate sufficient momentum to flex the prosthetic knee by "kicking" the prosthesis forward, there is a tendency to keep the COM over the heel of the stance limb. The posterior rotation of the pelvis and the increased hip flexion on the prosthetic side do not permit the smooth transition of the COM from the heel to toe on the stance limb. Instead, the COM remains over the heel for a longer period of time as the swing limb recovers from the upward thrust initiated to propel the prosthetic limb forward. To make up for the increased time spent on the heel, there is a need for a rapid transition over the midfoot to get to the toe in time as the prosthetic limb descends during terminal swing and the sound limb prepares to leave the ground.

■ Transfemoral amputees typically take a longer step with the prosthetic limb and demonstrate an increased stance time on the sound limb (James & Oberg, 1973; Murray et al., 1981; Skinner and Effeney, 1985; Zuniga et al., 1972). As previously discussed, the amputee has greater confidence during single-limb support over the sound limb and spends more time, allowing for a longer step with the prosthetic leg. The diminished ability to balance over the prosthesis produces a shorter step length with the nonprosthetic limb.

■ There is an increase in the double-support phase, indicating a need for additional stability (Jaegers et al., 1995; James & Oberg, 1973; Murray et al., 1981). To maintain balance, the amputee increases the period of double support before progressing to the next phase of single-limb support.

■ A slight increase in knee flexion on the nonprosthetic limb during stance may be present to assist in absorbing increased ground reaction forces (Jaegers et al., 1995; James & Oberg, 1973).

■ As with transtibial amputees, in transfemoral amputees Hungarford and Cockin (1975) found on radiographs of the nonamputated limb hip greater evidence of osteoporosis and joint space narrowing than in nonamputee controls and an absence of osteophytes. Only 10 percent of 54 transfemoral amputees had normal radiographs. Patellofemoral osteoarthritis in the sound limb was found to be considerably higher in the amputees than in nonamputees, with 63 percent of the transfemoral amputees, 41 percent of transtibial amputees, and only 22 percent of the control group demonstrating positive findings.

■ Transfemoral amputees have decreased velocity and cadence as compared with transtibial amputees and nonamputee ambulators (Godfrey et al., 1975; James, 1973b; Murray et al., 1981; Waters et al., 1976) (Table 10–4; see also Table 10–2). Interestingly, it has been suggested that walking speed is not related to residual limb length (Jaegers et al., 1995).

■ The metabolic cost of ambulation for the transfemoral amputees is also greater than that for the transtibial amputees and nonamputee (Table 10–5). Reducing the speed of ambulation assists in lowering the energy cost and heart rate (Huang et al., 1979; Waters et al., 1976). Moreover, each of the previously described variations from normal gait has some impact on the overall metabolic energy cost of walking. Therefore, the

TABLE 10–4

TRANSFEMORAL AMPUTEE MEAN VELOCITY, CADENCE, AND STRIDE LENGTH

Author	Cause	Velocity (m/min[±])	Cadence (steps/min[±])	Stride Length (m[±])
Murray et al. (1981)	D	60 (9.6)	97	1.36 (0.15)
Godfrey et al. (1975)	D	52	84	1.21
Waters et al. (1976)	D	36 (15)	72 (18)	1.00 (0.20)
Waters et al. (1976)	T	52 (14)	87 (13)	1.2 (0.18)
James (1973)	T	59 (7)	88 (5)	1.34 (0.14)
Jaegers et al. (1995)	T	60.6 (10.8)	89.4 (9)	1.33 (0.16)

D = Dysvascular; T = traumatic.

TABLE 10–5

TRANSFEMORAL AMPUTEE METABOLIC COST OF AMBULATION

Author	Type	Rate of Oxygen Uptake (ml/kg/min [±])	Net Oxygen Cost (ml/kg/m [±])	Heart Rate (beats/min [±])
Waters et al. (1976)	D	12.6 (2.9)	0.35 (0.06)	126 (17)
Waters et al. (1976)	T	12.9 (3.4)	0.25 (0.05)	111 (12)
Huang et al. (1979)	T	12.6	0.28	
Waters et al. (1988)	N	12.1	0.15	99

D = Dysvascular; N = nonamputee; T = traumatic.

need for reducing the extent of the deviations becomes paramount during the gait training and prosthetic fitting process.

Comprehension of the principles of gait permits the clinician to have greater insight into the variance that exists between normal and prosthetic gait, as well as the differences within the various levels of amputation. Moreover, once the cause of the deviation is identified, an appropriate treatment plan may be designed to address the specific needs of the individual. If the amputee lacks the physical strength, balance, or gait biomechanics to walk correctly, then these issues may be addressed. Conversely, if the prosthesis is at fault and requires an alignment adjustment or modification, then the necessary prosthetic action may be taken.

CRITICAL ELEMENTS OF GAIT WITH RESPECT TO LEVEL OF AMPUTATION AND PROSTHESIS

The causes for amputation in North America can be divided into four categories; however, estimates on the percentages do vary. Approximately 70 to 90 percent are the result of vascular disease, less than 20 percent are for traumatic reasons, approximately 4 percent are because of tumor, and 4 percent are congenital (Glattly, 1963; Glattly, 1964; Kerstein, 1974; Sanders, 1986; Tooms, 1980). During the period leading to amputation, there frequently exist secondary complications that could affect gait or function. Amputees with vascular disease commonly have problems associated with diabetes, heart disease, and other debilitating diagnoses. Traumatic amputees present with fractures, soft tissue injuries, or neuromuscular impairments associated with the accident. Congenital amputees may have more than one extremity involved or associated neuromuscular complications.

Age can influence the amputee's ability to ambulate with a prosthesis, just as age influences the gait of nonamputee ambulators. This is not to say that age alone dictates the amputee's capabilities. On the contrary, level of activity prior to amputation has a greater influence on the reha-

bilitation outcome than age, level of amputation, or number of limbs involved (Brodzka et al., 1990; Chan & Tan, 1990; Medhat et al., 1990; Nissen & Newman, 1992; Pinzur et al., 1992; Walker et al., 1994).

The level of amputation can have a significant impact on the amputee's ability to adjust to learning to ambulate with the prosthesis. There are several individual factors that must be considered when determining the expected gait for a particular level of amputation. The inability to adequately master any one of these contributing factors can prevent an amputee from reaching an optimal level of gait. Yet, an amputee with a high-level amputation who goes on to master each of the components of gait can achieve a higher-quality gait than an amputee with presumably greater potential who does not learn to walk properly for a multitude of reasons (Medhat et al., 1990; Pinzur et al., 1992). The following is a summary of the influencing elements associated with the level of amputation and prosthetic componentry. A brief statement of each element is followed by a sample question the clinician may want to consider when assessing the amputee.

- The degree of displacement of the COM over the BOS in all three planes of movement. Maintaining normal displacement of COM over BOS optimizes anatomic movement and metabolic cost of gait. Any alteration of COM displacement results in compensatory movements and increased metabolic cost (Engsberg et al., 1992; Peizer et al., 1969; Saunders et al., 1953).

    Can the amputee maintain the expected displacement of the COM over the BOS without compensatory movements such as unequal stance time, increased lateral trunk leaning, or decreased arm swing?

- Asymmetry of motion secondary to an imbalance of the muscle groups between the lower extremities (Breakly, 1976; Engsberg et al., 1992). Frequently, muscle groups become abnormally hyperactive during the gait cycle as a compensatory mechanism or to provide a sense of security to the amputee (Gitter et al., 1991; Winter & Sienko, 1988).

    Can muscle of the residual limb be reeducated to prevent unwarranted hyperactivity during certain phases and to create a smooth progression of the prosthetic limb, decreasing the need to rely on compensatory movements from the sound limb, trunk, and arms?

■ Diminished coordinated movement between the remaining anatomic joints secondary to the loss of proprioceptive feedback and absence of musculature on the prosthetic side (Mensch & Ellis, 1986; Skinner & Effeney, 1985; Waters et al., 1976).

Can the amputee move the prosthetic foot/ankle assembly, knee, and hip joint fluidly and efficiently with the remaining musculature and without proprioceptive feedback from the absent joints?

■ The loss of the normal biomechanics of the anatomic ankle and foot and the inability of the prosthesis to simulate specific movements. This would include the loss of not only muscle and joints but also their roles in gait, such as propelling the body forward during late stance or functioning as shock absorbers (Fisher & Gollickson, 1978; Radcliffe, 1962).

Will the amputee be able to compensate for this loss physically or with a prosthetic device?

■ Anatomic limitations of the residual limb or physiologic requirements result in a compromise in prosthetic design or alignment. The effect of the prosthetic design on the mechanics of gait may cause the amputee to deviate from a normal gait pattern (Murphy & Wilson, 1962; Radcliffe, 1955; Radcliffe, 1957; Radcliffe, 1961; Radcliffe, 1962).

Will the compensations made in prosthetic design because of predisposing physical abnormalities significantly affect the overall gait pattern?

■ The kinetic energy normally stored as potential energy in the anatomic limb during gait is absent (Ganguli et al., 1973; Gitter et al., 1991; Yoshihiro et al., 1993). The prosthetic limb offers limited kinetic energy return. More dynamic prosthetic components available today offer some mechanical potential energy storage; however, this varies tremendously between components, amputees, and a variety of other conditions.

Does the amputee have the ability to produce or receive maximum benefit from the kinetic energy return stored within the prosthetic limb?

■ The loss of the skeletal lever arm. The proximal muscle groups acting on the remaining bone must overcome a longer lever arm to control the entire lower extremity during the gait sequence (Ganguli et al., 1973; James, 1973c; Mensch & Ellis, 1986).

Does the amputee have the ability to sufficiently control the prosthesis with the remaining bone length?

■ The loss of contractile tissue results in diminished potential strength (Ganguli et al., 1973; James, 1973c; Mensch & Ellis, 1986; Winter & Sienko, 1988). The changes in insertions of the remaining musculature are altered, consequently changing

the functional capacity of the muscles (Klopsteg et al., 1968; Ryser et al., 1988).

Will the amputee be able to maximize the use of the remaining muscles that may have been altered in length, length-tension relationship, and by surgical technique?

■ The potential increase in body temperature secondary to loss of skin surface area disrupts the body's natural homeostasis. This leads to an overall increase in metabolic cost during all activities (Levy, 1983; Mensch & Ellis, 1986).

Will the amputee reach a level of cardiopulmonary fitness to overcome the physiologic deficit and minimize the metabolic cost of ambulation?

The amputee's gait can vary significantly depending on the cause of amputation, associated diagnoses, age, or level of amputation and the critical elements associated with each level of amputation. Because there are so many variables regarding amputee gait, it is difficult to identify one particular pattern that can be associated with a particular "type" of amputee. It is for this reason that normal gait may be used as the gold standard for all levels of amputation, realizing that in the majority of amputees, predisposing factors beyond their control limit their ability to obtain a "normal" gait pattern.

FUNCTIONAL GAIT ASSESSMENT OF THE AMPUTEE

Because amputee gait is complex and there are so many critical elements, the idea of observing an amputee's gait and simply identifying one or two causes for a particular deviation may result in a misdiagnosis or incomplete assessment. Therefore, it may be worth the evaluator's time to perform a more in-depth assessment in an attempt to gain greater insight into the "big picture."

Ambulation profiles are defined as clinical tests of locomotion skill (Craik & Oatis, 1995; Reimers, 1972; Wolf, 1979) or as quantitative methods of assessing ambulatory function (Craik & Oatis, 1995; Olney et al., 1979; Wolf, 1979). The information obtained from these tests can provide a more global view of the patient's ability to maintain standing balance, negotiate turns, and rise from a chair, and, in some cases, of physiologic factors such as decreased cardiorespiratory or muscular endurance. Used along with a standard gait evaluation, the ambulation profile tests can determine how a patient walks and what functional limitations may prevent him or her from reaching an optimal level of gait. The clinical administration requires only an assessment form, walkway, standard rehabilitation equipment, and minimal time and cost. Moreover, interrater reliability for ambulation profile tests generally is good. Currently, no one assessment tool exists to evaluate the amputee's locomotive function. However, in keeping with the concept of an ambulation profile or comprehensive evaluation of gait in terms of function, the reader is referred to Nelson (1974), Tinetti (1986), and Olney and associates (1979) for a comprehensive description of selected assessment tools. Although these evaluative tools were not specifically designed for the amputee and to date no data exist to demonstrate the validity of administering these tests to amputees, these tests appear to readily lend themselves to this population.

TEMPOROSPATIAL OBJECTIVE MEASURES

Optimal walk is defined as a walk of such speed and step frequency that the energy expenditure per meter walked is minimal (Zatsiorsky et al., 1994). When given the opportunity to choose a particular step frequency or cadence, people choose a speed that is most comfortable for them (Inman et al., 1981). Many amputees tend to adopt a gait pattern that has been described as asymmetric and slower than that of nonamputee ambulators. As the level of amputation increases, symmetry and velocity decrease. This is not to suggest that increased asymmetry is indicative of an optimal gait for the amputee; however, the evaluator must be aware of the common patterns of gait observed in amputees. The classic combination of events that compose the asymmetry in gait include the following:

Decreased stance time on the prosthetic limb, resulting in a faster, shorter step with the sound limb, with an increase in lateral leaning of the trunk over the prosthetic stance limb to decrease weight-bearing into the prosthesis.

Increased stride length with the prosthetic limb as a compensation for the shorter stride with the sound limb. The amputee attempts to maintain walking velocity by taking a longer stride with the prosthetic limb since maintaining sufficient stance time on the sound limb is possible.

Altered stride width in an attempt to maintain the body's center of gravity (COG) over a stable BOS— the amputee brings the sound limb to midline, more directly under the COG. Therefore, the sound limb becomes the primary BOS, having earned the amputee's trust as the more stable limb. To maintain some distance between the limbs, the prosthetic limb abducts slightly and acts as a strut or post over which the amputee advances during the prosthetic stance phase.

Reduced velocity can be attributed to several factors including, but not limited to, cause of amputation, ability to use the prosthesis, gait deviations, neuromuscular, skeletal, or cardiopulmonary limitations or pathology, general physical conditioning, and aerobic endurance.

TEMPOROSPATIAL ASSESSMENT

Objective measures of temporospatial gait characteristics can assist in documenting improvement in gait training or help to detect when there is a loss of quality of gait. Typically, temporospatial information is relatively easy to collect. Clinically feasible methods to objectively measure the temporospatial characteristics of a subject's gait can be used with inexpensive equipment. Simple items such as a stopwatch and a tape measure, masking tape to create a floor grid to measure length and width of stride, a number grid, powder or ink on the shoe to mark foot placement, or special paper designed to mark each step can be used to assist in the assessment of the amputee's walking pattern.

Velocity is easily measured by determining the time to cover a distance. As the amputee walks, the time to walk a given distance is measured with a stopwatch and divided by the total distance walked. Cadence is obtained by counting the number of steps taken per minute. Step length and width are measured after the amputee walks on a grid and the foot placement marked by an agent such as powder or ink. Robinson and Smidt (1981) describe a method by which the therapist walks behind the subject and records into an audio tape recorder each foot placement on a numbered grid.

FUNCTIONAL SCALES

Several authors have attempted to classify an amputee's functional ability by categorizing his or her abilities (Kegel et al., 1978; Medicare Region C Durable Medical Equipment Regional Carrier, 1995; Volpicelli et al., 1983). The focus of these scales is the ability to ambulate, the assistive device required for locomotion, and the environment that the patient is capable of negotiating. The merit of these scales is that allied health professionals familiar with the description of classes within the functional scale system can readily assume the functional level of the amputee identified with a particular functional level. As with any labeling system, there is a danger of forgetting that performance can improve or diminish and that reassessment on a regular basis is always a good idea.

The Functional Scale (Table 10–6) has been adopted by Medicare and the division of Durable Medical Equipment Regional Carriers (DMERC) (Medicare Region C Durable Medical Equipment Regional Carrier, 1995) as the indicator to determine what prosthetic components an amputee functioning at a particular level is qualified to receive. There is a strong possibility that most elderly amputees' rehabilitation potential will be assessed prior to initial prosthetic fitting, and they will be assigned a classification level.

TABLE 10–6

DURABLE MEDICAL EQUIPMENT REGIONAL CARRIER AMPUTEE FUNCTION LEVELS

Level 0	Does not have the ability or potential to ambulate or transfer safely with or without assistance, and a prosthesis does not enhance quality of life or mobility.
Level 1	Has the ability or potential to use a prosthesis for transfers or ambulation in level surfaces at fixed cadence. Typical of the limited and unlimited household ambulator.
Level 2	Has the ability or potential for ambulation with the ability to traverse low-level environmental barriers such as curbs, stairs, or uneven surfaces. Typical of the limited community ambulator.
Level 3	Has the ability or potential for ambulation with variable cadence. Typical of the community ambulator who has the ability to traverse most environmental barriers and may have vocational, therapeutic, or exercise activity that demands prosthetic utilization beyond simple locomotion.
Level 4	Has the ability or potential for prosthetic ambulation that exceeds basic ambulation skills, exhibiting high impact, stress, or energy levels. Typical of the prosthetic demands of the child, active adult, or athlete.

From Medicare Region C Durable Medical Equipment Regional Carrier. (1995). Supplier Update Workshops. Winter.

GAIT ASSESSMENT OF THE AMPUTEE

The most common variables described in gait are the joint angles or the kinematic events. Knowing the acceptable joint angles in relation to the appropriate phase of the gait cycle allows the evaluator to assess the quality of a particular individual's gait. If the joint angles do not fall within the established norms or fall out of expected phase of gait, then that deviation from "normal" gait must be identified and recorded. However, identifying abnormal temporal or kinematic patterns does not yield enough information to distinguish the cause of the deviation. For example, the joints of the lower limb and trunk of two different subjects may have near identical joint angles at a particular phase of gait. Yet the joint moment of force and musculoskeletal forces or mechanical power acting on each limb may be very different. Therefore, the forces that cause motion are the cause, and the kinematic and temporal events observed by the clinician become the result.

Winter (1985) puts forth additional difficulties in identifying the forces and EMG events that are acting on the limb. Two other problems face clinicians. First is indeterminacy (Seireg & Arvikar, 1975), or the fact that biomechanists do not have equations for all of the unknowns acting on a limb. Second, there is not a unique solution to the equation for moments of force at the ankle, knee, and hip (Winter, 1985). In other words, just because the knee and ankle angles are similar does not mean that the muscle patterns are the same (Winter, 1985). In most cases, a biomechanist with a full compliment of kinetic and EMG data will derive

a reasonable explanation for the kinematic events being observed. However, it is important to remember that even the most complete biomechanics laboratory will not make absolute statements concerning various events during gait. Moreover, clinicians performing observational gait assessments should proceed with even greater caution and be aware that there could exist multiple reasons for why a single event occurred.

Observational gait analysis (OGA) is often viewed as the most practical of assessment tools for the amputee during the gait training process. Although there appears to be only moderate reliability with OGA or videotaped OGA, this is currently the most pragmatic method for clinicians. Frame-by-frame slow-motion video analysis has improved the observer's ability to be consistent in gait assessment (Eastlack et al., 1991; Krebs et al., 1985). With the advent of personal computers and advanced video display capabilities, relatively inexpensive computer systems will offer a future of on-screen measurements providing kinematic and temporospatial information that may be objectively measured. Gait analysis has proven to be a useful tool for the study of prosthetics and amputee gait (Harris and Wertsch, 1994). The use of OGA in the clinic, while not the most reliable, is the most sensible because all it requires is simple observation of a subject's gait without the use of any equipment. Because the exact cause cannot always be correctly identified immediately owing to the absence of measurable kinetic, EMG, and kinematic data, an appropriate method of assessment would include a systematic evaluation of the subject's gait.

Observational gait analysis is best done by systematically concentrating on one body segment and then another. Perry's (1992) description of a well-organized method of gait evaluation permits clinicians to use a problem-solving approach to assess gait. The use of an itemized form can assist the clinician with identifying the presence, absence, or alteration of important events throughout the gait cycle (Observational Gait Analysis, 1993; Winter, 1985). Further application of reference materials aids in the identification of the underlying cause of the pathologic gait associated with commonly observed combinations of gait deviations. Limitations of OGA include identification of multiple events occurring at multiple body segments concurrently or simultaneously (Saleh & Murdoch, 1985). Gage and Õunpuu (1989) have illustrated that events occurring faster than $1/12$ of a second (83 msec) cannot be perceived by the human eye. As a result, the Rancho Los Amigos Medical Center staff recognizes that the traditional eight phases of gait may be an inappropriate method of analysis. Therefore, their gait assessment chart has been further simplified into the three basic tasks of gait: weight acceptance (initial contact to loading response), single-limb support (mid-stance to terminal stance), and limb advancement (preswing to terminal swing) (Perry, 1992).

As with any evaluative procedure, once the cause for the gait deviation has been identified, it must be appropriately treated. The degree to which the deviation is decreased or

GAIT ANALYSIS: FULL BODY

Rancho Los Amigos Medical Center, Physical Therapy Department

Reference Limb:

L ☐ R ☐

☐ Major deviation
▨ Minor deviation

		Weight Accept		Single-Limb Support		Swing Limb Advancement				MAJOR PROBLEMS:
		IC	LR	MSt	TSt	PSw	ISw	MSw	TSw	
Trunk	Lean: B/F									
	Lateral lean: R/L									
	Rotates: B/F									
Pelvis	Hikes									Weight Acceptance
	Tilt: P/A									
	Lacks forward rotation									
	Lacks backward rotation									
	Excess forward rotation									
	Excess backward rotation									
	Ipsilateral drop									
	Contralateral drop									
Hip	Flexion: limited									Single-Limb Support
	excess									
	Inadequate extension									
	Past retract									
	Rotation: IR/ER									
	Ad/Abduction: Ad/Ab									
Knee	Flexion: limited									
	excess									
	Inadequate extension									
	Wobbles									
	Hyperextends									Swing Limb Advancement
	Extension thrust									
	Varus/valgus: Vr/Vl									
	Excess contralateral flex									
Ankle	Forefoot contact									
	Foot-flat contact									
	Foot slap									
	Excess plantar flexion									
	Excess dorsiflexion									
	Inversion/eversion: Iv/Ev									Excessive UE Weight Bearing ☐
	Heel off									
	No heel off									
	Drag									
	Contralateral vaulting									Name _____
Toes	Up									
	Inadequate extension									
	Clawed									Diagnosis

© 1991 LAREI, Rancho Los Amigos Medical Center, Downey, CA 90242

FIGURE 10–1. Form for full-body gait analysis. (Courtesy of Rancho Los Amigos Medical Center, Physical Therapy Department.)

Prosthetic Observational Gait Assessment Form

Sagittal View	Weight Acceptance	Single-Limb Support		Swing
Foot/Ankle	foot flat	vaulting (excessive plantarflexion)		
	foot slap	increased dorsiflexion		
	external rotation			
Knee	hyperextension	decreased knee flexion		increased flexion or (excessive heel rise)
	increased flexion or (knee instability)			terminal impact
Hip		flexed		
Pelvis		posterior rotation		posterior rotation
		anterior rotation		
Trunk		lordosis		
		flexed		
Arm Swing	uneven			uneven
	decreased			decreased
Stride Length				increased
				decreased
Stance Time		increased		
		decreased		
Toe Clearance				increased
				decreased

Anterior/ Posterior View	Weight Acceptance	Single-Limb Support		Swing
Foot/Ankle	external rotation	walking on lateral border of foot		
		walking on medial border of foot		
Knee		valgus		medial whip
		varus		lateral whip
Hip		abducted		
		adducted		circumduction
Pelvis		pelvic drop off		pelvic rise
Trunk		lateral bending		
Arm Swing	uneven			uneven
	decreased			decreased
Stride Width		increased		increased
		decreased		decreased

FIGURE 10–2. Prosthetic observational gait assessment form. (From Gailey, R. S. (1996). *One step ahead: An integrated approach to lower extremity prosthetics and amputee rehabilitation.* Miami, FL: Advanced Rehabilitation Therapy.)

eliminated depends on whether the assessment was correct and the treatment appropriate and on the patient's ability to respond to the treatment. Consequently, there is a need for a confirmation of the original diagnosis, reassessment of the current treatment plan, and an appraisal for future treatment plans. The process of reassessment must be performed whether an elaborate motion analysis, EMG, and ground force gait evaluation are performed or if the therapist used OGA to evaluate and prepare the rehabilitation treatment.

PROSTHETIC OBSERVATIONAL GAIT ASSESSMENT

Assessment of the amputee's gait does not differ from the evaluation of any other patient diagnosis. A form such as Rancho Los Amigos Medical Center's Full Body Evalu-

ation (Fig. 10–1) is an excellent tool to assist the evaluator in systematically identifying the minor and major deviations that occur during each phase of gait. The evaluator must then determine the cause of the deviation(s). Four general categories—(1) impaired motor control, (2) abnormal joint range of motion, (3) impaired sensation (including balance), and (4) pain (Observational Gait Analysis, 1993)—are potential amputee causes, while one additional category—(5) prosthetic causes—must be included for amputee assessment. It should be emphasized that there are four major categories for potential cause of gait deviations that are amputee related and one that is prosthetic related. This is an important note because too frequently the prosthesis is distinguished as being at fault for the amputee's gait deviations. When attempts to adjust the prosthesis are performed and the deviation persists, becomes worse, or is replaced by another deviation, clinicians may want to further explore the potential amputee causes rather than persisting in modifying the prosthesis.

The Prosthetic Observational Gait Assessment Form (POGA) (Fig. 10–2) and the corresponding Prosthetic Gait Deviation Identification Charts (Tables 10–7 and 10–8) are designed to simplify the process of identifying a gait deviation and determining the cause of the deviation (Gailey, 1996). The assessment form lists the most common deviations observed with all levels of lower extremity amputees, and the corresponding Gait Assessment Charts suggest the possible causes for the observed gait deviations.

To use the assessment system, the evaluator systematically observes the various body segments from the ground

---

TABLE 10–7

TRANSTIBIAL AMPUTEE PROSTHETIC GAIT DEVIATION IDENTIFICATION CHART

Gait Deviation	Prosthetic Cause	Amputee Cause
Weight Acceptance (Initial Contact to Loading Response)		
Foot flat	1. Flexed socket > 5°–15° 2. Foot is dorsiflexed	1. Knee flexion contracture 2. Weak quadriceps 3. Poor balance or proprioception 4. Lack of confidence
Foot slap	1. Too soft a heel cushion or plantar flexion bumper 2. Too low a heel cushion 3. Too short a heel lever	1. Too-forceful driving of prosthesis into ground to ensure knee stability
External rotation of the prosthesis	1. Too hard or too high a heel cushion 2. Too much toe-out 3. Suspension too loose	1. Poor pelvic control 2. Weak internal rotators 3. Striking the ground with excessive force
Increased flexion of the knee	1. Too hard or too high a heel cushion 2. Socket set too far anterior to foot 3. Too long a heel lever 4. Flexed socket > 5°–15° 5. Foot is dorsiflexed 6. Suspension too loose 7. Prosthesis too long	1. Knee flexion contracture 2. Weak quadriceps
Hyperextension of the knee	1. Too soft or too low a heel cushion 2. Too short a heel lever 3. Socket set too far posterior to foot 4. Insufficient socket flexion 5. Foot is plantar flexed 6. Suspension too tight 7. Prosthesis too short	1. Weak quadriceps 2. Excessive extensor force
Single-Limb Support Phase (Mid-Stance to Terminal Stance)		
Walking on the lateral border of the foot	1. Abducted socket 2. Laterally leaning pylon 3. Inverted foot	
Walking on the medial border of the foot	1. Adducted socket 2. Medially leaning pylon 3. Everted foot	
Increased dorsiflexion	1. Foot too dorsiflexed 2. Insufficient socket flexion	
Decreased knee flexion	1. Socket set too posterior to foot 2. Posterior leaning pylon (socket in too much extension, foot too plantar flexed) 3. Too-hard dorsiflexion bumper 4. Restrictive suspension	1. Poor pelvic control 2. Weak knee flexors
Valgus moment at the knee	1. Outset foot 2. Excesive medial tilt of socket 3. Pain over fibular head 4. Too loose a socket or not enough socks	1. Short residual limb 2. Ligament laxity
Varus moment at the knee	1. Inset foot 2. Excessive lateral tilt of socket 3. Too loose a socket or not enough socks	1. Short residual limb 2. Ligament laxity
Abducted gait	1. Prosthesis too long 2. Outset foot	1. Poor balance 2. Adducted sound limb 3. Habit
Pelvic drop off	1. Toe lever too short 2. Excessive knee flexion 3. Foot too dorsiflexed 4. Socket set too anterior to foot	

TABLE 10–7

TRANSTIBIAL AMPUTEE PROSTHETIC GAIT DEVIATION IDENTIFICATION CHART *Continued*

Gait Deviation	Prosthetic Cause	Amputee Cause
Single-Limb Support Phase (Mid-Stance to Terminal Stance) *Continued*		
Pelvic posterior rotation Lateral bending of the trunk toward the prosthetic side	1. Pylon too short 2. Outset foot 3. Prosthetic pain	1. Inadequate transverse pelvic rotation 1. Inability to balance over prosthesis 2. Inability to fully bear weight in prosthesis 3. Muscle weakness (hip abduction) 4. Pain 5. Habit
Decreased stance time	1. Pain from socket	1. Inadequate weight-bearing 2. Poor balance 3. Insecurity
Increased stride width	1. Prosthesis too long 2. Outset foot	1. Poor balance 2. Abducted prosthetic limb 3. Habit
Decreased stride width		1. Adducted sound limb
Swing Phase (Preswing to Terminal Swing)		
Pelvic rise	1. Posterior leaning pylon 2. Toe lever too long 3. Insufficient socket flexion 4. Prosthesis too long	1. Poor pelvic control 2. Insufficient knee or hip flexion
Decreased stride length on prosthetic side	1. Anterior leaning pylon 2. Prosthesis too short 3. Inadequate suspension	1. Pain in the sound limb 2. Hip flexion contracture on sound side 3. Knee flexion contracture on prosthetic side
Increased stride length on prosthetic side	1. Painful socket 2. Prosthesis too long	1. Compensation for decreased stride with sound limb 2. Insecurity during prosthetic stance 3. Hip flexion contracture on prosthetic side 4. Knee flexion contracture on sound side
Decreased toe clearance	1. Prosthesis too long 2. Pistoning (inadequate suspension, insufficient socks, socket too large)	1. Improperly donned prosthesis 2. Muscle atrophy 3. Loss of weight 4. Weak hip or knee flexors
Increased toe clearance		1. Excessive hip or knee flexion 2. Vaulting
Lateral whip	1. Internally rotated socket 2. Inadequate suspension	1. Improperly donned prosthesis
Medial whip	1. Externally rotated socket 2. Inadequate suspension	1. Improperly donned prosthesis
Sound Limb and Arm Swing		
Adducted limb		1. Uses sound limb as principal base of support
Vaulting	1. Prosthesis too long 2. Inadequate suspension	1. Habit
Uneven arm swing	1. Poorly fitted socket causing pain or instability	1. Poor balance 2. Fear and insecurity 3. Habit
Extended rotation		1. Poor balance 2. Fear and insecurity 3. Habit
Increased stance time		1. Poor balance 2. Fear and insecurity 3. Habit

From Gailey, R.S. (1996). *One step ahead: An integrated approach to lower extremity prosthetics and amputee rehabilitation.* Miami, FL: Advanced Rehabilitation Therapy.

up as the amputee walks. Each of the three general phases of gait—weight acceptance, single-limb support, and swing—should be partitioned in the observer's mind to assist in isolating the deviation. Finally, the evaluator must consider both the sagittal and frontal views when perform-ing the evaluation. Without the necessary information from both planes, deviations may be missed or misinterpreted. Interestingly, Krebs and coworkers (1985) found greater reliability with sagittal view assessment, whereas Eastlack and colleagues (1991) found that frontal plane assessment

TABLE 10-8

TRANSFEMORAL AMPUTEE PROSTHETIC GAIT DEVIATION IDENTIFICATION CHART

Gait Deviation	Prosthetic Cause	Amputee Cause
Weight Acceptance Phase (Initial Contact to Loading Response)		
External rotation of the prosthesis	1. Anterior or medial brim pressure 2. Too-stiff heel cushion or plantar flexion bumper 3. Too long a heel lever 4. Too much built-in toe-out	1. Extension force too great 2. Poor residual limb muscle control 3. Improperly donned prosthesis
Knee flexion or instability	1. Knee axis too far ahead of TKA line 2. Insufficient socket flexion 3. Too-long heel lever arm 4. Too-stiff heel cushion or plantar flexion bumper 5. Too much dorsiflexion	1. Weak hip extensors 2. Severe hip flexion contracture 3. Altered height of shoes
Foot slap	1. Too-soft heel cushion or plantar flexion bumper 2. Too short a heel lever	1. Too-forceful driving of prosthesis to the ground ensuring knee stability
Single-Limb Support (Mid-Stance to Terminal Stance)		
Abducted gait	1. Prosthesis too long 2. Too-high medial wall 3. Improper relief for distal femur on lateral wall 4. Foot too much outset	1. Abduction contracture 2. Fear or habit
Pelvic lateral tilt	1. Inadequate adduction of the socket	1. Weak gluteus medius stance limb 2. Poor balance
Pelvic drop off (during late stance on the prosthetic side)	1. Toe lever too short 2. Anterior leaning pylon foot too dorsi-flexed 3. Socket set too anterior to foot	
Pelvic posterior rotation		1. Inadequate transverse pelvic rotation
Lateral bending of trunk	1. Inadequate adduction of the socket 2. Prosthesis too short 3. Too-high medial wall causing pain 4. Outset foot	2. Weak hip abductors 3. Abduction contracture 4. Painful residual limb 5. Very short residual limb 6. Inability to weight-bear 7. Habit or fear
Trunk lordosis	1. Insufficient socket flexion 2. Posterior wall promotes anterior pelvic tilt	1. Tight hip flexors 2. Weak hip extensors 3. Weak abdominals 4. Habit
Trunk flexion	1. Too much socket flexion	1. Flexion contracture 2. Poor proprioception 3. Habit
Decreased stance time	1. Pain from socket	1. Inadequate weight-bearing 2. Poor balance 3. Insecurity
Increased stride width	1. Prosthesis too long 2. Outset foot 3. Socket too abducted 4. Medial wall pressure 5. Medial-leaning pylon	1. Poor balance 2. Abduction contracture 3. Adducted sound limb 4. Habit
Swing Phase (Preswing to Terminal Swing)		
Increased knee flexion (excessive heel rise)	1. Insufficient knee friction	1. Too-strong hip flexion
Increased knee extension (terminal impact)	1. Insufficient knee friction	1. Too-vigorous hip flexion followed by strong hip extension 2. Security to ensure knee extension
Medial whip	1. Excessive external rotation 2. Too-tight socket 3. Excessive valgus of prosthetic knee 4. Scilesian belt too tight laterally	1. Improper donning of prosthesis 2. Excessive adipose tissue with poor muscle control

TABLE 10–8

TRANSFEMORAL AMPUTEE PROSTHETIC GAIT DEVIATION IDENTIFICATION CHART *Continued*

Gait Deviation	Prosthetic Cause	Amputee Cause
Swing Phase (Preswing to Terminal Swing) *Continued*		
Lateral whip	1. Excessive internal rotation 2. Too-tight socket 3. Excessive valgus of prosthetic knee	1. Improper donning of prosthesis 2. Excessive adipose tissue with poor muscle control
Circumduction	1. Too-long prosthesis 2. Too-thick medial brim 3. Too much knee stability (alignment or resistance 4. Improperly aligned pelvic band	1. Abduction contracture 2. Insecurity regarding knee control
Pelvic rise	1. Too-long toe lever arm 2. Too much knee stability (alignment or resistance)	
Pelvic posterior rotation		1. Inadequate transverse pelvic rotation
Decreased stride length on prosthetic side	1. Anterior-leaning pylon 2. Prosthesis too short 3. Inadequate suspension	1. Pain in the sound limb 2. Hip flexion contracture on sound side
Increased stride length on prosthetic side	1. Painful socket 2. Prosthesis too long	1. Compensation for decreased stride with sound limb 2. Insecurity during prosthetic stance 3. Hip flexion contracture on prosthetic side 4. Knee flexion contracture on sound side
Decreased toe clearance	1. Prosthesis too long 2. Pistoning (inadequate suspension, insufficient socks, socket too large) 3. Prosthesis too long	1. Loss of weight 2. Muscle atrophy 3. Improperly donned prosthesis 4. Weak hip or knee flexors
Increased toe clearance	1. Insufficient knee friction	1. Excessive hip flexion 2. Vaulting
Sound Limb and Arm Swing		
Adducted limb		1. Uses sound limb as principal base of support
Vaulting	1. Too-long prosthesis 2. Too much knee friction leading 3. Excessive built-in knee stability; knee joint too far posterior to TKA line	1. Limb not properly down in socket 2. Fear of stubbing prosthetic toe or of poor knee control 3. Weak hip flexors 4. Habit
Uneven arm swing	1. Poorly fitted socket causing pain or instability	1. Poor balance 2. Fear and insecurity 3. Habit
Unequal step length	1. Improperly fitted socket causing pain 2. Unaccommodated hip flexion contracture	1. Fear and insecurity 2. Poor balance 3. Weak residual limb musculature
Increased stance time		1. Poor balance 2. Fear and insecurity 3. Habit

From Gailey, R. S. (1996). *One step ahead: an integrated approach to lower extremity prosthetics and amputee rehabilitation.* Miami, FL: Advanced Rehabilitation Therapy.

was more reliable when performing OGA. Clinically, however, the evaluator should observe from both planes and in many cases must be aware of the amputee's endurance level to ensure that an accurate picture of the walking pattern can be observed before fatigue becomes a factor.

Once the gait deviation(s) have been identified by using the POGA form, the cause for the gait deviation should be confirmed by using the Prosthetic Gait Deviation Identification Chart. The evaluator must determine if the deviation is related to physical or prosthetic causes. The potential amputee and prosthetic causes for gait deviations most commonly observed for transtibial and transfemoral amputees are listed in the Prosthetic Gait Assessment Chart. Other excellent resources offer a more complete listing of potential deviations, many of which are rarely seen (Bowker & Michael, 1992; Lower-Limb Prosthetics, 1980; Mensch & Ellis, 1986; Sanders, 1986).

To confirm the assessment, the evaluator may want to attempt to correct the deviation by instructing the amputee on how to physically overcome the impairment or make the appropriate prosthetic adjustment. Unfortunately, when it comes to physical limitation, it is not always possible to correct the deviation immediately. In some cases, because of physical deconditioning, diagnosis, or other impairment, the amputee might have to adopt a less than satisfactory gait pattern. However, it is important to note that prosthetic componentry and gait training methods introduced over the last decade have offered many fit and motivated amputees the ability to learn how to walk with barely a detectable gait deviation.

CONCLUSIONS

The assessment of the amputee's gait can be a complex task when all the potential causes leading to a less than optimal gait pattern are considered. However, if a systematic approach to the evaluation process is employed, taking into account both the functional aspects of gait and the observable gait deviations, the reasons for an unfavorable gait pattern often become more clear. The clinician will find that regular assessments throughout the rehabilitation period not only assist in monitoring the progress of the amputee during the rehabilitation process but also aid in the design and modification of the treatment program.

GLOSSARY

Base of support (BOS)—The area of the body in contact with a resistive surface that exerts a reaction force against the body.

Cadence—The number of steps per minute.

Center of mass (COM)*—The point on a body that moves in the same way that a particle subject to the same external forces would move.

Displacement*—The change in body position.

Kinematic*—Describing motion.

Kinetics*—The study of forces that cause motion.

Oxygen cost—The amount of oxygen used per meter walked (milliliters/kilogram of body weight/meter walked).

Single-limb support[†]—Total weight-bearing on one lower extremity.

Stride length—The measurement from one initial contact to the ipsilateral initial contact.

Stride width—A measurement of distance from medial point of contact from the right metatarsal head to that of the left.

Swing[†]—The period in the gait cycle when the foot is not in contact with the floor.

Temporospatial—The relationship of time and space.

Transfemoral amputee—A person with an amputation site through the femur bone (above-knee amputee).

Transtibial amputee—A person with an amputation site through the tibial/fibula bone. The site must be above the malleoli but not past the knee joint (below-knee amputee).

Weight acceptance[‡]—The initial period in the gait cycle when body weight is dropped onto the limb. The phases of initial contact and loading response are involved.

REFERENCES

Bowker, J. H., & Michael, J. W. (1992). *Atlas of limb prosthetics* (2nd ed.). St. Louis: Mosby-Year Book.

Breakly, J. (1976). Gait of unilateral below-knee amputees. *Orthotics and Prosthetics, 30*(3), 17–24.

Brodzka, W. K., Thronhill, H. L., Zarapkar, S. E., et al. (1990). Long-term function of persons with atherosclerotic bilateral below-knee amputation living in the inner city. *Archives of Physical Medicine and Rehabilitation, 71,* 898–900.

Burke, M. J., Roman, V., & Wright, V. (1978). Bone and joint changes in lower limb amputees. *Annals of Rheumatic Disease, 37,* 252–254.

Cavanagh, P. R., & Henley, J. D. (1993). The computer era in gait analysis. *Clinics in Podiatric Medicine and Surgery, 10,* 471–484.

Chan, K. M., & Tan, E. S. (1990). Use of lower limb prosthesis among elderly amputees. *Annals of the Academy of Medicine, 19*(6), 811–816.

Craik, R. L., & Oatis, C. A. (1995). *Gait analysis: Theory and application.* St. Louis: Mosby-Year Book.

Czerniecki, J. M., Gitter, A., & Nunro, C. (1991). Joint moment and muscle power output characteristics of below knee amputees during running: The influence of energy storing prosthetic feet. *Journal of Biomechanics, 24*(1), 63–75.

Eastlack, M. E., Arvidson, J., Snyder-Mackler, L., Dandoff, J. V., & McGarvey, C. L. (1991). Interrater reliability of videotaped observational gait-analysis assessments. *Physical Therapy, 71*(6), 465–472.

Eberhart, H. D., & Inman, V. T. (1951). An evaluation of experimental procedures used in a fundamental study of human locomotion. *Annals of New York Academy of Sciences, 5,* 1213–1228.

Engsberg, J. R., MacIntosh, B. R., & Harder, J. A. (1990). Comparison of effort between children with and without below-knee amputation. *Journal of the Association of Children's Prosthetic-Orthotic Clinics, 25*(1), 1522.

Engsberg, J. R., Tedford, K. G., & Harder, J. A. (1992). Center of mass location and segment angular orientation of below-knee amputee and able-bodied children during walking. *Archives of Physical Medicine and Rehabilitation, 73,* 1163–1168

Fisher, S. V., & Gollickson, G. (1978). Energy cost of ambulation in health and disability: A literature review. *Archives of Physical Medicine and Rehabilitation, 59,* 124–133.

Gage, J. R., & Hicks, R. (1985). Gait analysis in prosthetics. *Clinical Prosthetics and Orthotics, 9*(3), 17–22.

Gage, J. R., & Õunpuu, S. (1989). Gait analysis in clinical practice. *Seminars in Orthopaedics, 4*(2), 72–87.

Gailey, R. S. (1996). *One step ahead: An integrated approach to lower extremity prosthetics and amputee rehabilitation.* Miami, FL: Advanced Rehabilitation Therapy.

Gailey, R. S., Wenger, M. A., Raya, M., Kirk, N., Erbs, K., Spyropoulos, P., & Nash, M. S.: Energy expenditure of trans-tibial amputees during ambulation at self-selected pace. *Prosthetics and Orthotics International, 18,* 84–91.

Ganguli, S., Datta, S. R., et al: Performance evaluation of an amputee-prosthesis system in below-knee amputees. *Ergonomics, 16*(6), 797–810.

---

*From Rodgers, M. M., & Cavanagh, P. R. (1984). Glossary of biomechanical terms, concepts, and units. *Physical Therapy, 64*(12).
[†]From Perry, J. (1992). *Gait analysis: Normal and pathological function.* Thorofare, NJ: Slack, Inc.

[‡]From Perry, J. (1992). *Gait analysis: Normal and pathological function.* Thorofare, NJ: Slack, Inc.

Gitter, A., Czerniecki, J. J., & DeGroot, D. (1991). Biomechanical analysis of the influence of prosthetic feet on below knee amputee walking. *American Journal of Physical Medicine and Rehabilitation, 70*(3), 142–148.

Glattly, H. W. (1963). A preliminary report on the amputee census. *Artificial Limbs, 7,* 5–10.

Glattly, H. W. (1964). A statistical study of 12,000 new amputees. *Southern Medical Journal, 57,* 1373–1378.

Godfrey, C. M., Jousse, A. T., Brett, R., & Butler, J. F. (1975). A comparison of some gait characteristics with six knee joints. *Orthotics and Prosthetics, 29,* 33–38.

Gonzalez, E. G., Corcoran, P. J., & Reyes, R. L. (1974). Energy expenditure in below-knee amputees: Correlation with stump length. *Archives of Physical Medicine and Rehabilitation, 55,* 111–119.

Hale, S. A. (1991). The effect of walking speed on the joint displacement patterns and forces and moments acting on the above-knee amputee prosthetic leg. *Journal of Prosthetics and Orthotics, 3*(2), 460–479.

Hannah, R. E., & Morrison, J. B. (1984). Prostheses alignment: Effect on the gait of persons with below-knee amputations. *Archives of Physical Medicine and Rehabilitation, 65,* 159–162.

Harris, G. F., & Wertsch, J. J. (1994). Procedures for gait analysis. *Archives of Physical Medicine and Rehabilitation, 75,* 216–225.

Huang, C. T., Jackson, J. R., & Moore, N. B. (1979). Amputation: Energy cost of ambulation. *Archives of Physical Medicine and Rehabilitation, 60,* 18–24.

Hungarford, D. S., & Cockin, J. (1975). Fate of the retained lower limb joints in Second World War amputees. *Proceedings and Reports of Universities, Colleges, Councils and Associations, 57-B*(1), 111.

Hurley, G. R. B., McKenny, R., Robinson, M., Zadrauec, M., & Pierrynowski, M. R. (1990). The role of the contralateral limb in below-knee amputee gait. *Prosthetics and Orthotics International, 14,* 33–42.

Inman, V. T., Ralston, H. J., & Todd, F. (1981). *Human walking.* Baltimore: Williams & Wilkins.

Jaegers, S., Hans Arendzen, J. H., & de Jongh, H. J. (1995). Prosthetic gait of unilateral transfemoral amputees: A kinematic study. *Archives of Physical Medicine and Rehabilitation, 76,* 736–743.

James, U. (1973a). Maximal isometric muscle strength in healthy active male unilateral above-knee amputees with special regards to the hip joint. *Scandinavian Journal of Rehabilitation Medicine, 5,* 55–66.

James, U. (1973b). Oxygen uptake and heart rate during prosthetic walking in healthy male unilateral above-knee amputees. *Scandinavian Journal of Rehabilitation Medicine, 5,* 71–80.

James, U. (1973c). Unilateral above-knee amputees. *Scandinavian Journal of Rehabilitation Medicine, 5,* 23–34.

James, U., & Oberg, K. (1973). Prosthetic gait pattern in unilateral above-knee amputees. *Scandinavian Journal of Rehabilitation Medicine, 5,* 35–50.

Kegel, B., Carpenter, M. L., & Burgess, E. M. (1978). Functional capabilities of lower extremity amputees. *Archives of Physical Medicine and Rehabilitation, 59,* 109–120.

Kerstein, M. D. (1974). Amputations of the lower extremity: A study of 194 cases. *Archives of Physical Medicine and Rehabilitation, 55,* 454–459.

Klopsteg, P. E., Wilson, P., et al. (1968). *Human limbs and their substitutes.* New York: Hafner Publishing Company.

Krebs, D. E., Edelstein, J. E., & Fishman, S. (1985). Reliability of observational kinematic gait analysis. *Physical Therapy, 65*(7), 1027–1033.

Lehmann, J. F., Price, R., Boswell-Bessette, S., Dralle, A., Questad, K., & deLateur, B. J. (1993). Comprehensive analysis of energy storing prosthetic feet: Flex Foot and Seattle Foot versus standard SACH Foot. *Archives of Physical Medicine and Rehabilitation, 74,* 1225–1231.

Levy, S. W. (1983). *Skin problems of the amputee.* St. Louis: Warren H. Green.

Lewallen, R., Dyck, G., Quanbury, A., Ross, K., & Letts, M. (1986). Gait kinematics in below-knee child amputees: A force plate analysis. *Journal of Pediatric Orthopedics, 6,* 291–298.

Lower-limb prosthetics. (1980). New York: New York University Medical Center, Prosthetics and Orthotics Department.

Medhat, A., Huber, P. M., & Medhat, M. A. (1990). Factors that influence the level of activities in persons with lower extremity amputation. *Rehabilitation Nursing, 13,* 13–18.

Medicare Region C Durable Medical Equipment Regional Carrier (1995). 1995 Supplier Update Workshops.

Mensch, G., & Ellis, P. M. (1986). *Physical therapy management of lower extremity amputations.* Gaithersburg, MD: Aspen Publishers.

Murphy, E. F., & Wilson, A. B. (1962). Anatomical and physiological considerations in below-knee prosthetics. *Artificial Limbs, 6*(2), 4–15.

Murray, M. P., Drought, B., & Kory, R. S. (1964). Walking patterns of normal men. *Journal of Bone and Joint Surgery, 46A*(2), 335–360.

Murray, M. P., Sepic, S. B., Gardner, G. M., & Mollinger, L. A. (1981). Gait patterns of above-knee amputees using constant friction knee components. *Bulletin of Prosthetic Research, 17*(2), 35–45.

Nelson, A. J. (1974). Functional ambulation profile. *Physical Therapy, 54*(10), 1059–1065.

Nissen, S. J., & Newman, W. P. (1992). Factors influencing reintegration to normal living after amputation. *Archives of Physical Medicine and Rehabilitation, 73,* 548–551.

Observational gait analysis. (1993). Downey, CA: Los Amigos Research and Education Institute, The Pathokinesiology Service and The Physical Therapy Department, Rancho Los Amigos Medical Center.

Olney, S. J., Elkin, N. D., Lowe, P. J., et al. (1979). An ambulation profile for clinical gait evaluation. *Physiotherapy Canada, 31,* 85–90.

Pagliarulo, M. A., Waters, R., & Hislop, H. (1979). Energy cost of walking of below-knee amputees having no vascular disease. *Physical Therapy, 59* (5), 538–542.

Peizer, E., Wright, D. W., & Mason, C. (1969). *Human locomotion. Bulletin of prosthetic research.* Washington, DC: Veterans Administration.

Perry, J. (1992). *Gait analysis: Normal and pathological function.* Thorofare, NJ: Slack.

Perry, J., & Shanfield, S. (1993). Effiency of dynamic elastic response prosthetic feet. *Journal of Rehabilitation Research and Development, 30*(1), 137–143.

Pinzur, M. S., Littooy, F., Daniels, J., et al. (1992). STAMP (Special Teams for Amputations, Mobility, Prosthetics/Orthotics) Center, Hines Veteran Administration Hospital. *Clinical Orthopaedics and Related Research, 281,* 239–243.

Powers, C. M., Torburn, L., Perry, J., & Ayyappa, E. (1994). Influence of prosthetic foot design on sound limb loading in adults with unilateral below-knee amputations. *Archives of Physical Medicine and Rehabilitation, 75,* 825–829.

Radcliffe, C. W. (1962). The biomechanics of below-knee prostheses in normal, level, bipedal walking. *Artificial Limbs, 6*(2), 16–24.

Radcliffe, C. W. (1957). The biomechanics of the Canadian-type hip-disarticulation prosthesis. *Artificial Limbs, 4*(2), 29–38.

Radcliffe, C. W. (1961). The biomechanics of the Syme prosthesis. *Artificial Limbs, 6*(1), 4–43.

Radcliffe, C. W. (1955). Functional considerations in the fitting of above-knee prostheses. *Artificial Limbs, 2*(1), 35–60.

Reimers, J. (1972). A scoring system for the evaluation of ambulation in cerebral palsy patients. *Developmental Medicine and Child Neurology, 14,* 332–335.

Robinson, J. L., & Smidt, G. L. (1981). Quantitative gait evaluation in the clinic. *Physical Therapy, 61*(3), 351–353.

Robinson, J. L., Smidt, G. L., & Arora, J. S. (1977). Accelerographic, temporal, and distance gait: Factors in below-knee amputee. *Physical Therapy, 57*(8), 898–904.

Rodgers, M. M., & Cavanagh, P. R. (1984). Glossary of biomechanical terms, concepts, and units. *Physical Therapy, 64*(12), 1886–1902.

Ryser, D. K., Erickson, R. P., & Cahlen, T. (1988). Isometric and isokinetic hip abductor strength in persons with above-knee amputations. *Archives of Physical Medicine and Rehabilitation, 69,* 840–845.

Saleh, M., & Murdoch, G. (1985). In defense of gait analysis. *Journal of Bone and Joint Surgery, 67B*(2), 237–241.

Sanders, G. T. (1986). *Lower limb amputations: A guide to rehabilitation.* Philadelphia: F. A. Davis.

Saunders, J. B., DeC. M., Inman, V. T., & Eberhart, H. D. (1953). The major determinants in normal and pathological gait. *Journal of Bone and Joint Surgery, 35,* 543–558.

Seireg, A., & Arvikar, R. J. (1975). The prediction of muscular load sharing and joint forces in the lower extremities during walking. *Journal of Biomechanics, 8,* 89–102.

Skinner, H. B., & Effeney, D. J. (1985). Special review gait analysis in amputees. *American Journal of Physical Medicine, 64*(2), 82–89.

Stokes, V. P., Andersson, C., & Forssberg, H. (1989). Rotational and translational movement features of the pelvis and thorax during adult human locomotion. *Journal of Biomechanics, 22*(1), 43–50.

Tinetti, M. E. (1986). Performance-oriented assessment of mobility

DIAGNOSIS	PURPOSE	PATIENT VARIABLES	ASSESSMENTS	DESIGN AND COMPONENTS	MATERIALS
			Upper Extremity Orthotics ROM Sensibility Strength Volume Pain Function Circulation Tissue Proximal stability	**Upper Extremity Orthotics** Single surface Circumferential Dynamic Serial static Static progressive Semiflexible Resilient components Outriggers Hinges External power	Plaster Leather Rubber and silicone Low-temperature plastic Foam Fabric High-temperature plastic Laminates Metal
Primary	**Upper Extremity Orthotics** Rest or protect Restore motion Restore function Prevention	Age Sex Cognition Socioeconomic Work history Avocation Expectations			
	Upper Extremity Prosthetics Replace grasp Extend control Body image ADL independence		**Upper Extremity Prosthetics** ROM Sensibility Muscle control Wound Immediate postoperative fitting Edema control Strength	**Upper Extremity Prosthetics** Body powered Myoelectric Cosmetic Terminal device Wrist unit Socket Hinges Elbow unit	

FIGURE 10–3. The decision tree is presented to assist the clinician through the process of determining and providing the optimal orthosis or prosthesis. Use of the decision tree is a hierarchic process whereby information at one branch leads the clinician to the next higher level of decision making.

questions must consider the status of skeletal involvement, soft tissue structures, and neurologic involvement.

A necessary question to be asked is "How long has it been since the onset of disease or trauma?" Soft tissue, including muscle, tendon, and skin, undergoes structural changes with the onset of trauma, edema, or long-term immobilization. With long-term flexion contractures, the shortening of the musculotendinous junctures, along with reabsorption of volar skin, may make reduction of a contracture with intermittent orthotic application unfeasible. Long-term posturing of the neurologically impaired hand may have led to functional contractures, which, if reduced, would lead to loss of function rather than functional gains.

In the case of the upper extremity prosthetic prescription, the diagnosis of partial hand, wrist disarticulation, long below-elbow, short below-elbow, elbow dislocation, long above-elbow, short above-elbow, or shoulder disarticulation amputation is only the description of the level of amputation. The diagnosis must also be considered in terms of the cause of the absence, be it traumatic or congenital. Upper extremity amputations can result from a variety of trauma, including avulsion or crush-type injury; thermal injury, including frostbite, electric burns, or chemi-

cal burns; vascular disease, including arteriosclerosis or vasospastic disease; tumors; infections; or neurotrophic disease, such as diabetes. In the case of congenital problems, terminal deficiency is the type seen more frequently; however, patients also present with terminal deformity and with permanent nerve loss, such as brachial plexus injury with flail arm.

PURPOSE—ORTHOTICS

It is wise to consider at this point in the decision process what an orthosis cannot do, as well as what it can do. An orthosis can provide mobility or stability to a joint but generally not both. An orthosis cannot provide dexterity, and it can generally supply only one type of prehension. It can provide gross strength but with little or no control over the amount of force applied. Although an orthosis can substitute for the natural protective padding of the hand to a degree, cushions or pads add bulk and may impede mobility. An orthosis can do virtually nothing to aid sensibility and in fact often hinders it by covering sensate surfaces. Finally, an orthosis can rarely substitute for the cosmesis and expressiveness of the hand. The end result of wearing an orthosis may be a more aesthetically pleasing and functional hand, but during the treatment process, these desirable features may be compromised.

The stated purpose of an orthosis must have a measurable outcome if one is to determine the effectiveness of the intervention. In determining purpose, assessments are suggested to clarify the pathology we seek to treat or alleviate. Many authors have described other categories for upper extremity orthotics (Brand, 1993; Fess & Philips, 1987; Redford, 1986; Rose, 1986). Although one could probably argue for the addition of several categories, four are identified here.

Rest or Protection for Pain Reduction

Orthoses that provide rest or protection to relieve or minimize pain are perhaps the most often prescribed upper extremity orthoses. A protective orthosis may be chosen in the event of an acute trauma such as a sprain or strain, for postoperative positioning, or in the presence of a long-term pathology such as rheumatoid arthritis.

Restore Joint Motion or Correct Deformity

Several orthotic designs are available when restoration of joint ROM is desired. Dynamic orthoses can be fabricated to restore motion through the use of resilient components, or a static progressive design may be indicated. Dynamic orthoses utilize a variety of mechanisms with which to provide traction, including springs, rubber bands, and woven or knitted elastic threads or straps (Fig. 10–4). Static progressive designs use nonresilient straps or buckle designs to apply traction (Fig. 10–5). Serial static designs rely on remolding by the clinician to reposition a joint at end range to facilitate tissue expansion. Orthoses with resilient or dynamic components are contraindicated in the presence of involuntary muscle contractions. For such patients, static progressive components may be useful, as they are designed to apply an adjustable static force against which the patient cannot move. In

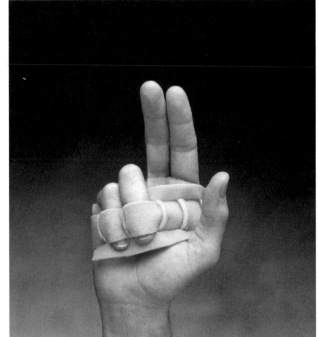

FIGURE 10–5. The nonelastic strapping employed here provides a static progressive stretch to the proximal and distal interphalangeal joints.

addition, this static force is not likely to facilitate an involuntary contraction. A serial static orthosis such as a cylindrical cast is an example of an orthotic application often indicated to correct a long-standing contracture when patient cooperation in an orthotics program is not feasible.

Restore or Augment Function

Orthoses fabricated to substitute for lost or impaired function span the spectrum from simple hinged orthoses that align or control motion to complex externally powered orthoses. Function may be supplied by one of three designs. First, the dynamic functional design uses external power or dynamic components to assist insufficient or replace absent muscle innervation. The externally powered orthosis is an example of this design. Second, an active functional orthosis can be designed to mechanically transfer power from one joint to another. A radial nerve palsy WHO with static MP assist 2–5 is an example of this (Fig. 10–6). Finally, a passive functional orthosis augments function through the stabilization of unstable joints, thereby positioning the hand to accomplish functional tasks.

Prevent Deformity or Cumulative Trauma

Muscle contractures that occur due to the paralysis or paresis of the antagonist may be prevented by positioning the muscle at its resting length to prevent shortening and reduction of muscle fibers. One example of a functional

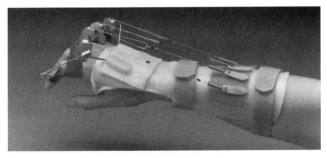

FIGURE 10–4. This dynamic orthosis consists of a static base, outrigger, and traction supplied by steel springs.

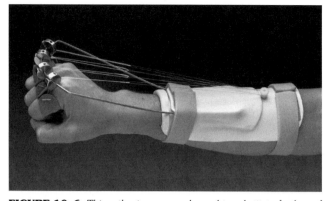

FIGURE 10–6. This orthosis, commonly used to substitute for loss of radial nerve function, employs tenodesis action to achieve finger extension on active wrist flexion.

preventative orthosis is a figure-of-eight hand orthosis that positions the hand in an intrinsic minus position to overcome intrinsic paralysis and to maintain mobility at the MP joints (Fig. 10–7). An example of a nonfunctional orthosis is a functional position WHO (commonly known as a resting pan splint) used in the presence of flaccid hemiplegia, also to maintain mobility at the MP joints (Fig. 10–8).

Orthoses are frequently being used in repetitive stress disorder prevention programs. The expanding field of ergonomics has brought a focus to positioning of the hand during the performance of vocational tasks. Advances in technology, particularly the proliferation of computers in the work place, have resulted in the development of semiflexible orthoses designed to limit specific ROMs, rather than to restrict all motion. Orthoses prescribed for prevention include those with gel cushions designed to absorb vibratory shock and orthoses fabricated from urethane foams or rubber and elastic materials that retain warmth and act to limit end ROMs, particularly at final

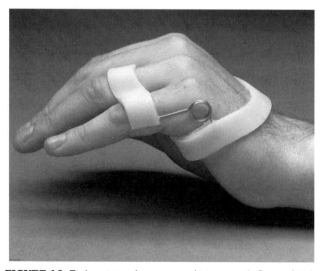

FIGURE 10–7. A spring coil incorporated into a simple figure-of-eight design holds the MP joint in flexion to allow action of the lumbricals on the proximal and distal interphalangeal joints to bring them into extension in the absence of ulnar nerve function.

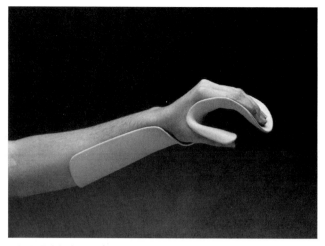

FIGURE 10–8. The functional position orthosis maintains the wrist and digits in midrange for rest and to prevent shortening of soft tissue structures following trauma or neurologic impairment.

ranges of wrist flexion and extension. This category of orthoses is not explored in depth here, as the prescription for an appropriate prevention program includes other ergonomic considerations aside from positioning of the upper extremity.

PURPOSE—PROSTHETICS

The purpose of the upper extremity prosthesis is
- To replace not the lost hand but the grasping function of the hand
- To extend the control of the residual limb through the prosthetic components to the terminal device
- To maintain or restore a positive body image
- To restore independent ADL performance by restoring bimanual performance ability (Fig. 10–9).

Like the upper extremity orthosis, the upper extremity prosthesis cannot provide dexterity. Each terminal device can, for the most part, provide only one type of prehen-

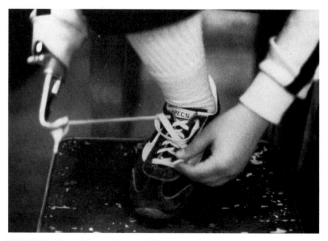

FIGURE 10–9. This 12-year-old boy was able to master shoe tying with the aid of his prosthesis with minimal training.

sion; however, terminal devices may be interchanged to accomplish various tasks. Some terminal devices do give the amputee a degree of control over the amount of force that is exerted through the terminal device. The prosthesis at its current technical level of development does not allow sensory feedback. The prosthesis does not improve sensibility, although some prosthetic wearers suggest that they are aware of sensory feedback through the prosthesis to the residual limb. The prosthesis rarely meets the cosmetic desires of the wearer.

PATIENT VARIABLES

The process of determining an optimal prosthetic or orthotic prescription must include assessment of patient variables. The ultimate outcome of this assessment process is the fitting of an external device. This device may have profound implications on a person's ability to perform those upper extremity tasks that help retain or restore functional independence. An orthosis or prosthesis is often accepted or rejected on the basis of its cosmesis. Upper extremity prostheses in particular may be viewed by the recipient as either completing their body image or so significantly altering it as to be unacceptable. Of ultimate concern here are those factors that must be assessed to determine the likelihood of compliance versus noncompliance with orthotic or prosthetic use.

The time and expense required for the fabrication of an orthosis or prosthesis are significant, and the assessment process may be stopped here if it is determined that the recipient is not yet willing or able to accept the device. There is no tool, save the skill and intuition of the evaluator, that can measure the readiness of a person to accept an orthosis or prosthesis.

The variables that follow are to be assessed both independently of one another and as a whole, as they create a total picture of the individual. It is this total picture that determines the ultimate requirements of an orthosis or prosthesis for a given individual.

Age

Age influences ability to cooperate with the wearing schedule and the tolerance to the forces applied by an orthosis or prosthesis. Young children are likely to accept a prosthesis or an orthosis that allows them to participate in play, even if it is not aesthetically appealing. The older person whose diagnosis of arthritis makes functional tasks difficult may be less accepting of an orthosis that assists function but is cosmetically unappealing. A study at Shriner's Hospital, Philadelphia unit, found that adolescents were more accepting of myoelectric prostheses that allowed them to look and feel more like other people than

of conventional cable-driven prostheses (Weaver et al., 1986).

Wright and Johns (1961), in their study of five types of stiffness in subjects with connective tissue diseases, found advancing age to be a significant factor in increased elastic joint stiffness. The results of this study are particularly important when considering the alternatives in orthotic application to restore motion in the hand of an older patient. Greater force may be required to achieve mobilization, but the skin and soft tissues may be less tolerant of this force due to the loss of their ability to sustain stress. The skin's normal protective mechanisms against ischemia are reduced with age. Restricted capillary flow, inflammation, diminished sensibility, and the reduction of the viscoelastic properties of the skin may all contribute to age-related intolerance of stress applied by either orthoses or prostheses.

In the case of the child amputee, age may preclude the fitting of an externally powered prosthesis because of the necessity of frequent replacement to accommodate growth. In addition to potential financial constraints, the use of an externally powered prosthesis may prevent the child from participating in activities such as age-appropriate water play without special precautions to prevent the destruction of the device. Like the child, the older amputee may be less of a candidate for the heavier externally powered device due to decreased strength.

Sex

Aside from the societal differences that may affect acceptance of an orthosis or a prosthesis for a man or woman, certain inherent biologic differences may alter the effectiveness of a chosen device. Wright and Johns (1961) cite a highly significant difference in normal joint stiffness between men and women. Men were found to have significantly greater joint stiffness than women. Although this may be viewed as a disadvantage to the clinician seeking to restore joint motion in a male patient, the greater bone and muscle mass in males allows for larger areas of pressure distribution and tolerance of externally applied mechanical force.

In the prescription of the upper extremity prosthesis, cosmesis is likely to be of greater concern to the female than the male patient. Therefore, in addition to attempting to meet the performance requirements of the female patient's vocational and avocational roles, cosmesis must be considered if the prosthesis is to be accepted. The female patient may be more likely to request, in addition to a functional prosthesis, a passive or cosmetic prosthesis for social use.

Cognition

General orientation to time, place, and person must be demonstrated if there is to be independent compliance with orthotic or prosthetic use. The cognitively impaired individual requires the assistance of a competent and motivated caregiver to ensure carryover with a prescribed wearing program. If a dedicated caregiver is not available, the choice of no orthosis or prosthesis, as opposed to one improperly applied or unused, may be in the best interest of the patient.

Socioeconomic Status

The economics involved in the fabrication of an initial orthosis or prosthesis and the cost of maintenance must be considered. The clinician may eschew more expensive, "high-tech" components when these are not economically feasible. In an environment of ever-rising restraints on reimbursement, the economics of necessary rehabilitation technology may be borne more and more by the recipient. Clinicians must be sensitive to the financial resources of their patients.

This again points to the situation of the child amputee who may do quite well with an externally powered prosthesis. Insurance may only pay for the initial fitting. The child will need adjustments on a yearly basis or perhaps even more frequently; therefore, unless the family can pay for the equipment or find another source to help, the child will not be kept in well-fitting devices.

Another consideration is the amputee who lives in a remote area or whose home does not have electricity. The battery-powered prosthesis requires access to electricity to charge the battery and to more regular maintenance to keep it in good working order. Where access to these services is questionable, body power is more reliable.

Work History

The motivation of a person wishing to return to gainful employment plays a major role in his or her acceptance or rejection of an orthosis or prosthesis. The clinician must not discount the possible societal or financial rewards for not returning to employment. The person motivated by the desire or the necessity of returning to work is likely to assist in the determination of which orthosis or prosthesis to fabricate. It is necessary to fully understand the demands of a person's job to choose the appropriate components that will ensure adequate force and maximal longevity for a given device. The component requirements for the carpenter are different than those for the office administrator.

The work history of the upper extremity amputee is important in making decisions related to prosthetic components, harnessing, and suspension and is a strong determinant in the choice of a body- versus electrically powered prosthesis. Special terminal devices are available for specific occupations, especially in the Dorrance series (Dorrance Company, Campbell, California). The individual whose job has several facets may require different prosthe-

ses or at least different terminal devices to meet his or her job demands.

Avocational History

The upper extremity prosthesis should provide the amputee with the ability not only to return successfully to employment but also, wherever possible, to return to his or her avocational life. This may require consideration of special terminal devices or other components to allow for task performance (Figure 10–10).

Patient Expectations

The traumatic amputee who has had no previous exposure to another amputee or to a prosthetic device is likely to have unrealistic expectations. He or she may have read about or seen a "bionic arm" and may expect to receive a "replacement arm." He or she may be fearful about the course of life without an arm or part of an arm. The sooner questions can be answered and correct infor-

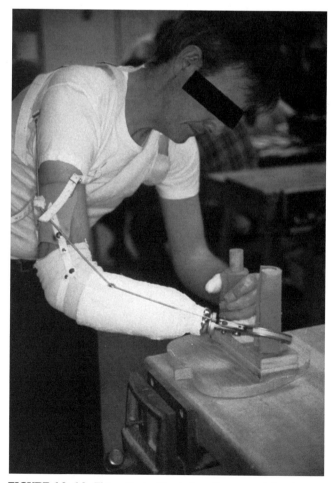

FIGURE 10–10. This patient with a below-elbow amputation is using a prehensile hand terminal device for his woodworking project. He uses a split hook for most activities.

mation provided, the more likely the patient is to let go of misinformation and unrealistic expectations.

Definitive orthoses, in contrast to prostheses, are generally fit farther along in the rehabilitation process. The patient may have already been fit with a temporary orthosis for the purpose of training as well as for determining the optimal functional position in which to fabricate the final orthosis. Generally, if an orthosis provides meaningful function—that is, meaningful to the recipient—it will be accepted. If the orthosis acts as a hindrance for those tasks the patient deems important, it will likely be rejected.

ASSESSMENTS

It is at this branch of the tree that the decision variables for orthotics and prosthetics diverge. It is the difference inherent in providing a replacement for a missing limb or in providing a support or assist for an existing part that necessitates this divergence. Although the ultimate objective may be the same—to restore function—the assessments necessary to achieve this objective vary. For clarity and ease of following the decision process, the branches of the orthotics decision tree are presented first, followed by the branches of the prosthetic decision tree. The final branch converges to present materials common to both orthotics and prosthetics.

ORTHOTICS

Once it has been determined that an orthosis is appropriate, that the patient is accepting of the need for an orthosis, and what it is that the clinician wishes to accomplish, the true work of gathering data begins. Each clinician must have a basic set of evaluation tools and a thorough knowledge base to use those tools properly. This text concerns itself with specific evaluation techniques, and the reader is referred to the appropriate chapters for greater detail and depth in technique. What is presented here is the rationale behind the use of a particular evaluation. The appropriate evaluation techniques and tools are discussed for each of the four defined orthotic purposes.

Rest or Protection for Pain Reduction

Range of Motion. Orthoses fabricated for the purpose of rest or protection, by their very definition, restrict motion. It is therefore necessary to determine precisely the degree and arc or motion one seeks to restrict. In the presence of acute trauma, it may not be possible to determine the origin of the pain or precisely which structures are involved. Careful recording of available ROM prior to providing

complete immobilization is required. It may not be possible or necessary to record the ROM of all involved joints at the initial visit. The clinician may simply establish a baseline for the joints included in the orthosis by recording the position of the joints within the orthosis. One certain mark of progress is the recovery of motion that allows for improved orthotic positioning, even as pain persists.

Pain caused by inflammation secondary to overuse is more easily assessed, and only the arc of motion in which the patient experiences the pain need be restricted. The advent of semiflexible orthoses that allow for midrange motion but increase their restriction as range increases requires that the clinician record two sets of measurements, available active ROM and pain-free active ROM.

Sensibility. In the presence of acute trauma, assessment of pain may be solely via subjective report from the patient. It is likely that in the most acute stages, the patient or clinician is unable to distinguish between subjective pain and objective sensibility. If pain is secondary to a diagnosis of nerve entrapment or localized inflammation, the clinician needs to establish some baseline measure of sensibility. It is suggested that a brief evaluation of light touch–deep pressure responses be performed using monofilaments. This assessment is suggested for the purpose of comparison rather than as a basis for treatment planning.

Strength Testing. When a resting orthosis is prescribed to reduce pain related to a chronic diagnosis, an abbreviated assessment of functional strength patterns may be indicated.

Volume. Volumetric assessment may be indicated in either acute or subacute trauma, as well as in the presence of chronic inflammatory disease. It is essential to record volume prior to the application of an orthosis, as any form of immobilization may exacerbate edema due to the decrease in active muscle function when the hand or limb is put at rest. Of particular interest to the treating clinician should be the effect of volume on pain. A volumetric reduction that is not accompanied by an expressed reduction in pain and increase in ROM may indicate more extensive tissue or skeletal involvement.

Subjective Pain Assessment. Pain is a subjective sensation and should be recorded in a consistent manner. The use of scales on which the patient indicates a level of pain may be used and reassessed over time (Merskey, 1973). A pain scale developed for clinical use by this author that measures how restrictive pain is in the performance of daily activities is suggested as one means of demonstrating progress to the patient (see Appendix A at the end of this chapter). The use of body charts may aid the clinician in distinguishing the site of injury from areas of referred pain and help to define the appropriate intervention. Each assessment of pain should be independent of the previous one. The patient should be given a clean recording form each time and not encouraged to compare levels from one assessment to the next. This limits the likelihood that symptom exacerbation will influence the choice of intervention.

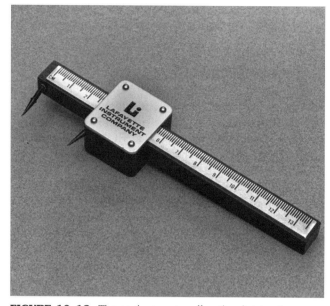

FIGURE 10–12. The aesthesiometer offers the clinician the convenience of a sliding scale for distance between two points of stimulation. (Courtesy of Lafayette Instrument, Lafayette, IN.)

a digitally self-calibrated dynamometer and pinch meter, raising the reliability and validity of strength testing (Fig. 10–14).

Manual muscle tests are suggested to assess the appropriateness of an orthotic prescription. If a patient has a muscle power grade of 0 or 1, this will not be adequate to utilize a wrist-driven tenodesis orthosis without an external power source. Insufficient muscle strength in one position may be increased if tested with the muscle in its lengthened posture. Testing of incompletely innervated muscles may be performed in positions other than those described as

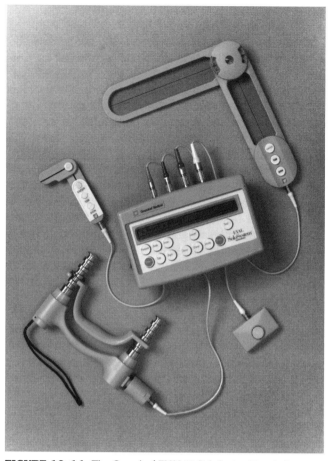

FIGURE 10–14. The Greenleaf EVAL™ SoloSystem™ includes computerized instrumentation for evaluation of grasp and pinch strength as well as ROM of the upper extremity. All instruments are self-calibrating for consistent, objective measures. (Courtesy of Greenleaf Medical Systems, Palo Alto, California.)

optimal in the literature (Kendall et al., 1971). Inadequate finger flexion force may be increased as the wrist is extended, and this determines how the clinician is to position adjacent joints in the orthosis to maximize function.

Tissue Extensibility. Soft tissue structures must be elastic enough to allow positioning without resistance. The neurologically impaired hand tolerates less force due to sensory deficits and atrophy of soft tissues. If the orthosis is fit against restricted tissues, the resultant forces may be intolerable.

Proximal Stability. The successful use of an orthosis by a person with neurologic impairment or spinal cord injury is often dependent on sufficient proximal function and stability. The person with C3 or C4 quadriplegia may lack the upper extremity placement and trunk stability required to use an externally powered orthosis. In fitting a mobile arm support to a person with multiple sclerosis, trunk or head and neck rigidity may preclude the motions necessary to ensure successful performance of activities. For the child with cerebral palsy, the clinician must be aware of sitting postures and restrictive seating devices that may require alternate setups for the successful completion of activities.

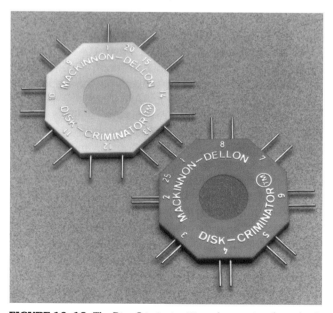

FIGURE 10–13. The Disc-Criminators™ employ a series of metal rods spaced from 2 mm to 25 mm apart for testing static and moving two-point discrimination. (Courtesy of Neuroregen, Lutherville, MD.)

Functional Task Performance. A full ADL assessment prior to and following fitting is indicated any time a functional orthosis is contemplated. A baseline must be established for performance of daily tasks that includes not only a patient's ability to complete the tasks but also the time necessary to complete the tasks. The classic example is the patient with rheumatoid arthritis who, because of loss of pinch strength, can button a blouse but takes 30 minutes to do so. The fitting of a thumb IP extension blocker that serves to improve stability may reduce the time necessary to complete the task. Presenting orthotic intervention as a means to perform tasks in a more time-efficient manner is more likely to be acceptable to the reluctant recipient.

Prevention

Range of Motion. The goal in preventative orthosing is to maintain ROM rather than to increase it. ROM assessment should include TAM and TPM. Hand and upper extremity orthoses should be directed at maintaining functional ROM. Functional ROM is considered to be midrange motion for each joint crossed. In the presence of hypertonicity, it is necessary to assess and record at what degree and in what position muscle tone increases.

Sensibility. Preventative orthoses are often fit for long wearing periods, and patients and caregivers must be cognizant of any areas of sensory deficit that require greater care and attention. In the upper extremity, it is important to test for response to light touch–deep pressure over any areas the orthosis will cover.

Strength. It may not be feasible or necessary to assess strength formally when fitting a preventative orthosis. Resisted strength assessment is contraindicated in the presence of hypertonicity. It is important, however, to assess and record the amount of force required and the length of time over which this force is applied to effect a reduction in tone. The result of this "strength of tone" assessment is necessary in determining optimal wearing schedules.

Tissue Extensibility. It should be assumed that soft tissue is pliable and no absolute restriction yet exists if an orthosis is defined as preventative. If either condition exists, the orthosis would be corrective and not preventative. Of concern here is the assessment of whether the patient or caregivers can provide an appropriately prescribed regimen of ROM exercise to augment the orthotic positioning.

Functioning Task Performance. We generally view preventative orthoses to be resting orthoses, which therefore act to impede rather than allow function. Of concern again is the ability of the patient or caregiver to properly don and doff the orthosis. In the case of nighttime positioning hand orthoses, the ability to manage night clothing and bedding should be assessed. Bilateral orthoses may make nighttime toileting impossible, and a schedule of alternating nights for each hand may be considered.

PROSTHETICS

Wound Healing

Wound healing is the primary goal of early postamputation management. The postoperative dressing may be soft, semirigid, or rigid. The type of postoperative dressing chosen by the surgeon affects every other aspect of the patient's early postoperative management.

The soft dressing provides a mechanical barrier between the wound and the environment. It is composed of a layer of sterile, nonadherent material and sterile gauze or fluff held in place with a gauze wrap. This system of management allows for frequent inspection of the postoperative wound site.

The semirigid or rigid dressing prevents frequent wound inspection. This dressing can be fabricated from a number of materials including Unna paste, plaster, or elastic plaster. It is applied over a sterile dressing. The dressing can be changed as needed to maintain gentle distal pressure and good support of the limb. This dressing can serve as a socket base for the early- or immediate-fit prosthesis discussed in the following section.

Regardless of the type of postoperative dressing chosen, wound shear must be avoided. This is accomplished by providing good, even compression with a firm fit in the rigid and semirigid dressing. Applying a layer of nonadherent gauze prior to application of the top dressing layers is also recommended. The soft dressing should be applied firmly but not so tight as to cause vascular compromise.

Immediate Postoperative Fit

When feasible, an immediate postoperative fit (IPOF) or early-fit prosthetic device is used following traumatic amputation. With IPOF, patient expectations are more likely to be realistic, and the healing process may be enhanced. The patient either wakes up from surgery with the immediate postoperative plaster socket in place or receives it shortly thereafter. The goals of early, i.e., within the first 2 weeks following amputation, or immediate postoperative fittings are

- To prevent the development of one-handed techniques for activity performance
- To control edema
- To decrease or prevent problems associated with phantom pain
- To allow for experimentation with prosthetic options prior to definitive prosthetic fitting

A plaster socket or rigid dressing is applied at the time of surgery. After 1 to 3 days, the other components of the early-fit device are applied, including a harness suspension system, the wrist unit (or elbow unit in the case of the above-elbow amputee), and the terminal device

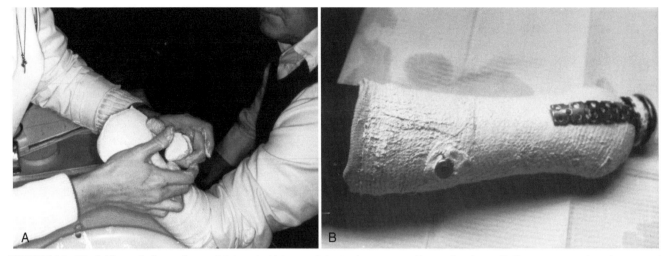

FIGURE 10–15. *A,* The early-fit prosthesis is fabricated with layers of elastic plaster covered by regular plaster. *B,* Components such as the wrist unit shown here are added to the plaster socket.

(Fig. 10–15). The rigid plaster dressing provides compression to assist with edema control. The compression provided by the dressing also helps with control of phantom pain. Although the mechanism through which phantom pain is reduced or relieved is not adequately understood, it is possible to provide anecdotal evidence of its reduction (Jacobs & Brady, 1975).

The patient who is fitted immediately after surgery does not have the opportunity to develop unilateral patterns of activity performance that the patient who has to wait several weeks or even months for a prosthesis to be fit is certain to develop. In addition, the patient has the opportunity to experiment with various terminal devices to familiarize himself or herself with what is available and to help in definitive terminal device selection.

Edema Control

Edema control is important in all postoperative management, but especially so in the amputee, as it affects the timing for the patient's definitive prosthetic fitting. Edema control may be addressed by elevation, regardless of the type of postoperative dressing chosen.

Where a soft dressing is chosen, the patient may also be instructed in the use of an elastic wrap or Compressogrip stockinette (Para Medical Distributors, Kansas City, Missouri) to provide assistance with edema control and with shaping of the residual limb. The elastic wrap is applied in a graded figure-of-eight fashion from distal to proximal (Fig. 10–16). If the limb is short, especially if it has been amputated at a short above-elbow level, it is very difficult to keep the wrap in place. Using a chest wrap with a figure-of-eight over the shoulder can help to maintain the position of the wrap. The Compressogrip, while it decreases control of pressure application, is less likely to slip and may be very useful for the patient or family member who is having difficulty applying the elastic wrap correctly.

The rigid or semirigid dressing itself serves as the means of external compression. The dressing must be changed to accommodate decreases in edema. As mentioned previously, edema measurements help to determine the patient's readiness for definitive prosthetic fitting. Edema measurements must be taken regularly and documented

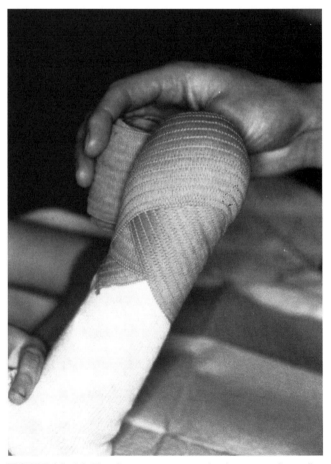

FIGURE 10–16. The elastic wrap assists with edema control as well as with shaping of the residual limb. The wrap is applied from distal to proximal in a graded figure-of-eight fashion.

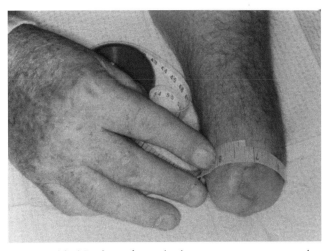

FIGURE 10–17. Circumferential edema measurements are taken frequently, as they help to determine the patient's readiness for his or her definitive prosthesis.

accurately to be meaningful (Fig. 10–17). The measurements should be taken at easily duplicatable landmarks and at specified points along the residual limb. When measurements have been stable for 2 weeks, it is generally safe to proceed with definitive conventional fitting. The myoelectric prosthesis requires a more intimate fit between the residual limb and the prosthetic socket for reliable prosthetic function. For this reason, definitive fitting of the myoelectric prosthesis should be delayed until circumferential measurements have been stable for 4 to 6 weeks.

Range of Motion

Active and passive ROM are assessed goniometrically on a regular basis. These measurements are taken without and later with a definitive prosthesis. This is one method that is used to determine if the definitive prosthesis has achieved a good fit.

Gentle active and passive ROM exercises are started as soon as possible following amputation surgery. Motion is much easier to maintain than it is to regain once it is lost. Pronation and supination are especially difficult to regain. Patients have a habit of posturing their residual limb in pronation and allowing the interosseous membrane to contract into a shortened position. As the level of amputation becomes higher, residual pronation and supination lessens. Effective elbow motion may also lessen at higher below-elbow levels. As a general rule, everything that can move should move, to ensure maximum functional ability following prosthetic fitting. Good shoulder and scapular motions are essential for operation of the body-powered prosthesis.

Sensibility

Most upper extremity sockets are fit as total-contact sockets; i.e., there is equal pressure distribution over the entire portion of the residual limb that is housed in the prosthetic socket. Areas of the residual limb that have decreased or absent residual sensibility, as identified through sensibility evaluation as described earlier, must be given special attention in terms of socket fit. Frequent inspection to prevent the development of skin breakdown and wound healing problems is recommended. These problems, should they be allowed to develop, could result in the amputee's needing to go without the prosthesis until healing is accomplished.

Just as diminished sensibility can present problems for the amputee, hypersensitivity or pain caused by a neuroma can present its own complications. A hypersensitive wound area or neuroma can prevent the amputee from tolerating the pressure of the prosthesis and severely limit wearing tolerance. Appropriate intervention is indicated in these cases.

Muscle Control

It is important to determine whether the patient has volitional control of the musculature of the residual limb. If the muscles are not under voluntary control, the patient may not be a candidate for a myoelectric prosthesis. New, more sensitive devices can use very small amounts of muscle power at as few as one site to power a myoelectric prosthesis, but the muscle function must be under voluntary control to allow the patient to open and close the terminal device in a functional way.

Strength

The patient must have adequate strength in his or her residual musculature to support prosthetic components and to power them successfully. Manual muscle testing is indicated to assess muscle strength. For example, in the case of the short below-elbow amputation, where a step-up hinge is needed to increase the effective range through which the patient is able to drive the prosthetic forearm, use of this hinge requires greater strength on the part of the amputee to achieve the motion. Additional componentry in the form of amplifiers may be needed to overcome any problem.

DESIGN AND COMPONENTS— ORTHOTICS
Rest or Protection to Reduce Pain

There are two design options for orthoses directed at rest and protection. One is the fabrication or fitting of a single-surface orthosis—one that covers only the palmar or

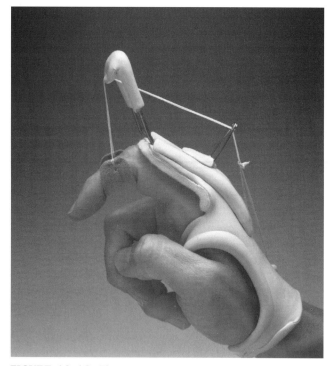

FIGURE 10–18. This outrigger is attached to the low-temperature thermoplastic base by the application of a second piece of thermoplastic heat bonded to the base.

dorsal surface of the hand or extremity or the ulnar or radial surface. Single-surface orthoses require straps or wrappings to create one or more three-point pressure systems to secure the orthosis in place. The second option is a circumferential design that wraps around the joint, creating equal pressure over all surfaces to limit motion. Strapping is needed only to maintain closure of the orthosis.

Single-surface orthoses are effective for support and rest of joints surrounded by weak or flaccid muscles, such as found following a CVA or peripheral nerve injury. In the absence of active motion, a single-surface design provides sufficient control and allows the clinician to readily adjust the force of the orthosis through adjustment or realignment of straps.

Circumferential designs offer the choice of using lighter-weight or thinner materials, as the additional contours of the design add strength to the orthosis. Circumferential designs are particularly applicable when the patient has active motion and will be using the orthosis during activity. The control that a circumferential orthosis provides helps to limit the shear forces that can be created when there is movement within or against the orthosis. These design qualities make the circumferential design most applicable in the presence of tendinitis or neuritis, as well as for the support or immobilization of unstable joints.

Restore Motion or Correct Deformity

The options for orthoses designed to restore motion fall into three categories: dynamic, serial static, and static

progressive. The choice of design is again dependent on the results of assessments related to patient variables; to purpose of the orthosis; and now, more importantly, to information gathered from assessments of ROM, tissue extensibility, sensibility, and vascular status.

By definition, a dynamic orthosis incorporates a resilient component (e.g., elastic, rubber bands, or springs) against which the patient can move. Dynamic orthoses restore motion by assisting a joint through its range and by applying traction force at the end of available range to promote tissue lengthening. This resilient component generally acts on the joint through attachment to an outrigger to secure the line of pull. The outrigger, in turn, is attached to a static base fit securely to the hand or extremity (Fig. 10–18).

A serial static orthosis restores motion through the static application of end-range stretch. The serial static orthosis relies on repeated remolding and repositioning to maintain the part at end range to achieve an increase in joint motion. This orthosis has no movable or resilient components. The classic example of a serial static orthosis is a serial plaster cast or circumferential thermoplastic orthosis fit to reduce a flexion contracture. Frequent remolding or replacement of the cast or orthosis places and holds the joint at its end range of motion to facilitate tissue lengthening (Fig. 10–19).

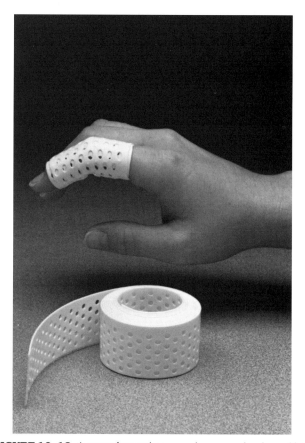

FIGURE 10–19. A circumferential wrap can be removed and remolded, placing the proximal interphalangeal joint in progressively greater extension.

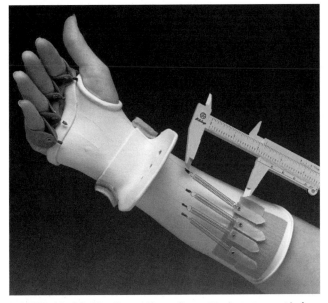

FIGURE 10–20. The Gyovai Finger Spring™ adjusts to provide force between 50 and 400 g. (Courtesy of North Coast Medical, San Jose, CA.)

Static progressive orthoses incorporate a static mechanism to adjust the amount or angle of traction acting on the joint. This static mechanism is most often a loop or cloth strapping material, a turn buckle, or a nonresilient nylon line. The mechanism itself is adjusted to progressively change the angle and amount of force directed to the joint. The base orthosis remains unchanged (see Fig. 10–5).

The resilient components used in dynamic orthoses are most commonly rubber bands or steel springs. The advantages of rubber bands are their universal availability and low cost. The disadvantages include their lack of uniformity, limited and variable shelf life, and inconsistent quality. Mildenberger and colleagues (1986) have created a force-enlongation values chart useful in helping to determine the spring constant for rubber bands. Spring constant is given by "the product of the cross-sectional area and the modulus of rubber band elasticity." Spring constant is defined as the "amount of force required to elongate the rubber band to twice its original length" (Mildenberger et al., 1986, p. 242). The chart offers a systematic approach to the selection of rubber bands used to supply traction.

An evaluation of commercially available SCOMAC steel springs by Roberson and colleagues (1988) found them to be linear and consistent with negative creep and minimal hysteresis. The springs are supplied in kits and are color coded and graded for force from 50 to 2000 g. The authors concluded that the use of SCOMAC springs offers the advantage of greater consistency and predictability when applying force with a dynamic orthosis. They do, however, suggest that as with rubber bands, the springs be measured and adjusted accordingly once they are attached to an orthosis. SCOMAC springs are available from S.G.M. (Codim, St. Etienne, France).

Graded springs are more readily available, the cost has diminished over time, and their design for convenient use

continues to improve. In addition to SCOMAC springs, Gyovai Finger Springs™ are available assembled with outrigger line and loop tabs for attachment to the base of an orthosis. The amount of force applied is a result of the distance the spring is stretched (Fig. 10–20).

When fabricating orthoses with components designed to restore motion, no other choice is as important as the choice of what force to use and how much force to apply. Although the materials described here each have limitations, it is the clinician's responsibility to obtain the most reliable information by using the appropriate tools. The assessment of rubber bands or springs can be readily performed in the clinic. The results can be easily checked and confirmed by the use of a simple spring scale when attaching components to an orthosis. The information gathered during the performance of torque ROM is meaningful only when the clinician incorporates the information appropriately and consistently to apply the predetermined degree of traction with the properly tested components.

Fess and Philips (1987) give a "safe force magnitude" table that suggests force parameters to be used when applying dynamic traction to the digits. Although this table offers no absolute values, it does offer the clinician a formula for determining force parameters. Taking the reading of the force gauge used in evaluating ROM and multiplying this reading by the distance from the point of traction to the axis of the joint gives a measurement for torque (torque equals force times distance). This measure must then be matched with the force and distance measures of the chosen resilient component to provide a known degree of force.

The two other components that make up a dynamic or static progressive orthosis are the outriggers employed in alignment of the force and hinges used to facilitate movement of the orthosis as it crosses a joint. The outrigger may be viewed as a nonmobile structural mechanism that acts solely as a pivot point from which to establish an angle of pull. A high-profile outrigger is one that is set at sufficient height above the joint being acted on that it can extend the resilient component to the length necessary to apply a predetermined measure of force (Fig. 10–21). A low-profile outrigger is one designed to act as a pivot point for a static line. The static line, once it has passed through or

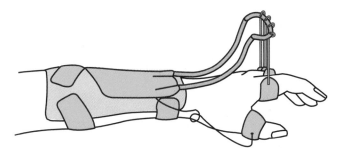

FIGURE 10–21. The high-profile outrigger is set at a height that allows the resilient component to apply its force in optimal midrange.

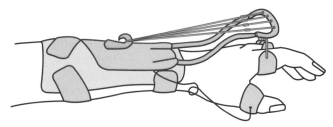

FIGURE 10–22. The low-profile outrigger acts as a pivot point for the static component of the traction line. Once the pivot point is established at 90 degrees to the part being acted on, the angle of pull of the resilient component may be directed as needed.

over the pivot point, is then attached to a resilient component for the application of force (Fig. 10–22).

In assessing the orthosis to be constructed, the choice of high- versus low-profile outrigger is determined in part by the skill of the fabricator, the overall length of the orthosis, and patient tolerance and convenience. The choice of outrigger height may be determined in great part by the size and length of the base orthosis. A finger-based or short hand-based orthosis may simply not have the length necessary to supply an attachment point and produce the optimal force range if a low-profile outrigger is used. A WHO or elbow wrist hand orthosis (EWHO) offers the clinician greater flexibility in establishing the necessary attachment sites for resilient components.

A variety of dynamic and static progressive designs rely on articulating hinged components to facilitate motion across a joint (Fig. 10–23). Consideration must be given to the alignment of hinges with the anatomic joint. Many of the joints of the upper extremity are multiaxial with alignment that deviates from pure anatomic planes. The wrist joint is one example of a complex joint with two axes of motion—one for flexion and extension and one for radial and ulnar deviation. In addition to these two axes, conjunct motions occur that are not in alignment with anatomic planes. Wrist extension combines with radial deviation and a slight degree of forearm supination. Wrist flexion combines with ulnar deviation and slight pronation.

No manufactured hinge is now available that duplicates these conjunct motions. Therefore, any orthosis designed

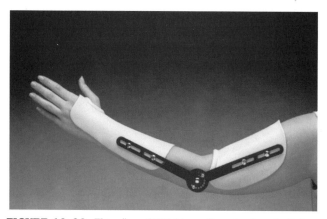

FIGURE 10–23. This elbow ROM hinge allows for free, limited, or blocked ROM at the elbow.

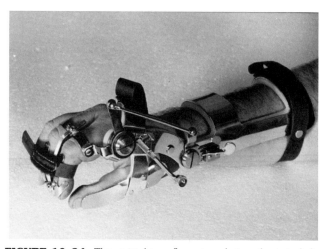

FIGURE 10–24. This wrist-driven flexor tenodesis orthosis includes locking ratchets for both the wrist and the digits to supply static prehension without sustained voluntary muscle contraction. (Courtesy of JAECO, Hot Springs, Arkansas.)

to apply force across a hinge in the expectation of restoring motion to a multiaxial joint must consider this limitation. Binding and friction will be created, despite the greatest care in axial alignment. The clinician must constantly reassess the alignment of any articular component and the fit of the base orthosis to reduce the deleterious effects of friction.

Restore or Augment Function

The broadest range of designs and components exist for this category of orthotic application. Designs range from the simple static figure-of-eight HO that positions the MP joints in flexion to substitute for lost intrinsic function (see Fig. 10–7), to the highly complex externally powered WHOs.

As was mentioned earlier, the fitting of an orthosis on the hand has the potential to limit, as well as to augment, function. Of the orthoses cited in the previous paragraph the figure-of-eight positions the hand to allow for full IP joint extension and improves grasp. It does so, however, at the expense of covering a portion of the palmar surface of the hand. Care must be taken when fabricating this HO to minimize the palmar surface covered, yet it must fit snugly to overcome the strength of the extrinsic extensors.

The wrist-driven tenodesis orthosis is commonly prescribed to augment function for the person with a spinal cord injury at levels C5 through C7. It is at these levels that the extensor carpi radialis longus and brevis (C5–8) and the extensor carpi ulnaris (C6–8) are innervated. This allows for active wrist extension and the accomplishment of a weak tenodesis grasp. The wrist-driven orthosis augments the tenodesis action through the posting of the thumb and the attainment of sustained pinch. Orthoses with a locking ratchet at the wrist allow for passively sustained wrist extension (Fig. 10–24). This further augments function by lessening the likelihood of extensor carpi radialis and ulnaris muscle fatigue.

The static MP extension assist WHO designed for use in the presence of radial nerve dysfunction makes it possible to use the hand without needing to use the substitute motions of forearm supination and pronation to facilitate grasp and release (see Fig. 10–6). The simple thumb IP extension blocker prevents IP joint hyperextension and can increase pinch strength by as much as 50 percent or more. For persons with severe arthritis in the thumb who may have a pinch measurement of only 2 to 3 lb, this increase is functionally significant.

Prevention

Orthoses designed to prevent deformity are often just one aspect of an ongoing program of prevention or maintenance, depending on the expectations for recovery of function. In the absence of motor function or in the presence of hypertonicity, a static-design orthosis is suggested. The choice of single-surface or circumferential orthosis is to be made by the clinician based on experience and preference.

In general, the design choice will be that of a static orthosis without hinged or resilient components. In situations where there is unopposed innervation of muscle groups, an orthosis may be designed to supply, or simply allow for, the absent motion. A drop-out–style elbow orthosis allows for passive elbow extension when there is relaxation of spastic flexors and therefore prevents contractures. Similarly, orthotic hinges are available that allow

for locking out degrees of range to prevent positioning that may result in contracture (Fig. 10–25).

Orthoses used in the prevention of cumulative trauma are chosen for their ease of donning and doffing and for their low-profile designs. Thin, lightweight circumferential designs are frequently the design of choice, as they lessen interference with activity. Components may include flexible stays or foam pads that limit end ranges of motion. Hinges may be indicated to block motion in undesirable planes; e.g., an ulnar-based wrist hinge allows free flexion and extension but prevents ulnar deviation. To be effective in preventing trauma, an orthosis must be designed to limit only undesirable motion without transferring stress onto adjacent structures.

DESIGN AND COMPONENTS— PROSTHESES

Upper extremity prosthetic components are chosen primarily to meet the functional needs and durability requirements of the individual with emphasis on restoration of prehension. The patient, surgeon, therapist, and prosthetist should work as a team to determine the optimal prosthesis based on the results of the assessment process. The three primary prosthetic systems available to the upper extremity amputee are as follows:

Body-powered or conventional systems: The body-powered or conventional prosthesis is controlled by motion from the amputee's body (Fig. 10–26). The harness transmits power through the control strap to the cable and eventually to the terminal device. Humeral flexion on the amputated side is the primary motion utilized for terminal device operation in the below-elbow patient.

External or myoelectric systems: Myoelectric prostheses are the popular version of the externally powered prosthesis. They rely on an external power source, a battery, to convert the electric signal from a muscle to motion through an electric appliance (Fig. 10–27). The muscle acts as a signal source. The signal is passed through electrodes embedded in the socket to the control system, which translates the signal into the desired action, i.e., opening or closing of the prosthetic appliance. Depolarization of the cell membrane of individual muscle fibers that occurs during muscle contraction is the origin of the myoelectric signal.

Cosmetic or passive systems: While these devices are most popular for the digital, partial hand, or hand amputee, endoskeletal designs may be fabricated for patients with higher levels of loss. These systems are dedicated to improving the cosmetic appearance of the amputated part and addressing the psychological needs of the person for whom a functional prosthesis

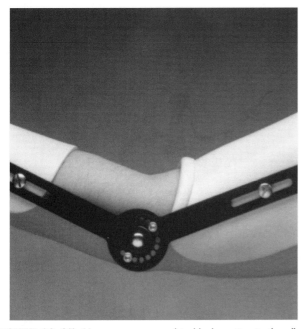

FIGURE 10–25. Hex screws are used to block motion in the elbow ROM hinge to allow for many combinations of free or limited elbow flexion and extension.

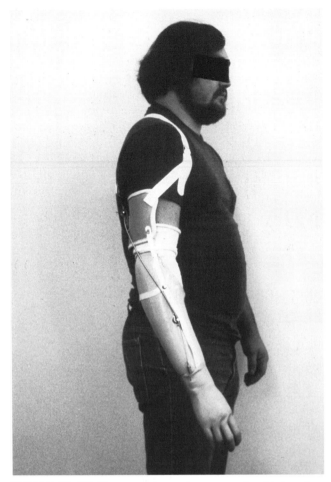

FIGURE 10–26. This patient is wearing a conventional below-elbow system with mechanical hand.

is not feasible (Fig. 10–28). A wide variety of cosmetic prostheses are available, from prefabricated gloves to those that are custom fit and custom colored. The price range is as varied as the options, and it often falls to the therapist to justify the cosmetic prosthesis to third-party payers. Patients are generally encouraged to look toward a functional prosthesis, either conventional or myoelectric, before the notion of a cosmetic prosthesis is introduced, since restoring function is our primary goal. In addition to the choices listed above, hybrids that combine aspects of several system types are also available.

Terminal Device

Every upper extremity prosthesis includes a terminal device. The terminal device may be either a hook or a hand that is either voluntary opening or voluntary closing. As the names imply, force is required either to open the terminal device to achieve prehension or to close the terminal device to maintain prehension. The terminal device may be manual (Fig. 10–29) or electric in operation (Fig. 10–30), de-

pending on the type of prosthesis that has been selected. Decisions regarding the most appropriate or necessary terminal devices may be made during the early-fit period when the patient may be experimenting with various devices during training. Considerations in terminal device selection include the patient's preinjury activity level, both vocationally and avocationally, residual limb length, residual limb strength, and general prosthetic choice.

Wrist Units

The wrist unit provides a point of attachment for the terminal device, allows for prepositioning of the terminal device in either pronation or supination, and allows for the exchange of terminal devices. Wrist units are available in either friction or locking type. Quick-disconnect components are available for rapid switching of terminal devices. A wrist flexion component is available for the amputee who has a bilateral injury or is unable to operate close to the body with the opposite arm; e.g., an individual with a wrist fusion on the opposite side (Fig. 10–31).

Prosthetic Socket

The prosthetic socket encases the residual limb. An extension is used to fill the space between the end of the socket and the wrist unit or between the end of the limb and the elbow unit in above-elbow patients. Socket design is dependent on the level of amputation, residual function, and prosthetic choice.

Special socket designs such as the split socket or Muenster socket may be necessary for individuals with very short below-elbow amputations. The Muenster socket has very high trim lines and encases the olecranon and condyles to provide additional stability. The disadvantage

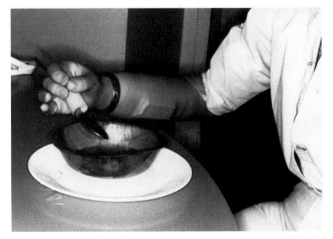

FIGURE 10–27. The below-elbow myoelectric system used by this patient has an electric hand.

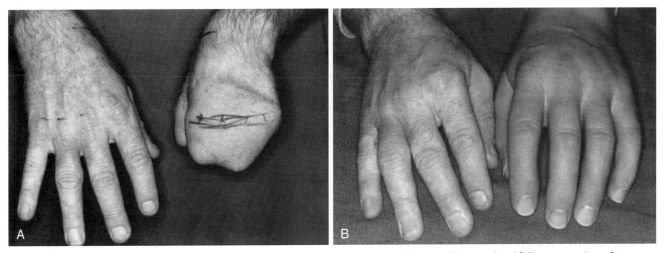

FIGURE 10–28. *A,* The patient's residual limb prior to fitting with a cosmetic prosthesis. *B,* The same hand following prosthetic fitting.

of this socket is that elbow flexion is limited, usually to about 70 degrees, because of these trim lines.

The split socket includes a socket that encases the residual limb and a separate forearm shell that includes the wrist unit and terminal device. This design may be used with step-up hinges discussed in the following section or with other modifications, such as an elbow lock.

Hinges

There are three primary types of hinges used with the below-elbow prosthesis. Flexible hinges fabricated from Dacron, leather, or other flexible material serve primarily a suspensory function. They are used mostly for wrist disarticulation and long below-elbow patients who retain pronation and supination.

Step-up hinges are used in combination with a split

socket, where residual elbow flexion is also limited. They step up the range of flexion through which the stump is able to drive the prosthetic forearm by either a 2 : 1 or 3 : 2 ratio; i.e., for every 1 degree of active elbow flexion, the forearm will move 2 degrees. As mentioned earlier, the disadvantage of using this device is that the strength required to achieve the same amount of flexion nearly doubles.

Elbow Units

Elbow units provide elbow flexion and locking in various degrees of flexion. There are two basic types of elbow units: the external elbow, used for the elbow disarticulation patient, and the internal elbow, used for above-elbow and shoulder patients. Both are controlled by a separate elbow lock mechanism and are available in manual and electric versions (Fig. 10–32).

Harness Systems

The most frequently used harnessing system is the figure-of-eight (Fig. 10–33). The below-elbow harness functions to suspend the prosthesis and to allow the patient to utilize body motions to operate the terminal device. The harness works to hold the socket firmly against the residual limb. The power of body motions is transmitted to the terminal device via the cable system. Other harnessing systems that are frequently used are the figure-of-nine and the chest strap with shoulder saddle. The less-cumbersome figure-of-nine harness is most appropriate for longer below-elbow amputations, as it provides a greater degree of freedom. In above-elbow harnessing, the system is meant to provide power to flex the elbow and to lock and unlock it.

The chest strap and shoulder saddle harnessing arrangement may be used for individuals who do frequent heavy

FIGURE 10–29. One example of a conventional terminal device is the Dorrance 5X. (Courtesy of Dorrance Company, Campbell, California.)

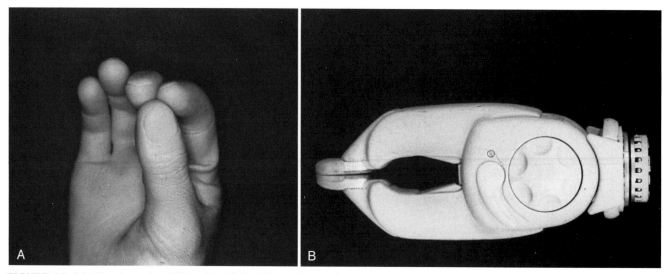

FIGURE 10–30. The electric hand (A) and the Griffer (B) are the most frequently used myoelectric terminal devices. (B, Courtesy of Otto Book, Minneapolis, Minnesota.)

lifting or for those who are unable to tolerate an axilla loop, perhaps due to nerve or skin irritation.

Control Systems

The below-elbow cable system is the Bowden system. The cable produces only one function in the below-elbow system—the operation of the terminal device. In this system, the cable slides through a single length of housing to achieve this function. In the above-elbow prosthesis, the cable system is required to perform two functions—

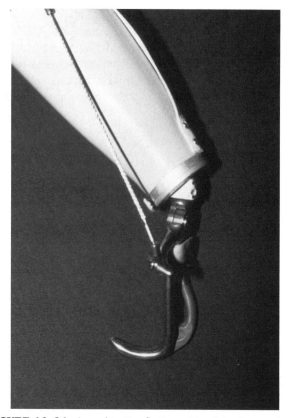

FIGURE 10–31. A combination flexion wrist unit is often used with bilateral amputees to improve their ability to perform tasks close to midline.

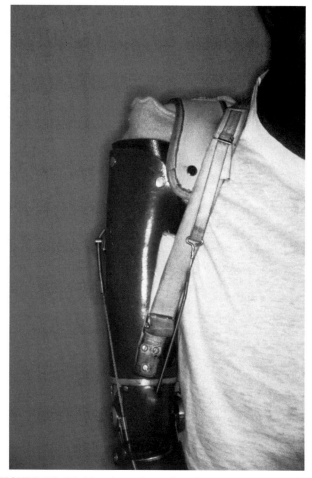

FIGURE 10–32. The above-elbow elbow lock mechanism runs from the harness to the elbow unit. It locks the elbow in the desired degrees of elbow flexion.

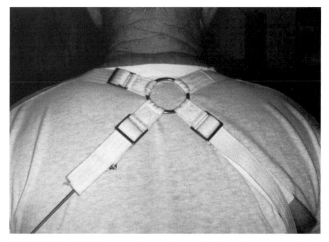

FIGURE 10–33. The most frequently used below-elbow harnessing is the figure-of-eight *(A)*, which includes an axilla loop on the uninvolved side, a suspensor strap, and control strap that attaches to the control cable on the involved side.

terminal device operation and elbow flexion. The above-elbow cable system is known as the fair lead or dual-cable system. It uses two lengths of cable housing to accomplish the two functions of elbow flexion and terminal device operation (Fig. 10–34).

MATERIALS

The materials used in orthotic and prosthetic fabrication span a broad spectrum from low-cost, readily available plaster-of-Paris bandage to expensive Kevlar®, Kingsley Manufacturing Company, Costa Mesa, California, and

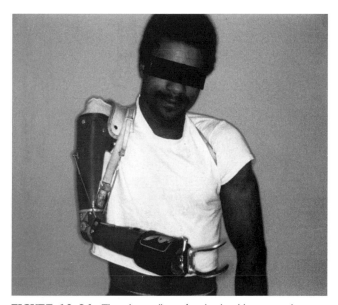

FIGURE 10–34. The above-elbow fair lead cable system has two lengths of cable housing. As the cable slides through the first, the elbow is brought into position. Once the elbow is locked, the cable is free to operate the terminal device. The terminal device cannot be operated without first locking the elbow.

carbon graphite. Today's clinician should have a basic understanding of the characteristics of available materials to make appropriate choices for a given prescription.

It is ever more important in an era of cost containment that clinicians choose those materials that will serve best for short- or long-term use of an orthosis. Orthoses fabricated to augment function for the spinal cord–injured patient are considered permanent and must be fabricated from long-lasting materials. Orthoses expected to be used intermittently or for a short time frame may be appropriately fabricated from lower-cost materials that have a known limited shelf life.

To facilitate the assessment process along the decision tree, at this point we present an explanation of materials and their properties and then offer suggestions for materials for each orthotic or prosthetic application.

Plaster-of-Paris

The ready availability, low cost, and ease of use of plaster-of-Paris continues to make it an appropriate material for many orthotic and prosthetic applications. Plaster-of-Paris is manufactured from calcium sulfate, more commonly known as gypsum. Plaster-of-Paris bandage is commercially available in loose dry plaster bandage and hard-coated bandages, and in elastic fabric impregnated with plaster (Prosthetic Orthotic Center).

Setting time can be manipulated by increasing or decreasing the water temperature. Water temperature should not be set above 150°F (65.5°C), as excessive temperature actually prevents rather than hastens setting time. When working with plaster bandage, the clinician should be aware that setting time and drying time are not equivalent. Setting is a relatively short process, while drying takes significantly longer and is not complete until the excess water has evaporated from the plaster. Drying may take anywhere from 8 hours to several days, depending on the size and thickness of the applied bandage.

Plaster-of-Paris is highly moldable, has excellent rigidity, can be used circumferentially or for single-surface applications, and is comparatively low in cost. This convenience and low cost continue to make plaster-of-Paris bandage a frequent choice for postsurgical positioning. Plaster is used as the initial model of the residual limb and as the basis for fabrication of the check socket in prosthetics. It is also the rigid component of the early-fit prosthesis.

Leather

Animal skins and hides are composed mainly of minute, intricately interlaced protein fibers. Tanned leather has tensile properties unmatched by any other material of equal weight. It can retain a molded shape permanently while maintaining flexibility and strength. Leather is highly puncture resistant yet maintains excellent porosity for ventilation. Leather can be cut, perforated, sewn, molded with water, laminated, and riveted.

Most of the leathers used in orthotic and prosthetic applications are vegetable tanned for a smooth texture and to prevent skin irritation. Calfskin and deer skin are used in upper extremity orthotic applications due to their light to medium weight. Weight is expressed in the number of ounces per square foot with light weight being 2 to 3 oz per square foot, and medium weight being 3.5 to 4 oz per square foot (Redford, 1986).

When wet, leather can be readily stretched and molded over a plaster or wood mold. Once dry, leather holds its molded shape permanently and continues to contour and mold to a body part over time. In upper extremity prosthetics, leather is frequently used in the fabrication of shoulder saddles and as portions of the harnessing system. For these applications, heavier horsehide and stretchable cowhide are used for their durability and strength.

Rubber and Silicone Elastomers

Natural and synthetic rubber is available in a variety of forms, all of which have the common characteristic of elasticity. Rubber and rubberlike compounds are highly resilient to pressure deformation and so have excellent shock-absorbing qualities. Silicone elastomers are now available for use in both orthotic and prosthetic fabrication (Haberman, 1995). Their use is suggested relative to the use of rubber due to their ease of application and ready availability.

Natural rubber is a highly elastic material with good tear and abrasion resistance. The disadvantage of the use of natural rubber in orthotic and prosthetic applications is its low resistance and tendency to degrade with exposure to sunlight, water, skin oils, and most solvents. Of the commonly used synthetic rubbers, Butyl rubber has greater resistance to heat, sunlight, and water but is not as resilient or elastic as natural rubber. Neoprene is one of the synthetic rubbers commonly used for orthotics today.

Neoprene combines excellent resistance to water, aging, and heat with good resistance to oil and solvents. Neoprene lacks the extreme resistance of rubber to deformation and requires the addition of plastic or metal stays to provide any significant degree of joint restriction (Redford, 1986).

Silicone elastomers are available in a variety of forms for the fabrication of flexible orthoses. Open-weave fabrics or bandages can be incorporated into the mold for greater strength and longevity. Silicone elastomers retain their flexibility and elastic qualities when molded and are often recommended when an orthosis is required during sporting events. Unlike rubber, silicone is stable in heat and in oxidizing environments and does not yellow with time. The elasticity and elongation of silicone are not equivalent to those of rubber, but silicone is a highly acceptable substitute.

Low-Temperature Thermoplastics

Low-temperature thermoplastics include synthetic rubber sheets, such as Orthoplast® (Johnson and Johnson, Piscataway, New Jersey), and polyester polycaprolactone sheets, such as NCM Clinic® (North Coast Medical, Inc., San Jose, California) and Polyform® (Smith & Nephew Rolyan, Germantown, Wisconsin). By definition, these thermoplastics require no more than 180°F (80°C) dry or wet heat to become moldable, and they may be shaped directly on the body part. Their principle use is in upper extremity orthotics, where rapid fabrication and frequent remolding for positioning are essential.

The array of available low-temperature thermoplastics is ever expanding. The clinician is referred to the thermoplastic charts available from distributors for specific characteristics of each material. Basic characteristics of low-temperature thermoplastics are given in Appendix B at the end of the chapter to assist the clinician in choosing the thermoplastic most appropriate for a given application.

Low-temperature plastics are susceptible to oxidation and crystallization that cause breakdown of the polymer structure over time. The level of resistance to crystallization varies among low-temperature plastics, and therefore the shelf life of plastics varies. Those thermoplastics that contain isoprene are known to be more susceptible to oxidation and experience yellowing and structural degradation more quickly.

Polyethylene Foams and Cellular Rubbers

The two basic classes of foams and cellular rubbers are open-cell and closed-cell structures. In open-cell foams and rubbers, fluids can flow through the holes. The holes in a closed-cell structure are separately sealed, preventing fluid transfer. Foam density is dependent on the size of individual cells, the ratio of cell space to volume, and the continuity or discontinuity of the cells (Redford, 1986).

Open-cell foams are softer and spongelike and allow for varying degrees of ventilation. Their use in orthotics is primarily as lining materials to assist in the distribution of shear stress and to act as a moisture wick. Closed-cell foams are firmer and nonabsorbent and can often be heat-molded to create a semiflexible orthosis. Plastizote (Kewell Converters Limited, Surrey, England) is a commonly used closed-cell polyethylene foam that is moldable when heated at 230°F to 285°F (110°C to 140°C). Plastizote can be used as a liner or incorporated with thermoplastic or leather to form a semiflexible orthosis.

Polyethylene foams have the disadvantage of rapid loss of their density and absorption capacity under pressure. This limits their usefulness to non–weight-bearing orthoses. Their lack of fluid absorption may also be seen as a disadvantage, as perspiration and heat tend to build up in the orthosis. Perspiration build-up may be alleviated by frequent changes of cotton lining, and heat may be somewhat dissipated by perforating the foam.

Woven and Knit Materials

Cotton duck, polyester and cotton woven with elastic threads, and a variety of vinyl-impregnated materials are in common use for upper extremity orthotics. Woven or knit materials are readily available, cost effective, and easily modified for custom fitting. The use of such materials for orthotic application is generally limited to short-term use due to the limited durability of these materials.

High-Temperature Thermoplastic

The designation of *high temperature* when applied to thermoplastics denotes materials that become moldable at 350°F to 450°F (176°C–232°C) and can only be molded over a model. High-temperature thermoplastics are highly resistant to stress and heat and are ideal for long-term use and for weight-bearing applications. Corrective forces can be incorporated into the model prior to vacuum forming the materials over the model for an exact fit.

Of the high-temperature plastics used in orthotics, polyethylene has the most application in upper extremity orthotics. Polyethylene is available in low-, medium-, or high-density formulas, each having a specific gravity and tensile strength. Low-density polyethylene is most commonly used in upper extremity orthotics and prosthetics due to its toughness and flexibility. Low-density polyethylene can be heated in a convection oven and then vacuum formed or hand formed on a plaster model. With care, polyethylene may be molded over a foam base directly on the patient. Polyethylene is used also in upper extremity prosthetics to make molded shoulder saddles and triceps cuffs.

The high-temperature thermoplastics are susceptible to both oxidation and crystallization that, over time, lead to structural failure. These plastics, however, have a significantly greater life span than the low-temperature plastics and are likely to last for up to 10 years.

Laminating Resins

A variety of polyester, acrylic, and epoxy resins are available for creating thin shell laminates for use in upper extremity orthotics and particularly for prosthetics. These shells are formed over plaster models, and some materials can then be heated, sanded, and reshaped as needed. Color can be added to certain resins to simulate skin tones.

The addition of nylon or carbon graphite into the resins gives the materials a greater strength-to-weight ratio. Kevlar® adds significant strength and decreases the weight of components significantly, but it does so at an increase in cost. The choice of laminates is dependent in good part on the stress tolerances needed, on funding availability, and on the experience of the prosthetist or orthotist.

Metals

The metals most commonly used in orthotics are stainless steel and aluminum. Metal alloys such as those with titanium or magnesium offer some distinct advantages in terms of decreased weight and density and increased tensile strength. Their disadvantage is high cost, which limits their use to small component parts.

The metals are chosen for their properties of strength; weight; resistance to deformation, fatigue, and corrosion; ease of fabrication; and cost. Aluminum is commonly used in upper extremity orthotics due to its high strength-to-weight ratio and its corrosion resistance. Aluminum is approximately one third the weight of steel, and its strength can be enhanced by heat treatment, the addition of small amounts of alloy metals, or by cold working to increase the tensile strength. Pure aluminum is a relatively soft metal that can be hammered and thinned to accommodate complex shapes without loss of strength or increase in brittleness (Redford, 1986).

Although resistant to corrosion, aluminum can be damaged by alkalis and acids. To counteract this, aluminum can be coated by anodizing or by exposing it to electrolytic action. This has the added advantage of giving aluminum parts a more attractive finish and allows the metal to be colored for a cosmetically pleasing appearance.

Materials Application

Although many materials may be useful for one application, and one material may be useful for many applications, there are choices to be made to choose the most appropriate material for a given application. Appendix C at the end of the chapter gives suggestions for material usage for the described orthotic and prosthetic applications. Durability, cost, availability, and fabrication experience all factor into the decision.

Prosthetic Checkout

Prosthetic checkout is performed to ensure that the completed device is fitting and operating well and that it adheres to clinic prescription. A few of the items evaluated at checkout include length, efficiency in various planes of motion, control system efficiency, ROM with and without the prosthesis, and suspension.

The length of the completed prosthesis should be close to that of the uninvolved arm. This becomes a problem in fitting a myoelectric prosthesis in the wrist disarticulation patient where limited space is available for componentry. The patient should be able to move through space to complete a task without the terminal device opening and closing involuntarily. The patient should be able to achieve maximum opening or closing of the terminal device with the forearm in 90 degrees of flexion at waist and at mouth levels.

For the conventional prosthesis, efficiency is evaluated with the elbow in 90 degrees of flexion. A small spring scale that registers up to 50 lb in 1-lb increments is required with adaptors to attach the scale to a hand, hook, or hanger. The control cable is disconnected from the terminal device, and the scale with appropriate adaptor is attached. A 0.5-inch–thick wood block is placed in the terminal device. The amount of force required to open the terminal device is recorded. The cable is reattached. Next, the scale with adaptor is attached at the hanger, the proximal end of the cable assembly through which the cable assembly attaches to the harness. Again, the evaluator pulls on the scale, and the amount of force required to open the terminal device is recorded. Efficiency is determined by multiplying force at the terminal device by 100 and dividing it by the force at the hanger. The prosthesis should be at least 80 percent efficient.

The patient should be able to achieve at least 50 percent of full available pronation and supination with the prosthesis in place. In a standard below-elbow socket, active elbow flexion with the prosthesis in place should be within 10 degrees of full available ROM. The prosthesis should not slip distally by more than 1 inch when a heavy axial load, 50 lb, is applied at the terminal device.

Orthotic Checkout

All custom-fit and custom-fabricated orthoses should be checked for fit and function. The wearer should be instructed in recommended wearing schedules and in the performance of regular skin checks. Orthoses fabricated from both high- and low-temperature thermoplastics should be checked regularly for signs of wear, particularly for any signs of potential fracture sites.

If an orthosis is fit to restore or augment motion, ongoing documentation should be performed to ensure that this purpose is in fact being met. Once the wearer has ceased to make gains, it must be determined whether an adjustment or realignment is necessary or if no further progress is possible. At that point, the orthosis should be discontinued, a retaining orthosis fabricated to consolidate the gains made, or an alternative intervention considered.

Any wearer of a long-term orthosis should arrange for follow-up with a therapist or orthotist for regular maintenance and reassessment of the continuing necessity of the orthosis. Patients will and do accommodate to the use of an orthosis that has long since ceased to bring them any benefit beyond that of a placebo. It is the health professional's responsibility to educate patients in the proper usage, including expected outcomes from use, of every orthosis he or she fits.

APPENDIX A

Pain Scales

ANALOG PAIN SCALE

Pain levels are marked on a linear pain scale and compared over time.

_____

No pain   Unbearable pain

Patients are given a clean, unmarked form to indicated their subjective pain level each time it is assessed in the clinic.

FUNCTIONAL PAIN SCALE

The focus is on how pain affects performance of functional tasks rather than on the severity or location of pain.

Indicate the statement that most accurately reflects how the pain you are experiencing affects you on a daily basis.

_____ I cannot accomplish any of my daily activities, even with medication.

_____ I require rest breaks at least every hour and regular medication to accomplish my daily activities.

_____ I can perform activities for 2 to 3 hours before pain interferes and I must rest or take medication.

_____ I can usually accomplish all my activities but I am aware of the pain several times a day and take medication at least once a day.

_____ I am aware of the pain occasionally but it does not stop my performance of daily activities. I do not require daily medication.

A clean, unmarked form is used with each assessment of pain levels.

Low-Temperature Thermoplastic Characteristics

The low-temperature thermoplastics currently available are frequently described by their handling characteristics—their handling when warm—and their finished characteristics—their qualities when cold. Given here is a brief explanation of the terms used to describe these characteristics, followed by a description of categories of available materials.

CHARACTERISTICS OF WARM OR MOLDABLE MATERIAL

Resistance to Stretch. This refers to the tendency of a material to stretch and thin with only the force of gravity pulling on it. Materials with low resistance to stretch tend to conform easily with only minimal effort on the clinician's part. Those materials that resist stretch even with manual force require and tolerate more aggressive handling to achieve conformability.

Conformability or Drape. Conformability has a direct correlation with resistance to stretch. If a material has low resistance to stretch, it will have a high degree of conformability. When laid on the body part, the material will conform intimately around the angles and configurations of that part. Materials with high resistance to stretch have a low degree of conformability and require handling on the clinician's part to achieve good conformability and fit, especially around small parts and bony prominences.

Memory. Memory is the ability or tendency for molded material to return to its original cut shape and thickness when reheated. Materials are available with varying de-grees of memory, from 100 percent to very slight memory or ability to regain size and thickness if stretched.

Self-Sealing Edges. This refers to the tendency of the cut edges of material to round and seal together when cut while warm. Scissors crimp warm material as they cut. Generally, materials that have little or no memory seal together and stay sealed even when reheated. Materials with high degrees of memory do not seal as firmly when cut and unseal if reheated.

CHARACTERISTICS OF COLD OR MOLDED MATERIAL

Rigidity Versus Flexibility. These terms describe the degree to which a molded material will resist deformation when force is applied. Materials with a high degree of resistance to deformation are considered to be rigid. Materials that give or deform with force are flexible. Low-temperature thermoplastics range from very flexible, highly perforated $\frac{1}{16}$ inch (1.6 mm) thick materials, to very rigid $\frac{1}{8}$ inch (3.2 mm) or $\frac{1}{16}$ inch (4.2 mm) materials.

Self-Adherence or Bonding. This describes the strength of the bond between two pieces of material pressed together when warm and cooled. The majority of materials available today are coated to resist accidental bonding and require a solvent to remove the coating to allow bonding. The strength of the bond varies between materials and is in part dependent on how hot the materials are when pressed together and whether a wet or dry heat band was used.

CATEGORIES OF LOW-TEMPERATURE THERMOPLASTIC

The low-temperature thermoplastics currently available fall generally into one of four categories of material depending on their chemical formulas.

The materials said to be *plasticlike* generally have excellent conformity and drape. When warm they stretch with only the force of gravity, which allows them to conform intimately over body parts with minimal effort on the clinician's part. When cold, plasticlike materials are very rigid and withstand the forces applied by outriggers and resilient components.

The *rubberlike* materials tend to resist stretch and have a low degree of conformability and drape. The resistance to stretch of the rubberlike materials allows them to be handled more aggressively to achieve good conformity without thinning or overstretching. When cold, the rubberlike materials generally are flexible and give when pressure is applied.

Combination *plastic and rubberlike* materials are available that have midrange characteristics. They do not stretch as readily as do the plasticlike materials, but they offer greater ease of conformability than do the rubberlike materials. Their resistance to deformation when cold is less than that of the plasticlike and greater than that of the rubberlike materials.

The fourth category of materials is the *elastics,* which have unique handling characteristics because of their memory. These materials can be handled and stretched aggressively to form circumferential orthoses, and they can be readily re-formed by reheating. When cold, these materials may be quite rigid if full thickness ($\frac{1}{8}$ in [3.2 mm]) or flexible if thin ($\frac{1}{16}$ in [1.6 mm]) and highly perforated.

APPENDIX C

Material Application

Orthotics

	Plaster	Leather	Silicone/Rubber	Low-Temperature Plastic	Foam	Fabric	High-Temperature Plastic	Laminates	Metal
REST AND PROTECTION	Short-term, posttrauma, postsurgical	Long-term use only	Cushioning Good for small protective orthoses	Short-term use, good adjustability	Liners for prefabricated or molded orthosis	For short-term or intermittent use	Long-term use only		
RESTORE MOTION, CORRECT DEFORMITY	Serial static designs		Liners to assist with scar management	Excellent due to easy remolding Attachments easy to add	Relieve or distribute pressure				Outriggers
RESTORE OR AUGMENT MOTION		Excellent for heavy use for cuffs	Protection over atrophied parts	Use for less than 1 y, use when functional return expected	Line cuffs for pressure distribution and comfort		Polyethylene, long-term use	For hand and forearm shells	Aluminum, composits for outriggers
PREVENTION	Postoperative use	Good durability for long-term use		Short-term use, trial positioning	For safety and comfort, prevent self-injury	Functional activities Semiflexible orthoses	Long-term positioning, polyethylene, polypropylene		For dynamic components

Prosthetics

	Plaster	Leather	Silicone/Rubber	Low-Temperature Plastic	Foam	Fabric	High-Temperature Plastic	Laminates	Metal
IPOF	IPOF sockets	For harness	Protect incision, scar management	May use for molding socket	Cushion and help achieve contact	Dacron or nylon for harness			Cable systems
HARNESS		Elk, horsehide, russet			Sleeve liners				
SOCKET	Check sockets		Liner sleeve for suspension				Shoulder saddles, triceps cuffs	Acrylic, epoxy polyester resins	

GLOSSARY

Creep—The phenomenon of tissue degradation over time with constant application of pressure.

Dynamic splint—A molded or contoured body support employing resilient components to produce motion.

Force—Any action of one object on another that results in a measurable effect on either or both objects.

Hysteresis—The lag or difference between the reaction of a resilient material being stretched or compressed as compared with the same material's response as it relaxes. The variance in response can be displayed graphically as a hysteresis loop.

Moberg pick-up test—Timed test of functional sensibility involving picking up and placing nine objects with and without visual assist.

Moment, or torque—A measurement of the effect of force given by multiplying force times the distance from the axis of a lever where that lever is capable of rotating at its axis.

Serial static splint—A molded or contoured body support that employs an adjustable static component to produce motion.

Static progressive splint—An adjustable molded support fabricated for the purpose of increasing joint ROM through frequent remolding and repositioning.

Thermoplastics—A group of polymer-based materials that become moldable with heat and that retain a molded shape when cooled.

REFERENCES

American Academy of Orthopaedic Surgeons. (1975). *Atlas of orthotics*. St. Louis, MO: C. V. Mosby Company.

American Society of Hand Therapists. (1992). *Splint classification system*. Chicago: American Society of Hand Therapists.

Ashbell, T., Kutz, J., & Kleinert, H. (1967). The digital Allen test. *Plastic and Reconstructive Surgery, 39*, 311.

Bell-Krotoski, J. A., Breger, D. E., & Beach, R. B. (1990). Application of biomechanics for evaluation of the hand. In *Rehabilitation of the hand: Surgery and therapy* (3rd ed.). St. Louis, MO: C. V. Mosby Company.

Bell-Krotoski, J. A. (1990). Light touch-deep pressure testing using Semmes-Weinstein monofilament. In *Rehabilitation of the hand: Surgery and therapy* (3rd ed.). St. Louis, MO: C. V. Mosby Company.

Brand, P. W. (1993). *Clinical mechanics of the hand* (2nd ed.). St. Louis, MO: C. V. Mosby Company.

Callahan, A. D. (1984). Sensibility testing: Clinical methods. In *Rehabilitation of the hand* (2nd ed.). St. Louis, MO: C. V. Mosby Company.

Dellon, A. L. (1981). *Evaluation of sensibility and reeducation of sensation in the hand*. Baltimore: Williams & Wilkins.

Fess, E. E., & Philips, C. A. (1987). Appendixes. In *Hand splinting principles and methods*. St. Louis, MO: C. V. Mosby Company.

Fess, E. E., & Philips, C. A. (1987). *Hand splinting principles and methods*. St. Louis, MO: C. V. Mosby Company.

Flowers, K. R., & Pheasant, S. D. (1988). The use of torque angle curves in the assessment of digital joint stiffness. *Journal of Hand Therapy, 1*(2), 69.

Gelberman, R. H., et al. (1983). Sensibility testing in peripheral nerve compression syndromes: An experimental study in humans. *Journal of Bone and Joint Surgery, 65A*, 632.

Guilford, A., & Perry, J. (1975). Orthotic components and systems. In *Atlas of orthotics: Biomechanical principles and application*. St. Louis, MO: C. V. Mosby Company.

Haberman, L. J. (1995). Silicone-only suspension with socket-lock and the ring for the lower limb. *Journal of Prosthetics and Orthotics, 7*(1).

Jacobs, R. R., Brady, W. M. (1975). Early post-surgical fitting in upper extremity amputations. *Journal of Trauma, 15*(22), 966–968.

Kendall, H. O., Kendall, F. P., & Wadsworth, G. E. (1971). *Muscles testing and function*. Baltimore: Williams & Wilkins.

Merskey, H. (1973). The perception and measurement of pain. *Journal of Psychosomatic Research, 17*, 251–255.

Mildenberger, L. A., Amadio, P. C., An, K. N. (1986). Dynamic splinting: A systematic approach to the selection of elastic traction. *Archives of Physical Medicine and Rehabilitation, 67*, 241–244.

Moberg, E. (1958). Objective methods for determining the functional value of sensibility in the hand. *Journal of Bone and Joint Surgery, 40B*, 454.

Nalebuff, E. A., Philips, C. A. (1984). The rheumatoid thumb. In *Rehabilitation of the hand* (2nd ed.). St. Louis, MO: C. V. Mosby Company.

Prosthetic Orthotic Center. (Undated). Upper limb orthotics for orthotists. *Manual for orthotics 721*. Chicago: Northwestern University Medical School.

Redford, J. B. (1986). Materials for orthotics. In *Orthotics etc*. (3rd ed.). Baltimore: Williams & Wilkins.

Roberson, L., Breger, D., Buford, W., & Freeman, M. J. (1988). Analysis of physical properties of SCOMAC springs and their potential use in dynamic splinting. *Journal of Hand Therapy, April-June 1*(2).

Rose, G. K. (1986). *Orthotics: Principles and practice*. London: William Heinemann Medical Books.

vonPrince, K., & Butler, B. (1967). Measuring sensory function of the hand in peripheral nerve injury. *American Journal of Occupational Therapy, 21*, 385.

Weaver, S. A., Lange, L. R., & Vogts, V. M. (1986). *Comparison of myoelectric and conventional prosthesis in adolescent amputees*. Philadelphia: Hospitals for Crippled Children.

Wright, V., & Johns, R. J. (1961). Quantitative and qualitative analysis of joint stiffness in normal subjects and in patients with connective tissue disease. *Annals of the Rheumatic Diseases, 20*, 36.

Yamada, H. (1970). In F. G. Evans (Ed.), *Strength of biological materials*. Baltimore: Williams & Wilkins.

BIBLIOGRAPHY

Burkhalter, W. E., Mayfield, G., & Carmona, L. S. (1976). The upper extremity amputee: Early and immediate post-surgical prosthetic fitting. *Journal of Bone and Joint Surgery, 58A* (1).

Childress, D. S. (1981). External power in upper limb prosthetics. In American Academy of Orthopaedic Surgeons, *Atlas of limb prosthetics, surgical and prosthetic principles*. St. Louis, MO: C. V. Mosby Company.

Day, H. J. (1981). The assessment and description of amputee activity. *Prosthetics and Orthotics International, 5*(1), 23–28.

Fryer, C. M. (1981). Upper limb prosthetic components. In American Academy of Orthopaedic Surgeons, *Atlas of limb prosthetics, surgical and prosthetic principles*. St. Louis, MO: C. V. Mosby Company.

Jacobsen, S. C., & Knutt, D. (1973). *A preliminary report on the Utah arm*. Salt Lake City, UT: University of Utah.

Lamb, D. W. (1993). State of the art in upper-limb prosthetics. *Journal of Hand Therapy 6*(1), 1–8.

Maiorano, L. M., & Byron, P. M. (1990). Fabrication of an early-fit prosthesis. In J. M. Hunter, L. H. Schneider, E. J. Mackin, & A. D. Callahan (Eds.), *Rehabilitation of the hand*. Philadelphia: C. V. Mosby Company.

New York University, Post Graduate Medical School. (1982). *Prosthetics and orthotics, upper limb prosthetics*. New York: New York University.

Olivett, B. L. (1990). Adult amputee management and conventional prosthetic training. In J. M. Hunter, L. H. Schneider, E. J. Mackin, & A. D. Callahan (Eds.), *Rehabilitation of the hand*. Philadelphia: C. V. Mosby Company.

Sanderson, E. R., & Scott, R. N. (1985). *UNB Test of Prosthetic Function: A test for unilateral upper extremity amputees*. New Brunswick, NJ: Bio-engineering Institute, University of New Brunswick.

UNIT THREE

Assessment of Central Nervous System Function of the Adult

of persons with stroke. This descriptive, longitudinal study of individuals with occlusive cerebrovascular accidents observed motor recovery of both upper and lower limbs but focused on function in the arm and hand. Twitchell noted that the patients studied progressed uniformly through a series of recovery stages. All patients began with total, flaccid paralysis of limb muscles. This was followed by the demonstration of positive stretch reflexes in selected muscles, and the influence of tonic neck reflexes on active movement and muscle tone in the arm and leg.

Patients whose recovery was not arrested at one of these early stages progressed to demonstrate active performance of gross, stereotypic movement patterns. Twitchell termed these gross patterns the flexor and extensor limb synergies. Patients who continued to progress eventually performed voluntary hand movements, as well as active arm and leg movements that deviated from the limb synergies. Of the 121 patients in Twitchell's study, 25 were observed until a comparatively stable condition had been reached. After 3 months, five patients demonstrated full recovery. The remaining participants varied in the levels of recovery they achieved.

The Brunnstrom Approach

Signe Brunnstrom (1970) applied Twitchell's findings and her own clinical experience to develop a program that would guide persons with hemiplegia through the following six stages toward motor recovery:

Stage 1: flaccidity
Stage 2: associated reactions/developing spasticity

TABLE 11–1

SYNERGIES OF THE UPPER AND LOWER LIMBS

Flexor Synergy: Upper Limb	Extensor Synergy: Upper Limb
Elbow flexion	Elbow extension
Forearm supination	Forearm pronation
Shoulder abduction (to 90 degrees)	Shoulder adduction (front of body)
Shoulder external rotation	Shoulder internal rotation
Shoulder girdle retraction	Shoulder girdle protraction
Shoulder girdle elevation	

Flexor Synergy: Lower Limb	Extensor Synergy: Lower Limb
Toe dorsiflexion	Toe plantarflexion
Ankle dorsiflexion and inversion	Ankle plantarflexion and inversion
Knee flexion	Knee extension
Hip flexion, abduction, and external rotation	Hip extension, adduction, and internal rotation

Data from Brunnstrom, S. (1970). Movement therapy in hemiplegia: A neurophysiological approach. New York: Harper & Row.

TABLE 11–2

HAND FUNCTION—SEQUENCE OF RECOVERY

Mass grasp
Hook grasp
Lateral prehension
Palmar prehension
Cylindric grasp
Spheric grasp
Release of grasp
Individual finger movements
Manipulative tasks
  Affected hand as an assist
  Affected hand as dominant

Data from Brunnstrom, S. (1970). Movement therapy in hemiplegia: A neurophysiological approach. New York: Harper & Row.

Stage 3: severe spasticity/active movement in synergy patterns
Stage 4: some movements deviating from synergy patterns
Stage 5: active movements isolated from synergy patterns
Stage 6: isolated active movement with near normal speed and coordination

Brunnstrom clearly categorized the flexor and extensor synergies of the hemiparetic arm and leg (Table 11–1). Other contributions included a postulated sequence of recovery in hand function (Table 11–2) and a clearly defined sequence of movement patterns hemiparetic individuals are expected to achieve as they recover the ability to perform movements that deviate from the gross limb synergies.

In addition, Brunnstrom (1970) superficially introduced the concept that balance and postural abnormalities are common motor residuals of stroke. Brunnstrom proposed that therapists evaluate balance impairments by (1) assessing patients' tendencies to list toward the affected side when sitting unsupported, and (2) observing patients' responses to forceful manual disturbance of their unsupported sitting posture.

Neurodevelopmental Treatment

While Brunnstrom's program sought to facilitate motor recovery by encouraging the development of primitive reflexes and active movement in synergy patterns, Berta Bobath's (1970, 1978) approach followed an opposite course. Neurodevelopmental treatment (NDT) for adults with hemiplegia was designed to minimize the development of spasticity and to prevent the learning of stereotypic patterns of movement.

Neurodevelopmental treatment viewed the motor impairments of stroke survivors from a broader perspective than Brunnstrom and Twitchell. In addition to limb paralysis, descriptions of hemiplegia were expanded to include specific disorders in posture, balance, and motor control of the head, trunk, shoulder, and pelvic girdles. Bobath (1970, 1978) introduced therapists to the roles of righting and equilibrium reactions for maintaining balance in upright positions. Furthermore, training in performance of gross transitional movements from one posture to another was included in the restorative treatment protocol. Previously, individuals with hemiplegia were taught only compensatory strategies for achieving mobility in rolling, achieving sitting, and rising to stand. The NDT approach considered improvements in the procedures used to perform such tasks to be indicative of motor recovery. Finally, NDT emphasized the interrelationships between positioning of specific body segments and motor control at other regions. For example, control of shoulder and elbow movements is facilitated by assumption of the supine position, as well as by enhanced mobility at the pelvis.

Bobath's (1970, 1978, 1990) treatment program for adults with hemiplegia differed significantly from Brunnstrom's approach in its use of closed kinematic chain movements, or weight bearing, in the therapeutic sequence toward motor recovery. Like the Rood (1954, 1956) and proprioceptive neuromuscular facilitation (PNF) (Knott and Voss, 1956) interventions, NDT recognized that activities in which the limbs served as distal supports for proximal movement (or weight shift) played an important developmental role in the acquisition of motor control. Bobath's treatment attempted to bypass movement in synergy patterns by teaching patients to exercise muscles in closed, rather than open, kinematic chains.

Neurodevelopmental treatment recognizes the need for mobility, or disassociation, between adjacent body segments, such as the scapula on the thorax or the thorax on the lumbar spine. Disassociation between spinal segments is demonstrated as trunk rotation.

Contemporary Theories of Motor Behavior

In the past several decades, interdisciplinary study in the neural sciences has generated new theories of motor control and motor learning (Mathiowetz & Bass-Haugen, 1994; Schmidt, 1992). A hierarchical view of the central nervous system has been replaced with distributed control, or dynamic systems, theories.

According to the hierarchical model (Jackson & Taylor, 1932), movements are centrally controlled in a top-down fashion. Muscular activity is influenced by alpha and gamma motoneurons, which are in turn controlled by spinal and brain stem mechanisms. These primitive levels of the motor system are held in check by control centers in the basal ganglia and cerebellum. Motor centers in the cerebral cortex exert executive influences on the entire system through their modulation of cerebellar and basal ganglia activity. The Brunnstrom, Rood, PNF, and early NDT approaches are based on a hierarchical model of motor control, which predicts that dysfunction in the motor cortex results in a release from inhibition of the brain stem and spinal networks. Subsequently, the major neuromotor sequelae of stroke are the positive symptoms of spasticity and reflex domination of muscle tone. Treatment focuses on decreasing abnormal reflex and primitive movement patterns to facilitate normal movement (Gordon, 1987; Poole, 1991).

According to dynamical systems theory, responsibilities for motor control are distributed among a number of structures in the central nervous system. Spinal-level structures are not completely dependent on higher centers for direct movement commands. Instead, the role of hemispheric structures is to tune and prepare the motor system to respond most efficiently to changing environmental and task demands (Carr & Shepherd, 1991).

Ecologic theories of movement are compatible with distributed control models and emphasize the interaction between the performer and the environment (Saltzman & Kelso, 1987). Motor behaviors emerge as a result of context or regulatory conditions in the environment (Bernstein, 1967; Gentile, 1972, 1987). A successful motor strategy for reaching forward with one arm varies, depending on several factors: the person's posture (sitting, standing, kneeling) and postural alignment; the shape and stability of the seat or supporting surface; how far away and in what direction the goal object is located; and the presence of any obstacles between the individual and the goal object. Skilled motor performance in any task is the ability to perform in a number of different ways, according to variations in environmental demands (Summers, 1989).

Contemporary understanding of postural control differs significantly from the viewpoints applied in the Brunnstrom, Rood, NDT, and PNF approaches. Assessments of balance using previous models assume that: (1) postural mechanisms occur in response to a stimulus (e.g., manual displacement by the examiner); and (2) stability, or the ability to maintain a static position without falling, is a necessary prerequisite to balance (Carr & Shepherd, 1990).

Balance is now understood to be controlled via feedforward, rather than feedback mechanisms. Postural adjustments (rather than responses) are anticipatory and ongoing. Prior to the onset of motor activities, widespread changes occur in the muscular organization of persons with intact central nervous systems (Brunia et al., 1985). These feed-forward adjustments occur simultaneously with the plan to move and prepare the person for performing the subsequent task. Well-organized postural adjustments prevent major displacements in an individual's center of gravity through a feed-forward mode of control. Postural adjustments are both task and context specific. Muscle activation patterns for balance control vary according to (1) the position of the person; (2) the task being performed; (3) the context in which the activity occurs; and (4) the person's perception of which body part is in contact with the more stable base of support (Nashner & McCollum, 1985).

Application of Contemporary Theories to Therapeutic Intervention for Persons with Hemiplegia

Refinements in theories of motor behavior have influenced the ways in which therapists observe and explain movement disorders demonstrated after stroke. The NDT and Brunnstrom approaches have evolved in response to these trends, and current practice reflects several of the changing views (Bobath, 1990; Davies, 1985, 1990; Sawner & LaVigne, 1992).

Individuals with hemiplegia continue to exhibit stereotypic patterns of active movement in the synergies described by Twitchell and Brunnstrom. Although some theorists view these abnormal movement constellations as direct results of the cerebrovascular accident, others (Carr, 1992; Carr & Shepherd, 1987a, 1987b) believe they are compensatory strategies that persons with hemiplegia develop as they attempt to move. Mechanical factors, such as muscle shortening, weakness, and fixation of body parts in response to postural insecurity are possible contributing factors to movement in abnormal patterns.

Ecologic theories of movement have led to an enhanced consideration of environmental and task-specific influences on the motor performance of individuals with hemiplegia (Jarus, 1994; Mathiowetz & Bass-Haugen, 1994; Sabari, 1991). Evaluation and treatment are increasingly administered in naturalistic environments, as patients perform movements in the context of functional tasks.

Finally, changing views about postural control have influenced assessment and treatment of balance dysfunction in individuals after stroke (Shepherd, 1992). Earlier tools evaluated patients' responses to rapid manual displacements that were intended to suddenly disturb their centers of gravity. Contemporary assessments of balance examine the person's adjustments to self-initiated displacements performed within the context of a functional task.

Carr and Shepherd's (1987a, 1987b) Motor Relearning Programme for Stroke applies current theories of motor control and motor learning to the evaluation and treatment of individuals with movement dysfunction due to stroke. This approach assesses motor performance in the context of functional tasks and teaches patients motor strategies rather than specific movements. The motor relearning approach views movement in synergy patterns as a maladaptive compensatory strategy that limits further motor recovery. Therefore, a major goal of intervention is to ensure that compensatory behavior is not learned as a substitute for optimal performance (Carr, 1992; Carr & Shepherd, 1989). Rather than performing exercises in isolation of functional goals, patients practice tasks that require mild variations in movement patterns during successive repetitions. Furthermore, limb movements and postural adjustments are always learned simultaneously, in the context of task performance.

Evaluation is a detailed analysis of the patient's performance of tasks within seven categories of daily activities:
Upper limb function
Orofacial function
Sitting up over the side of the bed
Balanced sitting
Standing up and sitting down
Balanced standing
Walking
Carr and Shepherd (1987b) provide a description of normal function and a list of essential components for performing each task based on published normative descriptive studies, as well as clinical experience. The therapist observes the patient as he or she performs each activity and then compares the patient's performance with the normal kinesiology associated with the task. A major focus of the analysis is to hypothesize the underlying reasons for the individual's development of the compensatory strategies he or she has chosen.

The patient is included as an active participant in the analysis of his or her performance. This allows the therapist to see how well an individual is able to detect his or her own movement problems. In addition, this encourages patients to develop insight and problem-solving skills about their own movement and helps them to understand the treatment goals.

AREAS OF MOTOR DYSFUNCTION IN INDIVIDUALS WITH HEMIPLEGIA DUE TO STROKE

Cerebrovascular accidents cause a broad variety and continuum of motor impairments. Each stroke survivor exhibits a unique constellation of problems and abilities. Depending on individual characteristics, therapists assess the following areas:
Muscle tone
Influence of primitive reflexes
Postural alignment in sitting and standing
Limitations and pain on passive range of motion
Postural control
Gross mobility
Somatosensory function
Active movement of the arm and leg
Functional hand skills
Ambulation

Muscle tone is generally assessed as the resistance felt when selected muscles are manually lengthened by the therapist (Wilcock, 1986). Hypertonus is felt as an increased resistance to passive movement and is often evaluated through quick stretch to the muscle to elicit a hyperactive stretch reflex. Hypotonus is demonstrated by too little or no resistance to the muscle lengthening, and the limb feels limp and floppy. Hypotonicity may also be assessed through placing, in which the therapist passively positions the head, trunk, or limb and observes whether the patient is able to momentarily hold the position against gravity.

Influence of primitive reflexes on muscle tone is evaluated by administering stimuli associated with the tonic neck, tonic labyrinthine, positive supporting, and grasp reflexes. The therapist assesses the amount of hypertonicity demonstrated when the reflex stimuli are present and compares this with the patient's muscle tone under neutral conditions (Davies, 1985; Sawner & LaVigne, 1992).

Longstanding debate continues about the nature and role of spasticity as an underlying factor in the motor dysfunction exhibited by individuals with hemiplegia (Sahrmann & Norton, 1977; Trombly, 1992). Therefore, some therapists question the value of these assessment procedures.

Visual observation of postural alignment of a person's head, scapula, trunk, pelvis, and limbs provides the therapist with qualitative information about muscle shortening, balance, and motor control that may be helpful in planning treatment. Therapists are particularly attentive to asymmetries in postural alignment between the patient's hemiplegic and nonhemiplegic sides.

Limitations and pain on passive range of motion are secondary impairments that significantly influence a person's functional potential. Goniometric measurements are generally not indicated because range of motion may fluctuate in patients with hemiplegia. However, it is useful for therapists to note limitations and determine whether these impairments are due to muscle shortening or to specific joint abnormalities.

Postural control over gravitational forces is assessed in a variety of procedures in which the therapist observes a person's righting and equilibrium adjustments when his or her body's center of gravity is displaced (Davies, 1985). This displacement may be achieved through passive movement of the patient on a stationary supporting surface, tilting of a mobile supporting surface, or active reaching in a variety of directions. Neck- and body-righting adjustments serve to align body parts with one another when one segment rotates around the body axis. Head-righting adjustments serve to orient the head and body in space in relation to the visual horizon. For example, normal head-righting maintains the eyes at a perpendicular position to the environment, even when the body is shifted laterally. Equilibrium adjustments include a variety of trunk and limb movements that serve to shift the body mass away from the direction of displacement, so that the body's center of gravity remains over its base of support. Protective extension is a primitive type of equilibrium adjustment, in which the upper extremity extends in the direction toward which the center of gravity has been displaced. This mechanism is used as a last resort when more subtle equilibrium responses are insufficient to counteract the effects of the displacing force (Sabari, 1994).

Gross mobility is assessed by observing a person's motor performance as he or she attempts to roll, sit up from supine, rise to standing, and sit from standing. The therapist compares the patient's performance with kinematic descriptions of normal task performance that have been determined through empirical research (Carr & Shepherd, 1987a, 1987b) or informal movement analysis (Bobath, 1990; Davies, 1985).

Somatosensory evaluation is often considered part of a comprehensive motor evaluation because tactile and proprioceptive awareness may contribute to functional limb movement. Stereognosis in the palmar surface of the hand facilitates manipulative skill in individuals who demonstrate active control over wrist and finger muscles.

Active movement in the arm and leg is a critical component of a motor assessment. Many therapists use Brunnstrom's postulated recovery stages as a framework for organizing their observations. Patients are first assessed to determine whether they can actively perform the gross flexion and extension synergies of the upper and lower limbs. Next, they are asked to perform movements that deviate from the basic synergies. Some examples of arm movements in this category are

1. Placing the hand behind the back, requiring internal rotation, adduction, and extension of the shoulder, combined with elbow flexion and forearm pronation
2. Forward flexion of the shoulder to 90 degrees with the elbow extended
3. Isolated forearm pronation and supination with the elbow flexed to 90 degrees (Sawner & LaVigne, 1992)

Lower extremity movements that require some deviation from the basic synergies can be tested with the patient sitting in a standard chair. The patient may be asked to flex his or her knee beyond 90 degrees, with the foot sliding backwards on the floor. Or the patient may perform a forward movement of the tibia over the weight-bearing foot to produce ankle dorsiflexion in a closed kinematic chain.

Relative independence of the basic limb synergies is tested by asking the patient to perform movements that equally combine elements of both flexion and extension synergies. Examples in the upper limb include (1) shoulder abduction to 90 degrees with the elbow extended; (2) overhead forward flexion of the shoulder with the elbow extended; and (3) reciprocal internal and external rotation at the shoulder with the elbow extended and the shoulder maintained at 90 degrees flexion or abduction. Lower extremity movements that require independence of the limb synergies include the ability to flex the knee with the hip extended in standing and dorsiflexing the ankle with the knee extended.

Advocates of the NDT or motor relearning approaches are generally uninterested in Brunnstrom's framework of synergy patterns or stages of recovery. Early motor recovery may be assessed through the patient's ability to support and shift proximal body weight over the affected arm or leg. Open chain upper extremity control is often

Name:	Date:	Score 1 or 0		
Arm				
1. Lying, protract shoulder girdle with arm in elevation. (Arm may be supported.)				
2. Lying, hold extended arm in elevation—some external rotation—for at least 2 seconds. (Physiotherapist should place arm in position and patient must maintain position with some external rotation. Do not allow pronation. Elbow must be held within 30° of full extension.)				
3. Flexion and extension of elbow with arm as in 2. (Elbow must extend to at least 20° full extension. Palm should not face outwards during any part of movement.)				
4. Sitting, elbow into side, pronation and supination. (¾ range is acceptable, with elbow unsupported and at right angles.)				
5. Reach forward, pick up large ball with both hands and put down again. (Ball should be on table so far in front of patient that he has to extend arms fully to reach it. Shoulders must be protracted, elbows extended, wrists neutral or extended and fingers extended throughout movement. Palms should be kept in contact with ball.)				
6. Stretch arm forward, pick up a tennis ball from table, release on mid-thigh on affected side, return to table, then release again on table. Repeat five times. (Shoulder must be protracted, elbow extended and wrist neutral or extended during each phase.)				
7. Same exercise as 6 with pencil. (Patient must use thumb and fingers to grip.)				
8. Pick up a piece of paper from table in front and release five times. (Patient must use thumb and fingers to pick up paper, not pull it to edge of table. Arm position as in 6.)				
9. Cut putty with a knife and fork on plate with non-slip mat and put pieces into a container at side of plate. (Bite size pieces.)				
10. (Stand on spot, maintain upright position, pat a large ball on floor with palm of hand for five continuous bounces.)				
Total				

FIGURE 11–1. *Continued*

Balance is indirectly assessed through active task performance; no manual displacements are provided.

The **leg and trunk** subscale reflects NDT's emphasis on the importance of dynamic weight bearing through the lower limbs. The half-bridging task requires weight bearing through both feet to elevate the pelvis when the person is lying supine. Two items require the person to maintain upright standing on the affected leg while releasing body weight from the other leg. In the scale's most difficult item, the individual is asked to control movement at the knee in a closed kinematic chain by flexing the affected knee while standing.

Tasks on the **arm** subscale clearly reflect an NDT perspective. In early items, the patient is tested in the supine position and asked to perform shoulder girdle protraction followed by external rotation of the shoulder and controlled elbow flexion and extension while maintaining the arm in an elevated position. Items progress to increasingly more difficult arm activities while sitting and then while standing. Patients are required to demonstrate the forward reach pattern (shoulder protraction, elbow extension, wrist and finger extension) advocated by Bobath as being integral to upper limb recovery. Use of the upper limb for dynamic weight bearing is assessed by requiring the person to stand with his or her affected arm abducted to 90 degress and the palm flat against a wall. While maintaining this position, the patient rotates his or her body in a closed chain on the weight-bearing hand. The final item on this

Name:	Date:	Score 1 or 0		
Arm, cont. 11. Continuous opposition of thumb and each finger more than 14 times in 10 seconds. (Must do movements in consistent sequence. Do not allow thumb to slide from one finger to the other.) 12. Supination and pronation onto palm of unaffected hand 10 times in 10 seconds. (Arm must be away from body, palm and dorsum of hand must touch palm of good hand. Each tap counts as one. This is similar to 4, but introduces speed.) 13. Standing, with affected arm abducted to 90°, with palm flat against wall. Maintain arm in position. Turn body towards wall and as far as possible towards arm; i.e., rotate body beyond 90°. (Do not allow flexion at elbow, and wrist must be extended with palm of hand fully in contact with wall.) 14. Place string around head, tie bow at back. (Do not allow neck to flex. Affected hand must be used for more than just supporting string. This tests function of hand without help of sight.) 15. Pat-a-cake 7 times in 15 seconds. (Mark cross on wall at shoulder level. Clap both hands together—both hands touch crosses—clap—one hand touches opposite cross—clap—other hand touches opposite cross. Must be in correct order. Palms must touch. Each sequence counts as one, give patient three tries. This is a complex pattern which involves coordination, speed and memory as well as good arm function.)				
Total of 1 to 10				
Total				

For information contact Dr. Nadina Lincoln, Department of Psychology, University of Nottingham, Nottingham NG7 ZRD, UK.

FIGURE 11–1. *Continued*

subscale incorporates coordination, speed, and memory as well as complex reciprocal arm function.

EVALUATION OF THE HEMIPLEGIC SUBJECT BASED ON THE BOBATH APPROACH: "THE MONTREAL EVALUATION"

This assessment was developed by a research team at the Montreal Rehabilitation Institute (Arsenault et al., 1988; Corriveau et al., 1988; Guarna et al., 1988). Since it is not the only evaluation based on the Bobath approach, this tool is referred to as "The Montreal Evaluation" throughout this chapter. Six parameters of function are scored on a four-point scale, ranging from 0 for most severe impairment to 3 for normal performance. Specific criteria are provided for scoring each test item (Corriveau et al., 1988).

The test requires a maximum of 20 minutes to administer, and the six parameters are always assessed in the following order:

Mental clarity (sensorium)

Muscle tone
Reflex activity
Voluntary movement
Automatic reactions
Pain

The Montreal Evaluation is surprisingly similar to the FMA in its reference to six stages of recovery: (1) initial recovery; (2) hypotonicity; (3) imbalanced tonicity; (4) hypertonicity; (5) relative recovery; (6) return to normal. The test also resembles the FMA in its use of ordinal scaling and a cumulative scoring system. However, a weakness of the Montreal Evaluation is its tendency to include multiple findings in each item scored. For example, the test of sensorium includes responses to verbal, nociceptive, olfactory, and tactile stimuli, as well as observations of the patient's ability to cooperate with testing procedures. All of these findings are reflected in only one score. This factor significantly limits an examiner's ability to use item scores for comparisons between individual patients.

Tests of **muscle tone**, **voluntary movement**, and **automatic reactions** are the most clearly influenced by

TABLE 11–6

THE MONTREAL EVALUATION

A: Muscle Tone: Upper Extremity

Procedures

Support is given at the elbow and wrist by examiner, and the following passive movements are performed
1. With the shoulder in external rotation and the elbow in extension, flex shoulder to a range from 0 to full flexion
2. With shoulder flexed at 90°, flex and extend elbow, bringing palm of hand to opposite shoulder and to the top of the head
3. With elbow flexed and palm of hand on opposite shoulder, flex and extend the shoulder
4. With elbow extended and shoulder flexed to 90°, protract the shoulder
5. With arm next to trunk, forearm and hand supported, and with the elbow flexed to 90°, pronate and supinate forearm
6. With elbow extended and shoulder at 90° (with forearm in neutral position and arm supported at elbow and wrist), flex and extend the wrist
7. With elbow extended, shoulder flexed at 90° with wrist and forearm in neutral position (arm supported at elbow and wrist) flex and extend fingers

Ratings

0 = Flaccidity: flaccidity noted in all the muscle groups including distal
1 = Mainly flaccid with some spasticity: this category includes the patients who have one of the following:
    Flaccidity in shoulder girdle and shoulder with spasticity in the fingers, wrists, and pronators
    Flaccidity distally and spasticity proximally
    Weakness and weak tendon reflexes
2 = Mainly spastic with some flaccidity: spasticity dominated in upper extremity with possibility of some specific muscle flaccidity
3 = Normal: normal tone with possible residual muscle weakness. The tendon reflexes are normal

B: Muscle Tone: Lower Extremity

Procedures

Support is given at the knee and toes by examiner, and the following passive movements are performed
1. With the knee flexed to 90° and ankle held in neutral position, flex and extend the hip
2. With ankle held in neutral, flex and extend the knee
3. With the knee flexed to 90° and the ankle held in neutral, abduct and adduct the hip
4. With the affected knee crossed over the unaffected knee, protract the pelvis on the affected side
5. With the knee flexed to 70° with the foot resting on the floor, dorsiflex and plantar flex the ankle; with the knee extended and the lower extremity supported, dorsiflex and plantar flex the toes
6. With the knee flexed to 70° and the foot resting on the floor, flex and extend the toes; with the knee extended and the lower extremity supported, flex and extend the toes

Ratings

0 = Flaccidity: flaccidity noted in all the muscle groups including distal
1 = Mainly flaccid with some spasticity: flaccidity dominates in lower extremity with possibility of some specific muscle spasticity
2 = Mainly spastic with some flaccidity: spasticity dominates in lower extremity with possibility of some specific muscle flaccidity
3 = Normal: normal tone with possible residual muscle weakness

C: Muscle Tone: Trunk and Neck

Procedures

TRUNK

Patient is sitting with fingers crossed, elbows extended, and shoulder flexed to 90°. Patient's arms cradled in therapist's forearms: passive rotation of upper trunk on lower trunk is performed

NECK

Patient is transferred in supine position later in the evaluation; patient's head cradled in therapist's hands: passive anterior flexion, lateral flexion and rotation of the neck is performed

Ratings

0 = Flaccidity
1 = Mainly flaccid with some spasticity
2 = Mainly spastic with some flaccidity
3 = Normal

From Corriveau, H., Guarna, F., Dutil, E., Riley, E., Arsenault, A. B., & Drouin, G. (1988). An evaluation of the hemiplegic subject based on the Bobath approach. Part II: The evaluation protocol. *Scandinavian Journal of Rehabilitation Medicine, 20,* 5–11.

NDT principles. Tests of **mental clarity**, **reflex activity**, and **pain** have little relationship to concepts of NDT.

Muscle tone and **voluntary movement** are evaluated through a series of patterned movements that resemble the reflex inhibiting patterns (or postures) espoused by Bobath in early writings (Bobath, 1978). In the muscle tone assessment (Table 11–6), the therapist passively moves the patient into these positions and notes excessive resistance to the passive muscle lengthening. In the assessment of voluntary movement (Table 11–7), the patient is required to actively reproduce these patterns.

Postural reactions are assessed in the sitting position. The therapist provides lateral displacement at the pelvis three times on each side and observes for the following reactions:

Head righting
Elongation of trunk and weight shift
Abduction-extension reactions of the extremities
Protective extension of the affected upper extremity

TABLE 11–7

THE MONTREAL EVALUATION—ACTIVE MOVEMENT

A: Active Movement: Upper Extremity

Procedures

1. All the same movements in the section on muscle tone but done actively
2. Opposition of fingers with arm by the side, elbow flexed, and wrist in neutral
3. Reaching for a ball in different directions and returning to the starting position

Ratings

0 = No movement or trace of active movement
1 = Voluntary movement present but executed with primitive synergies: a maximum of three movements are noted with half range or more
2 = Appearance of selective movements/decrease of influence of primitive synergies: four movements or more are noted
3 = Normal: all the selective movements are present, with strength and coordination being normal

B: Active Movement: Lower Extremity

Procedures

Same movements as in "muscle tone" section but done actively

Ratings

0 = No movement or trace of active movement
1 = Voluntary movement present but executed with primitive synergies: a maximum of three movements are noted with half range or more
2 = Appearance of selective movements/decrease of influence of primitive synergies: four movements or more are noted
3 = Normal: all the selective movements are present, with strength and coordination being normal

From Corriveau, H., Guarna, F., Dutil, E., Riley, E., Arsenault, A. B., & Drouin, G. (1988). An evaluation of the hemiplegic subject based on the Bobath approach. Part II: The evaluation protocol. *Scandinavian Journal of Rehabilitation Medicine, 20,* 5–11.

All these observations are reflected in one score, ranging from 0 to 3. If manual displacement fails to elicit reactions, the patient is asked to reach laterally for an object with the nonaffected hand. This reflects an understanding that the more subtle postural adjustments may be best elicited through active, rather than passive, shifts of body weight.

The Montreal Evaluation does not assess higher-level motor functions of dynamic weight bearing, ambulation, or step climbing. Evaluation of hand function is limited to one item, which requires the patient to oppose his or her thumb to the fingers.

ASHBURN'S PHYSICAL ASSESSMENT FOR STROKE PATIENTS

Ashburn's (1982) Physical Assessment for Stroke Patients provides an ordinal scale, divided into three major sections: **lower limb activities, upper limb activities, and balance and movement activities**. Items are scored on a three-point continuum, as in the FMA.

Three **lower limb activities** are assessed: hip and knee flexion while standing; isolated knee flexion from a prone position; and ankle dorsiflexion tested while the hip and knee are extended and when the hip and knee are flexed.

The ten **upper limb activities** include shoulder shrugging, arm thrusting, arm raising, forearm supination, wrist dorsiflexion, finger extension, and pinch grip. Clear illustrations on the test form facilitate correct testing of all limb items.

Eighteen **balance and movement activities** assess gross mobility; balance in sitting, standing, and kneel-standing; walking; and stair climbing.

Space is provided on the evaluation form for recording information about joint abnormalities, sensory loss, and muscle tone. These items, however, are ungraded and do not contribute to a total cumulative score.

Tests of Upper Extremity Function

A variety of assessments have been used for specifically assessing upper extremity function in individuals with stroke. The Action Research Arm Test (Lyle, 1981) is a hierarchically arranged evaluation of grasp, grip, pinch, and gross arm movement. The Arm Function Test (DeSouza et al., 1980) includes assessment of arm and trunk movement through evaluation of performance in turning a cranked wheel. Hand function is assessed through eight functional tasks. In addition, passive movement, muscle tone, and pain are evaluated.

FUNCTIONAL TEST FOR THE HEMIPARETIC UPPER EXTREMITY

The Functional Test for the Hemiparetic Upper Extremity (Wilson et al., 1984) assesses integrated arm and hand

FUNCTIONAL TEST FOR THE HEMIPARETIC UPPER EXTREMITY

Functional test for the hemiplegic/paretic upper extremity

Patient _____ RLAH # _____

LEVEL	TASK	GRADE	
1	Patient is unable to complete higher-level tasks		
2	A. Associated reaction		
	B. Hand into lap		
3	C. Shoulder abduction		
	D. Hold a pouch		
	E. Stabilize a pillow		
4	F. Stabilize a jar		
	G. Stabilize a package		
	H. Wringing a rag		
5	I. Hold a pan lid		
	J. Hook and zip a zipper		
	K. Fold a sheet		
6	L. Blocks and box		
	M. Box on shelf		
	N. Coin in coin gauge		
7	O. Cat's cradle		
	P. Light bulb		
	Q. Remove rubber band		
	DATE		
	EXAMINER		

FIGURE 11–2. Functional test for the hemiparetic upper extremity. (Reprinted by permission of the Occupational Therapy Department, Rehabilitation Engineering Center, Rancho Los Amigos Hospital, Downey, CA. Note: 40-page protocol booklet is available from Rancho Los Amigos Occupational Therapy Department, Rehabilitation Engineering Center, 7413 Golondrinas Street, Downey, CA 90242.)

function through the performance of 17 standardized tasks (Fig. 11–2). Like the Rivermead Motor Assessment, items are ordered hierarchically, according to their difficulty. Grading is on a pass-fail basis, and most activities are timed. Patients who do not successfully complete a task within the 3-minute prescribed period fail that item.

Items are grouped according to seven levels of upper extremity function, ranging from (1) absence of voluntary movement to (7) selective and coordinated movement. The patient earns a plus for successfully completing a task or a minus for failing at the task. After the assessment, the person is scored as functioning at the highest level in which he or she successfully completed all tasks. This categorization of performance by functional levels assists therapists in establishing treatment goals, and it allows for objective documentation of patient progress.

The seven levels of upper extremity function reflect influence by both Brunnstrom and NDT approaches. Items at early levels elicit associated reactions and gross synergy patterns. Subsequent levels require use of the hemiparetic arm as a gross assist for stabilizing objects during bimanual tasks. Mid- to high-level tasks require increasing amounts of finger dexterity, combined with proximal control.

There are strengths and weaknesses to the use of naturalistic tasks on an assessment of upper extremity function. One important asset is that the test score actually provides a direct indication of functional performance. In addition, the task-oriented instructions are easier for patients with cognitive and perceptual deficits to follow than test items that require performance of abstract movements.

The authors caution therapists about a drawback to the tool's clinical use. Since each task requires the integration of multiple skills (e.g., sensory awareness, shoulder control, grasp, coordination) a patient's score does not identify specific deficit areas. The examiner is responsible for qualitatively assessing which impairments have contributed to an individual's failure on a test item. This qualitative assessment, rather than the numeric score, guides therapeutic intervention. An additional weakness is that progression from one task to the next often requires significant improvements in function. The test may not be sensitive enough to reflect incremental achievements in upper extremity performance.

Carr and Shepherd's Motor Assessment Scale for Stroke Patients

Carr and Shepherd and colleagues (1985) developed this tool to reflect contemporary views about motor recovery after stroke. They offered the Motor Assessment Scale (MAS) as an alternative to other standardized assessments that are based on the assumptions that recovery is characterized by stereotyped movements in synergies and recovery proceeds in a proximal to distal sequence.

The MAS includes eight items representing the following areas of motor behavior:

Supine to side lying onto intact side
Supine to sitting over side of bed
Balanced sitting
Sitting to standing
Walking
Upper arm function
Hand movements
Advanced hand activities

Each item is scored on a seven-point scale from 0 to 6, according to the criteria listed in Table 11–8. The original version of the scale also included one item related to muscle tone on the affected side. The **general tonus** score is based on the examiner's continuous observation and handling throughout the assessment and is graded differently than other items.

Tests of gross mobility on the MAS deliberately omit assessment of rolling because Carr and Shepherd and their coworkers believe that rolling over is given excessive emphasis in many rehabilitation programs. Although rolling over is an important developmental milestone in babies, adults who are recovering from stroke do not need to follow a developmental sequence to achieve improved motor function.

Assessment of balanced sitting pays close attention to postural alignment during quiet sitting and functional movement. The person's ability to adjust to displacement of his or her center of gravity is tested through active movement, rather than the application of external force.

The **walking assessment** requires high-level function to achieve moderate and maximum scores. As in the Rivermead Assessment, patients are asked to walk with no aid and to perform a complex sequence including walking, turning, and retrieving an item from the floor. An individual receives the highest score if he or she is able to quickly ascend and descend steps without holding onto the rail.

Evaluation of **upper arm function** and **hand movements** is similar to that in the Rivermead Assessment. The major difference is that on the Rivermead, patients are not asked to demonstrate wrist or hand function unless they can accomplish earlier test items requiring shoulder, elbow, and forearm control. The MAS recognizes that some individuals may regain hand function before achieving recovery in proximal muscles.

The **advanced hand activities** item allows for assessment of higher-level grasp and manipulative skills. Unfortunately, no theoretical rationale is provided for the hierarchical scoring of patient performance. Loewen and Anderson (1988, 1990) developed the Modified Motor Assessment Scale (MMAS) by adapting the scoring criteria for advanced hand activities and eliminating the general tonus item.

PSYCHOMETRIC RESEARCH ON THE STANDARDIZED ASSESSMENT TOOLS

The Fugl-Meyer Assessment

Of all the available standardized tests of motor recovery after stroke, the FMA has been most rigorously analyzed for reliability and validity. Consequently, it is the most frequently chosen measure for clinical studies in which poststroke motor function is a dependent variable.

For the initial pilot study (Fugl-Meyer et al., 1975), 80 patients were evaluated with the FMA within 1 week of hospital admission for acute cerebrovascular accident. These individuals were examined at monthly intervals for 6 months and tested again at 1 year. The number of subjects remaining to completion of the study decreased to 15. Reasons for withdrawal included no finding of motor deficit on initial evaluation, new episodes of stroke or other illness, failure to cooperate with retesting, and death.

Longitudinal findings supported the postulated sequence

TABLE 11–8

MOTOR ASSESSMENT SCALE SCORING CRITERIA

1. Supine to Side Lying Onto Intact Side

1. Pulls self into side lying. (Starting position must be supine lying, legs extended. Patient pulls self into side lying with intact arm, moves affected leg with intact leg.)
2. Moves leg across actively, and the lower half of the body follows. Starting position as above. Arm is left behind.
3. Arm is lifted across body with other arm. Leg is moved actively, and body follows in a block. (Starting position as above.)
4. Moves arm across body actively, and the rest of the body follows in a block. (Starting position as above.)
5. Moves arm and leg and rolls to side but overbalances. (Starting position as above. Shoulder protracts and arm flexes forward.)
6. Rolls to side in 3 seconds. (Starting position as above. Must not use hands.)

2. Supine to Sitting Over Side of Bed

1. Side lying, lifts head sideways but cannot sit up. (Patient assisted to side lying.)
2. Side lying to sitting over side of bed. (Therapist assists patient with movement. Patient controls head position throughout.)
3. Side lying to sitting over side of bed. (Therapist gives stand-by help [see General Rules item 5] by assisting legs over side of bed.)
4. Side lying to sitting over side of bed. (With no stand-by help.)
5. Supine to sitting over side of bed. (With no stand-by help.)
6. Supine to sitting over side of bed within 10 seconds. (With no stand-by help.)

3. Balanced Sitting

1. Sits only with support. (Therapist should assist patient into sitting.)
2. Sits unsupported for 10 seconds. (Without holding on, knees and feet together, feet can be supported on floor.)
3. Sits unsupported with weight well forward and evenly distributed. (Weight should be well forward with hips flexed, head and thoracic spine extended, weight evenly distributed on both sides.)
4. Sits unsupported, turns head and trunk to look behind. (Feet supported and together on floor. Do not allow legs to abduct or feet to move. Have hands resting on thighs, do not allow hands to move onto plinth. Turn to each side.)
5. Sits unsupported, reaches forward to touch floor, and returns to starting position. Feet supported on floor. Do not allow patient to hold on. Do not allow legs and feet to move, support affected arm if necessary. Hand must touch floor at least 10 cm (4 in) in front of feet. Reach with each arm.
6. Sits on stool unsupported, reaches sideways to touch floor, and returns to starting position. (Feet supported on floor. Do not allow patient to hold on. Do not allow legs and feet to move, support affected arm if necessary. Patient must reach sideways not forward. Reach to both sides.)

4. Sitting to Standing

1. Gets to standing with help from therapist. (Any method.)
2. Gets to standing with stand-by help. (Weight unevenly distributed, uses hands for support.)
3. Gets to standing. (Do not allow uneven weight distribution or help from hands.)
4. Gets to standing and stands for 5 seconds with hips and knees extended. (Do not allow uneven weight distribution.)
5. Sitting to standing to sitting with no stand-by help. (Do not allow uneven weight distribution. Full extension of hips and knees.)
6. Sitting to standing to sitting with no stand-by help three times in 10 seconds. (Do not allow uneven weight distribution.)

5. Walking

1. Stands on affected leg and steps forward with other leg. (Weight-bearing hip must be extended. Therapist may give stand-by help.)
2. Walks with stand-by help from one person.
3. Walks 3 m (10 ft) alone or uses any aid but not stand-by help.
4. Walks 5 m (16 ft) with no aid in 15 seconds.
5. Walks 10 m (33 ft) with no aid, picks up a small sandbag from floor, turns around, and walks back in 25 seconds. (May use either hand.)
6. Walks up and down four steps with or without an aid but without holding on to the rail three times in 35 seconds.

6. Upper Arm Function

1. Supine, protract shoulder girdle with arm in 90 degrees of shoulder flexion. (Therapist places arm in position and supports elbow in extension.)
2. Supine, hold arm in 90 degrees of shoulder flexion for 2 seconds. (Therapist places arm in position and patient must maintain position with some [45 degrees] external rotation. Elbow must be held within at least 20 degrees of full extension.)
3. Supine, hold arm in 90 degrees of shoulder flexion, flex and extend elbow to take palm to forehead. (Therapist may assist supination of forearm.)
4. Sitting, hold extended arm in forward flexion at 90 degrees to body for 2 seconds. (Therapist should place arm in position, and patient maintains position. Patient must hold arm in midrotation [thumb pointing up]. Do not allow excess shoulder elevation.)
5. Sitting, patient lifts arm to above position, holds it there for 10 seconds, and then lowers it. (Patient must maintain position with some external rotation. Do not allow pronation.)
6. Standing, hand against wall. Maintain hand position while turning body toward wall. (Arm is abducted to 90 degrees with palm flat against the wall.)

TABLE 11-8

MOTOR ASSESSMENT SCALE SCORING CRITERIA *Continued*

7. Hand Movements

1. Sitting, extension of wrist. (Patient sits at a table with forearm resting on the table. Therapist places cylindric object in palm of patient's hand. Patient is asked to lift object off the table by extending the wrist. Do not allow elbow flexion.)
2. Sitting, radial deviation of wrist. (Therapist places forearm in mid–pronation-supination, i.e., resting on ulnar side, thumb in line with forearm and wrist in extension, fingers around a cylindric object. Patient is asked to lift hand off table. Do not allow elbow flexion or pronation.)
3. Sitting, elbow into side, pronation and supination. (Elbow unsupported and at a right angle. Three-quarter range is acceptable.)
4. Sitting, reach forward, pick up large ball of 14 cm (5 in) diameter with both hands, and put it down. (Ball should be placed on table at a distance that requires elbow extension. Palms should be kept in contact with the ball.)
5. Sitting, pick up a polystyrene cup from table and put it on table across other side of body. (Do not allow alteration in shape of cup.)
6. Sitting, continuous opposition of thumb and each finger more than 14 times in 10 seconds. (Each finger in turn taps the thumb, starting with index finger. Do not allow thumb to slide from one finger to the other, or to go backward.)

8. Advanced Hand Activities

1. Pick up the top of a pen and put it down again. (Patient reaches forward to arm's length, picks up pen top, releases it on table close to body.)
2. Pick up one jellybean from a cup and place it in another cup. (Teacup contains eight jellybeans. Both cups must be at arms' length. Left hand takes jellybean from cup on right and releases it in cup on left.)
3. Draw horizontal lines to stop at a vertical line 10 times in 20 seconds. (At least five lines must touch and stop at the vertical line. Lines should be approximately 10 cm in length.)
4. Hold a pen, make rapid consecutive dots on a sheet of paper. (Patient must do at least two dots a second for 5 seconds. Patient picks pen up and positions it without assistance. Pen must be held as for writing. Dots not dashes.)
5. Take a dessert spoon of liquid to the mouth. (Do not allow head to lower toward spoon. Liquid must not spill.)
6. Hold a comb and comb hair at back of head. (Shoulder must be externally rotated, abducted at least 90°. Head erect.)

Carr, J. H., Shepherd, R. B., Nordholm, L., & Lynne, D. (1985). Investigation of a new motor assessment scale for stroke patients. *Physical Therapy, 65,* 175–180.

of recovery assessed in the FMA. In all cases where the development of motor behavior could be followed, stage 2 behaviors preceded stage 3 behaviors, which preceded stage 4 behaviors, and so on. This provides strong support for the construct validity of the tool. Data indicated that balance did not necessarily follow the restoration of motor function of the limbs. However, full recovery of balance only occurred in patients who achieved maximum scores on the lower extremity subtest. Sensation scores did not correlate with either maximum motor behavior achieved at final test or slope of the recovery curve. This finding indicates that somatosensory function may not serve as a prognostic indicator of success in achieving motor recovery. Motor recovery of the shoulder-arm system was compared with recovery of lower extremity use through paired differences regression analysis. This yielded a mean correlation coefficient of 0.88, indicating a fairly strong relationship between amount of recovery in the arm and leg.

In subsequent piloting with 21 patients (Fugl-Meyer, 1980), patients were grouped for statistical analysis according to their cumulative scores for upper and lower extremity function. Scores between 50 and 84 were categorized as indicating severe impairment, scores between 85 and 95 as moderate impairment, and scores from 96 to 99 as minimal impairment. Contractures, which developed most frequently in the shoulder and ankle, were significantly more pronounced in patients with severe impairments than in those with moderate or minimal impairments. Motor function was significantly associated with balance, joint motion, and, inversely, with joint pain.

Intratester and intertester reliability were established in a study of 19 adult patients who had sustained cerebrovascular accidents at least 1 year before testing (Duncan et al., 1983). All participants had previously been discharged from occupational and physical therapy because of plateaued motor recovery. Four physical therapists with experience administering the FMA served as examiners.

For analysis of intratester reliability, one therapist administered the complete FMA three times to each patient at 3-week intervals. Two sets of correlation coefficients were determined: between tests 1 and 2 and between tests 2 and 3. Correlation coefficients for the total test were 0.984 and 0.988, indicating extremely high intrarater reliability. Intratester correlation coefficients for subtests ranged from 0.865 (joint range of motion and pain) to 0.996 (upper extremity motor function). Highest correlations were found on the upper extremity and lower extremity motor subscores, and lowest correlations were found for the balance and joint range of motion/pain subscores. All correlation coefficients were statistically significant at the 0.001 level. Analysis of variance of all total scores and subscores yielded no significant differences among the score distributions for first, second, and third testings.

For analysis of interrater reliability, participants performed only one section (upper or lower extremity motor performance) of the FMA on two additional occasions with two different examiners. Therefore, interrater reliability for the joint motion and pain, sensation, and balance subtests was not established. Scores from these two test sessions were correlated with one another, as well as with the corresponding scores received on the third testing of the intrarater reliability tests with the first examiner. Therefore, two sets of correlation coefficients were determined for total upper extremity function ($r = 0.984$ and 0.995), total lower extremity function ($r = 0.922$ and 0.953), and each of the subscores for upper and lower extremity function. Correlation coefficients for the subscores ranged from 0.833 (lower extremity coordination) to 0.997 (hand function). Analysis of variance revealed statistically significant differences in intertester scores for upper extremity coordination and reflex assessment. However, the authors attribute this to one examiner's misinterpretation of scoring instructions. No other statistically significant differences were found between intertester scores.

In summary, intratester reliability was established for the entire FMA, and intertester reliability was established for the upper and lower extremity components. Cumulative scores for upper and lower extremity motor function ranged from 50% to 98% of maximum performance, with a mean of 74%.

Concurrent validity of the FMA has been established through a series of studies that established strong relationships between scores on this test and on tests of other variables associated with motor recovery. It should be noted that the subtests of upper and lower extremity function are most commonly used in these studies. Therefore, no statements can be made about the validity of subscales of balance, sensation, or joint motion and pain.

Fugl-Meyer and associates found significant relationships when comparing the total motor score with independence in activities of daily living (Fugl-Meyer et al., 1975; Sjogren & Fugl-Meyer, 1982), participation in leisure activities and sexual intercourse (Sjogren & Fugl-Meyer, 1982), and scores on another test of arm control (Berglund & Fugl-Meyer, 1986). Kusoffsky and coworkers (1982) determined that somatosensory evoked potentials are predictive of Fugl-Meyer scores. Badke and Dunkan (1983) reported a statistically significant relationship between abnormalities in postural adjustments in standing with FMA scores on the lower extremity subscale.

The FMA has been used in a number of clinical studies about stroke rehabilitation. It was chosen as the tool for measuring outcome in a longitudinal study of motor recovery in a cohort of patients with an acute lesion in the carotid distribution (Duncan et al., 1992). FMA scores reflected the dependent variable in an experimental study comparing the effectiveness of EMG biofeedback, positional feedback with electrical stimulation, and proprioceptive neuromuscular facilitation in improving arm and hand function in stroke patients of more than 6 months duration (Kraft et al., 1992). In a study of functional recovery after discharge from inpatient stroke rehabilitation (Ferrucci et al., 1993), the FMA was used as a measure of neural impairment. Interestingly, the two latter studies found that FMA scores continued to improve when individuals were studied more than 1 year after their cerebrovascular accidents.

Standardized Assessments Based on the Neurodevelopmental Treatment Philosophy

THE RIVERMEAD MOTOR ASSESSMENT

Psychometric issues were a focus in the development of this tool. The order and instructions for test items in the final version were developed in response to pilot testing, which assessed interrater reliability and criteria for consideration as a Guttman scale. Initial piloting included 51 patients on a stroke rehabilitation unit. Seven physical therapists participated in reliability testing, which was based on videotapes of seven assessments.

The extent to which the data fit the Guttman scale model was evaluated by calculating coefficients of reproducibility and coefficients of scalability for each of the three sections (gross function, leg and trunk, and arm). Coefficients of reproducibility ranged from 0.90 (leg and trunk) to 0.98 (gross function). Coefficients of scalability ranged from 0.79 (leg and trunk) to 0.96 (gross function). Findings for all three sections met the criteria to be considered valid Guttman scales. The same statistical analyses were conducted with data from retesting 40 of the participants after a 4-week interval. Similar results were achieved. Test-retest reliability of the Rivermead's final version was established in a study of 10 hemiparetic individuals who were no longer participating in rehabilitation due to plateaus in motor recovery. Patients were assessed and then reassessed by the same examiner 4 weeks later. Correlation coefficients were 0.66 ($P < 0.05$) for gross function, 0.93 ($P < 0.001$) for leg and trunk, and 0.88 ($P < 0.001$) for arm. The test developers point out that the lower correlation between test and retest scores on the gross function scale was due to lack of variation of scores within the 10 patients.

Subsequent testing of the Rivermead's scalability indicated that the gross function and arm sections met Guttman scale criteria, with a sample of individuals presenting with acute strokes (Adams, 1993a). Recovery in these areas followed a hierarchic pattern on repeated testing, whereas recovery of leg and trunk function demonstrated a more uneven pattern, which did not correspond to the hierarchic listing of the items on the assessment. This finding, which is consistent with findings using the FMA, indicates that improvements of motor function in the arm follow a more predictable sequence during acute recovery than does improvement of trunk or leg function. In a study of nonacute stroke patients aged 65 or older (Adams, 1993b), only the gross function section retained the properties of a Guttman scale. This indicates that after the acute stage, patterns of further recovery are less likely to follow predictable sequences.

Further piloting of the Rivermead Assessment is needed. Firstly, establishment of interrater reliability would enable multiple examiners to compare their scores. Secondly, additional assessment of test-retest reliability, using a sample of individuals with greater variance in their gross functional abilities, might determine a higher estimate of stability for scores on this subtest. Finally, the scale's criterion-related validity needs to be determined. The Rivermead Motor Assessment has been used as an outcome measure in studies of rehabilitation for balance (deWeerdt et al., 1989) and functional abilities (Juby et al., 1994).

THE MONTREAL ASSESSMENT

Validity of subtests related to the upper extremity was established in a study of 62 individuals who participated in a 2-month inpatient stroke rehabilitation program (Arsenault et al., 1988). Participants were evaluated three times. They received a pretest on admission, an intertest after 1 month of NDT, and a posttest just before leaving the center after 2 months of NDT. Each evaluation included the following tests:

The nonstandardized Brunnstrom Evaluation (Brunnstrom, 1970)
The Upper Extremity Functional Test (Carroll, 1965)
The upper extremity section of the FMA, excluding tests of the wrist and hand
The Montreal Assessment

Friedman two-way ANOVA for ordinal data was used to determine differences in scores on all four tests across the three measurements taken during each patient's rehabilitation stay. All four evaluation protocols indicated statistically significant progress over time. Interestingly, this finding indicates that the FMA of the upper arm is a valid tool for measuring progress, even when patients receive Bobath-oriented intervention.

Spearman-rho correlations were determined between scores on each of the four assessments given at each testing. For this calculation, the authors correlated scores on a partial version of the Montreal Assessment, which excluded subtests of sensorium and pain. Pretest, intertest, and posttest scores on the partial Montreal Evaluation correlated significantly ($P < 0.001$) with corresponding scores on the other three assessments. Correlation coefficients with the FMA were 0.73 for the pretest, 0.62 for the intertest, and 0.85 for the posttest.

Content validity of the Montreal Evaluation was established through principal component analysis of scores for 38 hemiplegic subjects who were tested on admission, after 1 month of treatment, and just before discharge (Corriveau et al., 1992). Principal component analysis revealed three factors that correspond to the subsections of this tool:

Factor one: mobility—postural reactions and active movements
Factor two: muscle tone
Factor three: sensorium and pain

The statistical link between scores of postural reactions and active movements provides support for the NDT concept that limb movements can be improved through the development of enhanced postural reactions.

A reliability study of this tool (Corriveau et al., 1992)

yielded intraclass correlation coefficients for intrarater data of 0.95 for upper limb function and 0.97 for lower limb function. An interrater study yielded intraclass correlation coefficients of 0.79 and 0.77 for upper and lower limb function, respectively.

ASHBURN'S PHYSICAL ASSESSMENT FOR STROKE PATIENTS

Although this test has standardized instructions and yields a numeric score, no statistical analysis of scores has been reported. The test has been used clinically in a number of rehabilitation programs in England. A qualitative assessment of interrater reliability revealed few disagreements in scores when individuals were evaluated independently by 15 paired observers (Ashburn, 1982).

Tests of Upper Extremity Function

Since the Action Research Arm Test, like the Rivermead Motor Assessment, is a Guttman scale, coefficients of scalability and reproducibility are used as measures of validity. These coefficients range from 0.94 to 0.99 for the four subtests (Lyle, 1981). Interrater and test-retest reliabilities were established through pilot testing to be 0.99 and 0.98, respectively (Lyle, 1981). The tool's construct validity is supported by results from a study in which 53 individuals were assessed with this evaluation and the FMA at 2 weeks and at 8 weeks after the onset of stroke (deWeerdt & Harrison, 1985). Spearman rank correlation coefficients between scores on the two evaluations were extremely high ($r = 0.91$ at 2 weeks after stroke; $r = 0.94$ at 8 weeks after stroke).

Although descriptive measures have been reported from piloting of The Arm Function Test (DeSouza et al., 1980), no formal reliability or validity data are available.

FUNCTIONAL TEST FOR THE HEMIPARETIC UPPER EXTREMITY

The current version of The Functional Test was developed after several years of clinical use of an initial version, which was first developed in 1964 (Wilson et al., 1984). Notable revisions included removal of redundant items and changes in the order of tasks.

To establish interrater reliability, two occupational therapists tested 10 patients within 2 days. Each individual's scores between the two raters were within one item of each other, and the Spearman's rank correlation between the testers was 0.976.

A pilot study, including 82 individuals who participated in a stroke rehabilitation program, established concurrent validity of The Functional Test. In addition, analysis of scores provided support for the hierarchy of test items. Using multiple regression analysis, an objective test battery of subskills associated with upper extremity function were found to predict performance on The Functional Test. The objective test battery included evaluations of

1. Active, selective extension of the elbow, wrist, and index finger metacarpophalangeal joint
2. Active shoulder flexion and abduction
3. Isometric wrist extension torque
4. Two-point discrimination on the palmar distal phalanx of the index finger
5. Proprioception of the index finger, wrist, and elbow
6. Assessment of spasticity in the finger, wrist, and elbow flexors

This multiple regression data demonstrated that the composite scores from the test battery accounted for 86% of the variance of The Functional Test scores ($P < 0.001$) (Wilson et al., 1984). Stepwise regression analysis demonstrated that all tests on the objective battery contributed to variation in Functional Test scores, except for active extension of the elbow and index finger, two-point discrimination, and spasticity.

Indirect support for the validity of using functional hand tasks to assess upper extremity motor recovery after stroke is provided in an unrelated study of the hemiplegic arm (Wade et al., 1983). This highly referenced research used a series of seven tasks to assess arm function, but no reports exist in the literature of the test's reliability or validity. Future longitudinal studies of recovery in arm function would have stronger psychometric foundations if they used The Functional Test, rather than Wade and colleagues' assessment.

Further support for The Functional Test's concurrent validity was provided in a study of motor function and activities of daily living (Filiatrault et al., 1991). Scores on The Functional Test correlated highly with upper extremity scores on the FMA ($r = 0.96$). In addition, scores on The Functional Test increased between time of admission to a rehabilitation unit, 1 month later, and at time of discharge. Sensitivity to change, however, was greater for the FMA than for The Functional Test. Since this is probably due to the Functional Test's small global score (0–7), a French version has been adapted with a numeric scale (i.e., 0,1,2) for each task and a global score of 34 points (Dutil et al., 1990).

In summary, The Functional Test has well-established reliability and validity. Since individuals are scored on a pass-fail basis for each item, total scores range only from 0 to 7, and may not be sensitive to small improvements. If reliability can be established for the newer French version, the test may be even more useful as an outcome measure in clinical studies of upper extremity recovery after stroke.

Carr and Shepherd's Motor Assessment Scale for Stroke Patients

Test-retest reliability was established as 0.98 in a pilot study of 15 individuals after stroke who were tested by the same examiner twice within a 2-week period (Carr et al., 1985). High interrater reliability was determined in two separate studies. In the first study (Carr et al., 1985), one expert examiner assessed five individuals who were at various stages of motor recovery after stroke. Her assigned scores became the criterion ratings, and the assessment sessions were videotaped. After instruction and 3 weeks of practice implementing the MAS, 20 physical therapists and physical therapy students viewed the tapes and scored each patient's performance. (General tonus, item 9, was not included since this cannot be assessed by observation alone.) Spearman correlation coefficients between the rater's scores and the criterion ratings for each of the patients were calculated and averaged to yield a reliability coefficient of 0.95.

In a subsequent study (Poole & Whitney, 1988) two examiners observed actual assessments of 24 individuals after stroke and scored each subject independently. This yielded an interrater reliability coefficient for the total score of 0.99. All coefficients for individual items were high and statistically significant at the 0.001 level except general tone ($r = 0.29$).

Poole and Whitney (1988) also assessed concurrent validity by testing 30 subjects on both the MAS and the FMA and comparing scores. Spearman correlation coefficients could not be calculated for the supine to sidelying and supine to sitting activities since no comparable items are on the FMA. General tone was not included in calculating a total MAS score because this item, unlike all others, is not scaled ordinally. The correlation for the total scores on the MAS and the FMA was 0.88 ($P < 0.001$). All correlations for individual items were strong and significant at the 0.001 level, except for sitting balance ($r = 0.28$). The poor correlation between the balanced sitting item with scores on sitting balance in the FMA is not a negative finding for the MAS. The FMA's evaluation of balance is based on outdated principles and assesses static responses to sudden, external disturbances. The MAS assesses balance in the context of dynamic adjustments during active task performance. Furthermore, the sitting balance component on the FMA is psychometrically weak, with no evidence of either reliability or concurrent validity with other assessments of sitting balance.

Although correlation between scores on MAS's two items of hand function with the FMA's combined wrist and hand motor scores was high ($r = 0.92$), questions were raised about the validity of the scoring hierarchy for the MAS's advanced hand activities item (Poole & Whitney, 1988).

Loewen and Anderson's (1988, 1990) MMAS adapted the original MAS in response to concerns raised in earlier pilot testing. Specifically, they removed the general tonus item and reordered the scoring hierarchy for advanced hand activities. Interrater reliability of the MMAS was determined to be 0.96 through a Spearman rank-order correlation analysis of scores assigned by 14 trained physical therapists who watched videotaped assessments of seven individuals with hemiplegia due to stroke.

Intrarater reliability was assessed by comparing these 14 initial scores with scores assigned by the same therapists after watching the videotapes 1 month later. Spearman rank-order correlation coefficients ranged from 0.81 to 1.00, with a median of 0.98. Analysis of individual items showed correlations of 1.00 for all examiners on the hand movements and advanced hand activity items. Lowest intrarater correlations were found for the supine to side lying item. This is probably due to the fact that scoring on the hand assessments is based on the person's ability to succeed at a hierarchy of specific tasks. Scoring for the supine to side lying item is based on a qualitative assessment of the person's performance of one activity.

In summary, both the MAS and MMAS are highly reliable. Concurrent validity for the MAS, using the FMA as criterion, is also high. The scoring hierarchy for advanced hand activities on the MMAS seems to be an improvement to the original. However, its validity still needs to be established. The original MAS was used successfully as a measure of the dependent variable in a study of rehabilitation outcome following stroke (Dean & Mackey, 1992). Construct validity for the sit to stand item (Ada & Westwood, 1992) and the walking item (Nugent & Schurr, 1994) has been supported in clinical studies.

SUMMARY

Occupational and physical therapists often provide intervention to enhance motor function in individuals who are recovering from stroke. No doubt exists that stroke is a difficult disease to study because its clinical manifestations and extent of recovery vary widely between individuals (Lyden & Lau, 1991). However, it is hoped that the standardized tools described in this chapter can be used as outcome measures of motor function in well-designed research studies that examine the efficacy of selected approaches to stroke rehabilitation.

GLOSSARY

Associated reactions—Abnormal reflex movements that occur simultaneously with voluntary movement of another body segment and are accentuated by excessive effort or anxiety.

Balance—Ability to maintain an upright posture by maintaining one's center of gravity within the current base of support.

Coefficient of reproducibility—Statistic calculated to confirm the existence of a valid cumulative and unidimensional Guttman scale; gives the proportion of all item abilities correctly predicted from the knowledge of the number of each final score.

Coefficient of scalability—Statistic calculated to accept the validity of a Guttman scale; indicates the proportion of responses that can be correctly predicted from the total score, allowing for the relative frequency that different items are passed.

Closed kinematic chain—A system in which motion at one joint produces motion at all other joints in a predictable manner; occurs during human movement when the distal end of an extremity is fixed on a supporting surface.

Guttman scaling—Cumulative scales that present a set of items that reflect increasing intensities of the characteristic being measured.

Motor control—The mechanisms by which individuals regulate and coordinate actions to perform tasks.

Motor learning—The process by which individuals develop skilled control in performing motor tasks.

Muscle tone—A muscle's readiness to reflexively respond to stretch.

Open kinematic chain—A system in which body segments are free to move without causing motion at another joint; occurs during human movement when the distal end of an extremity moves freely in space.

Postural adjustments—Automatic, anticipatory mechanisms that enable an individual to maintain balance against gravity, optimal alignment between body parts, and optimal orientation of the head, trunk, and limbs with relation to the environment.

Postural control—Ability to maintain optimal postural alignment and balance in a variety of dynamic activities in changing environments.

Postural responses (reactions)—An older term used to describe postural adjustments; overlooks the automatic, anticipatory qualities of these mechanisms.

Primitive reflexes—Involuntary, often abnormal, changes in muscle tone in response to quick stretch of muscles or changes in the position or orientation of the head.

Reflex-inhibiting patterns—Combinations of movements designed to decrease tone in spastic muscles and facilitate active movement; advocated by NDT in the 1970s.

Spasticity—Hyperactive response to stretch in selected muscle groups.

REFERENCES

Ada, L., & Westwood, P. (1992). A kinematic analysis of recovery of the ability to stand up following stroke. *Australian Physiotherapy, 38,* 135–142.

Adams, S. A. (1993a). A study to test the scalability of the Rivermead Motor Assessment with acute stroke patients [Abstract]. *Physiotherapy, 79,* 506.

Adams, S. A. (1993b). A study to test the scalability of the Rivermead Motor Assessment with non-acute strokes over 65 [Abstract]. *Clinical Rehabilitation, 7,* 358.

Arsenault, A. B., Dutil, E., Lambert, J., Corriveau, H., Guarna, F., & Drouin, G. (1988). An evaluation of the hemiplegic subject based on the Bobath approach. Part III: A validation study. *Scandinavian Journal of Rehabilitation Medicine, 20,* 13–16.

Ashburn, A. (1982). A physical assessment for stroke patients. *Physiotherapy, 68,* 109–113.

Badke, M. B., & Duncan, P. W. (1983). Patterns of motor responses during postural adjustments when standing in healthy subjects and hemiplegic patients. *Physical Therapy, 63,* 13–20.

Berglund, K., & Fugl-Meyer, A. R. (1986). Upper extremity function in hemiplegia: A cross-validation study of two assessment methods. *Scandinavian Journal of Rehabilitation Medicine, 18,* 155–157.

Bernstein, N. (1967). *The coordination and regulation of movements.* Oxford: Pergamon Press.

Bobath, B. (1970). *Adult hemiplegia: Evaluation and treatment.* London: Heinemann Medical Books.

Bobath, B. (1978). *Adult hemiplegia: Evaluation and treatment* (2nd ed.). London: Heinemann Medical Books.

Bobath, B. (1990). *Adult hemiplegia: Evaluation and treatment* (3rd ed.). London: Heinemann Medical Books.

Brunia, C. H. M., Haagh, S., & Scheirs, J. G. M. (1985). Waiting to respond: Electrophysiological measurements in man during preparation for a voluntary movement. In H. Heuer, U. Kleinbeck, & K. Schmidt (Eds.), *Motor behavior: Programming, control and acquisition* (pp. 35–78). Berlin: Springer-Verlag.

Brunnstrom, S. (1970). *Movement therapy in hemiplegia.* New York: Harper & Row.

Carr, J. H. (1992). Compensatory and substitution movements following acute brain lesions: Useful or not? Proceedings of World Confederation for Physical Therapy (pp. 985–987), London.

Carr, J. H., & Shepherd, R. B. (1987a). A motor learning model for rehabilitation. In J. H. Carr, R. B. Shepherd, J. Gordon, A. M. Gentile, & J. M. Held (Eds.), *Movement science: Foundations for physical therapy in rehabilitation* (pp. 31–91). Rockville, MD: Aspen Systems Corp.

Carr, J. H., & Shepherd, R. B. (1990). A motor learning model for rehabilitation of the movement-disabled. In L. Ada & C. Canning (Eds.), *Key issues in neurological physiotherapy.* Oxford: Butterworth Heinemann.

Carr, J. H., & Shepherd, R. B. (1989). A motor learning model for stroke rehabilitation. *Physiotherapy, 75,* 372–379.

Carr, J. H., & Shepherd, R. B. (1987b). *A motor relearning program for stroke* (2nd ed.). Rockville, MD: Aspen Systems Corp.

Carr, J. H., Shepherd, R. B., Nordholm, L., & Lynne, D. (1985). Investigation of a new motor assessment scale for stroke patients. *Physical Therapy, 65,* 175–180.

Carroll, D. (1965). A quantitative test of upper extremity function. *Journal of Chronic Disease, 18,* 479–491.

Corriveau, H., Arsenault, A. B., Dutil, E., Besner, C., Dupuis, C., Guarna, F., & Lambert, J. (1992). An evaluation of the hemiplegic patient based on the Bobath approach: A reliability study. *Disability and Rehabilitation, 14,* 81–84.

Corriveau, H., Arsenault, A. B., Dutil, E., & Lepage, Y. (1992). *Disability and rehabilitation, 14,* 85–88.

Corriveau, H., Guarna, F., Dutil, E., Riley, E., Arsenault, A. B., & Drouin, G. (1988). An evaluation of the hemiplegic subject based on the Bobath approach. Part II: The evaluation protocol. *Scandinavian Journal of Rehabilitation Medicine, 20,* 5–11.

Davies, P. M. (1990). *Right in the middle: Selective trunk activity in the treatment of adult hemiplegia.* Berlin & New York: Springer-Verlag.

Davies, P. M. (1985). *Steps to follow—A guide to the treatment of adult hemiplegia.* Berlin & New York: Springer-Verlag.

Dean, C., & Mackey, F. (1992). Motor assessment scale scores as a measure of rehabilitation outcome follwing stroke. *Australian Physiotherapy, 38,* 31–35.

DeSouza, L. H., Langton Hewer, R. L., Miller, S. (1980). Assessment of recovery of arm control in hemiplegic stroke patients. Arm function tests. *International Rehabilitation Medicine, 2,* 3–9.

deWeerdt, W., Crossley, S. M., Lincoln, N. B., & Harrison, M. A. (1989). Restoration of balance in stroke patients: A single case design study. *Clinical Rehabilitation, 3,* 139–147.

deWeerdt, W., & Harrison, M. A. (1985). Measuring recovery of arm-hand function in stroke patients: A comparison of the Brunnstrom-Fugl-Meyer test and the Action Research Arm test. *Physiotherapy Canada, 37,* 65–70.

Duncan, P. W., & Badke, M. B. (1987). *Stroke rehabilitation: The recovery of motor control.* St. Louis: Year Book Medical.

Duncan, P. W., Goldstein, L. B., Matchar, D., Divine, G. W., & Feussner, J. (1992). Measurement of motor recovery after stroke: Outcome assessment and sample size requirements. *Stroke, 23,* 1084–1089.

Duncan, P. W., Propst, M., & Nelson, S. G. (1983). Reliability of the Fugl-Meyer Assessment of sensorimotor recovery following cerebrovascular accident. *Physical Therapy, 63,* 1606–1610.

Dutil, E., Filiatrault, J., DeSerres, L., Arsenault, A. B. (1990). *Evaluation of upper extremity function in subjects with hemiplegia* (in French). Montreal: University of Montreal Library.

Eggers, O. (1984). *Occupational therapy in the treatment of adult hemiplegia.* London: Heinemann Medical Books.

Ferrucci, L., Bandinelli, S., Guralnik, J. M., Lamponi, M., Bertini, C., Falchini, M., & Baroni, A. (1993). Recovery of functional status after stroke: A postrehabilitation follow-up study. *Stroke, 24,* 200–205.

Filiatrault, J., Arsenault, A. B., Dutil, E., & Bourbonnais, D. (1991). Motor function and activities of daily living assessments: A study of three tests for persons with hemiplegia. *American Journal of Occupational Therapy, 45,* 806–810.

Fugl-Meyer, A. R. (1980). Post-stroke hemiplegia: Assessment of physical properties. *Scandinavian Journal of Rehabilitation Medicine, 7*(Suppl.), 83–93.

Fugl-Meyer, A. R., Jaasko, L., Leyman, I., Olsson, S., & Steglind, S. (1975). The post-stroke hemiplegic patient: A method of evaluation of physical performance. *Scandinavian Journal of Rehabilitation Medicine, 7,* 13–31.

Gentile, A. M. (1987). Skill acquisition: Action, movement, and neuromotor processes. In J. H. Carr, R. B. Shepherd, J. Gordon, A. M. Gentile, & J. M. Held (Eds.), *Movement science: Foundations for physical therapy in rehabilitation* (pp. 93–154). Rockville, MD: Aspen Systems Corp.

Gentile, A. M. (1972). A working model of skill acquisition with application to teaching. *Quest, 17,* 3–23.

Gordon, J. (1987). Assumptions underlying physical therapy intervention: Theoretical and historical perspectives. In J. H. Carr, R. B. Shepherd, J. Gordon, A. M. Gentile, & J. M. Held (Eds.), *Movement science: Foundations for physical therapy in rehabilitation* (pp. 1–30). Rockville, MD: Aspen Systems Corp.

Gowland, C. A. (1990). Staging motor impairment after stroke. *Stroke, 21*(Suppl. II), II-19–II-21.

Guarna, F., Corriveau, H., Chamberland, J., Arsenault, A. B., Dutil, E., Drouin, G. (1988). An evaluation of the hemiplegic subject based on the Bobath approach. Part I: The model. *Scandinavian Journal of Rehabilitation Medicine, 20,* 1–4.

Guttman, L. (1944). A basis for scaling qualitative data. *American Sociological Review, 9,* 139.

Jackson, J. H., & Taylor, J. (Eds.). (1932). *Selected writings of John B. Hughlings, I and II.* London: Hodder & Stoughter.

Jarus, T. (1994). Motor learning and occupational therapy: The organization of practice. *American Journal of Occupational Therapy, 48,* 810–816.

Juby, L. C., Lincoln, N. B., & Berman, P. (1994). *The effect of stroke unit rehabilitation on functional and psychological outcome: A randomized controlled trial.* Stroke Research Unit, Nottingham City Hospital, Nottingham, England. Unpublished study.

Knott, M., & Voss, D. E. (1956). *Proprioceptive neuromuscular facilitation: Patterns and techniques* (2nd ed.), Philadelphia: Harper and Row.

Kraft, G. H., Fitts, S. S., & Hammond, M. C. (1992). Techniques to improve function of the arm and hand. *Archives of Physical Medicine and Rehabilitation, 73,* 220–227.

Kusoffsky, A., Wadell, I., & Nilsson, B. Y. (1982). The relationship between sensory impairment and motor recovery in patients with hemiplegia. *Scandinavian Journal of Rehabilitation Medicine, 18,* 155–157.

Lincoln, N., & Leadbitter, D. (1979). Assessment of motor function in stroke patients. *Physiotherapy, 65,* 48–51.

Loewen, S. C., & Anderson, B. A. (1990). Predictors of stroke outcome using objective measurement scales. *Stroke, 21,* 78–81.

Loewen, S. C., & Anderson, B. A. (1988). Reliability of the Modified Motor Assessment Scale and the Barthel Index. *Physical Therapy, 68,* 1077–1081.

Lyden, P. D., & Lau, G. T. (1991). A critical appraisal of stroke evaluation and rating scales. *Stroke, 22,* 1345–1352.

Lyle, R. C. (1981). A performance test for assessment of upper limb function in physical rehabilitation treatment and research. *International Journal of Rehabilitation Research, 4,* 483–492.

Mathiowetz, V., & Bass-Haugen, J. (1994). Motor behavior research:

Implications for therapeutic approaches to central nervous system dysfunction. *American Journal of Occupational Therapy, 48,* 733–745.

Nashner, L. M., & McCollum, G. (1985). The organization of human postural movements: A formal basis and experimental synthesis. *The Behavioral and Brain Sciences, 8,* 135–172.

Nugent, J. A., & Schurr, K. A. (1994). A dose-response relationship between amount of weight-bearing exercise and walking outcome following cerebrovascular accident. *Archives of Physical Medicine and Rehabilitation, 75,* 399–402.

Parker, V. M., Wade, D. T., & Langton-Hewer, R. (1986). Loss of arm function after stroke: Measurement, frequency and recovery. *International Rehabilitation Medicine, 8,* 69–73.

Poole, J. (1991). Motor control. In C. B. Royeen (Ed.), *AOTA self study series: Neuroscience foundations of human performance.* Rockville, MD, American Occupational Therapy Association.

Poole, J. L., & Whitney, S. L. (1988). Motor assessment scale for stroke patients: Concurrent validity and interrater reliability. *Archives of Physical Medicine and Rehabilitation, 69,* 195–197.

Portney, L. G., & Watkins, M. P. (1993). *Foundations of clinical research: Applications to practice.* Norwalk, CT: Appleton & Lange.

Rood, M. S. (1956). Neurophysiological mechanisms utilized in the treatment of neuromuscular dysfunction. *American Journal of Occupational Therapy, 10,* 220–225.

Rood, M. S. (1954). Neurophysiological reactions as a basis for physical therapy. *Physical Therapy Review, 34,* 444–449.

Sabari, J. S. (1991). Motor learning concepts applied to activity-based intervention with adults with hemiplegia. *American Journal of Occupational Therapy, 45,* 523–530.

Sabari, J. S. (1994). Normal postural adjustments. In *AOTA Resource Guide: CVA (Stroke)* (pp. 64, 65), Rockville, MD: American Occupational Therapy Association.

Sahrmann, S. A., & Norton, B. J. (1977). The relationship of voluntary movement to spasticity in the upper motor neuron syndrome. *Annals of Neurology, 2,* 460–465.

Saltzman E., & Kelso, J. A. S. (1987). Skilled actions: A task-dynamic approach. *Psychological Review, 94,* 84–106.

Sawner, K., & LaVigne, J. M. (1992). Brunnstrom's movement therapy in hemiplegia: A neurophysiological approach (2nd ed.). Philadelphia: J. B. Lippincott.

Schmidt, R. A. (1992). *Motor performance and learning: Principles for practitioners.* Champaign, IL: Human Kinetics.

Shepherd, R. B. (1992). Adaptive motor behaviour in response to perturbations of balance. *Physiotherapy Theory and Practice, 8,* 137–143.

Shepherd, R. B., & Carr, J. H.(1991). An emergent or dynamical systems view of movement dysfunction. *Australian Journal of Physiotherapy, 37,* 4, 5.

Sjogren, K., & Fugl-Meyer, A. R. (1982). Adjustment to life after stroke with special reference to sexual intercourse and leisure. *Journal of Psychosomatic Research, 26,* 409–417.

Summers, J. J. (1989). Motor programs. In D. Holding (Ed.), *Human skills* (2nd ed.) (pp. 49–69). New York: Wiley.

Trombly, C. A. (1992). Deficits of reaching in subjects with left hemiparesis: A pilot study. *American Journal of Occupational Therapy, 46,* 887–897.

Trombly, C. A. (1993). Observations of improvement of reaching in five subjects with left hemiparesis. *Journal of Neurology, Neurosurgery, & Psychiatry, 56*(1), 40–45.

Twitchell, T. E. (1951). The restoration of motor function following hemiplegia in man. *Brain, 74,* 443–480.

Wade, D. T., Langton-Hewer, R., Wood, V. A., Skilbeck, C. E., & Ismail, H. M. (1983). The hemiplegic arm after stroke: Measurement and recovery. *Journal of Neurology, Neurosurgery, and Psychiatry, 46,* 521–524.

Wilcock, A. A. (1986). *Occupational therapy approaches to stroke.* Melbourne: Churchill Livingstone.

Wilson, D. J., Baker, L. L., & Craddock, J. A. (1984). Functional test for the hemiparetic upper extremity. *American Journal of Occupational Therapy, 38,* 159–164.

Upper Motor Neuron Syndrome

James Agostinucci, ScD, OTR

SUMMARY   This subchapter briefly describes the available methods for assessing the symptoms related to upper motor neuron syndrome (UMNS). The procedures described are predominantly limited to more practical assessment techniques that physical and occupational therapists may use in evaluating UMNS clinically. More sophisticated, albeit not necessarily practical, evaluations are included if they are noninvasive and appear valid and reliable. In addition, semiquantitative evaluations, such as timed motor tasks, are not included because research does not support their use as a valid and reliable measure of UMNS.

The clinical importance for measuring symptoms is extremely important, especially as the health care system evolves. It would be inappropriate to focus treatment on a particular symptom (spasticity) if one could not accurately document change. This subchapter reviews many techniques used to evaluate the symptoms related to UMNS and spasticity. No one assessment stands out as being superior to others; some are more appropriate clinically, whereas others are more suited for research study. Furthermore, some evaluations are better at documenting change, whereas others are superior at quantifying intensity of symptoms. Therefore, clinicians need to choose the appropriate assessments that fit their needs. Knowledge of the assessment's advantages and disadvantages will help in this decision.

Upper motor neuron refers to central nervous system (CNS) cells whose axons form descending motor pathways that either directly or indirectly exert influences on lower motoneurons (Noback et al., 1991). The term *upper motor neuron* is often used interchangeably with *corticospinal* and *pyramidal neuron*. The pyramidal or the corticospinal system refers to those fibers that originate in the cerebral cortex and descend to the spinal cord through the medullary pyramids. Corticospinal fibers decussate in the lower medulla and enter the spinal cord as the lateral corticospinal and anterior corticospinal tracts. The corticospinal tracts are the only tracts that directly connect the cerebral cortex to the spinal cord. There are other descending cortical systems that travel to the spinal cord; however, they synapse in the brain stem before going to spinal levels. These other "extrapyramidal" tracts also are included in the term *upper motor neuron* (Carpenter, 1991; Kandel et al., 1991; Kuypers, 1981).

Lower motor neuron refers to motor neurons (alpha cells) that innervate and control voluntary skeletal muscle. Destruction of lower motor neurons results in a loss of voluntary and reflex responses of the denervated muscle. Afterward, the muscle rapidly atrophies, and flaccid paralysis ensues (Carpenter, 1991; Kandel et al., 1991; Kuypers, 1981).

In this subchapter, the term *upper motor neuron syndrome* denotes the spasticity resulting mainly from corticospinal lesions. It must be realized that most lesions of the CNS damage structures other than corticospinal pathways. They also involve various other "extrapyramidal" CNS structures. The functional loss following an upper motor neuron lesion, therefore, varies, depending on the structures involved.

Symptoms from upper motor neuron syndromes may be subdivided into two categories, abnormal behaviors (positive symptoms) and performance deficits (negative symptoms) (Table 11–9) (Katz & Rymer, 1989). Abnormal behaviors are defined as exaggerated movements that result from the release of descending inhibitory control. The symptoms that fall into this category are the Babinski reflex, loss of autonomic control, exaggerated flexor reflexes, increased proprioceptive reflexes, hypertonia, clonus, spasticity, and other synkinesias. These deficits are more likely observed in individuals with spinal cord injury, as these patients have lost the connections to higher control centers (Katz & Rymer, 1989).

Performance deficits (positive symptoms), on the other hand, are symptoms more likely seen in patients with cerebral vascular accident (CVA) or traumatic brain injury (TBI). In this group, patients usually exhibit muscle weakness, fatigability, and loss of dexterity. Several physiologic factors may contribute to these performance deficits. For a complete review, refer to Katz and colleagues (1992), Landau (1980), Giuliani (1991), Dohrmann and Nowack (1974), and Dimitrijevic and Nathan (1967). Performance deficits produce the functional disability seen in upper motor neuron syndromes, although more visually dramatic symptoms are identified with abnormal behaviors (Bishop, 1977; Hagbarth, 1993; Young & Wiegner, 1987).

The goal for all therapists is to have their patients achieve functional independence. The physical impairment that results from upper motor neuron disease usually jeopardizes a person's ability to perform many daily living tasks. Initially, the therapist must assess the patient's level of functioning and then develop a treatment plan that will improve or eliminate the factors that are hindering performance. As the course of rehabilitation proceeds, intermittent systematic assessments are conducted to objectively determine patient progress.

In today's changing world of health care distribution, the role of objective assessment is becoming as important as the therapy itself. With the rising cost of health care, insurance companies are demanding more objective assessment regularly. Previously, clinical assessment was based on observation. The therapist would use a checklist indicating whether a functional item could be accom-

---

TABLE 11–9

UPPER MOTOR NEURON SYNDROME

Abnormal behaviors (positive symptoms)
   Reflex release phenomena (pathologic reflexes)
   Hyperactive proprioceptive reflexes
   Increased resistance to stretch
   Relaxed cutaneous reflexes
   Loss of precise autonomic control
Performance deficits (negative symptoms)
   Decreased dexterity
   Paresis/weakness
   Fatigability

From Katz R. T., & Rymer, W. Z. (1989). Spastic hypertonia: Mechanisms and measurement. *Archives of Physical Medicine and Rehabilitation,* 70; 144–155.

plished. Assessments such as these are less sensitive than other techniques, invalid, and not reliable. The lack of effective objective measurement techniques has been restrictive for physical and occupational therapists, since quantification is necessary to evaluate various modes of treatment. Efforts to develop quantifiable assessments have been limited.

This subchapter discusses the assessment tools advocated to quantitatively evaluate the symptoms of upper motor neuron syndrome. Quantification of these symptoms has been a difficult and challenging problem.

POSITIVE SYMPTOMS—SPASTICITY (ABNORMAL BEHAVIORS)

Spasticity is defined as "a motor disorder characterized by a velocity-dependent increase in tonic stretch reflexes (muscle tone) with exaggerated tendon jerks, resulting from hyperexcitability of the stretch reflex, as one component of upper motor neuron syndrome" (Lance & Burke, 1974). Clinicians perceive spasticity as a major impairment for individuals with upper motor neuron lesions. Many therapists believe spasticity is the cause of the abnormal movements and poor dexterity observed following upper motor neuron lesions. Although debatable, research has shown that spasticity rarely causes movement abnormalities (Young & Wiegner, 1987). Indeed, spasticity has been useful in helping some patients stand, dress, and transfer.

The controversy over the dehabilitating effect of spasticity is partially due to the heterogeneity of its clinical status. The heterogeneity arises from the numerous different sites in the CNS that may be damaged, the time from the injury, and the nature of the reaction of the CNS to the injury (Dimitrijevic et al., 1989). This is probably one of the reasons spasticity is so hard to quantify. The need to quantify functional disability is important since therapists need to correlate rehabilitative procedures with functional progress. This section provides the reader with a critical review of the more common assessment techniques concerning spasticity.

Neurophysiologic Assessments

Increased motor neuron excitability (MNE) is found in patients with upper motor neuron lesions and hyperreflexia (Magladery et al., 1953). Clinically, monosynaptic reflexes provide a means for testing phasic stretch reflexes, a cardinal feature in spasticity. Physicians have routinely assessed the strength of patient's stretch reflexes as part of the neurologic examination. Increased strength and speed of the stretch reflex are hallmark responses in clinically diagnosing muscle spasticity (Greenberg et al., 1993; Pryse-Phillips & Murray, 1985).

This section describes the electrophysiologic procedures that measure the mechanical and electrical features of tendon jerks and muscle hypertonia.

TENDON REFLEXES

Tendon reflexes (T-reflexes) are based on a two-neuron or monosynaptic reflex arc. Slight stretching of a muscle activates the neuromuscular spindle, and the resultant excitation travels to the spinal cord via the large Ia muscle spindle afferents. Ia axons synapse on and excite alpha motor neurons, causing the stretched muscle to contract (Fig. 11–3). This reflex is considered a postural reflex, since muscle spindles monitor changes in muscle length. The stretch reflex is the basis of the T-reflex that is used in neurologic examinations. A hammer delivers a sharp blow (tap) to the muscle tendon, stretching the muscle and its spindles, resulting in reflex contraction of the homologous muscle. The level of spasticity is evaluated by subjectively assessing the degree of reflex muscle contraction. The results are recorded on an ordinal scale where 0 equals no response and +2 and +4 are normal and hyperactive responses, respectively. Between values represent variations in muscle tone activity (Greenberg et al., 1993).

Electromyography (EMG) is utilized when more objective and precise assessments are needed. T-reflex amplitudes are measured and compared with normative values obtained from a population of healthy people. Mean values equal to or greater than 2 standard deviations above normative values are considered abnormal and indicative of spasticity (Ottenbacher, 1986).

Another assessment procedure uses the ratio of supramaximal T-reflexes to the supramaximal direct motor response* (T_{max}/M_{max}). Since it is presumed that the maximal direct motor (M) response represents the total motor neuron pool activated by a maximal stimulus, the ratio of T_{max} to M_{max} represents the percentage of the motor neuron pool participating in the T-reflex. This method assumes that presynaptic inhibition by descending tracts is held constant. Patients with severe hyperreflexia have T_{max}/M_{max} ratios around 1, whereas the ratios of subjects with normal tone are much lower (Dimitrijevic & Nathan, 1967). Treatment effects are assessed by the ratio of posttreatment to pretreatment measurements (T-reflex$_{after}$/T-reflex$_{before}$). Decreasing ratios represent positive treatment outcomes.

The use of T-reflexes in quantifying spasticity has many disadvantages. Objective quantification of T-reflexes requires a constant testing environment (Bishop, 1977). Patient positioning and limb stabilization must be controlled to prevent these parameters from altering the response under study. A constant force striking the tendon

---

*The direct motor response or M-wave is a nonreflexive muscle contraction after stimulating a mixed nerve. Electrical stimulation initiates a nerve impulse in motor fibers that travels directly to the muscle without involving spinal cord neurons. The muscle contraction elicited occurs sooner than a reflex contraction because the nerve impulse travels a shorter distance and has no synaptic delay.

participation of individual mechanisms in spasticity is not equivalent. Each patient has his or her own pathophysiologic profile. This is probably why individually the neurophysiologic techniques described do not correlate well with spasticity's clinical picture. Each neurophysiologic assessment only assesses one spinal cord mechanism. Thus, neurophysiologic techniques should be used in combination. In so doing, a pathophysiologic profile or functional baseline will be established with which to compare all future assessments.

Clinical Assessments

Clinical evaluations have been used extensively to quantify spasticity. They are easy to perform, inexpensive, and usually can be conducted in a short time. More importantly, the examiner can account for the confounding influencing factors that affect the state of spasticity at any given moment. Factors such as level of stress, bladder distention, subject position, and the state of neighboring muscles can influence the degree of spasticity (Young & Wiegner, 1987). Neurophysiologic tests often cannot account for these extraneous confounding factors without employing regimented protocols that are tedious and time consuming to perform. Therefore, although subjective and not overly reliable, clinical assessments remain the method of choice to assess spasticity.

The following section describes the clinical assessments that are commonly used to quantify spasticity. Each assessment is briefly described.

MODIFIED ASHWORTH SCALE

Ashworth was the first to devise an objective means to assess the severity of spasticity. The Ashworth scale involves manually moving a limb through the range of motion to stretch specific muscle groups. The resistance encountered during the passive muscle stretch is documented on a five-point ordinal scale from 0 to 4, with 0 representing normal tone, and 4 depicting severe spasticity (Ashworth, 1964).

Bohannon and Smith (1987) investigated the interrater reliability of a modified version of the Ashworth scale. They tested elbow flexor muscle spasticity in 30 patients with intracranial lesion. The original Ashworth scale was modified because the lower end of the scale was indiscrete. Grade "+1" was added to render the scale more distinct (Table 11–11). Slight variations in the definitions were also made.

Bohannon and Smith's research showed that the modified Ashworth scale had a high interrater reliability (86.7% agreement between raters). Because of this study, the modified Ashworth scale has become the clinical testing protocol to which all newer tests are compared.

A major difficulty with the Ashworth scale and other tests like it is that with repeated testing, both high and low scores

TABLE 11–11	
MODIFIED ASHWORTH SCALE FOR GRADING SPASTICITY	

Grade	Description
0	No increase in muscle tone
1	Slight increase in muscle tone, manifested by a catch and release or by minimal resistance at the end of the range of motion when the affected part(s) is moved in flexion or extension
1+	Slight increase in muscle tone, manifested by a catch, followed by minimal resistance throughout the remainder (less than half) of the range of motion
2	More marked increase in muscle tone through most of the range of motion, but affected part(s) easily moved
3	Considerable increase in muscle tone, passive movement difficult
4	Affected part(s) rigid in flexion or extension

From Bohannon, R. W., & Smith, M. B. (1987). Interrater reliability of a modified Ashworth scale of muscle spasticity. *Physical Therapy, 67*(2), 206–207.

within an overall range of scores cluster toward the mean. This tendency for scores to migrate toward the mean is termed statistical regression. Statistical regression has been identified as a major source of secondary variation that may produce internal invalidity in an investigation or evaluation (Ottenbacher, 1986). Therefore, the evaluation's validity decreases as the number of times the test is given increases. Clinicians should be instructed to limit the administration of these tests to as few times as possible.

FUGL-MEYER SCALE OF FUNCTIONAL RETURN AFTER HEMIPLEGIA

An alternative evaluation method based on Brunnstrom's qualitative assessments of motor recovery was developed by Fugl-Meyer and colleagues (Fugl-Meyer et al., 1975). The Fugl-Meyer (FM) scale differs from that of Brunnstrom in that it is quantitative and can be statistically analyzed for both research and clinical work. The evaluation is based on the recovery stages after the onset of the ictus. The test requires the subject to perform motor acts graduated in complexity and requires increasingly fine neuromuscular control. The items assessed are muscle tone, state of motor recovery, movement pattern (synergy), movement speed, and prehension pattern of the limbs (Table 11–12). A cumulative numerical scoring system for measurement is used to quantify the level of motor recovery. The FM scale uses an ordinal scoring system in which each detail is rated 0 (cannot be performed), 1 (can be partly performed), or 2 (can be performed faultlessly). Maximum scores range from 0 (flaccidity) to 100 (normal motor function) (Duncan et al., 1983; Fugl-Meyer et al., 1975; Katz et al., 1992; Trombly, 1989).

The Fugl-Meyer scale has been demonstrated to be valid and reliable (intra- and intertester) in the assessment of motor function in people with hemiplegia, although not necessarily in those with spasticity. It is easy to perform and takes approximately 20 minutes to conduct. It is objective and accurate. More important, Katz and coworkers showed that the FM scale correlated well with other clinical measures of spasticity (e.g., the Ashworth scale) (Duncan et al., 1983; Katz et al., 1992).

TABLE 11–12

EXAMPLE OF FUGL-MEYER ASSESSMENT FOR THE UPPER LIMB

Classification and Progress Record

Shoulder and Elbow
Stage
  I. No movement initiated or elicited, flaccidity
  II. Synergies or components may be elicited, spasticity developing
     a. Flexor synergy
     b. Extensor synergy
  III. Synergies or components initiated voluntarily, spasticity marked
     a. Flexor synergy
        1. Shoulder movements
        2. Elbow
        3. Forearm
     b. Extensor synergy
        1. Shoulder girdle protraction
        2. Elbow
        3. Forearm
  IV. Movements deviating from basic synergies, spasticity decreasing
     a. Hand behind back
     b. Raise arm to forward-horizontal
     c. Pronation-supination, elbow at 90 degrees
  V. Relative independence of basic synergies, spasticity waning
     a. Raise arm to side-horizontal
     b. Raise arm forward overhead
     c. Pronation-supination, elbow extended
  VI. Movement coordinated and near normal, spasticity minimal

Wrist
Stage
  I. Wrist stabilization for grasp
     a. Elbow extended
     b. Elbow flexed
  II. Wrist flexion and extension, fist closed
     a. Elbow extended
     b. Elbow flexed
  III. Wrist circumduction (stabilize forearm)

Digits
Stage
  I. Flaccidity, no voluntary movement
  II. Little or no active finger flexion
  III. Mass grasp or hook grasp
  IV. Lateral prehension; release by thumb movement
     a. Semivoluntary mass extension—small range of motion
  V. Palmar prehension
     a. Voluntary mass extension—variable range of motion
     b. Spherical grasp (awkward)
     c. Cylindrical grasp (awkward)
  VI. All types of grasp with improved skill
     a. Voluntary finger extension—full range of motion
     b. Individual finger movements (do dexterity tests)

Trombly, C. (1989). Motor control therapy. In C. Trombly (ed.), *Occupational therapy for physical dysfunction,* 3rd ed. Baltimore: Williams & Wilkins.

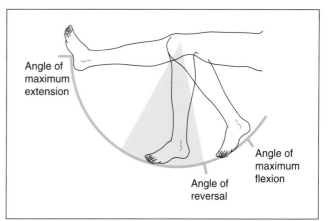

FIGURE 11–9. The pendulum-like movements (swinging back and forth) of the leg after it has been dropped from the extended position.

PENDULUM TEST

The pendulum test for spasticity is conducted by placing subjects in a comfortable supine position on a tilt table with both legs bent over the edge, hanging free at the knee. The thigh is supported distally. The examiner grasps the subject's ankle, raises it to full extension (horizontal position), and releases it, allowing the leg to fall freely. The leg swings back and forth like a pendulum for a short time before the motion is damped by the viscoelastic properties of the limb (Fig. 11–9) (Boczko & Mumenthaler, 1958; Bohannon, 1987).

Knee movement is recorded by an electrogoniometer. Hypertonicity is assessed by taking the angular difference between maximum knee flexion (angle a in Figure 11–10) and the angle of flexion at which the knee first reversed direction toward extension (angle d in Figure 11–10). Bohannon termed this difference (d–a) the "relative angle of reversal" (Bohannon, 1987).

An alternative method of calculation was described by Katz and colleagues and is illustrated in Figure 11–11. The amplitude of the limb motion as it fell from the fully

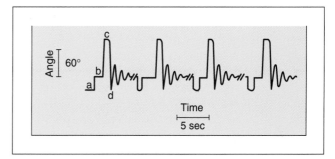

FIGURE 11–10. Goniometric tracings from a pendulum test of patients with intracranial lesions. Figure represents a normal pendulum test. (a = Angle of maximum possible knee flexion; b = angle of the knee with the leg hanging freely; c = knee fully extended; d = angle of flexion at which the knee first reverses direction after the leg is dropped. d–a = relative angle of reversal.) (Adapted from Bohannon, R. W., & Smith, M. B. [1987]. Interrater reliability of a modified Ashworth Scale of Muscle Spasticity. *Physical Therapy, 67*(2), 206–207, with the permission of the APTA.)

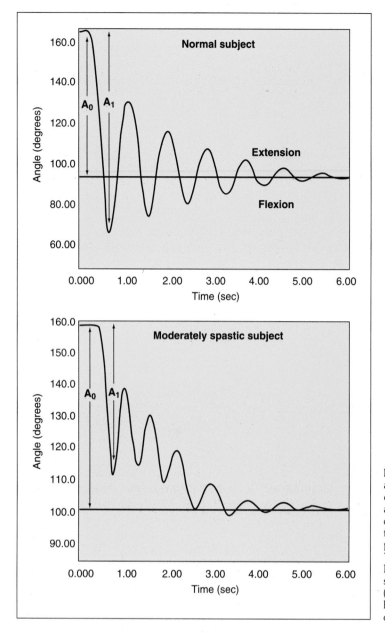

FIGURE 11–11. The pendulum movements of the lower limb after it is released from the extended position. Diagram also demonstrates a method to assess spastic hypertonia of the quadriceps and hamstring muscle groups. A_0 represents the amplitudes of the damped sinusoidal curve as the limb falls from the extended position to the final resting angle. A_1 represents the amplitude of the plotted waveform from full extension to its first absolute minimum. *Top,* A normal subject. *Bottom,* A moderately spastic subject. Note the marked damping of the altered sinusoidal curve in the spastic subject. (Refer to text for full explanation of assessment.) (From Katz, R. T., et al. [1992]. Objective quantification of spastic hypertonia: Correlation with clinical findings. *Archives of Physical Medicine and Rehabilitation, 70,* 339–347.)

extended position to the final resting angle was measured (A_0) and compared with the amplitude of limb motion from full extension to its first absolute minimum angle (A_1). They called this ratio the relaxation index (RI = A_1/A_0). Since in neurologically healthy individuals, the RI is generally more than 1.6, a correction factor was introduced to the RI equation (CRI), where CRI = $A_1/1.6A_0$. A CRI value greater than 1 signifies a nonspastic limb, and a CRI less than 1 signifies various degrees of spasticity (Katz et al., 1992). Katz and colleagues used this calculation method of the pendulum test in the quantification of spasticity. They demonstrated that the pendulum test accurately identified a spastic limb in all of their subjects who had clinical evidence of spasticity. Furthermore, intrasubject and intersubject variability was stable, and the test correlated significantly with their clinical scale.

These results strongly endorse the pendulum test as a measure of spasticity. The pendulum test is an accurate and reliable means of quantifying spasticity; however, one shortcoming is that it can only be performed manually on the lower extremity quadriceps muscle group. Another weakness in the manually performed pendulum test is that the undamped acceleration of the leg when dropped may exceed a limb acceleration of greater than 300 degrees per second. Since spasticity is velocity dependent and accelerations of this magnitude are not physiologic, the test becomes less sensitive and unimportant.

Biomechanical equipment can be used to simulate the pendulum test (Bohannon & Larkin, 1985). One such system is the Cybex II isokinetic dynamometer. The Cybex II system allows the examiner to precisely measure the reflexive induced muscle resistance while the muscle is stretched at various predetermined rates. Furthermore, large muscle groups from all four extremities can be tested.

Bohannon (1987) studied the between-trial variability and reliability of the pendulum test performed with the Cybex II isokinetic dynamometer. Using the relative angle of reversal method (RAR) of calculation, he demonstrated no significant difference in the RAR among four leg drops in 30 patients with spasticity. Bohannon concluded that the test performed on the Cybex II isokinetic dynamometer was reliable (r = 0.96). The variability in the testing procedure over long times (days to weeks), however, was not examined and remained questionable.

TORQUE/ELECTROMYOGRAM CURVES—RAMP AND HOLD

The ramp and hold technique measures the amount of torque produced during a specified passive joint movement. Threshold angle, the angle at which a significant increase occurs in torque or EMG activity, is also measured (Katz & Rymer, 1989; Katz et al., 1992; Myklebust et al., 1989; Powers et al., 1988; Powers et al., 1989).

The subject usually is connected to a device that is coupled to a servo-controlled torque motor (Fig. 11–12). The torque motor applies a force to the device that passively moves the limb though a specified horizontal displacement at different velocities (i.e., 0.25, 0.5, 1.0 radians per second). Angular position and velocity are measured by a potentiometer and tachometer attached to the motor shaft. The torque generated by the subject is measured by a torque meter. The EMG activity is recorded in the agonist and antagonist muscle groups. The degree of spastic hypertonia is measured by assessing the magnitude of torque evoked in response to the stretch. The threshold angle is determined by a change in the slope of the torque recording and the onset of EMG activity due to activation of the stretch reflex.

Figure 11–13 is an example from a subject with hemiparesis. The responses are from the unaffected side (N) and the side of hemiparesis (S). The subject was asked to relax while a series of elbow extension movements were administered to the limb. Each trial consisted of extending the limb through an arc of 1 radian (57.3 degrees) at a constant angular velocity of 0.5 radians per second (Powers et al., 1988).

Initial torque deflections observed in Figure 11–13 are relatively constant between the two limbs. This is because the initial ramp phase is due to the limb's inertia and should be the same between the left and right limbs. The torque, therefore, remains relatively low and constant during the initial portion of the lengthening movement. Torque and EMG activity begin to increase, compared with those of the unaffected limb, once the onset of reflex-mediated EMG activity develops. This increase occurs approximately one third of the way through the ramp phase.

Powers and colleagues (1988) used the ramp and hold technique to investigate the relative contributions of the stretch reflex threshold to stretch evoked torque in subjects

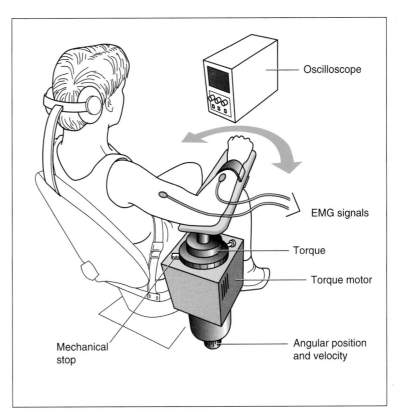

FIGURE 11–12. A servo-controlled motorically driven device, which applies ramp and hold movements to the upper extremity. Such an apparatus allows measurement of angular position and velocity in the horizontal plane. Electromyographic activity in the biceps brachialis, brachioradialis, and lateral triceps muscles can be measured with surface electrodes. (From Katz, R. T., & Rymer, W. Z. [1989]. Spastic hypertonia: Mechanisms and measurement. *Archives of Physical Medicine and Rehabilitation, 70,* 144–155.)

with spasticity. Comparisons of ramp and hold measures were correlated with clinical measures of hypertonia. The clinical measure was based on a 1 to 5 ordinal scale, where 1 and 2 corresponded to mild spasticity, and 4 and 5 related to severe spasticity. The authors demonstrated that subjects with clinical ratings less than 3 tended to have low values of stretch-evoked torque (0.9 to 4.7 Nm) and high threshold values (0.26 to 1.00 Nm). Subjects with high clinical ratings had higher torque values (3.3 to 4.7 Nm) and low thresholds (0.05 to 0.34 Nm). Intermediate ratings were more variable. On the basis of these findings, Powers and associates concluded that there was a definite correlation, although broad, between the ramp and hold technique and the clinical assessment of spasticity.

Two other studies that investigated the use of the ramp and hold technique to quantify spasticity showed similar results. Significant correlations were noted between ramp and hold torque measurements and threshold angles and the Ashworth and Fugl-Meyer scales of hypertonicity. Intrasubject and intersubject variability were nonsignificant even when the clinical perception of spasticity changed. The authors concluded that the ramp and hold test is consistently related to clinical measures of spastic hypertonia and is more accurate than other clinical measures presently used (Katz et al., 1992; Katz & Rymer, 1989).

The disadvantage of the ramp and hold technique is with the stretch stimulus that evokes the reflex. The stretch stimulus consistency varies with stretch velocity, enhancing as velocity increases and diminishing when velocity decreases (a reason for using isokinetic devices that allow a maintained constant rate of stretch). On the other hand, when velocity is held constant over an angular range, the stimulus again varies due to the differences in the mechanical advantage of muscles at different joint angles.

SPASTICITY MEASUREMENT SYSTEM—SINUSOIDAL OSCILLATION

To avoid the difficulties of the ramp and hold method just mentioned, an alternative method to quantify spasticity can be used. This method uses sinusoidally oscillating motions imposed on a joint as the stimulus to evoke muscle responses. Sinusoidal oscillations are claimed to produce more repeatable and controllable stimulus parameters than the ramp method (Lehmann et al., 1989).

Subjects are positioned prone on a padded plinth, with the knee straight, the foot secured to a footplate, and the ankle aligned with the footplate shaft. A motor randomly imposes sinusoidal oscillating motions on the joint at frequencies ranging from 3 to 12 Hz. The torque is measured in response to the oscillating movement through a 5-degree arc. Figure 11–14 demonstrates schematically the device used to move and record data from the lower limb.

Fourier analysis techniques are used to measure the amplitude and phase shift of the torque waveform, relative to the displacement waveform, to characterize spasticity (Agarwal & Gottlieb, 1977; Lehmann et al., 1989; Price et al., 1991; Rack et al., 1984). This system was termed the spasticity measurement system (SMS) and is shown sche-

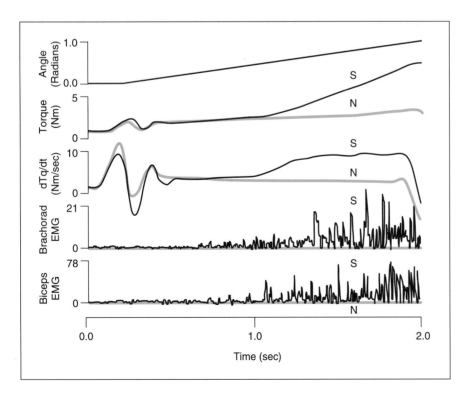

FIGURE 11–13. Stretch responses from a healthy arm and an arm with spasticity. Each elbow began in a position of 120 degrees (–2 radians) of flexion and was extended one radian at 0.5 radians per second. *Top,* Elbow angle (radians). *Second from top,* Torque (newton-meters [Nm]). *Middle,* Time derivative of the torque tract ([dTq/dT, which provides a measure of stiffness]). Rectified EMG recorded from the brachialis *(second from bottom)* and biceps *(bottom)* muscles. (From Powers, R. K., et al. [1988]. Quantitative relations between hypertonia and stretch reflex threshold in spastic hemiparesis. *Annals of Neurology, 23,* 115–124.)

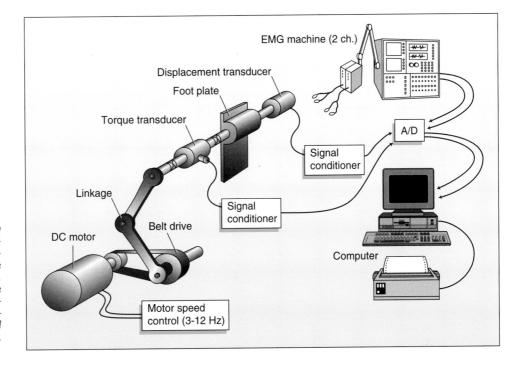

FIGURE 11-14. The Spasticity Measurement System: The assessment set-up used to measure spasticity by sinusoidally oscillating the limb. (From Lehmann, J. F., et al. [1989]. Spasticity: Quantitative measurements as a basis for assessing effectiveness of therapeutic intervention. *Archives of Physical Medicine and Rehabilitation, 70,* 6–15.)

matically in Figure 11–15. It was designed to characterize the response of the ankle to a passive, controlled stretch on the triceps surae muscle group (Lehmann et al., 1989; Price et al., 1991).

The ankle's response to sinusoidal displacements is expressed in terms of net stiffness after limb inertia and equipment drag have been eliminated. The term *stiffness* represents the ratio of the net torque to displacement (T/D) and is composed of two quantities, elastic and viscous stiffness. Elastic stiffness is similar to a torsional spring that represents the elasticity of the gastroc-soleus-Achilles tendon complex. It is in phase with the displacement of the ankle, and the force produced is proportional to the angular displacement and the stiffness of the spring

(Lehmann et al., 1989; Price et al., 1991; Rack et al., 1984).

The viscous component is comparable to a damper that is 90 degrees out of phase with the displacement. It will produce a resisting force in proportion to the velocity applied and the viscosity of the damper. Therefore, the total stiffness can be observed in graphic form by plotting the vector sum of the elastic and viscous stiffness components. The arc tangent of the ratio of the viscous to the elastic stiffness is the phase angle (see Fig. 11–15C) that is expressed as a function of frequency in a Nyquist diagram. To express the responses over the frequency spectrum of 3 to 12 Hz with a single value, a "pathlength" calculation is performed. Phase angles and vector amplitudes are

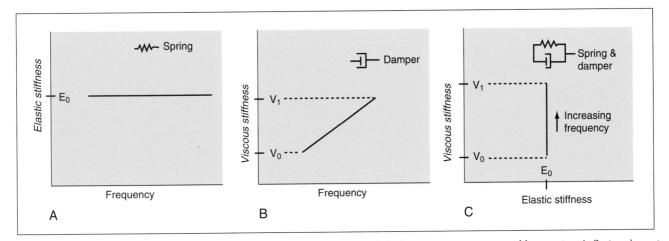

FIGURE 11-15. Stiffness response of idealized mechanical elements to sinusoidal displacements over spectrum of frequencies. *A,* Spring element. *B,* Damper element. *C,* Spring element in parallel with damper element. (From Price, R., et al. [1991]. Quantitative measurement of spasticity in children with cerebral palsy. *Developmental Medicine and Child Neurology, 33,* 585–595.)

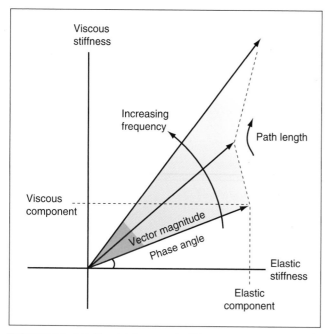

FIGURE 11–16. Nyquist diagram of stiffness, its components, and a demonstration of pathlength generation. (From Price, R., et al. [1991]. Quantitative measurement of spasticity in children with cerebral palsy. *Developmental Medicine and Child Neurology, 33,* 585–595.)

calculated and plotted sequentially from frequency to frequency (Fig. 11–16). (Refer to Lehmann and colleagues [1989] for a complete discussion of the method.)

In subjects without neurologic impairment, the stiffness vector for a given frequency (the viscous-to-elastic stiffness) will be a straight vertical line, moving upward with increasing frequency (see Fig. 11–15C). In spasticity, however, the behavior of the viscous-to-elastic stiffness vector is different, since both stiffness quantities vary nonlinearly with frequency. The stiffness vector plot will not be a straight vertical line but rather a distorted C. Therefore, simple measurement of the distance around the distorted vertical vector provides a descriptor of the amount of spasticity a subject demonstrates (see Fig. 11–16). Simply, the pathlength of the Nyquist diagram

measures the gain of the spastic response (Lehmann et al., 1989; Price et al., 1991).

Pathlength calculation as a quantifying measure for spasticity was shown to have a high test-retest reliability at the higher frequencies (r = 0.907). Intra- and intersubject variability was small. The authors concluded that the pathlength calculation clearly distinguished spastic from normal functioning muscles (p ≤ 0.0001). The technique's advantage is that the pathlength is independent of the increases in passive elastic properties that occur as the result of contracture (Lehmann et al., 1989). The ramp and hold method is not sensitive to these changes in passive elastic properties and therefore cannot be as accurate (Price et al., 1991).

ISOKINETIC DYNAMOMETRY

Firoozbakhsh and others (1993) proposed a new method for quantifying spasticity, which is simple and reliable. An isokinetic dynamometer is used to passively move the leg at different velocities (30, 60, and 120 degrees per second) though a range of motion of 60 degrees. Resistance to passive movement was determined by recording the torque versus angular position of the knee during each of the three angular velocities. Maximum torque (T_{max}) and the sum of four consecutive torque amplitudes (ΣT) was measured in Newton meters during both flexion and extension displacement. Figure 11–17 shows a typical torque-angular displacement curve recorded from a subject. The figure also shows the four consecutive ΣT used in the analysis (Firoozbakhsh et al., 1993).

Firoozbakhsh and colleagues (1993) showed that serial summation of the resisting ΣT during passive movements was capable of differentiating healthy subjects from subjects with spasticity. The authors emphasized that their assessment did not use maximum resisting torque, as did previous studies (Powers et al., 1989; Powers et al., 1988), to determine the magnitude of spasticity. The authors claim this is an advantage because the maximum resisting

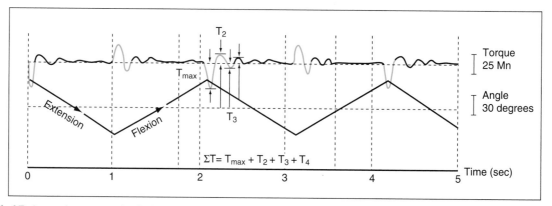

FIGURE 11–17. A typical torque-angular displacement curve displaying the 5-s midtest period. T_{max} and the four consecutive ΣT also are shown. (From Firoozbokhsh, K. K., et al. [1993]. Isokinetic dynametric technique for spasticity assessment. *American Journal of Physical Medicine and Rehabilitation, 72,* 379–385.)

torque includes the inertia of the leg and its compliant coupling to the lever arm of the dynamometer. Furthermore, the initial torque value is also affected by the rate of acceleration and deceleration of the limb. Serial summation of consecutive resisting torques, avoid this shortcoming by measuring damped oscillations whose values depend on the passive viscoelastic properties of the paretic muscles (Firoozbakhsh et al., 1993).

The disadvantages of this technique are twofold. First, an expensive isokinetic dynamometer is required to perform the examination. Second and more importantly, because of the assessment novelty, it has not undergone stringent validity and reliability testing. Further studies are needed before its use in the quantification of spasticity can be sanctioned.

NEGATIVE SYMPTOMS (PERFORMANCE DEFICITS)

As stated previously, the symptoms of weakness, fatigability, and poor dexterity are more serious functional deficits affecting patients' movements than is spasticity. Evidence shows that reducing spasticity does not improve function; however, it continues to be identified by clinicians as an important factor associated with movement dysfunction (Gordon, 1989; Landau & Hunt, 1990; Young & Wiegner, 1987). Since functional improvement is usually the therapeutic goal, emphasis should be placed on enhancing movement performance rather than decreasing spasticity.

Few studies have looked at the effect of occupational and physical therapy on enhancing movement performance. A reason for the paucity of movement analysis may be due to the few evaluation techniques that are available to reliably assess movement performance. A reliable measure would need to detect both qualitative and quantitative changes of a particular movement (Fetters, 1991; Kluzik et al., 1990).

Quantitative components are fundamental to all movements and are therefore more obvious of scrutiny during evaluation. Characteristically these include movement amplitude, duration, and trajectory. The qualitative components are less obvious but just as important. For example, movement qualities such as biomechanical alignment, proper synergistic patterns, proximal stability, and head control all assist in movement refinement. Deterioration in any of these associative reactions will decrease motor performance. Rarely are these qualities considered in the treatment or evaluation of motor disorders. It is paradoxical that so much attention is place on the positive symptoms of upper motor neuron syndrome rather than the more debilitating symptoms. This section describes the few techniques that are known to evaluate the negative symptoms (movement performance) resulting from upper motor neuron syndrome.

Kinematic Analysis

Fetters (1991) and Kluzik and colleagues (1990) advocate assessing purposeful movement rather than the magnitude of the disorder's symptoms. These authors stress that this approach is needed because therapeutic interventions on abnormal behaviors have not been too successful in the treatment of patients. Their approach uses kinematic and videotape recordings to analyze reaching movements in three-dimensional space. This method has the advantage of looking at complex human movement as it occurs in life situations by assessing both the quantitative and qualitative components involved in a purposeful movement.

Reaching movements are recorded using a motion analysis and recording system. Two infrared light-emitting diodes are attached: one on the skin over the ulna's styloid process and the other on the target. Two cameras record the infrared light emitted by the diodes as the arm moves through space. Kinematic data are collected and then averaged. The data are further simplified by combining the three-dimensional movement components into a single displacement coordinate for each movement frame. The distance that the infrared diodes traveled during the reaching movement is calculated by determining the distance that the diode moves between consecutive frames. Acceleration and deceleration are also calculated (Kluzik et al., 1990).

Statistical analysis for individuals uses the two standard deviation band method described earlier. Briefly, two horizontal lines are drawn above and below the mean baseline data. Statistical significance is shown if two successive data points occur outside the two standard deviation band (Ottenbacher, 1986).

Qualitative data are recorded using videotape that has a frame-by-frame analysis capability. Quantitative criteria are established for each of the qualitative components so that the data can be analyzed and compared. For example, Fetters (1991) looked at associated reactions (AR) by calculating the amount of time the nonreaching hand remained on the table (tnr) and dividing it by the sum of movement time (smt) and reaction time (rt) (AR = tnr/[smt + rt]). Evaluation results were shown to be reliable, valid, and sensitive for describing change in both quantitative and qualitative movement parameters (Kluzik et al., 1990).*

A disadvantage of this assessment technique is the expense of the digital motion analysis system equipment and video cameras required to complete the assessment. Additionally, depending on the level of equipment, motion analysis can be time consuming. Another obstacle, which is similar to the drawbacks with electrophysiologic assessments, is the plethora of kinematic variables that may be

---

*The WATSMART motion analysis system used in these experiments was shown to be valid and reliable (ICCs > 0.99). Validity and reliability may be compromised if adherence to accurate experiment setup is not performed (Scholz, 1989).

TABLE 11–13

SUMMARY OF TECHNIQUES TO EVALUATE UPPER MOTOR NEURON SYNDROME

Technique	Advantages	Disadvantages
Positive Symptoms		
NEUROPHYSIOLOGIC ASSESSMENTS		
1. Tendon reflexes	Easily administered and analyzed	Needs a constant testing environment Limb stabilization must be controlled for Tendon striking force must be constant Sensitive recording equipment is required Intersubject variability is high Poor correlation with clinical assessments
2. H-reflexes	Easily administered and analyzed Stimulus stability controlled for	Needs a constant testing environment Limb stabilization must be controlled for Sensitive recording equipment is required Intra- and intersubject variability is high Poor correlation with clinical assessments Can only be elicited from antigravity extensor muscles
3. H-reflex recovery curves	Same as H-reflex technique above	Same as H-reflex technique above
4. Presynaptic inhibition	Same as H-reflex technique above	Same as H-reflex technique above Weak correlation with clinical assessments
5. F-waves	Easily administered and analyzed Can be elicited from many muscles including the hand Reflex reflects only motor neuron activation May assist in differentiating pathologic from normal states of MNE	Supramaximal stimulus is required to elicit response Sensitive recording equipment is needed Response occurrent is intermittent Poor correlation with clinical assessments
6. Long latency stretch reflexes	May reflect suprasegmental structures	Sophisticated equipment is required for eliciting response and recording Reflexes are unpredictable Poor understanding of the reflexes Poor correlation with clinical assessments
7. Tonic vibration reflex	Easily administered and analyzed	No literature on the validity or reliability of the reflex
8. Flexor reflexes	Easily administered Provides a means of assessing spinal cord interneurons	Response elicited with noxious stimulus (painful) Sophisticated recording equipment is required Poor correlation with clinical assessments
CLINICAL ASSESSMENTS		
1. Modified Ashworth scale	Very easily performed Inexpensive Examiner can account for confounding influencing factors High interrater reliability	Subjective Validity decreases upon repeated usage Limited sensitivity
2. Fugl-Meyer scale	Very easily performed Inexpensive Examiner can account for confounding influencing factors High interrater reliability More objective than modified Ashworth scale Can be statistically analyzed Demonstrated to be valid and reliable Correlates well with other clinical measures	Same as above but to a lesser degree
3. Pendulum test	Easily performed Intra- and intersubject variability is stable Good correlation with other clinical tests Shown to be accurate and reliable	When performed manually, only tests the quadriceps muscles Sensitivity of test may be a problem due to accelerations of limb above physiologic values To increase sensitivity expensive biomechanical equipment is needed (i.e., Cybex II dynamometer)
4. Ramp and hold	Correlates with clinical measures, although broadly More objective and accurate than other clinical measures Intra- and intersubject variability varies nonsignificantly	Sophisticated and expensive equipment needed Stretch stimulus varies, depending on limb position Not sensitive to changes in passive elastic properties

TABLE 11-13

SUMMARY OF TECHNIQUES TO EVALUATE UPPER MOTOR NEURON SYNDROME *Continued*

Technique	Advantages	Disadvantages
5. Sinusoidal oscillation	Stimulus parameters are considered more repeatable and controlled than ramp methods Pathlength is independent of increases in passive elastic properties of muscle; therefore, more accurate than ramp method	Sophisticated and expensive equipment needed Analysis and calculation more sophisticated and harder to understand
6. Isokinetic dynamometry	Simpler than ramp and hold and sinusoidal methods of testing Shown to be reliable	Expensive isokinetic dynamometer is required Has not undergone stringent validity and reliability testing
Negative Symptoms		
1. Kinematic analysis	Evaluates purposeful movements rather than magnitude of symptoms Looks at complex movement physiologically, not under laboratory conditions Results are reliable, valid, and sensitive for both quantitative and qualitative movements parameters	Expensive digital motion analysis system needed Analysis can be time consuming Plethora of kinematic variables that are used in analysis
2. Integrative EMG assessment	Tests purposeful volitional movements Characterizes total activity of movements Results can be graphically illustrated for comparison purposes Characterizes the subject's functional motor status	Sophisticated EMG equipment needed Recording parameters are very strict Required trained technologists to perform and score the maneuvers Does not correlate with other clinical scales

Reflex—Involuntary movement elicited by a stimulus applied to the periphery, transmitted to the CNS, and directed back out to the periphery.

Reliability—A reliable assessment is one that measures the parameter under study consistently, whether more than one person evaluates the parameter (interrater reliability) or the same evaluator scoring the tests at subsequent times (test-retest reliability).

Sensitivity—The ability of an assessment to detect the smallest increment of change that would be considered significant for the purpose of the examination.

Spasticity—A motor disorder characterized by a velocity-dependent increase in tonic stretch reflexes with exaggerated tendon jerks resulting from hyperexcitability of the stretch reflex.

Stretch reflex—Also known as myotatic reflex or monosynaptic reflex. Tonic contraction of muscles in response to a stretching force. The reflex is initiated by muscle proprioceptors (i.e., muscle spindles).

Tendon reflex (T-reflex)—Similar to the myotatic reflex except the reflex is elicited by a hammer strike to a tendon.

Torque—Muscle force (F) times the perpendicular distance. The perpendicular distance is defined as the distance from the fulcrum (A) (joint) to the muscle's line of pull at right angles (F'). Torque = F × F'A.

Upper motor neuron—Refers to the descending motor pathways within the CNS that either directly or indirectly exert influences on lower motor neurons.

Validity—A valid assessment is one that measures what it is purported to measure.

REFERENCES

Adams, R. D., & Victor, M. (1993). *Principles of neurology* (5th ed.). New York: McGraw-Hill.

Agarwal, G. C., & Gottlieb, G. L. (1977). Oscillation of the human ankle joint in response to applied sinusoidal torque on the foot. *Journal of Physiology, 268,* 151–176.

Angel, R. W., & Hofmann, W. W. (1963). The H-reflex in normal, spastic, and rigid subjects. *Archives of Neurology, 8,* 591–596.

Ashworth, B. (1964). Preliminary trial of carisoprodol in multiple sclerosis. *Practitioner, 192,* 540–542.

Bischoff, C., Schoenle, P. W., & Conrad, B. (1992). Increase F-wave duration in patients with spasticity. *Electromyography Clinics of Neurophysiology, 32,* 449–453.

Bishop, B. (1977). Spasticity: Its physiology and management: Part 1. Neurophysiology of spasticity: Classical concepts. *Physical Therapy, 57*(4), 371–376.

Bishop, B. (1977). Spasticity: Its physiology and management. Part III. Identifying and assessing the mechanisms underlying spasticity. *Physical Therapy, 57*(4), 385–393.

Boczko, M., & Mumenthaler, M. (1958). Modified pendulousness test to assess tonus of thigh muscles in spasticity. *Neurology, 8,* 846–851.

Bohannon, R. W. (1987). Variability and reliability of the pendulum test for spasticity using a Cybex II isokinetic dynamometer. *Physical Therapy, 76*(5), 659–661.

Bohannon, R. W., & Larkin, P. A. (1985). Cybex II isokinetic dynamometer for the documentation of spasticity. *Physical Therapy, 65*(1), 46–47.

Bohannon, R. W., & Smith, M. B. (1987). Interrater reliability of a modified Ashworth scale of muscle spasticity. *Physical Therapy, 67*(2), 206–207.

Burke, D., Andrews, C. J., & Lance, L. W. (1972). Tonic vibration reflex in spasticity, Parkinson's disease, and normal subjects. *Journal of Neurology, Neurosurgery, and Psychiatry, 35,* 477–486.

Burke, D., Hagbarth, K-E., Lofstedt, L., & Wallin, B. G. (1976). The responses of human muscle spindle endings to vibration of non-contracting muscles. *Journal of Physiology, 261,* 673–711.

Carpenter, M. B. (1991). *Core text of neuroanatomy* (4th ed.). Baltimore: Williams & Wilkins.

Curry, E. L., & Clelland, J. A. (1991). Effects of the asymmetric tonic neck reflex and high-frequency muscle vibration on isometric wrist extension strength in normal adults. *Physical Therapy, 61*(4), 487–495.

Delwaide, P. J. (1973). Human monosynaptic reflexes and presynaptic inhibition. An interpretation of spastic hyperreflexia. In J. E. Desmedt (Ed.), *New developments in electromyography and clinical neurophysiology.* Vol. 3 (pp. 508–522). New York and Basel: S. Kager.

Desmedt, J. E. (1973). A discussion of the methodology of the triceps surae T- and H-reflexes. In J. E. Desmedt (Ed.), *New developments in electromyography and clinical neurophysiology.* Vol. 3 (pp. 773–780). New York and Basel: S. Kager.

Dimitrijevic, M. R. (1973). Withdrawal reflexes. In J. E. Desmedt (Ed.), *New developments in electromyography and clinical neurophysiology.* Vol. 3 (pp. 744–750). New York and Basel: S. Kager.

Dimitrijevic, M. M., Dimitrijevic, M. R., Sherwood, A. M., & Vanderlinden, C. (1989). Clinical neurophysiological techniques in the assessment of spasticity. *Physical Medicine and Rehabilitation, 3*(2), 64–83.

Dimitrijevic, M. R., & Nathan, P. W. (1967). Studies of spasticity in man: Some feature of spasticity. *Brain, 90*(1), 1–42.

Dohrmann, G. J., & Nowack, W. J. (1974). Relationship between various clinical signs in lesions of the descending motor system. *Diseases of the Nervous System, 35,* 375–377.

Duncan, P. W., Propst, M., & Nelson, S. G. (1983). Reliability of the Fugl-Meyer assessment of sensorimotor recovery following cerebrovascular accident. *Physical Therapy, 63*(10), 1606–1610.

Eisen, A., & Odusote, K. (1979). Amplitude of the F-wave: A potential means of documenting spasticity. *Neurology, 29,* 1306–1309.

Eklund, G., & Hagbarth, K. E. (1966). Normal variability in tonic vibration reflexes in man. *Experimental Neurology, 16,* 80–92.

Fellows, S. J., Domges, F., Topper, R., Thilmann, A. F., & Noth, J. (1993). Changes in the short- and long-latency stretch reflex components of the triceps surae muscle during ischemia in man. *Journal of Physiology, 472,* 737–748.

Fellows, S. J., Ross, H. F., & Thilmann, A. F. (1993). The limitations of the tendon jerk as a marker of pathological stretch reflex activity in human spasticity. *Journal of Neurology, Neurosurgery, and Psychiatry, 56,* 531–537.

Fetters, L. (1991). Measurement and treatment in cerebral palsy: An argument for a new approach. *Physical Therapy, 71*(3), 244–247.

Firoozbakhsh, K. K., Kunkel, C. F., Scremin, A. M. E., & Moneim, M. S. (1993). Isokinetic dynamometric technique for spasticity assessment. *American Journal of Physical Medicine and Rehabilitation, 72,* 379–385.

Fisher, M. A. (1978). Assessing segmental excitability after acute rostral lesions: I. The F response. *Neurology, 28,* 1265–1271.

Fisher, M. A. (1983). F response analysis of motor disorders of central origin. *Journal of Neurological Sciences, 62,* 13–22.

Fisher, M. A. (1988). F/M ratios in polyneuropathy and spastic hyperreflexia. *Muscle & Nerve, 11,* 217–222.

Fisher, M. A. (1992). H-reflexes and F-waves: Physiology and clinical indications. *Muscle & Nerve, 15,* 1223–1233.

Fisher, M. A., Bhagwan, T., Shahani, T., & Young, R. R. (1979). Electrophysiologic analysis of the motor system after stroke: The flexor reflex. *Archives of Physical Medicine and Rehabilitation, 60,* 7–11.

Fugl-Meyer, A. R., Jaasko, L., Leyman, I., Olsson, S., & Steglind, S. (1975). The post-stroke hemiplegic patient: 1. A method for evaluation of physical performance. *Scandinavian Journal of Rehabilitation Medicine, 7,* 13–31.

Garcia-Mullin, R., & Mayer, R. F. (1972). H reflexes in acute and chronic hemiplegia. *Brain, 95,* 559–572.

Gassel, M. M. (1973). An objective technique for the analysis of the clinical effectiveness and physiology of action of drugs in man. In J. E. Desmedt (Ed.), *New developments in electromyography and clinical neurophysiology.* Vol. 3 (pp. 342–359). New York and Basel, S. Kager.

Gassel, M. M. (1969). Monosynaptic reflexes (H-reflex) and motor neurone excitability in man. *Developmental Medicine and Child Neurology, 11,* 193–197.

Giuliani, C. A. (1991). Dorsal rhizotomy for children with cerebral palsy: Support for concepts of motor control. *Physical Therapy, 71*(3), 248–259.

Gordon, J. (1989). Assumptions underlying physical therapy intervention: Theoretical and historical perspectives. In C. H. Carr & R. B. Shepard (Eds.), *Movement science: Foundations for physical therapy in rehabilitation.* Rockville, MD: Aspen.

Greenberg, D. A., Aminoff, M. J., & Simon, R. P. (1993). *Clinical neurology* (2nd ed.). Norwalk, CT: Appleton & Lange.

Hagbarth, K. E. (1993). Microneurography and applications to issues of motor control: Fifth annual Stuart Reiner memorial lecture. *Muscle & Nerve, 16,* 693–705.

Hagbarth, K. E., & Eklund, G. (1968). The effects of muscle vibration in spasticity, rigidity, and cerebellar disorders. *Journal of Neurology, Neurosurgery, and Psychiatry, 31,* 207–213.

Hagbarth, K. E., & Finner, B. L. (1963). The plasticity of human withdrawal reflexes to noxious stimuli in lower limbs. In G. Moruzzi, A. Fessard, & H. H. Jasper (Eds.), *Brain Mechanisms. (Progress in Brain Research Series)* Amsterdam: Elsevier, *1,* 65–78.

Hallett, M. (1985). Spasticity: Assessment and pathophysiology (modification of long-latency reflexes). In P. J. Delwaide & R. R. Young (Eds.), *Clinical neurophysiological spasticity.* New York: Elsevier.

Hugon, M. (1973). Methodology of the Hoffmann reflex in man. In J. E. Desmedt (Ed.), *New developments in electromyography and clinical neurophysiology.* Vol. 3 (pp. 277–293). New York and Basel: S. Kager.

Hultborn, H., Meunier, S., Pierrot-Deseilligny, E., & Shindo, M. (1987). Changes in presynaptic inhibition of Ia fibers at the onset of voluntary contraction in man. *Journal of Physiology, 389,* 757–772.

Iles, J. F., & Roberts, R. C. (1986). Presynaptic inhibition of monosynaptic reflexes in the lower limbs of subjects with upper motor neuron disease. *Journal of Neurology, Neurosurgery, and Psychiatry, 49,* 937–944.

Jabre, J. F. (1981). Surface recording of the H-reflex of the flexor carpi radialis. *Muscle & Nerve, 4,* 435–438.

Kandel, E. R., Schwartz, J. H., Jessell, T. M. (1991). *Principles of neural science* (3rd ed.). New York: Elsevier.

Katz, R. T., Rovai, G. P., Brait, C., & Rymer, Z. (1992). Objective quantification of spastic hypertonia: Correlation with clinical findings. *Archives of Physical Medicine and Rehabilitation, 73,* 339–347.

Katz, R. T., Rymer, W. Z. (1989). Spastic hypertonia: Mechanisms and measurement. *Archives of Physical Medicine and Rehabilitation, 70,* 144–155.

Kimura, J., Yanagisawa, H., Yamada, T., Mitsudome, A., et al. (1984). Is the F wave elicited in a select group of motor neurons? *Muscle & Nerve* 7:392–399.

Kluzik, J., Fetters, L., Coryell, J. (1990) Quantification of control: A preliminary study of effects of neurodevelopmental treatment on reaching in children with spastic cerebral palsy. *Physical Therapy, 70*(2), 65–78.

Koelman, J. H. T. M., Bour, L. J., Hidgevoord, A. A. J., van Bruggen G. J., & Ongerboer de Visser, B. W. (1993). Soleus H-reflex tests and clinical signs of the upper motor neuron syndrome. *Journal of Neurology, Neurosurgery, and Psychiatry,* 56:776–781.

Kuypers, H. G. J. M. (1981). Anatomy of the descending pathways. In V. Brooks (Ed.), *Handbook of physiology.* Vol II, Part 1. Bethesda: American Physiological Society.

Lance, J. W., & Burke, D. (1974). Mechanisms of spasticity. *Archives of Physical Medicine and Rehabilitation, 55,* 332–336.

Landau, W. M. (1980). Spasticity: What is it? What is it not? In R. G. Feldman, R. R. Young, W. P. Koella (Eds.), *Spasticity: Disordered motor control.* Chicago: Mosby-Year Book.

Landau, W. M., & Hunt, C. C. (1990). Dorsal rhizotomy: A treatment of unproven efficacy. *Journal of Child Neurology, 5,* 174–178.

Lee, R. G., & Tatton, W. G. (1975). Motor responses to sudden limb displacements in primates with specific CNS lesions and in human patients with motor system disorders. *Canadian Journal of Neurological Science, 2,* 285–293.

Lehmann, J. F., Price, R., deLateur, B. J., Hinderer, S., & Traynor, C. (1989). Spasticity: Quantitative measurements as a basis for assessing effectiveness of therapeutic intervention. *Archives of Physical Medicine and Rehabilitation, 70,* 6–15.

Levin, M. F., & Hui-Chan, C. (1993). Are H and stretch reflexes in hemiparesis reproducible and correlated with spasticity? *Journal of Neurology, 240,* 63–71.

Magladery, J. W., & McDougal, D. B. (1950). Electrophysiological studies of nerve and reflex activity in normal man. I. Identification of certain reflexes in the electromyogram and the conduction velocity of peripheral nerve fibers. *Bulletin of Johns Hopkins Hospital, 86,* 265–290.

Magladery, J. W., Porter, W. E., Park, A. M., & Teasdall, R. D. (1951).

Electrophysiological studies of nerve and reflex activity in normal man. IV. The two-neurone reflex and identification of certain action potentials from spinal roots and cord. *Bulletin of Johns Hopkins Hospital, 88,* 499–519.

Magladery, J. W., Teasdall, R. D., Park, A. M., & Languth, H. W. (1953). Electrophysiological studies of reflex activity in patients with lesions of the nervous system: I. A comparison of spinal motorneurone excitability following afferent nerve volleys in normal persons and patients with upper motorneurone lesions. *Bulletin of Johns Hopkins Hospital, 91,* 219–244.

Marsden, C. D., Merton, P. A., & Morton, H. B. (1983). Rapid postural reactions to mechanical displacement of the hand in man. In J. E. Desmedt (Ed.), *Motor control mechanisms in health and disease* (pp. 509–539). New York: Raven Press.

Matthews, P. B. C. (1966). The reflex excitation of the soleus muscle of the decerebrate cat caused by vibration applied to its tendon. *Journal of Physiology, 184,* 450–472.

Meinck, H. M., Beneche, R., & Conrad, B.(1985). Spasticity and the flexor reflex. In P. J. Delwaide & R. R. Young (Eds.), (1985). *Clinical neurophysiology in spasticity.* Vol. 4. New York: Elsevier. 41–53.

Milanov, I. G. (1992). F-wave for assessment of segmental motorneurone excitability. *Electromyography Clinical Neurophysiology, 32,* 11–15.

Milanov, I. G. (1992). Flexor reflex for assessment of common interneurone activity in spasticity. *Electromyography Clinical Neurophysiology, 32,* 621–629.

Morin, C., Pierrot-Deseilligny, E., & Hultborn, H. (1984). Evidence for presynaptic inhibition of muscle spindle Ia afferents in man. *Neuroscience Letters, 44,* 137–142.

Myklebust, J. B., Myklebust, B. M., & Gottlieb, G. L. (1989). Techniques for evaluating spasticity: Joint mechanics and EMG in spasticity. *Physical Medicine and Rehabilitation, 3*(2), 96–110.

Noback, R. C., Strominger, N. L., & DeMarest, R. J. (1991). *The human nervous system: Introduction and review* (4th ed.). Philadelphia: Lea & Febiger.

Ottenbacher, K. J. (1986). *Evaluating clinical change: Strategies for occupational and physical therapists.* Baltimore: William & Wilkins.

Palmer, F. B., Shapiro, B. K., Wachtel, R. C., et al. (1988). The effects of physical therapy on cerebral palsy. *New England Journal of Medicine, 31,* 803–808.

Parette, H. P., Biocca, Z., DeCremer, G., et al. (1984). Quantitative analysis of the effectiveness of pediatric therapy. Emphasis on the neurodevelopmental treatment approach. *American Journal of Occupational Therapy, 38,* 462–468.

Powers, R. K., Campbell, D. L., & Rymer, W. Z. (1989). Stretch reflex dynamics in spastic elbow flexor muscles. *Annals of Neurology, 25*(1), 32–42.

Powers, R. K., Marder-Meyer, J., & Rymer, W. Z. (1988). Quantitative relations between hypertonia and stretch reflex threshold in spastic hemiparesis. *Annals of Neurology, 23*(2), 115–124.

Price, R., Bjornson, K. F., Lehmann, J. F., McLaughlin, J. F., & Hays, R. M. (1991). Quantitative measurement of spasticity in children with cerebral palsy. *Developmental Medicine and Child Neurology, 33,* 585–595.

Pryse-Phillips, W., & Murray, T. J. (1985). *Essential neurology* (4th ed.), Norwalk, CT: Appleton & Lange.

Rack, P. M. H., Ross, H. F., & Thilmann, A. F. (1984). The ankle stretch reflexes in normal and spastic subjects: The response to sinusoidal movement. *Brain, 107,* 637–654.

Sax, D. S., & Johnson, T. L. (1980). Spinal reflex activity in man, measurement in relation to spasticity. In R. G. Feldman, R. R. Young, & W. P. Koella (Eds.), *Spasticity: Disordered motor control* (pp. 301–313). Miami: Symposia Specialists.

Schiller, H. H., & Stalberg, E. (1978). F responses studies with single fibre EMG in normal subjects and spastic patients. *Journal of Neurology, Neurosurgery, and Psychiatry, 41,* 45–53.

Scholz, J. P. (1989). Reliability and validity of the WATSMART three-dimensional optoelectric motion analysis system. *Physical Therapy, 69,* 679–689.

Shahani, B. T., & Young, R. R. (1973). Human flexor spasms. In J. E. Desmedt (Ed.), *New developments in electromyography and clinical neurophysiology.* Vol. 3 (pp. 744–750). New York and Basel, S. Kager.

Sherrington, C. S. (1903). Qualitative difference of spinal reflex corresponding with quantitative difference of cutaneous stimulus. *Journal of Physiology, 30,* 39–46.

Sherwood, A. M. (1993). Characterization of upper motor neuron dysfunction: Motor control profile. *Proceedings, 15th International Conference of the IEEEE EMBS, 15,* 1227.

Sherwood, A. M., Priebe, M. M., Markowski, J., Kharas, N. F., & Ambatipudi, R. (1994). Assessment of spasticity in spinal cord injury: A comparison of clinical and neurophysiological measures. In N. F. Sheppard, M. Eden, & G. Kantor (Eds.), *Engineering advances: New opportunities for biomedical engineers, 16,* 462–463.

Somerville, J., & Ashby, P. (1978) Hemiplegic spasticity: Neurophysiologic studies. *Archives of Physical Medicine and Rehabilitation, 59,* 592–596.

Taborikova, H., & Sax, D. S. (1968). Motoneurone pool and the H-reflex. *Journal of Neurology, Neurosurgery, and Psychiatry, 31,* 354–361.

Tardieu, C., Lacert, P. L., Lombard, M., Truscelli, D., & Tardieu, G. (1977). H reflex and recovery cycle in spastic and normal children: Intra- and inter-individual and inter-groups comparisons. *Archives of Physical Medicine and Rehabilitation, 58,* 561–567.

Tarkka, I. M. (1986). Short and long latency reflexes in human muscles following electrical and mechanical stimulation. *Acta Physiologica Scandinavica Supplement, 128,* 5–32.

Taylor, S., Ashby, P., & Verrier, M. (1984). Neurophysiological changes following traumatic spinal lesions in man. *Journal of Neurology, Neurosurgery, and Psychiatry, 47,* 1102–1108.

Thilmann, A. F., Fellows, S. J., & Garms, E. (1990). Pathological stretch reflexes on the "good" side of hemiparetic patients. *Journal of Neurology, Neurosurgery, and Psychiatry, 53,* 208–214.

Trombly, C. (1989). Motor control therapy. In C. Trombly (Ed.), *Occupational therapy for physical dysfunction* (3rd ed.). Baltimore: Williams & Wilkins.

Yap, C. B. (1967). Spinal segmental and long-loop reflexes on spinal motor neurone excitability in spasticity and rigidity. *Brain, 90,* 887–889.

Young, R. R., & Wiegner, A. W. (1987). Spasticity. *Clinical Orthopedics & Related Research, 219,* 50–62.

Zander Olsen, P. Z., & Diamantopoulos, E. (1967). Excitability of spinal motor neurones in normal subjects and patients with spasticity, parkinsonian rigidity and cerebellar hypotonia. *Journal of Neurology, Neurosurgery, and Psychiatry, 30,* 325–331.

CHAPTER 12

Sensory Processing

Introduction to Sensory Processing

Julia Van Deusen, PhD, OTR/L, FAOTA

SUMMARY   Because the neural processing of sensory input is very complex, the assessment for functioning (or dysfunctioning) in this area is necessarily complex. Sensory processing involves many modalities including somatosensory, visual, auditory, gustatory, and olfactory. Assessment includes not only the many kinds of sensation but also the many skill levels manifested in this processing. We have divided this discussion of assessment of sensory processing into three major areas typically addressed by occupational and physical therapists: evaluation of the sensory receptive component (sensory deficits), assessment of the integrative component (perceptual dysfunction), and assessment of the more complex integrative component (conceptual dysfunction). Because of their relevance to physical and occupational therapists' activities, the modalities emphasized are the somatosensory (i.e., touch, temperature, pain, and proprioception) and the visual. The language pathologist or audiologist is typically responsible for in-depth auditory assessment, and olfactory and gustatory sensation is less vital for the performance of most daily activities.

Many models exist elaborating complex sensory processing. Luria's model has been shown to be useful in rehabilitation (Abreu & Toglia, 1987; Purisch, 1993). As described by Purisch (1993), this model proposes three units involved in brain-behavior relationships. Unit I functions for the modulation of arousal and selective attention so that damage results in dysfunction in these areas. Biologic and environmental sources of arousal are processed by the Ascending Reticular Activating System; intentional arousal is initiated by cortical structures. Unit II involves the cortical functions of reception, coding, and storage of sensory input from internal and external sources. Unit II consists of three zones, one for projection, a second for projection-association, and the third for association. Dysfunction from damage to these areas involves progressively more complex sensory processing skills. Unit III (anterior cerebral cortex) involves the most complex aspects of sensory processing, including intention, regulation, evaluation, and modification of behavior; therefore, damage can affect motor skills, speech, attitudes, and cognition. According to Purisch (1993), three principles apply to brain-behavior relationships: 1) hierarchic organization within the brain, 2) diminishing specificity of the sensory modality, and 3) progressive lateralization. The Luria-Nebraska Neuropsychological Battery is the test battery based on the Luria model. Although this battery is not appropriately used by occupational or physical therapists, these professionals do use the Luria model to guide their own assessments of sensory processing dysfunction.

A second model showing the complexity of sensory processing is the Reitan-Wolfson Model of Neuropsychological Functioning (Reitan & Wolfson, 1988). This model serves as the framework for assessment with the Halstead-Reitan Neuropsychological Test Battery, again a battery not appropriate for use by occupational or physical therapists. However, this model can conceptualize the sequencing for the assessments that are a part of the occupational and physical therapy process. According to the Reitan-Wolfson Model, processing occurs at five levels: 1) input; 2) attention, concentration, and memory; 3) language and visuospatial skills; 4) concept formation, reasoning, and logical analysis; and 5) output. A third model, that of Moore (Warren, 1993), which is directed specifically to the visual system, involves the same kind of hierarchic processing, with minor differences. The foundational level is responsible for quick, accurate, and complete receipt of information by the central nervous system (oculomotor control, visual fields, visual acuity). The next skill level is visual attention, influenced strongly by global attention, a reticular system function. Next is scanning, with a systematic, sequential information-seeking function. After pattern identification, this hierarchy includes the storage and retrieval of visual images (visual memory), as preceding the highest forms of visual processing (visuocognition followed by adaptation). One of the emphases of occupational therapy based on this model is that the foundational visual skills such as visual acuity and visual attention are of primary importance and must be treated before higher-level functions can be addressed. Thus, it is crucial to initially assess these foundational skills.

Such specialists as the neuropsychologist, the neurologist, and the optometrist have special expertise in the evaluation of sensation. If current reports are available on the patient's sensory processing status, the occupational and physical therapist typically use these reports and do their own as a part of their other therapeutic assessments, such as in the activities of daily living evaluation. In settings where sensory reports are not available, it may be necessary to assess sensory processing status directly.

REFERENCES

Abreu, B. C., & Toglia, J. P. (1987). Cognitive rehabilitation: An occupational therapy model. *American Journal of Occupational Therapy, 41,* 439–448.

Purisch, A. D. (1993, December). *Brain-behavior relationships.* Paper presented at the Introduction to the Luria-Nebraska Neuropsychological Battery Workshop of the Neuropsychological Associates of California, Orlando, FL.

Reitan, R. M., & Wolfson, D. (1988). The Halstead-Reitan Neuropsychological Test Battery and REHABIT. *Cognitive Rehabilitation, 6,* 10–17.

Warren, M. (1993). A hierarchical model for evaluation and treatment of visual perceptual dysfunction in adult acquired brain injury, Part 1. *American Journal of Occupational Therapy, 47,* 42–54.

Sensory Deficits

Julia Van Deusen, PhD, OTR/L, FAOTA

with

Joanne Jackson Foss, MS, OTR

SUMMARY   This section of Chapter 12 addresses the assessment of sensibility, specifically in the visual and somatosensory domains. Basic sensibility must be assessed before higher levels of sensory processing can be evaluated. Among the procedures recommended by occupational therapists for basic visual assessments are contrast sensitivity function testing, confrontational testing, use of such tests as the King-Devick for saccadic eye movements, and cancellation tasks. If financially feasible, computerized automated perimetry can be used by therapists. The main reasons for basic visual assessment by occupational or physical therapists are for functional decisions and appropriate referrals to vision specialists.

Assessment for somatosensory deficits is necessary for patients with either peripheral nerve or central nervous system dysfunction. Many tests are used in either direct patient service or for research. Therapists commonly assess proprioception and touch or pressure, and, more rarely, temperature and vibration. Among the more useful tests are the Semmes-Weinstein Monofilament Test, the Disk-Criminator, and the Automated Tactile Tester.

From the behavioral responses observed by occupational and physical therapists, one cannot define patient dysfunction as perceptual or conceptual unless deficits in primary sensation first have been ruled out. Cooke (1991) cited literature clarifying the difference between sensation and sensibility. Sensibility is the conscious appreciation and interpretation of the stimulus that produced sensation, which is the actual activation of the afferent receptors. If a person cannot appreciate touch, he or she certainly cannot differentiate various objects by means of touch; that is, tactile perception cannot be assessed. If a person has limited visual acuity, it would be difficult to assess his or her visual perceptual performance. Thus, it is vital to have adequate information on the patient's primary or foundational sensory status before progressing to the assessment of more complex sensory processing functions.

VISUAL DEFICITS

The primary or foundational visual deficits include problems with visual acuity, visual field deficits, and oculomotor dysfunction. Visual acuity screening is by means of a Snellen letter chart or similar test. Results of this type of testing have long served as the standard for prescription of corrective lenses (Warren, 1993a). In the opinion of Warren, a Snellen test should be supplemented by contrast sensitivity function testing, which incorporates the variables of contrast, target size, and luminosity.

Foss (1993) has described clinical screening for other primary visual deficits. The following four paragraphs have been taken, with permission, from Foss. Although Foss has addressed the patient with cerebrovascular accident (CVA), the information is applicable to any patient with potential sensory processing dysfunction.

A comprehensive visual screening enables the rehabilitation professional to make a decision to refer patients who have medical histories identifying them as being at risk for primary visual deficits to a vision specialist. A qualified vision specialist may administer a complete visual assessment; however, a nonstandardized visual screening device used by a rehabilitation professional should include activities that provide information about visual attention, oculomotor movements (scanning and saccadic movements), visual fields, and visual neglect (Zoltan, 1990). Similar testing items also may be used by other professionals as part of a general neurologic examination, but these screening procedures commonly are used clinically by rehabilitation professionals.

Zoltan and associates (1986) describe screening items that can be used to evaluate these areas. A suspended orange ball can be used to evaluate visual attention and ocular pursuits. When the ball is held static, the rehabilitation professional can record how long the patient is able to attend to the stimulus after being told to watch it. Observations of convergence and fixation also can be made. When the ball is moved horizontally, vertically, diagonally, clockwise, and counterclockwise, ocular pursuits are evaluated. The quality and range of eye movements, ability to cross the midline, and visual overshooting can be observed.

The King-Devick Test can be used when evaluating saccadic eye movements (Lieberman et al., 1983). This test consists of cards with randomly spaced lines of numbers connected by arrows. The patient calls out the numbers as fast as possible, following the order indicated by the arrows. The fact that this test requires the patient's ability to call out numbers assumes a level of verbalization and conceptualization that may limit the usefulness of this task with the CVA population. Letter or symbol cancellation tasks often are used to identify visual scanning and visual field deficits. These tasks require the patient to find and cross out a targeted letter or symbol from among other letters or symbols on a page (Weinberg et al., 1977). Observations of other visual deficits such as visual neglect also may be observed during this task.

Evaluation of visual field deficits such as homonymous hemianopsia in the CVA patient often is accomplished by the use of confrontational testing (Bouska et al., 1990). As the patient fixates on a targeted area, such as the examiner's nose or forehead, a stimulus target is moved in an arc from the periphery. The patient then indicates the point at which the stimulus comes into view. Poor depth perception, another common visual deficit observed in stroke patients, also can be evaluated through the use of confrontational testing. The patient identifies the closest of two targets. These tests can be performed with or without an eye patch (Zoltan et al., 1986). The CVA patient may exhibit visual neglect with or without the presence of a visual field cut; therefore, it is important to test for both deficits.

Because the assessment of visual neglect has been addressed elsewhere in this book, we do not discuss it here. Besides visual acuity, discussed in the previous paragraphs, Warren (1993b) also is concerned with assessing the foundational visual deficits of visual field and oculomotor function. She cites evidence supporting the idea that the finger confrontation visual field test is sensitive only to gross deficits. Warren recommends that occupational therapists measure visual field deficits by means of computerized automated perimetry to identify potential patient problems with activities such as driving. Unfortunately, a perimeter is costly and serves a limited patient population. Warren also suggests the following observations of activities of daily living indicative of field deficits if visual inattention or neglect is known to not be present: missing or misreading the beginnings or ends of words, consistently bumping objects to one side, and obviously moving the head to view objects in a certain plane.

Warren (1993b) believes that occupational therapists often are the first professionals to observe patient oculomotor dysfunction. She suggests the use of simple screening tests such as that described by Bouska and coworkers (1990). The purposes of the occupational therapy screening in this complex visual area are to describe the functional effect of the deficit and to refer the patient appropriately for evaluation by a vision specialist. The interested therapist can obtain considerable information about oculomotor function from Warren's articles (1993a, 1993b).

SOMATOSENSORY DEFICITS

In peripheral nerves, motor and sensory fibers can be clearly distinguished. Motor and sensory *function* is not as clearly differentiated. As Marsh and Smith (1986, p. 82) have so aptly stated, "The motor system is actively used in gathering sensory information and the afferent system is used in control of motor performance." Limited evidence from research and case histories does indicate the relation between impaired fine motor control and impaired sensation (Bell-Krotoski et al., 1993; Marsh & Smith, 1986).

Thus, assessment of somatosensory deficits is pertinent to some kinds of hand function, such as the picking up of small objects; however, a recent study of stroke patients (Robertson & Jones, 1994) showed no relation between sensation and a hand test involving simulated eating, object manipulation, and other functional hand activities, and Jerosch (1993) showed that results of sensibility assessment did not predict activities of daily living results in those with peripheral nerve injury. He suggested compensatory functioning as the explanation because all subjects were evaluated at least 2 years after surgical repair. Clinically, if time is a major problem, somatosensory testing could consist only of a functional measure such as the Moberg (Trombly & Scott, 1989) involving the picking up of small objects. There are many reasons why therapists recommend more extensive somatosensory assessment.

Primary somatosensory deficits include those of proprioception, pain, temperature, and the tactile mode (light touch, pressure, vibration, two-point discrimination). A wide variety of problems require somatosensory assessment. As previously stated, to evaluate other levels of sensory processing in persons with central nervous system lesions, it is necessary first to assess sensibility deficits. Even the patient emerging from coma is assessed for responses to tactile stimulation. In the instrument developed by Crosby and Parsons (1989), responses to tactile stimuli are rated as part of their neurologic assessment of persons in coma to aid in detecting changes in the comatose state.

The hand therapist is intimately concerned with somatosensory assessment. Cooke (1991) provided eight reasons why occupational and physical therapists complete a systematic sensibility evaluation following peripheral nerve injury of their patient. Many of these reasons are similar to those we have had for our sensibility assessment of patients with central nervous system lesions. An asterisk has been put before those reasons typically applicable to both types of problems.

*Assess extent of sensory loss
Evaluate its recovery after nerve repair
Aid in diagnosis of peripheral nerve injury
*Determine functional impairment
Compare effectiveness of different surgical procedures
Contribute data for legal purposes
*Provide data pertinent to patient precautions
*Determine the best time for sensory reeducation and evaluate its effectiveness

We have described tests often used clinically by therapists, supplemented by samples of tests appropriate for research. Usually, at least part of the testing necessitates occluded vision. Although vision can be blocked with a sheet of cardboard, the preferred method is use of a cut-out box similar to that included with the Benton tactile perceptual tests (Benton et al., 1994, p. 96). When assessing elders, interpretation of the results of sensibility testing should take into consideration the data showing they have higher somatosensory thresholds than younger persons (Evans et al., 1992; Horch et al., 1992).

Proprioception

Trombly and Scott (1989) described clinical testing for proprioception or position sense. Holding the involved part laterally, the therapist passively positions the joint to be tested. This positioning is done slowly, 10 degrees per second, and the patient is asked to reproduce it with the opposite uninvolved part or to describe the position. Joints may be tested singly or in combination, but large joints are tested separately from the small ones. Each joint is scored independently.

Dannenbaum and Jones (1993) addressed evaluation of the proprioceptive system specifically by the flexion or extension of the patient's proximal or distal interphalangeal joint of each finger. Typically, 10 trials are allowed per finger. The patient responds to the flexed or extended joint by indicating "up" or "down." Normative data are available for this test.

Carey and colleagues (1993) described a method for assessment of proprioception appropriate for research. Only the wrist position was used in their project. This proprioceptive discrimination test used a pointer on top of a protractor scale as the response mechanism for the subject. The subject's hand was passively moved to 20 different wrist positions in random sequence. The test score was the mean absolute error between the actual measured wrist position and the subject's estimate with the pointer. Carey and associates showed by use of quasiexperimental single-subject design with four subjects that this test was sensitive to improvement following a discrimination training program. Other tests for proprioception have also been shown to be useful for experimental work (Dannenbaum & Jones, 1993).

Pain and Temperature

Assessment of the primitive or protective sensibilities of pain and temperature is accomplished by evaluating sharp versus dull and warm versus cold responses. Among those describing clinical methods for pain and temperature assessment are Cooke (1991), Harlowe and Van Deusen (1985), and Trombly and Scott (1989). Traditionally, pain is assessed by randomly applying to the patient's skin the blunt and sharp ends of a pin for appropriate identification. Temperature is assessed by test tubes of hot and cold water, first applied to the therapist's own skin for the determination of approximate temperature and then applied randomly to the patient's skin. Therapists assess pain and temperature sensibility less frequently than they evaluate touch and proprioception for several reasons: (1) the traditional methods of assessment are not very satisfactory, especially for temperature (Cooke, 1991; Harlowe and Van Deusen, 1985); (2) pain and temperature sensibility recover first, so that satisfactory performance on other tests of sensibility implies no need to test pain and temperature (Cooke, 1991; Marsh & Smith, 1986); and

(3) recent, more sophisticated tests (Horch et al., 1992; Verdugo & Ochoa, 1992) typically require an inappropriate amount of therapist time or expense, especially since thermal assessment has not been found to be clinically useful for quantifying hand function or predicting its recovery (Dellon, 1993). Cooke (1991) suggested a set of assessment tools that excluded pain and temperature for use by the therapist treating peripheral nerve injuries; however, some early-stage patients may need pain and temperature evaluations so that return of protective sensation can be monitored. The idea that results from testing only one modality (e.g., temperature) in stroke patients could provide information on the other primitive senses was not supported (Harlowe & Van Deusen, 1985); therefore, if persons with central nervous system lesions show need for such testing, all modalities need to be included.

We recommend for research purposes the Automated Tactile Tester (ATT), a computer-controlled device used to measure temperature and pain as well as touch and vibration (Horch et al., 1992). This instrument is described later in this section of Chapter 12. Physical therapists also might use in research the Quantitative Somatosensory Thermotest (QST) described by Verdugo and Ochoa (1992). This test allows rigorous assessment of warm and cold sensation and heat and cold pain. Normal control values for thermal-specific and thermal pain thresholds for hand and foot are provided for the QST, as is information on various kinds of sensory pathology.

Touch and Pressure

The Semmes-Weinstein Monofilament Aesthesiometer Test (Bell-Krotoski et al., 1993), the weighted touch-pressure aesthesiometer (Sieg & Williams, 1986), the Disk-Criminator™ (Robertson & Jones, 1994), and the Automated Tactile Tester (Horch et al., 1992) are all possible instruments for assessing touch and pressure sensitivity. We have not reviewed the tests for texture discrimination and object recognition (stereognosis), often discussed with tests of sensibility, since we agree with the position (Cooke, 1991; Dannenbaum & Jones, 1993) that these functions require a high degree of perceptual-cognitive ability as well as sensitivity and we believe tests for texture and object recognition are therefore more appropriately addressed in discussions of higher-level sensory processing assessment. Although reliable assessment of responses to high- and low-frequency vibration has been demonstrated with the ATT (Horch et al., 1992; Jimenez et al., 1993), some therapists do not consider vibration testing to be of vital importance clinically in either peripheral nerve (Bell-Krotoski et al., 1993) or CNS injury (Dannenbaum & Jones, 1993). Vibration testing might be eliminated in the clinic when intervention time is at a premium. It should be incorporated in research involving sensibility assessment.

Semmes-Weinstein Monofilaments. The Semmes-Weinstein monofilament aesthesiometer (available from Sammons Preston, 1-800-323-5547), as discussed by Bell-Krotoski and coworkers (1993), by Cooke (1991), and by Trombly (1989), is used to evaluate light touch and deep pressure. It consists of nylon monofilaments in rods, each of which can be held perpendicular to the skin so that the filament touches the skin (see figures, Chapter 10). The filaments are graded as to length and thickness and bend when a peak-force threshold has been achieved in contact with the skin. The filaments maintain a constant force with only minor amounts of variation. According to Bell-Krotoski and associates (1993), the mini-kit of five filaments is time-saving and appropriate for most clinical testing. For upper extremity sensory abnormality screening, only one filament is necessary (pressure rating, 2.83). To track sensory function, the use of at least five filaments is required. The lightest filament is applied first, with subsequent application of the more forceful filaments in order. Although this application differs from the original method for the test, it has been found to be time saving and reliable by clinical users. Formal reliability for this test was established in a rigorous study in which the complete set of filaments (20, all new) was used. Care in application and regular calibration of the filaments are necessary for objectivity. Although there are limited normative data for this test, it is typically used with patients who have peripheral nerve injuries in only one extremity, so the other limb can be used for control data. Normative data are essential if used in assessing sensibility of persons diagnosed with only unilateral brain injury since both hands are often affected (Dannenbaum & Jones, 1993). This Semmes-Weinstein monofilament tool is being widely and successfully used clinically and apparently is considered the best available tool for assessing tactile sensibility.

Weighted Touch-Pressure Tool. A less delicate device was used in research by Sieg and Williams (1986) to assess touch-pressure sensibility. These researchers found the use of a metal capsule into which graded weights could be inserted to be effective. Weights of 0.5, 1, and 2 oz were used. The blunt point of the capsule was applied to the skin, and its handle allowed for control of stimulus weight for any desired duration.

Disk-Criminator™. A common clinical method of the assessment of tactile sensibility is through reports of two-point discrimination. The underlying neuromechanism for two-point discrimination is responsible for sensory experiences (tactile-spatial) that are more complex than for the protective, primitive modalities. Thus, assessment of two-point discrimination is the highest level sensory ability assessed in this section. Two-point discrimination is evaluated by use of moving and static stimuli; however, one researcher (Jerosch, 1993) found a correlation of $r = 0.90$ between scores for static and moving two-point discrimination for 14 subjects with peripheral nerve injury and concluded that only the static procedure need be used.

The Disk-Criminator™ (developed by A.L. Dellon, MD, and available from Sammons Preston, 1-800-323-5547) is an octagonally shaped disk for measuring static and moving two-point discrimination of fingers and toes. Holding the Disk-Criminator, the examiner places the points on the skin of the patient. The distance between the points is adjustable, and the subject indicates whether he or she feels one or two points (Robertson & Jones, 1994). Major concerns have been raised about the reliability and validity of data from hand-held tools used for assessing two-point discrimination (Bell-Krotoski et al., 1993).

Automated Tactile Tester. The ATT (Horch et al., 1992; Jimenez et al., 1993) is an automated device for assessing touch-pressure, high- and low-frequency vibrations, warmth, sharpness, and two-point discrimination. Each stimulus delivery is precisely controlled by computer. The ATT uses the "staircase" method to establish thresholds, calculation of which is also done by computer. A stimulus threshold is defined as the minimal stimulus level required to produce an awareness of sensation. In the "staircase" method, once the stimulus has been detected by the subject, its intensity is reduced until it is no longer detected when it is raised until again detected. This procedure is continued until at least five reversals from detection to nondetection have occurred, and the results are then averaged. Horch and collaborators (1992) and Jimenez and others (1993) reported a study of 62 "normal" subjects (aged 9 to 83 y), which they considered to establish the validity, intertester reliability, and test-retest reliability for the ATT. "Age-related norms were established that could be used for future patient studies" (Jimenez et al., 1993, p. 125).

Three studies showed that the ATT can be successfully used to assess sensation of patients with burns and carpal tunnel syndrome (Jimenez et al., 1993). The authors reported that light touch and low-frequency vibration were the most important modalities for tracking recovery after intervention. Although much more research is needed, including replication with large numbers of "normal" subjects as well as continued patient research, the ATT has shown excellent promise as a research tool. Perhaps the ATT is not yet practical for use in many clinics, but it may well be a widely used clinical tool in the future for somatosensory assessment.

GLOSSARY

Aesthesiometer—An instrument for measuring tactile sensibility.

Oculomotor—Pertaining to scanning and saccadic movements of the eyes.

Proprioception—Sensibility of bodily movement and position mediated by receptors mainly in muscles, tendons, and the labyrinth.

Saccadic movements—The series of simultaneous, involuntary "jerks" of both eyes in changing the point of fixation.

Sensation—Activation of afferent receptors.

Sensibility—The conscious appreciation of sensation.

Sensory processing functions—A comprehensive term encompassing the entirety of the reception of and the progressively more complex levels of central nervous system integration of sensory input.

Somatosensory deficits—Inadequacies in proprioceptive, tactile, thermal, or pain sensation.

Tactile—Pertaining to touch.

Vibration testing—Traditionally, a procedure in which a tuning fork, randomly activated or not activated, is applied to the subject's skin for his or her report of feelings of vibration.

Visual acuity—Sharpness of vision; myopia (nearsightedness) is an example of impaired acuity.

Visual field deficits—Poor vision or blindness in part of the visual field. A common manifestation is hemianopsia after CVA, in which patients are unable to visually appreciate objects in the half of the visual field contralateral to the site of the brain lesion.

REFERENCES

Bell-Krotoski, J., Weinstein, S., & Weinstein, C. (1993). Testing sensibility, including touch-pressure, two-point discrimination, point localization, and vibration. *Journal of Hand Therapy, 6,* 114–123.

Benton, A., Sivan, A., des. Hamsher, K., Varney, N., & Spreen, O. (1994). *Contributions to neuropsychological assessment* (2nd ed.). New York: Oxford University Press.

Bouska, M. J., Kaufman, N. A., & Marcus, S. E. (1990). Disorders of the visual perceptual system. In D. A. Umphred (Ed.), *Neurological rehabilitation: Vol. 1* (2nd ed.) (pp. 705–740). St. Louis, MO: C. V. Mosby Company.

Carey, L. M., Matyas, T. A., & Oke, L. E. (1993). Sensory loss in stroke patients: Effective training of tactile and proprioceptive discrimination. *Archives of Physical Medicine and Rehabilitation, 74,* 602–611.

Cooke, D. (1991). Sensibility evaluation battery for the peripheral nerve injured hand. *The Australian Occupational Therapy Journal, 38,* 241–245.

Crosby, L., & Parsons, L. C. (1989). Clinical neurologic assessment tool: Development and testing of an instrument to index neurologic status. *Heart and Lung, 18,* 121–129.

Dannenbaum, R., & Jones, L. (1993). The assessment and treatment of patients who have sensory loss following cortical lesions. *Journal of Hand Therapy, 6,* 130–138.

Dellon, A. L. (1993). A numerical grading scale for peripheral nerve function. *Journal of Hand Therapy, 6,* 152–160.

Evans, E., Rendell, M., Bartek, J., Bamisedun, O., Connor, S., & Glitter, M. (1992). Current perception thresholds in ageing. *Age and Ageing, 21,* 273–279.

Foss, J. (1993). Cerebral vascular accident: Visual perceptual dysfunction. In J. Van Deusen (Ed.), *Body image and perceptual dysfunction in adults* (pp. 11–38). Philadelphia: W. B. Saunders Company.

Harlowe, D., & Van Deusen, J. (1985). Evaluating cutaneous sensation following CVA: Relationships among touch, pain, and temperature tests. *Occupational Therapy Journal of Research, 5,* 70–72.

Horch, K., Hardy, M., Jimenez, S., & Jabaley, M. (1992). An automated tactile tester for evaluation of cutaneous sensibility. *Journal of Hand Surgery (Am), 17,* 829–837.

Jerosch, H. (1993). Measuring outcome in median nerve injuries. *Journal of Hand Surgery (Br), 18,* 624–628.

Jimenez, S., Hardy, M., Horch, K., & Jabaley, M. (1993). *Journal of Hand Therapy, 6,* 124–129.

Lieberman, S., Cohen, A., & Rubin, J. (1983). NYSOA King Devick Test. *Journal of the American Optomological Association, 54,* 631–637.

Marsh, D., & Smith, B. (1986). Timed functional tests to evaluate sensory recovery in sutured nerves. *British Journal of Occupational Therapy, 49,* 79–82.

Robertson, S., & Jones, L. (1994). Tactile sensory impairments and left-hemisphere cerebral lesions. *Archives of Physical Medicine and Rehabilitation, 75,* 1108–1117.

Sieg, K. W., & Williams, W. (1986). *Occupational Therapy Journal of Research,* 195–206.

Trombly, C., & Scott, A. D. (1989). Evaluation and treatment of somatosensory sensation. In C. A. Trombly (Ed.), *Occupational therapy for physical disabilities* (pp. 41–54). Baltimore: Williams & Wilkins.

Verdugo, R., & Ochoa, J. (1992). Quantitative somatosensory thermotest. *Brain, 115*(Pt. 3), 893–913.

Warren, M. (1992a). A hierarchical model for evaluation and treatment of visual perceptual dysfunction in adult acquired brain injury, part 1. *American Journal of Occupational Therapy, 47,* 42–54.

Warren, M. (1992b). A hierarchical model for evaluation and treatment of visual perceptual dysfunction in adult acquired brain injury, part 2. *American Journal of Occupational Therapy, 47,* 55–66.

Weinberg, J., Diller, L., Gordon, W. A., et al. (1977). Visual scanning training effect on reading-related tasks in acquired right brain damage. *Archives of Physical Medicine and Rehabilitation, 58,* 479–486.

Zoltan, B. (1990). Evaluation of visual, perceptual, and perceptual motor deficits. In L. Pedretti & B. Zoltan (Eds.), *Occupational therapy practice skills for physical dysfunction* (3rd ed.) (pp. 194–201).

Zoltan, B., Siev, E., & Freishtat, B. (1986). *Cognitive dysfunction in the adult stroke patient: A manual for evaluation and treatment* (2nd ed.). Thorofare, NJ: Slack.

Assessment of Perceptual Dysfunction in the Adult

Sharon A. Cermak, EdD, OTR/L

Keh-Chung Lin, ScD, OTR

SUMMARY This section of Chapter 12 addresses the assessment of the integrative component of sensory processing. Various approaches and assessment tools are discussed in relation to neuropathology. Additional factors related to asessment of visual perception are discussed. Finally, suggestions on how to choose an assessment are given.

Brain damage, depending on its severity and location, can be responsible for various deficits in perceptual function. Perceptual deficits are present in many individuals with differing neurologic conditions. Perceptual problems are most characteristic of individuals with right cerebrovascular accident lesions (Gouvier & Cubic, 1991; Hier et al., 1983) but are also found in individuals with left cerebrovascular accident lesions (Okkema, 1993; Zoltan et al., 1986). Perceptual deficits have also been reported in individuals with Alzheimer's disease (Eslinger & Benton, 1983; Henderson et al., 1989; Mendez et al., 1990; Nebes, 1992; Ska et al., 1990; Swihart & Pirozzolo, 1988; Zec, 1993), multiple sclerosis (Fennell & Smith, 1990), and Parkinson's disease (Brown & Marsden, 1986, 1988; Cummings & Huber, 1992; Grossman et al., 1993). Although the deficits after head injury are most often reported in the cognitive domain in the areas of memory, problem solving, and judgment (Lezak, 1995), individuals may also show perceptual deficits (Gianutsos & Matheson, 1987; Neistadt, 1988, 1992). In addition to perceptual impairment in individuals with known neurologic disorders, there has been a reported decline in visuospatial and constructional abilities in the normal aging population (Howieson et al., 1993; Ogden, 1990; Schaie, 1994; Spreen & Strauss, 1991).

Deficits in perceptual abilities can greatly impact the life of a patient with brain damage, and their presence is one of the major disruptive factors impeding rehabilitation success (Barer, 1990; Bernspang et al., 1987, 1989; Campbell et al., 1991; Chen Sea et al., 1993; Denes et al., 1982; Friedman, 1990a, 1990b, 1991; Hartman-Maeir, 1995; Kinsella et al., 1993; Maeshima et al., 1990; Nogak, 1992; Shiel, 1989; Stone et al., 1993; Sunderland et al., 1987; Sundet et al., 1988; Taylor et al., 1994; Towle & Lincoln, 1991a; Wiart et al., 1994).

Perceptual dysfunction is a particularly likely explanation in cases in which the patient fails to fully participate in self-care activities and in retraining for reasons other than deficits in sensation, comprehension, or lack of motor ability (Arnadottir, 1990). The patient should not be dismissed as uncooperative or cognitively impaired.

Rather, the patient should be carefully assessed for perceptual deficits. Over the past years, a number of assessment procedures have been developed for evaluation of specific types of these deficits. These procedures rely heavily on neuropsychological tests (Benton et al., 1994), that is, the elicitation of specific behavioral responses to specific stimuli under controlled conditions (Benton, 1994). The purpose of this discussion is to review these developments, particularly with reference to their implications for clinical application and theoretical accounts of these deficits.

The assessment of perceptual dysfunction is probably one of the most difficult areas of investigation for the practicing rehabilitation clinician. Unlike aphasic disorders, perceptual deficits often go unnoticed by the patient and care providers and come to light only when directly evaluated. More often than not, individuals with aphasia present with relatively clear dissociations in a number of psycholinguistic processes (Goodglass & Kaplan, 1983), thereby allowing the development of reliable taxonomies of aphasias. In contrast, selective disruption of spatioperceptual components after brain damage has been more difficult to isolate and measure (Delis et al., 1988a). The primary reason is probably that spatioperceptual structure does not contain temporally discrete entities such as phonemes and words but must be inferred from perceptual judgments and visuospatial constructions (Delis et al., 1988b). To further complicate the issue, it is difficult to give a clear and concise account for the organization of perceptual functions in the brain (Beaumont & Davidoff, 1992). Although we are getting increasingly detailed anatomic and physiologic maps, especially of the visual pathways in the brain, and increasingly sophisticated accounts of perceptual deficits after circumscribed brain lesions, there is still a long way to go in putting it all together into a coherent theory (Corballis, 1994).

Despite this difficulty, numerous assessment techniques have been developed in the past two or three decades to allow clinically and theoretically relevant descriptions of the problems. In the following, we attempt to summarize some of the more common test procedures available for use. Although perceptual deficits can be found in a variety of sensory domains (e.g., vision, hearing, touch, smell, taste and kinesthesis), our discussion is centered on perceptual deficits in the visual domain. Perceptual dysfunctions in the auditory domain are not addressed because they are conventionally within the expertise area of speech and language pathologists. Specific deficits to be dealt with here include visuoperceptual disorders, constructional disorders, and unilateral neglect because they are most commonly noted by occupational therapists (Grieve, 1993).

Acquired visuoperceptual disorders involve changes in visual and perceptual functioning after cerebral insult. The disabilities may be reflected behaviorally in a variety of performance deficits: in failure to discriminate between objects; in defective discrimination of complex stimulus configuration (e.g., combinations of figures or forms); and in faulty localization of objects in space and defective topographic orientation (Benton & Tranel, 1993). Constructional disorders, according to Benton (1967), refer to "an impairment in combinatorial or organizing activity, in which details must be clearly perceived and in which the relationships among the component parts of the entity must be apprehended if the desired synthesis of them is to be achieved." Unilateral neglect is clinically characterized by the inability to perceive or respond to stimuli presented to the contralesional space, despite the absence of significant sensory or motor deficits (Heilman et al., 1993).

APPROACHES TO PERCEPTUAL ASSESSMENT

Occupational therapists use a variety of approaches to assess perception in the adult with brain injury. Whereas some therapists assess primarily functional activities, others assess the components of performance, including aspects of visual perception. Still others are primarily interested in examining a patient's potential for learning so they can identify the type of rehabilitation strategies that will be most effective. These three approaches to assessment are functional assessment, assessment of performance components, and dynamic assessment (Table 12–1).

Functional Task Assessment

The approach used by many occupational therapists is to assess functional activities and identify the tasks with which an individual has difficulty (Neistadt, 1988, 1994a, 1994b; Okkema, 1993). For example, the therapist may perform an assessment of activities of daily living (ADL) (e.g., dressing oneself) and rate the accuracy, the amount of verbal cueing needed, and the speed needed to complete the activity or the therapist may rate the patient's ability to complete each of the specific steps of the activity (e.g., put sleeve in coat). In all cases, the specific perceptual skills underlying performance are not specified, although the therapist may make assumptions or hypotheses about perceptual abilities or deficits. Examples of assessments of this type include the Functional Independence Measure (FIM) (Dodds et al., 1993; Granger et al., 1993; Keith et al., 1987), the Barthel Index (Mahoney & Barthel, 1965; Wade & Collin, 1988), the Klein-Bell (Klein & Bell, 1982), the Ribideau Kitchen evaluation (Neistadt, 1994b, 1994c), and other functional assessments described in Unit Five of this text. A limitation of many of these assessments is that they do not differentiate between physical and cognitive components of an activity for the adult with brain injury (Toglia, 1989). The majority of functional assessments used in physical disabilities emphasize motor skills and do not evaluate the perceptual or cognitive components of the tasks. This is problematic because there is a growing use of

TABLE 12–1

THREE APPROACHES TO PERCEPTUAL ASSESSMENT

Approach	Description	Advantage	Disadvantage
Functional	Assessment of specific functional tasks and ADL	Knowledge of patient performance on relevant tasks Readily understandable to patient and family	Does not provide insight regarding the underlying problems causing the functional performance deficit
Performance components	Assessment of the perceptual and constructional abilities believed to contribute to adequate functional performance	Identification of clients strengths and weaknesses to design treatment strategies	Multiple deficits are frequently found Training of deficit components may not result in improved functional performance
Dynamic assessment	Assessment that analyzes the patient's response to cues, task modifications, and characteristics of the task	Provides information about client's learning ability and therefore provides guidance in selecting appropriate intervention strategies	Experienced clinician needed Scores not standard

From Su, C. Y., et al. (1995). Performance of older adults with and without cerebrovascular accident on the test of visual-perceptual skills. *American Journal of Occupational Therapy, 49*(6), 495. Copyright 1995 by the American Occupational Therapy Association, Inc. Reprinted with permission.

ADL assessments as a major measurement tool to evaluate progress and set criteria for admission and discharge in rehabilitation facilities (Toglia, 1989). Moreover, the influence of perceptual disorders on the performance of an individual is often not readily apparent (Foss, 1993).

Recently, several assessments have been developed to identify the processing characteristics of performance in functional tasks (e.g., Park et al., 1994; Toglia, 1991a, 1991b). In the Assessment of Motor and Process Skills (AMPS) (Park et al., 1994), the therapist observes a client performing ADL and instrumental ADL tasks and assesses the client's specific motor and process skills that comprise performance in that task. Although the AMPS does not assess specific perceptual processes (e.g., spatial abilities, constructional abilities, memory), it assesses observable behaviors that reflect operations such as choosing the appropriate tools and materials.

Recognizing the close relationship between performance on ADL tasks and the deficits in the performance components, Arnadottir (1990) developed an instrument, the Arnadottir OT-ADL Neurobehavioral Evaluation (A-ONE) that simultaneously relates functional performance in ADL to neurobehavioral components. The tool includes (1) a Functional Independence Scale that determines the level of assistance needed on five ADL domains: dressing, grooming, hygiene, mobility, and feeding and communication with each of these domains having subcomponents that are assessed separately; (2) a Specific Neurobehavioral Scale, which assesses the type and amount of interference of 10 specific neurobehavioral impairments on each of the subcategories within each ADL domain; and (3) a Pervasive Neurobehavioral Scale that determines the presence or absence of other neurobehavioral impairments. Using clinical reasoning,

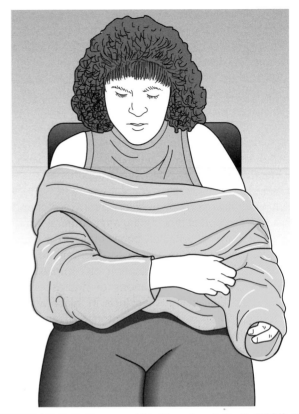

FIGURE 12–2. Putting on a shirt. (From Arnadottir, G. [1990]. The brain and behavior. Assessing cortical dysfunction through activities of daily living. St. Louis, MO: C. V. Mosby.)

the therapist observes the patient as he or she performs ADL, observing for possible neurobehavioral deficits during that specific activity rather than testing for each deficit separately (Fig. 12–1). For each ADL activity, Arnadottir describes performance that would reflect difficulty in a variety of areas. For example, in dressing, grabbing the shirt or sock but having difficulty adjusting grasp according to needs may reflect motor apraxia; not knowing what to do with the shirt, socks, or pants may reflect ideational apraxia; not pulling the shirt all the way down on the affected side may indicate unilateral neglect; putting the legs into the armholes may reflect somatoagnosia; inability to differentiate between the front from the back of the clothes may indicate a spatial relations disorder; attempting to button many buttonholes onto the same button may indicate perseveration; and not including all the steps of the activity such as not completing the fastenings may indicate organization and sequencing problems (Fig. 12–2).

Evaluation of Performance Components

An alternative approach to assessment is to evaluate specific perceptual abilities to identify the aspects that are believed to interfere with functional activity. An advantage to assessment of specific perceptual abilities is to enable the

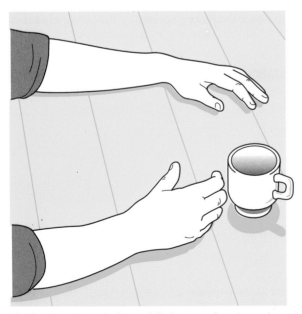

FIGURE 12–1. Spatial relation difficulties manifested in underestimation of distances when reaching for a cup. (From Arnadottir, G. [1990]. The brain and behavior. Assessing cortical dysfunction through activities of daily living. St. Louis, MO: C. V. Mosby.)

therapist to identify the client's strengths and weaknesses to better design appropriate intervention techniques and strategies that may include remediation of the deficits and capitalizing on the client's strengths.

Evaluation of individual cognitive skills and components such as orientation, attention, organization, and problem solving and reasoning are discussed in the next section of this text. Here we discuss the evaluation of visual perceptual and visual motor disorders under the categories of visuoperceptual disorders, constructional disorders, and unilateral neglect.

Assessment of basic visual skills is critical but is not discussed in this section. Warren (1993a, 1993b, 1994) presents a hierarchical model of visual perception and examines skills that she believes are the foundation of and prerequisites for higher level perceptual abilities. These foundation skills include visual acuity, visual fields, oculomotor control, and visual attention and scanning (see Section 2 of this chapter, Sensory Deficits, for a description of the assessment of these foundation abilities).

Assessment of specific perceptual abilities is intended to enable the therapist to better understand the nature of the deficit, to identify the patient's strengths, and to identify those deficits that are believed to interfere with function and then to use that information to develop treatment strategies. For example, in a study on driving, visuoperceptual test scores explained 64 percent of the variance in the driving assessment (Galski et al., 1992, 1993). The research group noted that use of the perceptual tests identified performance deficits that could be amenable to remediation or compensation for driving skill. However, it is important to recognize that improving the component abilities may not automatically result in improved performance in functional tasks (see Neistadt, 1995). In addition, in patients with brain damage, multiple impairments are common and it is often difficult to precisely differentiate factors that interfere with function (Toglia, 1989). Similarly, some patients who may show impairment on specific tests may perform adequately on functional tasks because they are able to perform the task using other abilities. Thus, it is important to incorporate both functional assessment and assessment of components.

Dynamic Assessment

Toglia (1989, 1991a, 1991b, 1992) advocates a dynamic investigative approach to supplement conventional measures of performance components as a means of analyzing the patient's processing strategies and determining his or her potential for learning. This approach includes analyzing the patient's response to cues and task modifications to be able to assess his or her potential for learning. The characteristics of the task include the modality of stimulus presentation, the number of stimuli, the number of task steps, and the familiarity of the task. Additional factors may include the rate and duration of stimulus presentation, the type of feedback (before activity, during an activity, on

completion of an activity), and the individual's error detection/correction (self-generated or externally generated). Toglia (1992) emphasizes that dysfunction is not task specific but is related to the characteristics of the task and the environment. This approach is detailed in several articles (Abreu, 1995; Toglia, 1989; 1991a, 1991b, 1992). Kaplan (1990) also supports the use of dynamic assessment, which she refers to as the process approach and argues that in addition to knowing whether a patient passes or fails a task, it is critical to know how a patient approaches a task. The advantage of the dynamic or process approach is that it provides more information that is relevant for treatment than traditional assessment. This approach, however, places greater demand on the therapist's clinical experience and ingenuity.

NEUROPATHOLOGY AND RESEARCH ON THE ASSESSMENT TOOLS

In the following section, we discuss the neuropathology of three major categories of perceptual disorders—visuoperceptual disorders, constructional disorders, and unilateral neglect—and review relevant research on their assessment.

Visuoperceptual Disorders

A basic division of visuoperceptual disorders pertains to the difference between defects in the identification of the formal characteristics of objects and defects in the localization of these objects in space (Benton & Tranal, 1993). Identification of the neuroanatomic correlates has led to the identification of two cortical visual systems: a ventral system (inferior occipitotemporal pathway) subserving object recognition (the "what" system) and a dorsal system (occipitoparietal pathway) subserving the appreciation of spatial relationships (the "where" system) (see Levine et al., 1985; Mishkin et al., 1983; Post & Liebowitz, 1986; Trevarthen, 1968) (Fig. 12–3).

The occipitotemporal system, also known as focal or attentive vision, involves attending to the salient features of an object to discriminate the details. This enables an individual to identify objects and differentiate them from other objects. It enables the reader to distinguish between a "b" and a "d." The occipitoparietal system involves peripheral or ambient vision and is concerned with detection of events in the environment and their location in space and relation to the individual. Visual input must be integrated with other sensory information, including tactile, auditory, kinesthetic, vestibular, and proprioceptive perceptions, to provide this information (Warren, 1993a, 1993b). Both systems working in concert contribute to efficient perceptual processing and to visual memory (Mishkin et al., 1983). In fact, it has been pointed out that

Parallel-distributed processing of the visual system

Sequence of synaptic and axonal flow in the cerebral cortex: input into 1° and 2 ° visual cortex, then via several parallel-distributed pathways and circuits:
1. Superior circuit ⟶ Superior parietal lobe and prefrontal lobe + FEF. ⎤
2. Inferior circuit ⟶ Post temporal lobe and prefrontal lobe + FEF. ⎦ *1
3. To limbic cortex especially temporal lobe components *2 & cingulate gyrus.
4. To the kinetic system to obtain a visual-manual and/or visual-motor program.
5. To the synergic system to obtain a coordinated-sequential programs for desired (goal oriented) movements involved in activities including visual movements.
*1. Prefrontal lobes: anticipatory executive, including judgement, of the CNS including (FEF) frontal eye fields for controlling visual movements in all skilled activities.

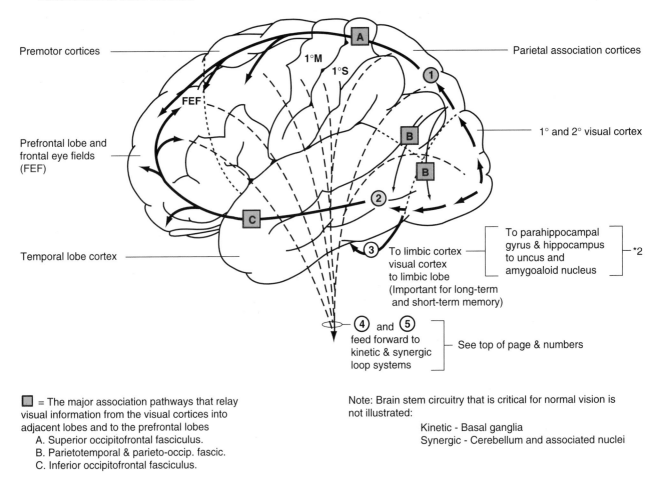

= The major association pathways that relay visual information from the visual cortices into adjacent lobes and to the prefrontal lobes
    A. Superior occipitofrontal fasciculus.
    B. Parietotemporal & parieto-occip. fascic.
    C. Inferior occipitofrontal fasciculus.

Note: Brain stem circuitry that is critical for normal vision is not illustrated:
    Kinetic - Basal ganglia
    Synergic - Cerebellum and associated nuclei

Area ① noted above is in the posterior part of the superior parietal lobule: MAJOR FUNCTIONS include visuospatial orientation, sensory appreciation of the external environment including an internal memory map of the environment and body-image map plus movement detection.

Area ② noted above is in the posterior temporal lobe: MAJOR FUNCTIONS include visuo-object and color recognition, orientation of objects and detailed serial processing of environment stimuli.

FIGURE 12–3. Two visual systems: parallel-distributed processing. (Courtesy of Josephine Moore, Vermillion, SD.)

damage to either system can result in spatial disorientation, although this occurs for different reasons (Lezak, 1995).

Perceptual processes include the structuring and organization of information: recognition, identification and classification; discrimination; and the extraction of meaning (Giles & Clark-Wilson, 1993). Under this rubric congregates a heterogeneous collection of disorders because the spectrum of performances that can be distorted as a consequence of defective visuoperceptual function is very large. Table 12–2 describes many of the commonly used tests of visual perception.

VISUAL ANALYSIS AND SYNTHESIS

Visuoperceptual skills considered to involve analysis and synthesis include making visual discriminations, differentiating foreground from background (figure ground), recognizing objects on the basis of incomplete information

TABLE 12–2

TESTS OF VISUAL PERCEPTION

Title	Author	Description	Source
Hooper Visual Organization Test	Hooper, 1958; revised 1983	The test consists of 30 line drawings of simple objects that have been cut into pieces and rearranged. The subject must verbally identify what the object would be if the pieces were put back together.	Western Psychological Services, 12031 Wilshire Boulevard, Los Angeles, CA 90025-1251; see Lezak, 1995, pp. 409–411.
Visual Form Discrimination	Benton, 1983	Book of 16 line drawings in which a stimulus and an array of choices are presented simultaneously. The subject must discriminate among the four response choices.	Psychological Assessment Resources (PAR), P.O. Box 998, Odessa, FL 33556; see Benton et al., 1994, pp. 65–72.
Visual Object and Space Perception (VOSP)	Warrington & James, 1991	To assess specific impairments of cognitive function after brain damage. The VOSP is designed to reflect specificity of right hemisphere lesions. Nine tests are included: 1 test (shape detection screening test) screens out patients for whom the VOSP is inappropriate; 4 tests assess object perception (incomplete letters, silhouettes, object decision, progressive silhouettes); 4 tests assess space perception (dot counting, position discrimination, number location, cube analysis).	Western Psychological Services, 12031 Wilshire Boulevard, Los Angeles, CA 90025-1251; see Lezak, 1995, pp. 408–409.
Motor-Free Visual Perception Test—Revised	Colarusso & Hammill, 1996; Bouska & Kwatny, 1983	Visual perception test with 36 items in which the subject is shown a line drawing and is asked to match the stimulus from a multiple-choice set of other drawings; originally standardized for children by Calorusso and Hammill; normative data and scoring system for use with adults is presented by Bouska and Kwatny.	Academic Therapy Publications, 20 Commercial Blvd, Novato, CA 94947-6191; see Bouska & Kwatny, 1983.
Test of Visual Perceptual Skills	Gardner, 1982	A nonmotor test of visual perception that assesses seven visual areas: discrimination, memory, spatial relationships, form constancy, sequential memory, figure ground, and closure; originally designed and standardized for children; normative data recently available for adults.	Psychological and Educational Publications, 147 Rollins Rd., Burlingame, CA 94010; see Su et al., 1995.
Judgement of Line Orientation	Benton, 1983	Subject is required to match one or two lines with those showing the same inclination on an array of lines presented on the same card.	Psychological Assessment Resources (PAR), P.O. Box 998, Odessa, FL 33556; see Benton et al., 1994, pp. 53–64.
Picture Completion	Weschsler, 1981	Identification of details within a picture to identify the missing feature.	Psychological Corporation, 555 Academic Ct., San Antonio, TX 78204-2498.
Raven's Progressive Matrices	Raven	A series of three nonverbal tests of varying ability level that assess mental ability by requiring the subject to solve problems presented in abstract visual figures and designs.	Psychological Corporation, 555 Academic Ct., San Antonio, TX 78204-2498.

Table continued on following page

TABLE 12–2

TESTS OF VISUAL PERCEPTION *Continued*

Title	Author	Description	Source
Embedded Figures Test	Spreen & Benton, 1969	Test consists of 16 line drawings used as stimulus figures and presented in left half of test booklet. The right half of each sheet is a complex figure drawing in which the stimulus figure is embedded. Subjects must search for and trace the stimulus figure in the embedded design using a pencil. Healthy adults make few errors on this test.	Neuropsychology Laboratory, University of Victoria, Victoria, British Columbia, VSW 3P5 Canada; see Spreen & Strauss, 1991, pp. 291–296.
Visual Figure Ground	Ayres, 1966	A test of the Southern California Sensory Integration Tests; originally developed for children; normative data is available for adults in the American Journal of Occupational Therapy.	Western Psychological Services, 12031 Wilshire Boulevard, Los Angeles, CA 90025-1251.
Test of Facial Recognition	Benton et al., 1983	Examines ability to recognize faces without a memory component; subject matches identical front views, front views with side views, and front views taken under different lighting conditions.	Psychological Assessment Resources (PAR), P.O. Box 998, Odessa, FL 33556; see Benton et al., 1994, pp. 35–52.
Minnesota Paper Form Board Test, Revised 1969	Likert & Quasha, 1970	Spatial task involving high level perceptual ability and analytical processing; involves ability to perceive fragments as wholes.	Psychological Corporation, 555 Academic Ct., San Antonio, TX 78204-2498; see Lezak, 1995, pp. 362–363.
Corsi Block Tapping Test	Milner, 1971 (research tool)	Memory for sequence of spatial locations. Nine black 1½-inch cubes are fastened in a random order to a blackboard. Examiner taps blocks in a prearranged order and the subject copies the tapping pattern.	

(visual closure), and synthesizing disparate elements into a meaningful whole (Efferson, 1995). Some tests of perceptual abilities include only one element. Examples of these tests include the Visual Organization Test, which assesses visual organization (Hooper, 1983) (Fig. 12–4), or the Visual Form Discrimination Test (Benton et al., 1983), which assesses the ability to analyze the critical features of forms and decides which of the response stimuli are the same as the target stimuli (Fig. 12–5). The Visual Form Discrimination Test is a multiple choice test of visual recognition. There are 16 items, each consisting of a target set of stimuli and four stimulus sets below the target. The distractors contain small variations of displacement, rotation, or distortion. Approximately two thirds of the control subjects received at or near ceiling scores. Lezak (1995) noted that patients with left anterior lesions, right parietal lesions, and bilateral diffuse lesions were associated with the highest percentages of impaired performance on this test.

In contrast to tests that assess a single aspect of visual perception, other tests such as the Visual Object and Space Perception Test (VOSP) (Warrington & James, 1991), the Motor-Free Visual Perception Test (MVPT) (Colarusso &

Hammill, 1972; Bouska & Kwatny, 1983), and the Test of Visual Perceptual Skills (TVPS) (Gardner, 1982) assess a variety of different perceptual skills. Whereas the VOSP includes several subtests, each of which assesses a discrete aspect of visual perception, the MVPT assesses a combination of visuoperceptual abilities.

The Visual Object and Space Perception Test (Warrington & James, 1991) was designed to reflect specificity of right hemisphere lesions and includes a set of nine different tests that were originally designed for research with adults with brain damage (Table 12–3, Fig. 12–6). The first test, a shape detection screening test, is used to screen out patients for whom the VOSP is inappropriate. Four tests assess aspects of object perception (incomplete letters, silhouettes, object decision, progressive silhouettes), and four tests assess aspects of space perception (dot counting, position discrimination, number location, cube analysis). Normative data and cut scores are provided for each test individually so that the tests can be used either individually or as a battery.

The Motor-Free Visual Perception Test (MVPT) (Colarusso & Hammill, 1972) and The Test of Visual Perceptual Skills (Gardner, 1982) were originally designed for children but have also been used with adults. The MVPT is a 36-item test of overall visuoperceptual abilities that includes items in the areas of spatial relationships, visual discrimination, figure-ground, visual closure, and visual memory. The test was originally standardized for children aged 4 through 8 years. The test has just been revised (The Motor-Free Visual Perception Test–Revised [MVPT-R]) (Colarusso & Hammill, 1996) (Fig. 12–7) and includes 4 additional and more difficult items. Normative data on the MVPT-R are presented for children aged 4 to 11. The authors state that because "Maturation of the human visual perceptual system is considered to be completed (i.e., "adult") by 10-11 years of age" (p. 13), the MVPT-R can be used with adults as well as children (Colarusso & Hammill, 1996). The MVPT will also be available in a format with stimuli arranged vertically rather than horizontally as with the MVPT and the MVPT-R. This new format will present the stimuli at visual field midline to allow assessment of visual perception in both children and adults without the confounding effects of visual field deficits. Bouska and Kwatny (1983) have used the MVPT (1972 version) with adults and provide normative data for adults aged 18 to 80 years old. Several measures can be computed from the test administration with adults: raw score, average time per item, response behavior for left-sided figures, response behavior for right-sided figures, performance behavior for left-sided figures, and performance behavior for right-sided figures. This scoring system was developed with particular application for use with stroke patients in an effort to separate problems in visual perception from unilateral neglect.

Another test that was originally designed for children but

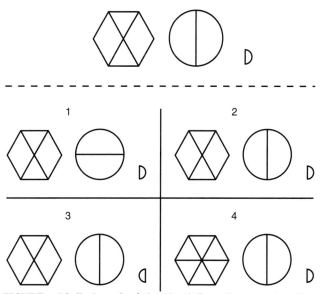

Visual form discriminiation

FIGURE 12–5. Item 9 of the Visual Form Discrimination Test. 1 = rotation of major figure; 2 = correct response; 3 = rotation of peripheral figure; 4 = distortion of other major figure. (From *Contributions to Neuropsychological Assessment: A Clinical Manual*, 2/e by Arthur L. Benton, Abigail B. Sivan, Kerry de S. Hamsher, Nils R. Varney, and Otfried Spreen. Copyright © 1994 by Oxford University Press, Inc. Reprinted by permission.)

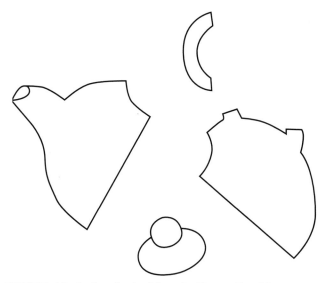

FIGURE 12–4. Stimulus (cup) from the Hooper Visual Organization Test. The individual must synthesize visual information to picture the object after viewing its parts. (Stimulus from the *Hooper Visual Organization Test* copyright © 1983 by Western Psychological Services, original edition copyright © 1958 H. Elston Hooper. Reprinted with permission of the publisher, Western Psychological Services, 12031 Wilshire Boulevard, Los Angeles, CA 90025. All rights reserved.)

that has been normed for adults is the Test of Visual Perceptual Skills (TVPS) (Non-Motor) (Gardner, 1982). The TVPS contains 112 items that involve the use of two-dimensional configurations. It is divided into seven subtests of visual perception: Visual Discrimination, Visual Memory, Visual Spatial Relationships, Visual Form Constancy, Visual Sequential Memory, Visual Figure Ground, and Visual Closure (*note:* although each test is designed to assess a specific aspect of visual perception, there is overlap among the subtests). Each subtest has a practice test plate that is followed by 16 items arranged in order of increasing difficulty. Subjects respond by indicating one of four or five options on each item that matches the test sample (Fig. 12–8). Hung and colleagues (1987) used the test to examine visuoperceptual skills in young adults with learning disabilities and found the test to discriminate between individuals with and without learning disabilities. Normative data have been published for 155 normal adults, aged 45 to 84 (Table 12–4) (Su et al., 1995). The researchers found that performance decreased with increasing age; education was also a significant factor. In addition, the authors found that the test discriminated between individuals with and without stroke, with individuals with stroke performing more poorly than normal controls. The scores on two subtests, Visual Form Constancy and Visual-Spatial Relationships, contributed significantly to the discriminant function between the control and stroke groups. There was no difference in performance of individuals with left compared with right cere-

TABLE 12-3

THE VISUAL OBJECT AND SPACE PERCEPTION BATTERY (VOSP)

Area Assessed	Name of Test	Description	Task
Screening	Shape Detection Screening	Consists of 20 cards; half the cards display an overall pattern with an embedded degraded X that the subject must identify.	Screens out subjects who are not appropriate for this test
Object Perception	Incomplete Letters	Subject must identify a letter that has been degraded.	Measures ability to identify degraded letter stimuli and is sensitive to right posterior lesions
	Silhouettes	Consists of the rotated and blackened shape of 15 objects and 15 animals; the subject names or describes each object.	Measures degree of impairment in object recognition
	Object Decision	Subject sees a set of 20 cards, each with four black silhouette shapes that have been rotated. Of these, one is a real object and three are distractors. The subject must identify the shape that is a silhouette of a real object.	Distinguishes word-finding problems from perceptual processing deficits
	Progressive Silhouettes	Objects presented in silhouette, initially distorted (elongated) and rotated, with increasingly closer approximations to the object. The number of silhouettes needed to correctly identify the object is recorded.	Assesses recognition threshold by presenting silhouettes of the same object from various angles
Space Perception	Dot Counting	Subject sees an array of 5 to 9 black dots randomly distributed on a white card. Subject must identify the number of dots in each of 10 arrays.	Measures spatial scanning and ability to localize a single point
	Position Discrimination	Subject sees a set of 20 cards, each with two squares next to each other. One square has a black dot exactly centered; the other is slightly off center. The subject must identify the picture with the dot in the center.	Assesses ability to discriminate between different positions in space
	Number Location	Two squares, one above the other, are presented on each of 10 cards. The top square has randomly placed numbers 1 to 9. The bottom square has a single dot in a different position. The subject must identify the number that corresponds to the position of the dot.	A more complex test of spatial discrimination
	Cube Analysis	This is a 10-item block counting task. The subject sees an outline representing a three-dimensional arrangement of blocks and must identify the number of blocks in the picture.	Measures perception of complex spatial relationships

brovascular accident lesions, although the sample size was quite small (11 subjects in each group).

SPATIAL PERCEPTION

Spatial orientation, one component of visual perception, refers to "the ability to relate to the position, direction, or movement of objects or points in space" (Lezak, 1995, p. 344). Disorders of spatial orientation may occur for different reasons. As illustrative examples, disorders of line orientation perception and topographic orientation are depicted because of their theoretical interest and functional significance.

Disorder of Line Orientation Perception. Disturbances of appreciation of the directional orientation of lines are among the salient visuoperceptual disorders after brain disease, particularly disease of the right hemisphere (Benton et al., 1994). A frequently used test to evaluate this ability, the Judgment of Line Orientation Test, was designed by Benton and colleagues (1978). In this test, the subject is required to match one or two lines with those showing the same inclination on an array of lines presented on the same card (Fig. 12–9).

The Judgment of Line Orientation Test has been described in detail and includes normative data for individuals aged 16 to 74 (Benton et al., 1994). Data are also included for individuals with brain damage. Forty percent of right brain–damaged patients showed impaired performance on this test, as compared with only 6 percent of patients with left brain damage, none of whom showed a remarkably poor performance. More recent studies (Hamsher et al., 1992; Trahan, 1991) confirmed that patients with right hemisphere lesions performed more poorly on the task than patients with left hemisphere lesions. Further evidence in support of the association between judgment of line orientation and right hemispheric function came from a positron emission tomographic scan study (Gur et al., 1987). An increase in cerebral blood flow in the right hemisphere was found during performance on this task.

By electrical stimulation mapping in awake patients undergoing neurosurgery, Fried and associates (1982) identified the loci of the right hemisphere where stimulation disrupted line orientation perception. These loci are located in the parieto-occipital junction and in a small region of the posterior frontal cortex, the homologue of Broca's area. Although the perception of directional orientation is mediated primarily by the right hemisphere in right-handed subjects, evidence has also been provided suggestive of a left hemisphere contribution to judgments

of line orientation when the standard matching-to-sample format is used (Kim et al., 1984; Mehta et al., 1987).

Disorder of Topographic Orientation. Topographic disorientation is a disturbance of the ability to find the way around an environment (Henderson, 1992-1993a; Paterson & Zangwill, 1945). The lesion responsible for topographic disorientation is frequently bilateral when the disorder is not secondary to unilateral neglect (McFie et al., 1950). Descriptions of the disorder include the inability to describe the spatial layout of objects in a room or of buildings and landmarks in large-scale spaces. Topographic disorientation is often manifested by the patient who gets lost in the hospital and cannot find the way back to his or her room. The central disability is primarily a disorder of the relationship of two or more objects in space, resulting in the loss of the sense of direction and of the ability to establish a spatial scheme or map to localize objects and describe routes (Henderson, 1992-1993b).

Most assessments of topographic orientation are obser-

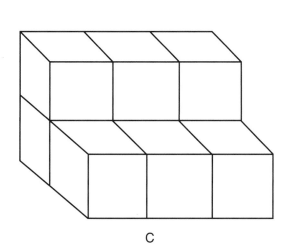

FIGURE 12–6. Items from selected subtests of the Visual Object and Space Perception Test. *A*, Two items (camel and frog) from the Silhouettes subtest. *B*, Multiple-choice item from the Object Decision subtest. *C*, An item from the Cube Analysis subtest. (Copyright E. Warrington & M. James, Thames Valley Test Co., Suffolk, England.)

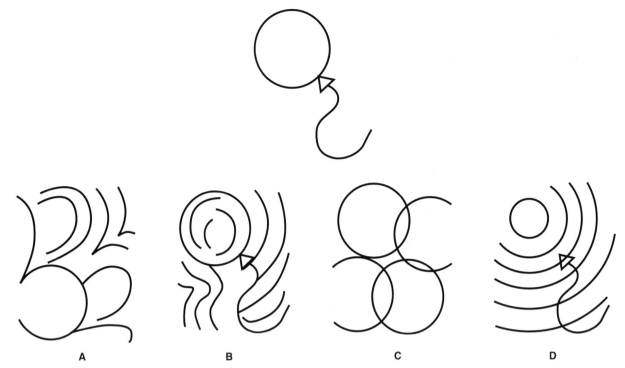

FIGURE 12–7. An item from the Motor-Free Visual Perception Test–Revised. (Courtesy of Academic Therapy Publications, Novato, CA.)

vational and are not standardized. Frequently the patient is assessed by observing his or her movement within an environment in response to directional cues (e.g., go to the Occupational Therapy Department; tell me how you would go to the Occupational Therapy Department; draw a map to show how you would go to the Occupational Therapy Department; or draw a map of the layout of your home).

When assessing topographic orientation, it is critical to assess the patient in familiar as well as unfamiliar environments. Familiar environments should include the patient's home; and if it is expected that the patient will be able to move independently within the community (i.e., drive to work, take the bus, walk to the corner store, or go to the bank), this ability should be assessed as well.

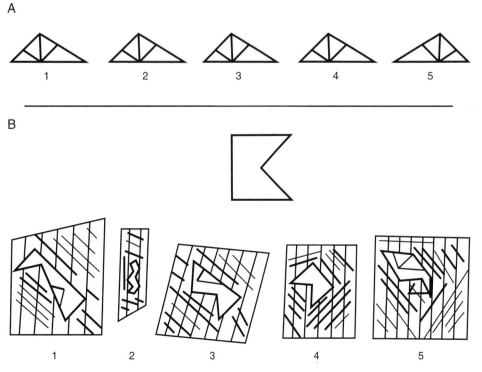

FIGURE 12–8. *A,* An of item from the Visual Spatial Relations subtest of the TVPS. The individual must identify the form that is going in a different way. *B,* An approximation of item from the Visual Form Constancy subtest of the TVPS. The individual must find the upper form in one of the five choices. (From the Test of Visual Perceptual Skills by M. Gardner © 1982, Psychological and Educational Publications, Burlingame, CA.)

DESCRIPTIVE STATISTICS FOR TOTAL TVPS TIME SCORE (SECONDS) AND ACCURACY SCORES FOR TVPS TOTAL AND SUBTESTS BY GROUP

TVPS	Control Subjects (n = 155)					Subjects with CVA (n = 22)
	Total	*45–54 Years*	*55–64 Years*	*65–74 Years*	*75–84 Years*	
Total-T						
M	1750.01	1196.44	1331.74	1746.68	2095.52	1916.82
SD	563.64	289.82	355.72	571.32	546.68	629.75
Total-A						
M	76.10	85.64	79.00	73.07	65.33	59.91
SD	15.98	13.89	13.32	14.31	16.54	14.54
VD						
M	11.94	13.11	12.87	11.15	10.33	10.27
SD	2.83	1.92	2.17	3.12	3.15	2.81
VM						
M	9.79	10.97	10.33	9.40	8.21	7.86
SD	2.82	2.40	2.74	2.65	2.87	2.77
VSR						
M	12.07	13.53	12.00	12.03	10.64	9.14
SD	2.81	2.31	2.58	2.58	3.18	2.78
VFC						
M	10.37	11.39	10.48	10.33	9.15	7.14
SD	2.81	3.27	2.68	2.44	2.49	2.64
VSM						
M	10.35	12.33	10.76	9.85	8.21	8.09
SD	2.71	2.37	2.02	2.33	2.67	3.12
VFG						
M	10.58	12.36	10.93	10.00	8.85	8.36
SD	2.75	2.45	2.652	2.25	2.72	2.90
VC						
M	11.01	11.94	11.63	10.33	9.94	9.05
SD	2.83	2.44	2.70	2.89	2.87	3.18

Total-A = Total accuracy score of TVPS. Total-T = Total time score of TVPS. TVPS = Test of Visual-Perceptual Skills. VC = Visual closure. VD = Visual discrimination. VFC = Visual form constancy. VFG = Visual figure-ground. VM = Visual memory. VSM = Visual sequential memory. VSR = Visual-spatial relationships.
From Su, C. Y., et al. (1995). Performance of older adults with and without cerebrovascular accident on the test of visual-perceptual skills. *American Journal of Occupational Therapy, 49*(6), 491–499. Copyright 1995 by the American Occupational Therapy Association, Inc. Reprinted with permission.

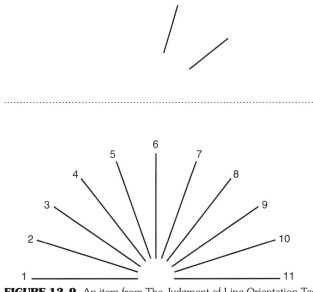

FIGURE 12–9. An item from The Judgment of Line Orientation Test. The individual must visually match the two stimulus lines oriented at different angles to the stimulus array. (From *Contributions to Neuropsychological Assessment: A Clinical Manual,* 1/e by Arthur L. Benton, Kerry de S. Hamsher, Nils R. Varney, and Otfried Spreen. Copyright © 1983 by Oxford University Press, Inc. Reprinted by permission.)

Constructional Disorders

The term *constructional praxis* is a broad concept and has been applied to different types of activities whose common characteristic involves requiring the individual to assemble, join, or draw parts to form a single unitary structure (Benton et al., 1994). According to Lezak, "constructional performance combines perceptual activity with motor response and always has a spatial component" (1995, p. 559). Constructional tasks encompass two classes of activities: (1) drawing (graphomotor), and (2) building or assembling. These can be further subdivided into two-dimensional and three-dimensional tasks.

Although there is no consensus as to whether constructional disorders are more specifically associated with one cerebral hemisphere than the other, the right hemisphere has more often been implicated (Binder, 1982; Black & Bernard, 1984; Mack & Levine, 1981; Piercy & Smyth, 1962). A recent meta-analysis (i.e., quantitative literature review) of 20 relevant studies (Lin & Tickle-Degnen, 1991) revealed that, on the average, patients with right hemispheric lesions performed more poorly on constructional

Drawings by individuals with right and left hemisphere damage

Copies   Spontaneous

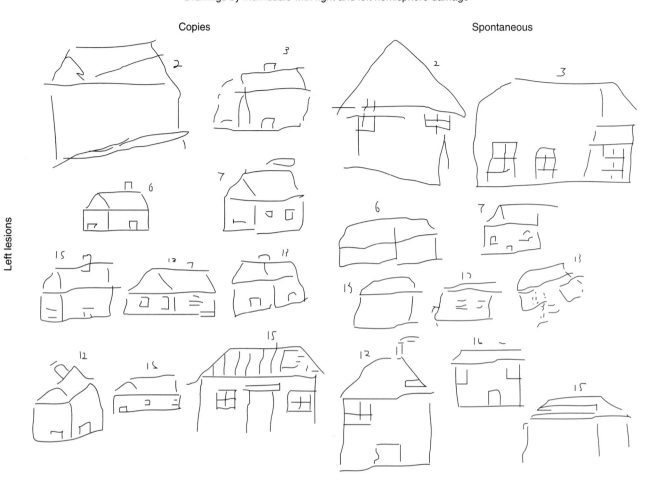

Copies   Spontaneous

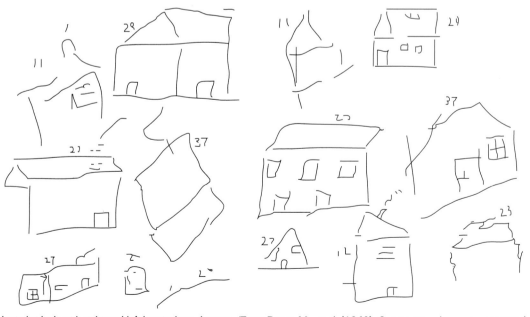

FIGURE 12–10. Drawings by individuals with right and left hemisphere damage. (From Percy, M., et al. [1960]. Constructional apraxia associated with unilateral cerebral lesions—left and right sided compared. *Brain, 83,* 225–242. By permission of Oxford University Press.)

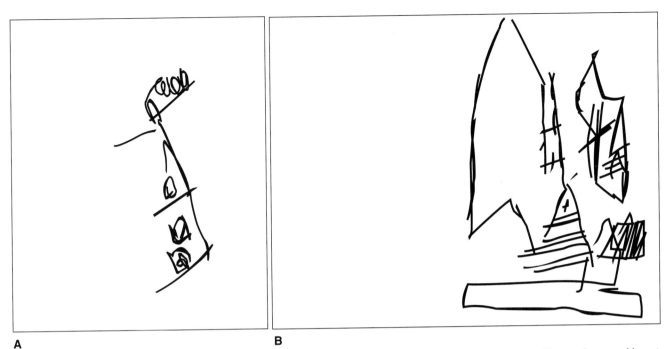

A   **B**

FIGURE 12–11. Drawings of a house by individuals after a right cerebrovascular accident. *A,* Severe neglect and mild to moderate problems in constructional abilities are shown. *B,* Severe neglect and severe problems in constructional abilities are shown.

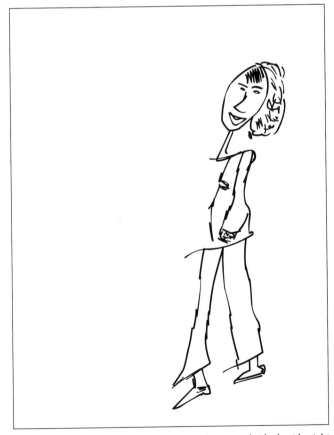

FIGURE 12–12. Drawing of a person by an individual with right cerebrovascular accident. Severe neglect with intact constructional abilities is shown.

with damage to the right hemisphere produced much less accurate copies than patients with left cerebrovascular accidents lesions, who in turn performed more poorly than controls. Individuals with left cerebrovascular accident lesions and aphasia were less accurate than individuals with left lesions without aphasia. In copying the drawing, patients with lesions in the left hemisphere tended to break up the design into smaller units than are normally perceived whereas patients with lesions in the right hemisphere tend to omit elements. On recall, the patients with left hemisphere lesions used a more configural approach, whereas patients with right hemisphere lesions continued to draw poorly integrated figures. Patients with right hemisphere lesions and neglect tended to omit details on the left side

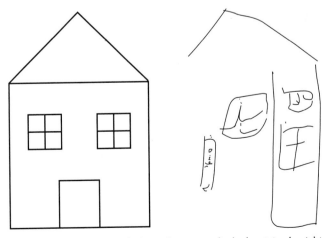

FIGURE 12–13. Copy of a house by a man who had sustained a right cerebrovascular accident that resulted in neglect.

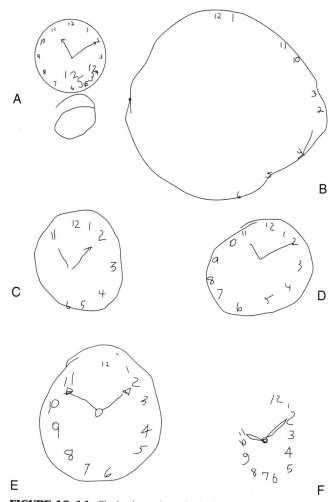

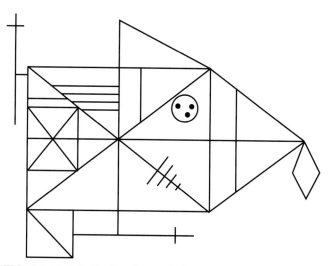

FIGURE 12–16. The Rey Osterrieth Complex Figure. (Adapted from *Archives de Psychologie* 1994; 30:206–356, Université de Genève.)

ASSEMBLY TASKS

Assembly or building tasks may be divided into two-dimensional constructional tasks such as block designs (Wechsler, 1981), parquetry blocks (Niestadt, 1989), stick pattern constructions (Goodglass & Kaplan, 1983), or three-dimensional constructions such as building from photographs or models (Benton & Fogel, 1962; Benton et al., 1994; Critchley, 1953). Table 12–7 identifies many of the commonly used tests of constructional abilities that involve assembling or building.

One of the most commonly used and researched tests of three-dimensional block construction is that described by Benton and associates (1994) (Fig. 12–18). This standardized, objectively scored test requires the subject to reproduce three block models of increasing complexity, using 6, 8, and 15 blocks from an assortment of 29 blocks on a tray. A comparable but more difficult form using photographs of the same block constructions is provided. The time taken for the construction of each model is recorded in seconds, although accuracy rather than speed is emphasized (Spreen & Strauss, 1991). Scoring is the total number of blocks correctly assembled with a time correction factor. Recording of the types of errors is also included. A more complete description of the test and accompanying normative data is described in several sources (Benton et al., 1994; Lezak, 1995; Spreen & Strauss, 1991).

In a study by Benton and associates (1979) using the three-dimensional block construction task, 54 percent of patients with right hemisphere lesions scored lower than 95 percent of the controls whereas 23 percent of individuals with left hemisphere lesions scored at that level. In another study, among patients with left hemisphere lesions, constructional deficits were most commonly seen in individuals with receptive aphasia (Benton et al., 1994).

Recently, Neistadt (1989) developed the Parquetry Block Test. This test of constructional ability involves constructing four block designs of 32 blocks each from model design cards. The materials for this test include a set

FIGURE 12–14. Clocks drawn by individuals with a *(A)* lesion in the posterior region of the right hemisphere, illustrating spatial disorganization of numbers and omission of hands on copy task; *(B)* lesion in posterior right hemisphere showing spatial disorganization of numbers and left hemi-inattention; *(C)* and *(D)* lesion in right parietal lobe showing spatial disorganization (i.e., left neglect) on the copy version *(C)* but not on command *(D)*; *(E)* and *(F)* right temporal lobe lesion illustrating more spatial disorganization (i.e., omission of outer configuration and inattention to spatial layout of number) on the command condition *(F)* than on the copy condition *(E)*. (From Clock Drawing: A Neuropsychological Analysis by Morris Freedman, Larry Leach, Edith Kaplan, Gordon Winocur, Kenneth I. Shulman, and Dean C. Delis. Copyright © 1994 by Oxford University Press, Inc. Reprinted by permission.)

(Fig. 12–17). The reader is referred to Lezak (1995, pp. 569–578) for a review of scoring systems and to D'Elia and associates (1995) and Spreen and Strauss (1991) for comprehensive norms on this test.

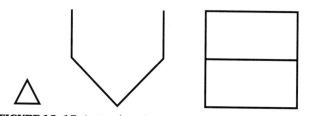

FIGURE 12–15. An item from the Benton Visual Retention Test. (From Benton Visual Retention Test: 5th Edition. Copyright © 1991 by The Psychological Corporation. Reproduced by permission. All rights reserved.)

of wooden parquetry blocks available from Learning Resources. These designs for which normative data are available are shown in order of easiest to hardest in Figure 12–19 (Neistadt, 1989), which also includes the average times that healthy college students, aged 18 to 35 years, took to accurately complete the designs. In addition to time to complete the design, error ratio scores are calculated that consist of the number of incorrectly and unplaced blocks in the design(s) completed divided by the total number of blocks used in the design(s). This test, which is described more fully in several publications (Neistadt, 1989; 1991; 1994b), has been shown to be reliable (test-retest coefficient of $r = 0.92$) and shows a high and significant correlation with the WAIS-R Block Design test ($r = 0.84$), a frequently used measure of constructional ability. Neistadt has used this test extensively with individuals with head injury and has suggested guidelines for type of intervention (functional or remedial) based on the client's performance on the test and his or her response to training.

Another test that can be used to assess constructional abilities and that involves assembly is the Tinker Toy Test (Lezak, 1982, 1995). Although this test is used primarily to assess executive abilities (the ability to formulate a goal and to plan, initiate, and carry out the activity to achieve the goal), the test evaluates an interplay of constructional abilities and executive abilities. The Tinkertoy Test includes 50 pieces from the standard Tinkertoy set. The patient is told to make whatever he or she wants. This test requires the ability to manipulate pieces with both hands. Scoring is based on complexity, including whether the patient made a structure, the total number of pieces used in the construction, whether the patient appropriately named the structure, whether there were moving parts, whether it had three dimensions, and whether it was free standing. Points are subtracted for specific types of errors. This test is described more fully in Lezak (1995, pp. 659–665).

CONSTRUCTIONAL ABILITIES: A UNITARY DISORDER?

Research has indicated that often an individual with brain damage fails on some constructional tasks but not on others. In a classic study addressing this issue, Benton and Fogel (1962) analyzed the interrelations among the performances of 100 brain-damaged patients on four constructional tasks (copying designs, stick-construction, three-dimensional block construction, and block designs). It was found that the intertest correlations were never very high, though statistically significant due to the large sample size. The finding indicated that both common and different abilities were involved in various constructive tasks. In a subsequent study using the aforementioned four tasks, Benton (1967) noted that the degree of communality between failure in copying designs and the other three tests was consistently lower than the degree of communality of failure among the other three tests. It is conceivable that the graphomotor element in copying designs may have endowed the test with a specific character that is not shared by the other three tests requiring assembling abilities. Beyond this, because the degree of concurrence among the other three tests was far from close, it was evident that intraindividual variation in performance level on these tests exists. The immediate implication of this finding is that it is unsatisfactory to use failure on any one test as the sole operational definition of constructional impairment be-

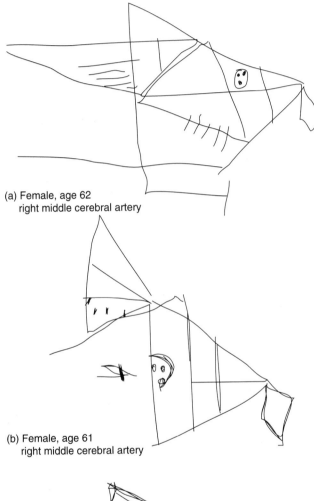

(a) Female, age 62
   right middle cerebral artery

(b) Female, age 61
   right middle cerebral artery

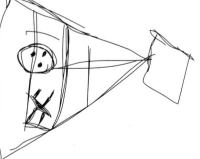

(c) Male, age 71
   right parietal-temporal infarct

FIGURE 12–17. Copy of the Rey Osterrieth Complex Figure by three individuals with right cerebrovascular accident and neglect. A, Female, age 62, right middle cerebral artery lesion. B, Female, age 61, right middle cerebral artery lesion. C, Male, age 71, right parietal-temporal infarct.

cause such a practice runs the risk of committing a false-negative error in diagnosis. As Critchley (1953) has found, assessment on a three-dimensional constructional task appeared to be necessary because some patients with parietal lesions who had no difficulty on the commonly employed two-dimensional tests displayed gross abnormalities of construction when the test moved into the third dimension.

Benton and Fogel (1962) emphasize that each constructional test used to measure constructional praxis skills may not be measuring the same skill. Tests may vary in regard to degree of difficulty, whether two or three spatial dimensions are required, degree of executive function required, and how much overall motor skill is necessary. Therefore, the various tests used to measure constructional abilities may yield different results even though each test purports to be measuring the same skill (Benton & Fogel, 1962). To provide a plausible typology of constructional performances, future research may attempt factor analysis to determine the underlying dimensions (or characteristics) being measured by various constructional tests.

The question remains as to whether constructional impairment as disclosed by failure on these tasks is in fact a unitary deficit. According to some authors (Benson &

TABLE 12–7

TESTS OF BUILDING OR ASSEMBLING

Name of Test	Author	Description	Source
Three-Dimensional Block Construction	Benton	There are two equivalent forms of the test in which the subject is presented with three block models (6 blocks, 8 blocks, and 15 blocks), one at a time, and required to construct an exact replica by selecting the appropriate blocks from a set of 29 blocks on a tray. A version in which the subject must replicate the constructions based on photographs of the model is also present.	Psychological Assessment Resources (PAR), P.O. Box 998, Odessa, FL 33556; see Benton, et al. 1994, pp. 115–136.
Parquetry Blocks Test	Neistadt, 1989*	Subject is required to construct four block designs of 32 blocks each. Time and accuracy are recorded, and error ratio scores are calculated.	Parquetry blocks available from Learning Resources; see Neistadt, 1989, 1994.
Tinker Toy	Lezak, 1983, 1995*	Subject is given 50 pieces of a standard Tinkertoy set and told to make whatever he or she wants; scored for complexity of construction according to specified criteria; assesses executive and planning abilities as well as construction.	See Lezak, 1995, pp. 659–665.
Block Design	Wechsler, 1981	Subtest of the WAIS-R in which the subject is given four or nine red and white blocks and must reproduce block designs made by the examiner and from a card in which the designs are printed in smaller scale than the blocks.	Psychological Corporation, 555 Academic Ct., San Antonio, TX 78204-2498.
Object Assembly	Wechsler, 1981	Subtest of the WAIS-R that contains four cut-up figures of familiar objects: manikin, profile, hand, and elephant. Responses are scored for time and accuracy.	Psychological Corporation, 555 Academic Ct., San Antonio, TX 78204-2498.
Stick Construction	Goodglass and Kaplan, 1983*	Subject is asked to construct matchstick geometric figures from memory. Each of 14 designs is first assembled before the subject. Each design is exposed for 10 seconds and then removed, and the subject is asked to reproduce it.	See Goodglass and Kaplan, 1983.
Constructional Praxis Test	Ayres, 1989	A subtest of the Sensory Integration and Praxis Tests. Subject constructs two different models of varying complexity. Test is standardized for children but has been used with adults with cerebrovascular accident.	

*Not commercially available.

A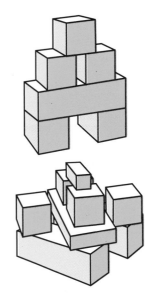 C

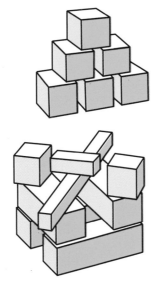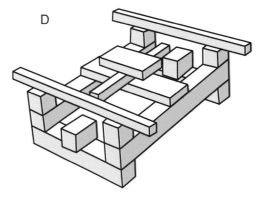

FIGURE 12–18. Schematic representation of *(A)* Models I and II, Form A; *(B)* Model III, Form A; *(C)* Models I and II, Form B; and *(D)* Model III, Form B. (From *Contributions to Neuropsychological Assessment: A Clinical Manual,* 2/e by Arthur L. Benton, Abigail B. Sivan, Kerry de S. Hamsher, Nils R. Varney, and Otfried Spreen. Copyright © 1994 by Oxford University Press, Inc. Reprinted by permission.)

B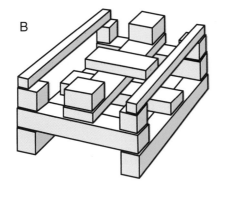 D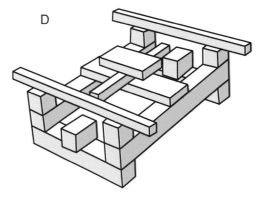

Full detail designs

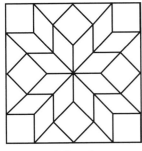

Pattern 1   Pattern 2   Pattern 3

Partial detail designs

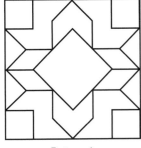

FIGURE 12–19. Design card patterns. (From Neistadt, M. [1989]. Normal adult performance on constructional praxis training tasks. *American Journal of Occupational Therapy, 47* [7], 450. Copyright 1987 by the American Occupational Therapy Association, Inc. Reprinted with permission.)

Pattern 1   Pattern 2   Pattern 3

Barton, 1970; McFie & Zangwill, 1960), two separate pathogenetic mechanisms underlie constructional disorders: a manifestation of a disturbance at the executive or planning level in the constructional act in left hemisphere–lesioned patients and a secondary consequence of a disturbance of visuoperception following right hemisphere damage.

Unilateral Neglect

Unilateral neglect is a common neurobehavioral disorder that occurs after brain damage and has important functional implications. This disorder is more common after a right hemisphere lesion (Heilman et al., 1985), although some recent studies (e.g., Ogden, 1987; Stone et al., 1993) have indicated that neglect may occur more commonly in left hemisphere stroke than previously reported. The incidence of unilateral neglect after right hemisphere stroke varies greatly, ranging from 12 percent (Smith et al.,

1983) to 90 percent (Schenkenberg et al., 1980). The variation in incidence may reflect the sensitivity of the tests used for diagnosis (Ogden, 1987) and the selection criteria for the subject cohorts (Sunderland et al., 1987). Although the majority of lesions causing neglect occur in the temporoparietal lobe (Cappa et al., 1991), lesions of the frontal lobe (Mesulam, 1985), inferior parietal lobe, lateral frontal lobe, cingulate gyrus, thalamus, and striatum may also result in the disorder (Heilman et al., 1993).

Although unilateral neglect may occur for visual, auditory, olfactory, or tactile modalities, the majority of neglect assessments tap the visuospatial aspect of the syndrome. Some of the most commonly used tests (for either clinical or research purposes) include line bisection tests, copying or drawing tests, cancellation tests, and reading tests (Cermak & Lin, 1994). Table 12–8 summarizes many of the tests used to evaluate neglect. Besides their clinical usefulness, these tests have been used for research on neglect mechanisms and therapy. A brief review of relevant research is provided below.

TABLE 12–8

TESTS OF UNILATERAL NEGLECT

Title	Author	Description	Source
Line Bisection Test	Schenkenberg, et al., 1980*	Line bisection of 20 lines of three different line lengths on a single page; Scoring involves the number and position of omitted lines as well as the deviation of the bisections from the midpoint.	Schenkenberg et al., 1980. See Lezak, 1995, pp. 390–392.
Cancellation Tests	Mesulam, 1985	A set of four cancellation tests, two that involve letters and two that involve symbols. A structured and a random array are presented for each type of stimulus. The subject is asked to cancel a particular target.	
The Bells Test	Gauthier, 1989*	A variation of the cancellation test in which the target stimuli are bells.	See Gauthier, et al., 1989.
Random Chinese Cancellation Test	Chen Sea, et al., 1993*	A variation of the cancellation test in which the stimuli are Chinese words. Normative data are available for Chinese subjects.	See Chen Sea, et al., 1993.
Unilateral Inattention Test	Toglia, 1991*	Assessment of neglect using a dynamic approach.	See Toglia, 1991.
The Indented Paragraph Test	Caplan, 1987*	The subject is asked to read a paragraph out loud in which the left margin is variably indented.	See Caplan, 1987. See Lezak, 1995, pp. 393–394.
Behavioral Inattention Test	Wilson et al., 1987	Test consists of six conventional paper and pencil tests of neglect including cancellation tests, a line bisection test, and drawing tests. There are also nine behavioral tests designed to simulate ADL: picture scanning, telephone dialing, menu reading, article reading, telling and setting time, coin sorting, address and sentence copying, map navigation, and card sorting.	

*Not commercially available.

TESTS OF LINE BISECTION

A number of tests of line bisection have been developed. A common feature of these tasks is that the subject is required to identify and bisect the midpoint of a line or a series of lines. Deviation toward the ipsilesional side indicates neglect. A variety of line bisection tasks have been described that vary in the number and position of lines on a page. Schenkenberg et al. (1980) designed and standardized a version of this task with 20 lines of three different lengths drawn on a single page (Fig. 12–20) . The test can be scored two ways: (1) by counting the number and position of omitted lines and (2) by calculating the deviation of the subject's bisection of each of the lines from the true center using the following formula:

$$\text{Bias index} = \frac{\text{Number of millimeters deviated from true center}}{\text{Half the line length in mm}}$$

In a study (Black et al., 1990) of neglect tasks administered at bedside to patients with right and left cerebrovascular accident (including line drawings, bisection of horizontal lines, cancellation of lines, letters, designs arrayed on a page, and a visual search of pictures on a large board), line bisection was found to be the most sensitive task, with 76 percent of subjects with right cerebrovascular accident and 30 percent of subjects with left cerebrovascular accident showing some abnormality. Besides its clinical popularity for diagnosis of the presence and severity of visual neglect, the line bisection test provides a useful instrument for research on how the neglect phenomenon may be modified through experimental manipulation of task demands or stimulus parameters such as the length of the line (Schenkenberg et al., 1980), anchors or cues at the end of the line (Lin et al., in press; Nichelli & Rinaldi, 1989; Riddoch & Humphreys, 1983), direction of visual scanning or manual control (Halligan & Marshall, 1989a, 1989b; Lin, 1994a; Reuter-Lorenz & Posner, 1990; Samuelsson, 1990), different orientations of the lines (Burnett-Stuart et al., 1991), and different positions in space (Nichelli & Rinaldi, 1989).

CANCELLATION TESTS

Various visual search tasks examine the ability to locate and cancel target stimuli from among a series of stimuli. More omissions on the contralesional side compared with the ipsilesional side are considered indicative of neglect. Commonly administered cancellation tests are line crossing (Albert, 1973), letter cancellation (Mesulam, 1985; Weintraub & Mesulam, 1985, 1988), star cancellation and number cancellation (Friedman, 1992; Halligan et al., 1992), Random Chinese Word Cancellation Test (Chen Sea et al., 1993), and the Bells Test (Gauthier et al., 1989).

Mesulam (1985) developed a set of four cancellation tests, two that involve letters and two that involve symbols (Fig. 12–21). A structured and a random array are presented for each type of stimulus. Normative data have indicated that performance on the tasks is age related. Normal adults younger than the age of 50 years can complete each of the four test conditions within 2 minutes without error. Over the age of 50 years, the omission of one target from each visual field is considered within normal limits, whereas over the age of 80 years, as many as four targets in each visual field may be omitted. A computerized version of this test has been published by Food for Thought.

As with the line bisection tests, a variety of formats of cancellation tasks have been administered to individuals with neglect. These variations use different stimuli such as bells (Gauthier et al., 1989), stars (Wilson et al., 1987a, 1987b), or Chinese words (Chen Sea et al., 1993). In some instances, different variations of the test have been developed, in part, to examine the different theories of neglect (Eglin et al., 1989; Mark et al., 1988; Rapscak et al., 1989; Weintraub & Mesulam, 1988).

Cancellation tests can also provide information about how an individual attends to and explores his or her environment. As the patient performs the task, the examiner has a similar sheet and numbers the order in which a patient cancels items. By recording the sequence of the cancellations and then connecting the lines (scanpath), the therapist can have a graphic representation of the patient's visual search and scanning patterns (Fig. 12–22). Mesulam (1985) described the visual search strategy used to locate target stimuli on cancellation tests. Typical English-speaking adults conduct a systematic search beginning on the left and proceeding to the right in horizontal or vertical rows, even in random arrays, whereas patients with right hemisphere lesions begin the search in either the center or on the extreme right side of the page. Although more targets are neglected with a random array compared with a structured array, the scanning strategy for individuals with

FIGURE 12–20. The Line Bisection Test, which requires that the individual put a mark at the center of each line. (From Schenkenberg, T., et al. [1980], *30,* 509. Copyright © 1980 AvanStar Communications, Inc.)

neglect tends to be erratic regardless of the stimulus array (Mesulam, 1985).

It has been suggested that because paper and pencil tasks are usually limited in space, the therapist should also examine the patient's scanning strategies in a larger space (Warren, 1993a, 1993b, 1994). In a typology of spatial abilities, Henderson (1992-1993a, 1992-1993b) also em-

phasized the distinction between peripersonal space and extrapersonal space.

READING TESTS

Because reading is a functional skill and is easy to measure, a variety of studies have used reading to assess

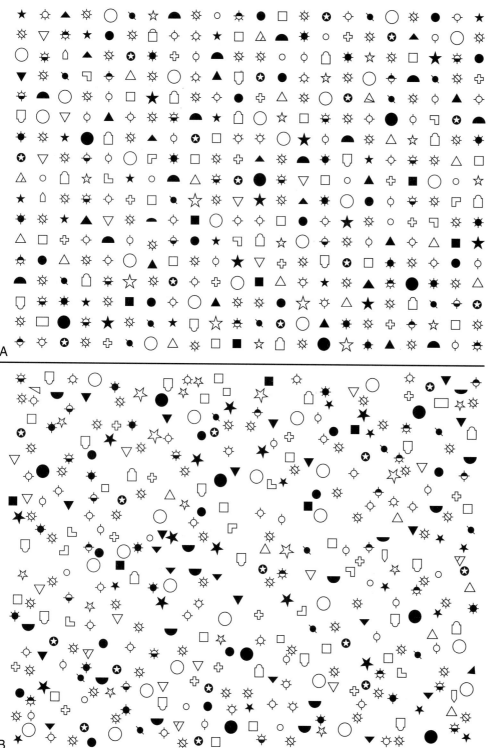

FIGURE 12–21. Symbol Cancellation Tests. (Approximation of test items.) *A,* Structured stimulus array. *B,* Random stimulus array. (From Weintraub, S., & Mesulam, M. M. [1985]. Mental state assessment of young and elderly adults in behavioral neurology. In M. M. Mesulam [Ed.], Principles of behavioral neurology [pp. 71–123]. Philadelphia, F. A. Davis.)

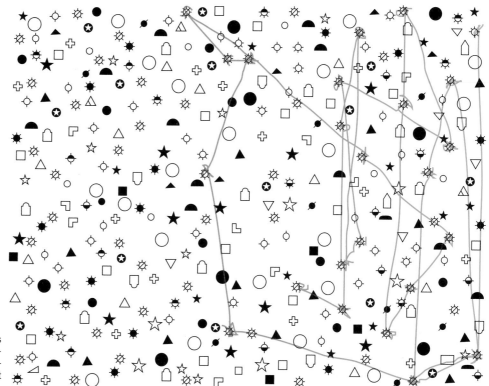

FIGURE 12–22. Scanpath reflects the order in which the subject, a 71-year-old man with a right cerebrovascular accident lesion, cancelled target stimuli.

neglect and to examine the outcome of various stimulus manipulations and intervention procedures (Butter & Kirsch, 1992; Gordon et al., 1985; Lin, 1994b; Pizzamiglio et al., 1992; Robertson et al., 1988; Robertson et al., 1990; Robertson & North, 1994; Weinberg et al., 1977, 1979; Young et al., 1983). Clinical observation has indicated that neglect patients tend to ignore one side of the page or word when reading. Battersby and coworkers (1956) developed a reading test that consisted of 10 large-printed phrases on cards. Kinsbourne and Warrington (1962) reported that patients with neglect commit two basic varieties of reading errors: (1) they may omit or misread the first letters of a particular word; (2) because of difficulty refixating from the end of the line to the beginning of the next, they may fail to read the first word(s) on a given line. Riddoch (1990) has presented a detailed analysis of the errors in reading observed in patients with neglect. Caplan (1987) developed the Indented Paragraph Test in which the left margins of the paragraph are variably indented (Fig. 12–23). The author suggests that this test identifies more subtle levels of left-sided neglect than text with a predictable format, although this was not supported by Towle and Lincoln (1991b), who examined performance on a reading task containing the same material but with different layouts.

THE BEHAVIORAL INATTENTION TEST

The Behavioral Inattention Test (BIT) is designed to include both conventional tests of neglect as well as a sampling of performance of everyday skills to provide more comprehensive information for developing rehabilitation programs (Halligan et al., 1991; Wilson et al., 1987a, 1987b). This standardized test battery consists of six conventional subtests that have traditionally been used to assess unilateral neglect. These subtests include three visual search (cancellation) tasks, a figure copying task, a line bisection task, and a drawing task (Table 12–9). The BIT also includes nine behavioral subtests that are designed to enable identification of the types of functional problems the patient may experience in everyday life. The subtests simulate ADL and include tasks such as scanning pictures and naming the objects in the pictures (e.g., a bathroom and a hospital room), dialing a telephone, reading a menu, reading a short article, and telling and setting time on a clock (Table 12–10).

The BIT was standardized on 80 patients with stroke (Halligan et al., 1991; Wilson et al., 1987a, 1987b). The scores of 50 British controls between the ages of 19 and 82 were used to establish the limits of normal performance on the conventional and behavioral subtests. The interrater reliability of the instrument was established by having two independent raters score 13 subjects after stroke (r = 0.99). Parallel form reliability for the behavioral subtests was determined by giving two alternate versions of the test to 10 patients (r = 0.91). Test-retest reliability was calculated by testing 10 patients on two separate occasions, about 15 days apart (r = 0.99). This instrument, therefore, appears to be reliable. This is especially true for test-retest reliability because patients with brain damage are characterized by spontaneous fluctuations in performance on such tests.

INDENTED PARAGRAPH TEST

Trees brighten the countryside and soften the harsh lines of city
streets. Among them are our oldest and largest living
things. Trees are the best-known plant and man's experience. They are
graceful and a job to see. So it is no wonder that people want
to know how to identify them. A tree is a woody
plant with a single stem growing to a height of ten
feet or more. Shrubs are also woody, but they are usually
smaller than trees and tend to have many stems growing
in a clump. Trees are easiest to recognize by their leaves. By
studying the leaves of trees it is possible to
learn to identify them at a distance. One group of trees has simple leaves
while others have compound leaves in which the blade is
divided into a number of leaflets. The leaf blade may have a
smooth uncut edge or it may be toothed. Not
only the leaves but also the flowers, fruit, seeds, bark,
buds, and wood are worth studying. When you look at a tree, see it as a
whole; see all its many parts; see it as a living
being in a community of plants and animals. The oldest trees live
for as long as three or four thousand years. Some grow almost
as tall as a forty story sky-scraper. The largest
trees contain enough wood to build dozens of average size
houses. Trees will always be one of the most important natural
resources of our country. Their timber, other
wood products, turpentine and resins are the great value. They also are
valuable because they hold the soil, preventing floods. In
addition, the beauty of trees, the majesty of forests,
and the quiet of woodlands are everyone's to
enjoy. Trees can be studied at every season, and they should be. Each
season will show features that cannot be seen at other times.
Watch the buds open in spring and the leaves unfold.

FIGURE 12–23. The Indented Paragraph Test. (From Caplan, B. [1987]. Assessment of unilateral neglect: A new reading test. *Journal of Clinical and Experimental Neuropsychology, 9,* 359–364.)

TABLE 12–9

CONVENTIONAL SUBTESTS OF THE BEHAVIORAL INATTENTION TEST

Subtest	Description	Scoring
Line Crossing	Present page containing 40 one-inch lines in a variety of orientations on the page. Subject is instructed to make an "X" through each line.	18 left, 18 right, 4 center lines that are not scored; maximal score = 36.
Letter Cancellation	Present page containing five rows of capital letters. Subject is instructed to make an "X" through each "R" and "E."	20 left, 20 right "R"s and "E"s; maximal score = 40.
Star Cancellation	Present page containing randomly arranged small stars, large stars, letters, and words. Subject is instructed to make an "X" through each small star.	27 left, 27 right small stars; maximal score = 54.
Figure and Shape Copying	Two parts: (A) Present page containing line drawings of star, cube, and daisy arranged vertically on left side of page. Subject is instructed to copy each on the corresponding right side of page. (B) Present page containing a group of simple geometric shapes. Subject is instructed to copy the three drawings on one separate sheet of paper.	(A) One point is given for each complete drawing. Failure is lack of any major component of drawing; maximal score = 3. (B) One point is given only if all shapes are complete; maximal score = 1.
Line Bisection	Present page containing 3 horizontal 8-inch lines. Subject is instructed to mark the center of each line.	3 points for each line bisected within one-half inch to right or left of center; 2 points for within three-fourths inch; 1 point for within 1 inch. Maximal score = 9.
Representational Drawing	Present blank sheet of paper. Subject is instructed to make three drawings on it. A clock face, a man or a woman, and a butterfly.	1 point is given for each complete drawing; maximal score = 3.

*Points are given for correct performance; thus, higher scores reflect better performance. Overall maximal score = 146; scores below 129 indicate neglect. (Data from Wilson, B., et al. [1987a]. Behavioral inattention test. Hants, England: Thames Valley Test Company.)

TABLE 12-10

BEHAVIORAL SUBTESTS FOR THE BEHAVIORAL INATTENTION TEST

Subtest	Description
Picture Scanning	Present picture of meal on plate, then wash basin, then view of room, one at a time. While viewing each photo, subject is instructed to point out and name all objects in the picture.
Telephone Dialing	Present disconnected telephone and cards with phone numbers to be dialed. Phone numbers increase in length from five to seven digits.
Menu Reading	Present menu. Subject is instructed to read it aloud.
Article Reading	Present page containing news article printed in three columns on the page. Subject is instructed to read it aloud.
Telling and Setting the Time	(A) Present three photographs of a digital clock, one at a time. Subject is instructed to read each time aloud; (B) Present large cardboard analogue clock with movable hands. Examiner sets three times, and subject is instructed to read each time aloud; (C) On same cardboard clock, subject is instructed to set three specific times.
Coin Sorting	Present coins arranged on board. Subject is instructed to point out all coins of a specific type when each is named by examiner.

Scoring: Each subtest has a maximum score of nine. Points are subtracted from the maximum score for errors/omissions by a formula specified for each subtest.

The validity of the BIT has also been examined and supported in several recent studies. Halligan and colleagues (1989) examined the performance of 80 patients with a diagnosis of unilateral stroke on the six conventional subtests of the BIT to analyze the relationship among these subtests. It was found that the six subtests all intercorrelated highly. A subsequent principal component analysis showed that all tests loaded significantly on one underlying component (eigen value = 4.36, percentage of variance explained = 72.6). The results provided preliminary evidence of factorial validity of the conventional subtests.

The authors of the instrument evaluated the concurrent, criterion-related validity of the behavioral subtests in two ways. First, the relationship between total scores on the behavioral subtest and total scores on the conventional subtests was studied for 80 patients with initial diagnoses of unilateral stroke, yielding a correlation of 0.92 (Wilson et al., 1987a). The authors believe that the strong correlation between the conventional subtests and the behavioral subtests helps establish the validity of the latter subtests because the conventional subtests were selected from previously published studies and are considered valid

measures of unilateral neglect (Wilson et al., 1987b). The second method of validation reported by the authors involved the correlation of the behavioral scores with the responses to a short ADL questionnaire completed by the occupational therapist when the assessment was administered ($r = 0.67$). The reader is referred to Chapter 8, which also includes a discussion of unilateral neglect.

ADDITIONAL ASPECTS TO CONSIDER IN ASSESSING VISUAL PERCEPTION

Awareness of Disability

Awareness of ability and disability is a key to accurate perceptual processing. Normally, we know when a task is difficult and we pay more attention to the information, enabling us to extract the important details. Crosson and coworkers (1989) identified three types of awareness:

1. *Intellectual awareness:* The patients have knowledge of a deficit but do not know how to use this knowledge in their functioning and are not aware of the consequences of the deficit to their daily functioning. An example is the patient who can tell you that he has a problem "doing things on the left side" but who then proceeds to eat only the food on the right side of his tray or shave the right side of his face.
2. *Emergent awareness:* The patients have a global recognition that something is wrong. When they perform a task and make an error, they realize that something is wrong and can, at times, self correct. For example, if a patient with neglect reads an article, he may realize it does not make sense and will then search for words on the left.
3. *Anticipatory awareness:* The patients with this level of awareness can specifically anticipate a problem before it occurs and can plan strategies before making an error.

If a patient is not aware that he or she has perceptual problems, then he or she cannot anticipate when tasks will be difficult. Therefore, the patient does not use increased attention to task. Thus, assessing awareness of performance is critical to evaluation of perceptual abilities.

The Importance of Context

Different aspects of perception have been viewed as separate subskills. Some researchers have suggested that these subskills form a hierarchical continuum (e.g., Warren, 1993a, 1993b, 1994), whereas others have suggested a conceptualization that analyzes the interaction among the task characteristics, environment, and individual to best understand perceptual function and dysfunction (e.g., Toglia, 1992). Toglia (1991a, 1992) emphasizes that dysfunction is not task specific but is related to the characteristics of the task and the environment. Research has clearly indicated that visual perception is influenced by context, including the characteristics of the task and the environment (Abreu, 1995; Gibson, 1988; Neistadt, 1994a; Trombly, 1995).

Moving Versus Stable Environments

Most often, visual perception is tested in a stable environment with the patient stable (seated in a chair) and the environment stable (paper on the table). However, in everyday life, it is often the case where the individual is moving (e.g., walking down the aisle in a grocery store) or the environment is moving (e.g., cars in the road) or both the individual and the environment are moving (crossing a busy street). In these instances, the individual must make ongoing perceptual judgments, many that involve anticipation. It is critical to examine a patient's performance in these situations. Often patients who can develop strategies to compensate and perform adequately on paper and pencil tasks have difficulty in the real world because of these issues.

Computer-Based Assessment

There have been an increasing number of assessments of perceptual abilities that have been computerized. Many of these are highly similar to the paper and pencil version. An example of this is the computerized version of Mesulam's cancellation tests. The Boston (Mesulam) Cancellation Test (BCT), distributed by Food for Thought, is available for the IBM (or equivalent) computer and requires a drawing tablet with cordless pen. An advantage to this test is that scoring can be done more quickly and information about subject performance can be more detailed (e.g., the reaction time of responses on the left vs. the right side of the page can be provided and a scan path can be drawn).

Examples of tests that are not available in a paper and pencil version is the Software for the Assessment of Visual Analysis and Synthesis (SRT) and the Software for the Assessment of Motor Functioning (MAB). Both tests are distributed by Food for Thought and are available for the IBM (or equivalent) computer. The SRT assesses visual and spatial functioning. It assesses right brain or frontal deficiencies and includes two- and three-dimensional figure testing, intensive error analysis, and spatial operations analysis. The test has three parts. First, subjects compare a complex graphic model to alternative shapes with systematic variations. Second, subjects reconstruct the model using object pieces and active reconstruction including object movement, rotation, and mirroring. Third, subjects compare stationary and moving three-dimensional objects in a more sophisticated test version.

The MAB includes seven tests that require perceptuo-motor abilities. These tests include Digit Speed and Hand Steadiness, Visuomotor Pursuit, Ballistic Visuomotor Movement, Visuomotor Sequences, Fine Motor Coordination, Visuomotor Scanning, and Visuomotor Learning. As with the Boston Cancellation Test, a drawing tablet with cordless pen is required.

There are many issues to consider in deciding whether to use a computer-based assessment. Advantages are that variables may be manipulated systematically, examiner scoring time is reduced, scoring can be more detailed, scoring errors can be reduced, and the assessment may be more motivating for the subject. Disadvantages are often cost. In addition, if the subject is not familiar with using a computer, this may present a new learning situation and his or her performance may not be valid.

SELECTING AN ASSESSMENT

There are literally hundreds of measures of perceptual and perceptuomotor abilities. Some emphasize perceptual discrimination; others emphasize constructional abilities. Some tests have been well standardized, providing data on normative performance as well as reliability and validity; others have minimal psychometric data.

Research has indicated that performance in many of these tests does not correlate highly, indicating that perception is multifaceted. This means that it may be necessary for a therapist to select more than one assessment. Given the large numbers of assessments of perceptual and constructional abilities, the therapist needs to know how to select a particular assessment(s).

The approach to assessment and the selection of specific assessments should reflect the purpose of the assessment (Schenkman, 1994). If the therapist is primarily interested in the assessment of clinically relevant naturalistic behavior, then a functional approach may be the most appropriate model. If, on the other hand, a therapist is interested in identifying why a patient may be having difficulty with particular tasks, then examination of the performance components may be useful. Finally, if the therapist is primarily interested in identifying factors that facilitate performance, then use of a dynamic model may be the most relevant.

A model suggested by Trombly (1993) involves an integration of these approaches in a top-down fashion. Trombly believes that the "occupational therapy assessment procedure should reflect our conceptualization of occupational therapy and that there should be congruence among goals, assessments, and treatment" (p. 256). Because occupational therapists are experts in occupational functioning, Trombly suggests starting the assessment process with inquiry into role competency and meaningfulness. The advantages of this approach are that it "helps the client to connect abilities (components of function) with occupational performance" (p. 253).

Wood-Dauphinee and colleagues (1994) discuss categorizing assessments in terms of the World Health Organization (WHO) International Classification of Impairments, Disabilities and Handicaps (ICIDH). Schenkman (1994) emphasizes the need to identify whether the assessment evaluates impairment, performance, disability, or some combination. Using the WHO classification system, the majority of assessments traditionally used to assess perceptual and constructional abilities would be categorized as assessing at the impairment level. This is comparable to the components of performance described by the American Occupational Therapy Association (1989). Some assessments may reflect both the impairment and the disability level. For example, in a driving assessment, aspects of the evaluation that look at factors such as reaction time provide information about the impairment level whereas actual "on the road" evaluations are at the disability level.

CONCLUSION

Accurate assessment is a key to appropriate intervention. It is critical for the therapist to accurately document the patient's abilities or disabilities to plan intervention and to monitor change. This is becoming increasingly important as third-party payers demand evidence of patient progress. There is no one "right" approach to assessment. Rather, the focus of the assessment and the selection of appropriate tools varies with the clinical picture of the patient, the focus of the rehabilitation program, and the philosophy of the facility. Whereas some therapists advocate a bottom-up approach (i.e. Warren, 1993a, 1993b, 1994), others advocate a top-down approach (i.e., Toglia, 1992; Trombly, 1993). Both approaches, however, emphasize the importance of discussing the results of assessment in terms of the client's occupational functioning.

GLOSSARY

Anticipatory awareness—Level of awareness in which the patient can specifically anticipate a problem before it occurs and can plan strategies before making an error.

Aphasia—A neurologically central disturbance of language characterized by paraphasias, word-finding difficulty, and variably impaired comprehension.

Constructional disorder—Refers to an impairment in combinatorial or organizing activity in which details must be clearly perceived and in which the relationships among the component parts of the entity must be apprehended if the desired synthesis of them is to be achieved.

Emergent awareness—Level of awareness in which the patient has a global recognition that something is wrong. When the patient who performs a task makes an error, he or she realizes that something is wrong and can, at times, self-correct.

Figure ground—Differentiating between foreground and background forms and objects.

Ideational apraxia—A disruption in the sequential organization of the gestures required to carry out a complex performance, owing to the disintegration or inadequacy of the plan of action.

Intellectual awareness—Level of awareness in which the patient has knowledge of a deficit but does not know how to use this knowledge in his or her functioning and is not aware of the consequences of the deficit to his or her daily functioning.

Motor apraxia—Condition in which the person's ability to perform skilled, purposeful movement is impaired.

Spatial orientation—Refers to the ability to relate to the position, direction, or movement of objects or points in space.

Unilateral neglect—A disorder usually associated with stroke, which results in a neglect or lack of attention to one side of space, usually, but not exclusively, the left.

Visual closure—Identifying forms or objects from incomplete presentations.

Visual form constancy—Recognizing forms and objects as the same in various environments, positions, and sizes.

REFERENCES

Abreu, B. (1995). The effect of environmental regulations on postural control after stroke. *American Journal of Occupational Therapy, 49* (6), 517–525.

Albert, M. L. (1973). A simple test of visual neglect. *Neurology, 23,* 658–665.

American Occupational Therapy Association (1989). Uniform terminology for occupational therapy (2nd ed.). *American Journal of Occupational Therapy, 43,* 808–815.

Arnadottir, G. (1990). *The brain and behavior: Assessing cortical dysfunction through activities of daily living.* St. Louis: C.V. Mosby.

Barer, D. H. (1990). The influence of visual and tactile inattention on predictions for recovery from acute stroke. *Quarterly Journal of Medicine, 74,* 21–32.

Battersby, W. S., Bender, M. B., Pollack, M., & Kahn, R. L. (1956). Unilateral "spatial agnosia" ("inattention") in patients' cerebral lesions. *Brain, 79,* 68–93.

Beaumont, J. G., & Davidoff, J. B. (1992). Assessment of visuoperceptual dysfunction. In J. R. Crawford, D. M. Parker, & W. W. McKinlay (Eds.), *A handbook of neuropsychological assessment* (pp. 115–140). Hillsdale, NJ: Lawrence Erlbaum.

Benson, D. F., & Barton, M. I. (1970). Disturbances in constructional ability. *Cortex, 6,* 19–46.

Benton, A. L. (1967). Constructional apraxia and the minor hemisphere. *Confinia Neurologica, 29,* 1–16.

Benton, A. L. (1994). Neuropsychological assessment. *Annual Review of Psychology, 45,* 1–23.

Benton, A. L., et al. (1979). Visuospatial judgment: A clinical test. *Archives of Neurology, 35,* 364–367.

Benton, A. L., & Fogel, M. L. (1962). Three-dimensional constructional praxis: A clinical test. *Archives of Neurology, 7,* 347–354.

Benton, A. L., Sivan, A. B., Hamsher, K. dsS., Varney, N. R., & Spreen, O. (1983). *Contributions to neuropsychological assessment.* New York: Oxford University Press.

Benton, A. L., Sivan, A. B., Hamsher, K. dsS., Varney, N. R., & Spreen, O. (1994). *Contributions to neuropsychological assessment* (2nd ed.). New York: Oxford University Press.

Benton, A. L., & Tranel, D. (1993). Visuoperceptual, visuospatial, and visuoconstructive disorders. In K. M. Heilman & E. Valenstein (Eds.), *Clinical neuropsychology (3rd ed.).* (pp. 165–213). New York: Oxford University Press.

Benton, A. L., Varney, N. R., & Hamsher, K. (1978). Visuospatial judgement: A clinical test. *Archives of Neurology, 35,* 364–367.

Bernspang, B., Asplund, K., Eriksson, S., & Fugl-Meyer, A. R. (1987). Perceptual and motor impairments in acute stroke patients: Effects on ADL-ability. *Stroke, 18,* 1081–1086.

Bernspang, B., Viitanen, M., & Eriksson, S. (1989). Impairments of perceptual and motor functions: Their influence on self-care ability 4 to 6 years after a stroke. *Occupational Therapy Journal of Research, 9,* 27–37.

Binder, L. M. (1982). Constructional strategies on complex figure drawing after unilateral brain damage. *Journal of Clinical Neuropsychology, 4,* 51–58.

Black, F. W., & Bernard, B. A. (1984). Constructional apraxia as a function of lesion locus and size in patients with focal brain damage. *Cortex, 20,* 111–120.

Black, S. E., Martin, B., & Szalai, J. P. (1990). Evaluation of a bedside battery for hemispatial neglect in acute stroke. *Journal of Clinical and Experimental Neuropsychology, 12,* 109.

Bouska, M. J., & Kwatny, E. (1983). *Manual for Application of the Motor-Free Visual Perception Test to The Adult Population.* Philadelphia: Temple University Rehabilitation Research and Training Center, No 8.

Brown, R. G., & Marsden, C. D. (1986). Visuospatial function in Parkinson's disease. *Brain, 109,* 987–1002.

Brown, R. G., & Marsden, C. D. (1988). "Subcortical dementia": The neuropsychological evidence. *Neuroscience, 25,* 363–387.

Burnett-Stuart, G., Halligan, P. W., & Marshall, J. (1991). A Newtonian model of perceptual distortion in visuo-spatial neglect. *Neuroreport, 2*(5), 255–257.

Butter, C. M., & Kirsch, N. L. (1992). Combined and separate effects of eye patching and visual stimulation on unilateral neglect following stroke. *Archives of Physical Medicine and Rehabilitation, 73,* 1133–1139.

Campbell, A., Brown, A., Schildroth, C., Hastings, A., Ford-Booker, P., Lewis-Jack, O., Adams, C., Gadling, A., Ellis, R., Wood, D., Dennis, G., Adeshoye, A., Weir, R., & Coffey, G. (1991). The relationship between neuropsychological measures and self-care skills in patients with cerebrovascular lesions. *Journal of the National Medical Association, 83,* 321–324.

Caplan, B. (1987). Assessment of unilateral neglect: A new reading test. *Journal of Clinical and Experimental Neuropsychology, 9,* 359–364.

Cappa, S., Guariglia, C., Messa, C., Pizzamiglio, L., & Zoccolotti, P. (1991). Computed tomography correlates of chronic unilateral neglect. *Neuropsychology, 5,* 195–204.

Cermak, S., & Lin, K. C. (1994). Assessment of unilateral neglect in individuals with right cerebral vascular accident. *Topics in Geriatric Rehabilitation, 10,* 42–55.

Chen Sea, M. J., Cermak, S., & Henderson, A. (1993). Performance of normal Chinese adults and right CVA patients on the Random Chinese Word Cancellation Test. *Clinical Neuropsychologist, 7,* 239–249.

Chen Sea, M. J., Henderson, A., & Cermak, S. A. (1993). Patterns of visual spatial inattention and their functional significance in stroke patients. *Archives of Physical Medicine and Rehabilitation, 74,* 355–360.

Colarusso, R. P., & Hammill, D. D. (1972). *MVPT. Motor-Free Visual Perception Test.* Novato, CA: Academic Therapy Publications.

Colarusso, R. P. & Hammill, D. D. (1996). *MVPT-R. Motor-Free Visual Perception Test–Revised.* Novato, CA: Academic Therapy Publications.

Corballis, M. C. (1994). Neuropsychology of perceptual functions. In D. W. Zaidel (Ed.), *Neuropsychology* (pp. 83–104). San Diego, CA: Academic Press.

Critchley, M. (1953). *The parietal lobes.* London: Arnold.

Crosson, B., Barco, P., Velozo, C., et al. (1989). Awareness and compensation in post-acute head-injury rehabilitation. *Journal of Head Trauma Rehabilitation, 4,* 46–54.

Cummings, J. L., & Huber, S. J. (1992). Visuospatial abnormalities in Parkinson's disease. In S. J. Huber & J. L. Cummings (Eds.), *Parkinson's disease: Neurobehavioral aspects.* New York: Oxford University Press.

D'Elia, L. F., Boone, K. B., & Mitrushina, A. M. (1995). *Handbook of normative data for neuropsychological assessment.* New York: Oxford University Press.

Delis, D. C., Kiefner, M. G., & Fridlund, A. J. (1988a). Visuospatial dysfunction following unilateral brain damage: Dissociations in hierarchical and hemispatial analysis. *Journal of Clinical and Experimental Neuropsychology, 10,* 421–431.

Delis, D. C., Robertson, L. C., & Balliet, R. (1988b). The breakdown and rehabilitation of visuospatial dysfunction in brain-injured patients. *International Journal of Rehabilitation Medicine, 5,* 132–138.

Denes, G., Semenza, C., Stoppa, E., & Lis, A. (1982). Unilateral spatial neglect and recovery from hemiplegia: Follow-up study. *Brain, 105,* 543–552.

Dodds, T. A., Martin, D. P., Stolov, W. C., & Deyo, R. A. (1993). A validation of the Functional Independence Measure and its performance among rehabilitation subjects. *Archives of Physical Medicine and Rehabilitation, 74,* 1291–1294.

Efferson, L. (1995). Disorders of vision and visual perceptual dysfunction. In D. Umphred (Ed.), *Neurological rehabilitation* (3rd ed.) (pp. 769–801). St. Louis: C. V. Mosby.

Eglin, M., Robertson, L., & Knight, R. (1989). Visual search performance in the neglect syndrome. *Journal of Cognitive Neurosciences, 1,* 372–385.

Eslinger, P. J., Benton, A. L. (1983). Visuoperceptual performances in aging and dementia: Clinical and theoretical implications. *Journal of Clinical Neuropsychology, 5,* 213–220.

Fennell, E. B., & Smith, M. C. (1990). Neuropsychological assessment. In S. M. Rao (Ed.), *Neurobehavioral aspects of multiple sclerosis.* New York: Oxford University Press.

Food for Thought. Nine Trafalgar Square. Nashua, New Hampshire 03063. Telephone 603-882-9900, Fax 603-886-2890.

Foss, J. J. (1993). Cerebral vascular accident: Visual perceptual dysfunction. In J. Van Deusen (Ed.). *Body image and perceptual dysfunction in adults* (pp. 11–37). Philadelphia: W. B. Saunders.

Freedman, M., Leach, L., Kaplan, E., Winocur, G., Shulman, K. I., & Delis, D. C. (1994). *Clock drawing: A neuropsychological analysis.* New York: Oxford University Press.

Fried, I., Mateer, C., Ojemann, G., Wohns, R., & Fedio, P. (1982). Organization of visuospatial functions in human cortex: Evidence from electrical stimulation. *Brain, 105 (pt 2),* 349–371.

Friedman, P. J. (1990a). Gait recovery after hemiplegic stroke. *International Disability Studies, 12,* 119–122.

Friedman, P. J. (1990b). Spatial neglect in acute stroke: The line bisection test. *Scandinavian Journal of Rehabilitation Medicine, 22,* 101–106.

Friedman, P. J. (1991). Clock drawing in acute stroke. *Age and Ageing, 20,* 140–145.

Friedman, P. J. (1992). The star cancellation test in acute stroke. *Clinical Rehabilitation, 6,* 23–30.

Galski, T., Bruno, R. L., & Ehle, H. T. (1992). Driving after cerebral damage: A model with implications for evaluation. *American Journal of Occupational Therapy, 46,* 324–332.

Galski, T., Bruno, R. L., & Ehle, H. T. (1993). Prediction of behind-the-wheel driving performance in patients with cerebral damage: A discriminant function analysis. *American Journal of Occupational Therapy, 47,* 391–396.

Gardner, M. F. (1982). *Test of Visual-Perceptual Skills (Non-motor) Manual.* Burlingame, CA: Psychological and Educational Publications.

Gauthier, L., DeHaut, F., & Joanette, Y. (1989). The Bells Test: A quantitative and qualitative test for visual neglect. *Journal of Clinical Neuropsychology, 11,* 49–54.

Gianutsos, R., & Matheson, P. (1987). The rehabilitation of visual perceptual disorders attributable to brain injury. In M. J. Meier, A. L. Benton, & L. Diller (Eds.), *Neuropsychological rehabilitation.* Edinburgh: Churchill Livingstone.

Gibson, E. J. (1988). Exploratory behavior in the development of perceiving, acting and the acquiring of knowledge. *Annual Review of Psychology, 39,* 1–41.

Giles, G. M., & Clark-Wilson, J. (1993). *Brain injury rehabilitation: A neurofunctional approach.* San Diego, CA: Singular Publishing Group.

Goodglass, H., & Kaplan, E. (1983). *The assessment of aphasia and related disorders.* Philadelphia: Lea & Febiger.

Gordon, W., Hibbard, M. R., Egelko, S., Diller, L., Shaver, P., Lieberman, A., & Ragnarson, L. (1985). Perceptual remediation in patients with right brain damage: A comprehensive program. *Archives of Physical Medicine and Rehabilitation, 66,* 353–359.

Gouvier, W. D., & Cubic, B. (1991). Behavioral assessment and treatment of acquired visuoperceptual disorders. *Neuropsychology Review, 2 (1),* 3–28.

Granger, C. V., Cotter, A. C., Hamilton, B. B., & Fielder, R. C. (1993). Functional assessment scales: A study of persons after stroke. *Archives of Physical Medicine and Rehabilitation, 74,* 133–138.

Grieve, J. (1993). *Neuropsychology for occupational therapists: Assessment of perception and cognition.* Oxford, UK: Blackwell.

Grossman, M., Carvell, S., Peltzer, L., et al. (1993). Visual construction impairment in Parkinson's disease. *Neuropsychology, 7,* 536–547.

Gur, R. C., Gur, R. E., Obrist, W. D., Skolnick, B. E., & Reivich, M. (1987). Age and regional cerebral blood flow at rest and during cognitive activity. *Archives of General Psychiatry, 44,* 617–621.

Halligan, P. W., Burn, J. P., Marshall, J. C., & Wade, D. T. (1992). Visuospatial neglect: Qualitative differences and laterality of cerebral lesion. *Journal of Neurology, Neurosurgery, and Psychiatry, 55,* 1060–1068.

Halligan, P. W., Cockburn, J., & Wilson, B. (1991). The behavioral assessment of unilateral neglect. *Neuropsychologic Rehabilitation, 1,* 5–32.

Halligan, P. W. & Marshall, J. C. (1989a). Laterality of motor response in visuospatial neglect: A case study. *Neuropsychologia, 27,* 1301–1307.

Halligan, P. W. & Marshall, J. C. (1989b). Perceptual cueing and perceptuo-motor compatibility in visuospatial neglect: A single case study. *Cognitive Neuropsychology, 6,* 423–435.

Halligan, P. W., Marshall, J. C., & Wade, D. T. (1989). Visuospatial neglect: Underlying factors and test sensitivity. *Lancet, 2,* 908–911.

Hamsher, K., Capruso, D. X., & Benton, A. (1992). Visuospatial judgement and right hemisphere disease. *Cortex, 23,* 493–496.

Hanson, C. S. (1993). Traumatic brain injury. In J. Van Deusen (Ed.). *Body image and perceptual dysfunction in adults* (pp. 39–63). Philadelphia: W. B. Saunders.

Hartman-Maeir, A. (1995). Validity of the Behavioral Inattention Test (BIT): Relationships with functional tasks. *American Journal of Occupational Therapy, 49* (6), 507–516.

Heilman, K. M., Valenstein, E., & Watson, R. T. (1985). The neglect syndrome. In J. A. Fredrick (Ed.), *Handbook of clinical neurology* (3rd ed., pp. 153–183). New York: Elsevier.

Heilman, K. M., Watson, R., & Valenstein, E. (1993). Neglect and related disorders. In K. M. Heilman & E. Valenstein (Eds.), *Clinical neuropsychology* (3rd ed., pp. 279–336). New York: Oxford University Press.

Henderson, A. (1992–1993a). A functional typology of spatial abilities and disabilities: Part I. *Sensory Integration Quarterly, 20*(3), 1–5.

Henderson, A. (1992–1993b). A functional typology of spatial abilities and disabilities: Part II. *Sensory Integration Quarterly, 20* (4), 1–5.

Henderson, V. W., Mack, W., & Williams, B. W. (1989). Spatial disorientation in Alzheimer's disease. *Archives of Neurology, 46,* 391–394.

Hier, D. B., Mondlock, J., & Caplan, L. R. (1983). Behavioral abnormalities after right hemisphere stroke. *Neurology, 33,* 337–344.

Hooper, H. E. (1983). *Hooper Visual Organization Test.* Los Angeles, CA: Western Psychological Services.

Howieson, D. B., Holm, L. A., et al. (1993). Neurologic function in the optimally healthy oldest old: Clinical neuropsychological evaluation. *Neurology, 43,* 1882–1886.

Kaplan, E. (1990). The process approach to neuropsychological assessment of psychiatric patients. *Journal of Neuropsychiatry and Clinical Neuroscience, 2,* 272–287.

Katz, N. (1994). Cognitive rehabilitation: Models for intervention and research on cognition in occupational therapy. *Occupational Therapy International, 1,* 49–63.

Keith, R. A., Granger, C. V., Hamilton, B. B., & Sherwin, F. S. (1987). The Functional Independence Measure: A new tool for rehabilitation. *Advances in Clinical Assessment, 1,* 6–18.

Kim, Y., Morrow, L., Passafiume, D., & Boller, F. (1984). Visuoperceptual and visuomotor abilities and locus of lesion. *Neuropsychologia, 22,* 177–185.

Kinsbourne, M., & Warrington, E. K. (1962). A variety of reading disabilities associated with right hemisphere lesions. *Journal of Neurology, Neurosurgery, and Psychiatry, 25,* 339–344.

Kinsella, G., Oliver, J., Ng, K., Packer, S., & Stark, R. (1993). Analysis of the syndrome of unilateral neglect. *Cortex, 29,* 135–140.

Klein, R. M., & Bell, B. (1982). Self-care skills: Behavioral measurement with the Klein-Bell ADL scale. *Archives of Physical Medicine and Rehabilitation, 62,* 335–338.

Levine, D. N., Warach, J., & Farah, M. (1985). Two visual systems in mental imagery: Dissociation of "what" and "where" in imagery disorders due to bilateral posterior cerebral lesions. *Neurology, 35,* 1010–1018.

Lezak, M. D. (1995). *Neuropsychological assessment* (3rd ed.). New York: Oxford University Press.

Lin, K. C. (1994a). *Modulation of unilateral neglect: A motor-response-based approach.* Research poster presented at the Canadian-American Occupational Therapy Association Annual Conference. Boston, MA.

Lin, K. C. (1994b). *Use of sensorimotor cueing in reducing unilateral neglect.* Paper presented at the 11th International Congress of the World Federation of Occupational Therapists, London, UK.

Lin, K. C., Cermak, S. A., Kinsbourne, M., & Trombly, C. A. (in press). Effects of left-sided movements on line bisection in post-stroke patients with unilateral neglect. *Journal of the International Neuropsychological Society.*

Lin, K. C., & Tickle-Degnen, L. (1991). *Laterality effects on constructional performances in post-stroke patients: A meta-analysis.* Poster presented at the national stroke rehabilitation conference, Cambridge, MA.

Mack, J. L., & Levine, R. (1981). The basis of visual constructional disability in patients with unilateral cerebral lesions. *Cortex, 17,* 515–532.

Maeshima, S., Hyoutani, G., Terada, T., Nakamura, Y., Yokote, H., Hayashi, S., Komai, N., & Dohi, N. (1990). [Effect of thalamic neglect on activities of daily living]. *Sogo Rehabilitation, 18,* 445–450.

Mahoney, F. I., & Barthel, D. (1965). Functional evaluation: The Barthel Index. *Maryland State Medical Journal, 14,* 61–65.

Mark, V. W., Kooistra, C. A., & Heilman, K. M. (1988). Hemispatial neglect affected by non-neglected stimuli. *Neurology, 38,* 1207–1211.

McFie, J., Piercy, M. F., & Zangwill, O. L. (1950). Visual-spatial agnosia associated with lesions of the right cerebral hemisphere. *Brain, 73,* 167–190.

McFie, J., & Zangwill, O. L. (1960). Visual-constructive disabilities associated with lesions of the left hemisphere. *Brain, 83,* 243–260.

Mehta, Z., Newcombe, F., & Damasio, H. (1987). A left hemisphere contribution to visual spatial processing. *Cortex, 23,* 447–461.

Mendez, M. F., Mendez, M. A., Martin, R., et al. (1990). Complex visual disturbances in Alzheimer's disease. *Neurology, 40,* 439–443.

Mesulam, M. M. (1985). Attention, confusional states, and neglect. In M. M. Mesulam (Ed.), *Principles of behavioral neurology* (pp. 125–168). Philadelphia: F. A. Davis.

Mishkin, M., Ungerleider, L., & Macko, K. (1983). Object vision and spatial vision: Two cortical pathways. *Trends in Neuroscience, 6,* 414–417.

Nebes, R. D. (1992). Cognitive dysfunction in Alzheimer's disease. In F. I. M. Craik & T. A. Salthouse (Eds.), *The handbook of aging.* Hillsdale, NJ: Laurence Erlbaum.

Neistadt, M. (1988). Occupational therapy for adults with perceptual deficits. *American Journal of Occupational Therapy, 42,* 434–439.

Neistadt, M. (1989). Normal adult performance on constructional praxis training tasks. *American Journal of Occupational Therapy, 43,* 448–455.

Neistadt, M. (1991). *Occupational therapy treatments for constructional deficits.* Unpublished doctoral dissertation. Boston University, Boston.

Neistadt, M. (1992). Occupational therapy treatments for constructional deficits. *American Journal of Occupational Therapy, 46,* 141–148.

Neistadt, M. (1994a). Using research literature to develop a perceptual retraining treatment program. *American Journal of Occupational Therapy, 48* (1), 62–72.

Neistadt, M. (1994b). Perceptual retraining for adults with diffuse brain injury. *American Journal of Occupational Therapy, 48* (3), 225–233.

Neistadt, M. (1994c). A meal preparation treatment protocol for adults with brain injury. *American Journal of Occupational Therapy, 48* (5), 431–441.

Neistadt, M. (1995). Relation of perceptual and body image dysfunction to activities of daily living of persons after stroke. *American Journal of Occupational Therapy, 49* (6), 551–559.

Nichelli, P., & Rinaldi, M. (1989). Selective spatial attention and length representation in normal subjects and in patients with unilateral spatial neglect. *Brain and Cognition, 9,* 57–70.

Nogak, H. (1992). [A statistical analysis of factors influencing standing balance activity of daily living and ambulation in hemiplegic patients]. *Nippon Ronen Igakkai Zassh, 29,* 285–292.

Ogden, J. A. (1987). The "neglected" left hemisphere and its contribution to visuospatial neglect. In M. Jeannerod (Ed.), *Neurophysiological and neuropsychological aspects of spatial neglect.* Amsterdam, North Holland: Elsevier.

Ogden, J. A. (1990). Spatial abilities and deficits in aging and age-related disorders. In F. Boller & J. Grafman (Eds.), *Handbook of neuropsychology,* Vol. 4. Amsterdam: Elsevier Science Publishers.

Okkema, K. (1993). *Cognition and perception in the stroke patient: A guide to functional outcomes in occupational therapy.* Gaithersburg, MD: Aspen Publishers.

Park, S., Fisher, A., & Velozo, C. (1994). Using the Assessment of Motor and Process Skills to compare occupational performance between clinic and home settings. *American Journal of Occupational Therapy, 48* (8), 697–709.

Paterson, A., & Zangwill, O. L. (1945). A case of topographical disorientation associated with a unilateral cerebral lesion. *Brain, 68,* 188–212.

Piercy, M., & Smyth, V. O. G. (1962). Right hemisphere dominance for certain non-verbal intellectual skills. *Brain, 85,* 775–790.

Pizzamiglio, L., Berego, C., Halligan, P. W., & Homeberg, V. (1992). Factors affecting the clinical measurement of visuospatial neglect. *Behavioral Neurosciences, 5,* 233–240.

Post, R. B., & Liebowitz, H. W. (1986). Two modes of processing visual information: Implications for assessing visual impairment. *American Journal of Optometry and Physiological Optics, 63,* 94–96.

Rapscak, S. Z., Verfaellie, M., Fleet, S., & Heilman, K. M. (1989). Selective attention in hemispatial neglect. *Archives of Neurology, 46,* 178–182.

Reuter-Lorenze, P., & Posner, M. (1990). Components of neglect from right hemisphere damage: An analysis of line bisection. *Neuropsychologia, 28,* 327–333.

Riddoch, J. (1990). Neglect and the peripheral dyslexias. *Cognitive Neuropsychology, 7,* 369–389.

Riddoch, M., & Humphreys, G. (1983). The effect of cueing on unilateral neglect. *Neuropsychologia, 21,* 589–599.

Robertson, I., Gray, J., & McKenzie, S. (1988). Microcomputer-based cognitive rehabilitation of visual neglect: Three multiple-baseline single-case studies. *Brain Injury, 2,* 151–163.

Robertson, I., Gray, J., Pentland, B., & Waite, L. J. (1990). Microcomputer-based rehabilitation for unilateral left visual neglect: A randomized controlled trial. *Archives of Physical Medicine and Rehabilitation, 72,* 663–668.

Robertson, I., & North, N. (1994). One hand is better than two: Motor extinction of left hand advantage in unilateral neglect. *Neuropsychologia, 32,* 1–11.

Samuelsson, H. (1990). Unilateral spatial neglect after right brain damage expressed in a line-bisecting task. *Goteb Psychol Rep, 20,* 31–38.

Schaie, K. W. (1994). The course of adult intellectual development. *American Psychologist, 49,* 304–313.

Schenkenberg, T., Bradford, D., & Ajax, E. (1980). Line bisection and unilateral visual neglect in patients with neurological impairment. *Neurology, 30,* 509–517.

Schenkman, M. (1994). Evaluation and measurement considerations for physical rehabilitation of patients who have neurologic deficits. *Topics in Geriatric Rehabilitation, 10* (2), 1–21.

Shiel, A. M. (1989). *An investigation into the relationship between unilateral neglect and A.D.L. dependency in right hemisphere stroke patients (Thesis).* Southampton University, Southampton, UK.

Sivan, A. B. (1991). *The Benton Visual Retention Test (5th ed.).* San Antonio: Psychological Corporation.

Ska, B., Poissant, A., & Joanette, Y. (1990). Line orientation judgment in normal elderly and subjects with dementia of Alzheimer's type. *Journal of Clinical and Experimental Neuropsychology, 12,* 695–702.

Smith, C., Akhtar, A., & Garraway, W. (1983). Proprioception and spatial neglect after stroke. *Age and Aging, 12,* 63–69.

Spreen, O., & Strauss, E. (1991). *A compendium of neuropsychological tests.* New York: Oxford University Press.

Stone, S. P., Patel, P., & Greenwood, R. J. (1993). Selection of acute stroke patients for treatment of visual neglect. *Journal of Neurology, Neurosurgery, and Psychiatry, 56,* 463–466.

Su, C. Y., Chien, T. H., Cheng, K. F., & Lin, Y. T. (1995). Performance of older adults with and without cerebrovascular accident on the Test of Visual-Perceptual Skills. *American Journal of Occupational Therapy, 49* (6), 491–499.

Sunderland, A., Wade, D. T., & Hewer, R. L. (1987). The natural history of visual neglect after stroke: Indications from two methods of assessment. *International Disabilities Studies, 9,* 55–59.

Sundet, K., Finset, A., & Reinvang, I. (1988). Neuropsychological predictors in stroke rehabilitation. *Journal of Clinical and Experimental Neuropsychology, 10,* 363–379.

Swihart, A. A., & Pirozzolo, F. J. (1988). The neuropsychology of aging and dementia: Clinical issues. In H. A. Whitaker (Ed.), *Neuropsychological studies of nonfocal brain damage.* New York: Springer-Verlag.

Taylor, D., Ashburn, A., & Ward, C. D. (1994). Asymmetrical trunk posture, unilateral neglect and motor performance following stroke. *Clinical Rehabilitation, 8,* 48–53.

Toglia, J. P. (1989). Approaches to cognitive assessment of the brain-injured adult: Traditional methods and dynamic investigation. *Occupational Therapy Practice, 1* (1), 36–57.

Toglia, J. P. (1991a). Generalization of treatment: A multicontext approach to cognitive perceptual impairment in adults with brain injury. *American Journal of Occupational Therapy, 45,* 505–516.

Toglia, J. P. (1991b). Unilateral visual inattention: Multidimensional components. *Occupational Therapy Practice, 3,* 18–34.

Toglia, J. P. (1992). A dynamic interactional approach to cognitive rehabilitation. In N. Katz (Ed.). *Cognitive rehabilitation: Models for intervention in occupational therapy* (pp. 104–143). Andover, MA: Andover Medical Publishers.

Towle, D., & Lincoln, N. B. (1991a). Development of a questionnaire for detecting everyday problems in stroke patients with unilateral visual neglect. *Clinical Rehabilitation, 5,* 135–140.

Towle, D., Lincoln, N. B. (1991b). Use of the indented paragraph test with right hemisphere–damaged stroke patients. *British Journal of Clinical Psychology, 30,* 37–45.

Trahan, D. E. (1991). Judgment of line orientation in patients with unilateral vascular lesions or severe head trauma. *Journal of Clinical and Experimental Neuropsychology, 13,* 23–24.

Trevarthen, C. (1968). Two mechanisms of vision in primates. *Psychologische Forschung, 31,* 299–337.

Trombly, C. (1993). The issue is—Anticipating the future: Assessment of occupational function. *American Journal of Occupational Therapy, 47* (3), 253–257.

Trombly, C. A. (1995). *Eleanor Clarke Slagle lectureship—Occupation: purpose and meaning as therapeutic mechanisms.* Presented at the 75th annual conference of the American Occupational Therapy Association, Denver, CO.

Wade, D. T., & Collin, C. (1988). The Barthel ADL Index: A standard measure of physical disability? *International Disabilities Study, 10,* 64–67.

Warren, M. (1993a). A hierarchical model for evaluation and treatment of visual perceptual dysfunction in adult acquired brain injury, Part I. *American Journal of Occupational Therapy, 47* (1), 42–53.

Warren, M. (1993b). A hierarchical model for evaluation and treatment of visual perceptual dysfunction in adult acquired brain injury, Part II. *American Journal of Occupational Therapy, 47* (1), 55–66.

Warren, M. (1994). Visual spatial skill. *American Occupational Therapy Association Self Study Series on Cognitive Rehabilitation.* Rockville, MD: American Occupational Therapy Association.

Warrington, E., & James, M. (1991). *Visual Object and Space Perception Test.* Suffolk, England: Thames Valley Test Co.

Wechsler, D. (1981). *Wechsler Adult Intelligence Scale—Revised manual.* New York: Psychological Corporation.

Weinberg, J., Diller, L., Gordon, W., Gerstman, L., Lieberman, A., Lakin, P., Hodges, G., & Ezrachi, O. (1977). Visual scanning training effect on reading-related tasks in acquired right brain damage. *Archives of Physical Medicine and Rehabilitation, 58,* 479–486.

Weinberg, J., Diller, L., Gordon, W., Gerstman, L., Lieberman, A., Lakin, P., Hodges, G., & Ezrachi, O. (1979). Training sensory awareness and spatial organization in people with right brain damage. *Archives of Physical Medicine and Rehabilitation, 60,* 491–496.

Weintraub, S., & Mesulam, M. M. (1985). Mental state assessment of young and elderly adults in behavioral neurology. In M. M. Mesulam (Ed.). *Principles of behavioral neurology* (pp. 71–123). Philadelphia: F. A. Davis.

Weintraub, S., & Mesulam, M. M. (1988). Visual hemispatial inattention: Stimulus parameters and exploratory strategies. *Journal of Neurology, Neurosurgery, and Psychiatry, 51,* 1481–1488.

Wiart, L., Dartigues, J. F., Richard, I., Giroire, J. M., Debelleix, X., Mazaux, J. M., & Barat, M. (1994). [Left hemiplegic's affective disorders: Hemineglect's role and therapeutic implications]. *Annales de Readaptation et de Medecine Physique: Revue Scientifique, 37,* 15–23.

Wilson, B., Cockburn, J., & Halligan, P. (1987a). Behavioral inattention test. Hants, England: Thames Valley Test Company.

Wilson, B., Cockburn, J., & Halligan, P. (1987b). Development of a behavioral test of visuospatial neglect. *Archives of Physical Medicine and Rehabilitation. 68,* 98–102.

Wood-Dauphinee, S., Berg, K., & Daley, K. (1994). Monitoring status and evaluating outcomes: An overview of rating scales for use with patients who have sustained a stroke. *Topics in Geriatric Rehabilitation, 10,* 22–41.

Young, G., Collins, D., & Hren, M. (1983). Effect of pairing scanning training with block design training in the remediation of perceptual problems in left hemiplegics. *Journal of Clinical Neuropsychology, 5,* 201–212.

Zec, R. F. (1993). Neuropsychological functioning in Alzheimer's disease. In R. W. Parks, R. F. Zec, and R. S. Wilson (Eds.), *Neuropsychology of Alzheimer's disease and other dementias.* New York: Oxford University Press.

Zoltan, B., Siev, E., & Frieshtat, B. (1986). *The adult stroke patient: A manual for evaluation and treatment of perceptual and cognitive dysfunction* (2nd ed.). Thorofare, NJ: Slack.

Cognition

Barbara Haase, MHS, OTR/L

SUMMARY This section of Chapter 12 is designed to provide the physical or occupational therapist with an understanding of the areas that constitute the assessment of cognition. A general overview of cognition, how cognition is assessed in various settings, and general comments introduce this section of Chapter 12. Each aspect of cognition is addressed with a definition and a theoretical overview. Problems associated with deficits in areas of cognition are reviewed. Assessment tools and strategies pertaining to each cognitive domain are discussed, including both subjective and standardized tests. Many assessments cover several different cognitive domains. The remainder of this section of the chapter provides a brief overview of standardized cognitive assessment instruments. It is hoped that this section of Chapter 12 will provide the clinician with the tools needed to develop a framework for assessing cognition in his or her own setting.

Cognition allows each of us to take in information and use the information to plan meaningful interactions with others and with the environment. It is the ability to understand and to be aware of the environment (Zoltan, 1990). The assessment of cognitive functioning needs to be taken into account and is necessary for the development and implementation of intervention plans, regardless of the patient's diagnosis.

CONTEXT FOR ASSESSMENT

The depth and breadth of the cognitive assessment performed is generally based on the therapist's discipline,

the patient's diagnosis, and the facility. In many settings, cognitive assessment is performed by the occupational therapist and/or speech-language pathologists. More in-depth assessments may be completed by psychologists and neuropsychologists, when available. Health care practitioners, whether physicians, nurses, or therapists, need an understanding of cognitive processes and the impact that impairment of these processes has on the general well-being and independent functioning of the patient. The patient's cognitive level influences his or her ability to follow through with medical care and can determine whether he or she is able to maintain his or her lifestyle and to live independently (Cohen & Mapau, 1988). Many diagnoses have accompanying cognitive deficits. These include cerebrovascular accidents (CVAs), traumatic brain injury (TBI), abilities. A combination of standardized assessment and observation of performance may often provide the clinician with information about a patient's executive functioning. Assessment of judgment and insight is important with any cognitive deficit. Patients who lack insight into their capabilities may continue to perform tasks such as driving that put them at risk. There are no quantitative measures for assessing insight. Assessment of insight is achieved primarily through the interview process of a cognitive assessment (Feher et al., 1989). When the cognitive assessment is completed, the information obtained is measured against the response of the patient for consistency. Judgment is assessed primarily through informal methods, such as interpretation of proverbs and incorporation of safety principles.

Lezak (1985) notes that few assessments have been developed to assess executive functioning. The Wisconsin Card Sorting Test has the patient sorting 128 cards according to specified piles. The examiner tells the patient whether he or she is correct. The patient must determine the concepts being used to sort the cards, such as color, shape, or number. Toglia (1993b) has designed an assessment using multicolored and multidesign tableware. This assessment examines the patient's ability to form relationships, organize, and solve problems. Other informal assessments include mazes, modified Stroop tests, and sequencing cards (Morse, 1986). The examiner will want to know whether the patient is aware of planning problems, how many steps in an occupation he or she is able to sequence, how he or she handles change, and whether he or she is able to problem-solve (Zoltan, 1990). Most assessments have the examiner observe for performance errors.

Many standardized tests are available. Refer to Table 12–12 (All tests in the table are reviewed in the chapter.) This table does not reflect all areas assessed by a specific test but only the components related to executive functioning.

Mental Status

Mental status tests are often used to assess mental functioning in dementia patients (Winograd, 1984) and psychiatric patients (Folstein et al., 1975). Examples of mental status tests are the Short Portable Mental Status Questionnaire (Pfeiffer, 1974) and the Mini-Mental State Exam (Folstein et al., 1975). Items included in mental status exams are usually questions of orientation, calculation, attention, and memory. Most are short and take about 10 minutes to administer. This makes these assessments valuable to quickly screen patients for cognitive deficit or the need for further assessment in a variety of settings. These settings may include acute care, psychiatric, nursing home, home health, and rehabilitation. Mental status tests were developed out of a need to assess more patients with cognitive dysfunction in a quick, reliable manner. This was needed to avoid overburdening neuropsychologists and to

TABLE 12–12	
ASSESSMENT OF EXECUTIVE FUNCTIONING	
Test	**Component Assessed**
Allen Cognitive Level Test	Ability to learn new information
Allen Cognitive Level Test—Problem Solving	Problem solving, ability to learn new information
Bay Area Functional Performance Evaluation	Ability to abstract and ability to detect errors
Cognitive Assessment of Minnesota	Following directions, foresight and planning, concrete problem solving, abstract reasoning
Cognitive Behavior Rating Scale	Abstract reasoning, need for routine
Cognitive Performance Test	Information processing
Loewenstein Occupational Therapy Cognitive Assessment	Thinking operations
Mini-Mental State Exam	Following directions
Neurobehavioral Cognitive Status Examination	Reasoning
Raven's Progressive Matrices	Ability to formulate constructs
Rey Complex Figure Test	Organization and problem solving
Short Category Test	Problem solving and abstract concept formation
Wisconsin Card Sorting Test	Abstract reasoning, problem solving, the ability to shift cognitive strategies

decrease cost. In addition, many chronically ill patients could not tolerate the length of standard neuropsychological tests (Schmitt et al., 1989).

Despite significant correlation with more formalized assessments of mental status, it is important to utilize these mental status assessments for clinical measurement and not for the diagnosis of organic impairments (Folstein et al., 1975). These assessments may be of particular benefit when mental status should not be a concern based on the diagnosis, but the subject is presenting with cognitive changes. Since promoting independence and limiting loss of function is a goal in geriatric medicine, in which most of these assessments are utilized, it is appropriate to objectively assess patients' functioning (Ham, 1992). Patients with deficits such as dementia often confabulate answers to questions on mental status examinations (DeLima, 1991), especially when they may be aware that something is wrong with their mental status. Patients with depression, on the other hand, will state that they do not know a response; however, when pursued, they will generally retrieve the correct response.

There are several assessments listed in the next section that assess overall cognitive function. Many have been developed to determine decline in cognitive function. These assessments include
- Dementia Rating Scale
- Short Portable Mental Status Questionnaire
- Middlesex Elderly Assessment of Mental State
- Severe Impairment Battery
- Cognitive Assessment of Minnesota
- Mini-Mental State Exam

STANDARDIZED COGNITIVE ASSESSMENTS

The following is a compilation of instruments that are available for use by therapists experienced in cognitive assessment. The following assessments may be utilized by occupational therapists more than physical therapists owing to the nature of their professional background and experience. An effort has been made to include only the assessments therapists are authorized to administer.

Note that practitioners should, when obtaining assessments, review the user qualifications required by the publisher. Several tests such as the Dementia Rating Scale and the Stroop Color and Word Test are available and may be administered to patients by occupational therapists. Interpretation must be completed by qualified psychological professionals. To order some assessments, documentation of these qualifications is necessary. Some assessments such as The Train Making Test are designed to be sold to and administered by psychologists only.

ALLEN TESTS

Several assessments developed by Claudia Allen, MA, OTR, FAOTA are utilized in the assessment of cognitive function. Several of these assessments were originally designed to assess the cognitively impaired psychiatric patient, including the geropsychiatric patient. Allen's theory, described in Chapter 7, has recently been applied to patients with physical disabilities. Allen originally designed the assessments to measure cognitive abilities through the sensorimotor actions of the individual (Allen & Allen, 1987). She defined cognitive disability in terms of deficits of sensorimotor actions in routine task behaviors due to physical or chemical changes in the structure of the brain. The Allen assessments differ from psychiatric assessments because the latter assessments are based on verbal responses. The Allen assessments are based on motor responses of a nonverbal type. The therapist is able, from observation, cueing, and rating the assessments, to make inferences about the type of sensory cues the patient needs to be able to perform and to maintain attention. Information based on these assessments has been used to predict the patient's ability to function in the community and vocationally. Allen and Reyner (no date) also describe therapy interventions, based on the Allen levels, including games and crafts. Allen and Reyner (no date) also provide a list of the cognitive levels at which a patient needs to be functioning to utilize various types of adaptive equipment, which is helpful when working with physically impaired patients who also demonstrate cognitive deficits. The list may assist, for example, in determining why patients with hip fractures and associated cognitive changes may not be able to learn how to utilize adaptive equipment, which

TABLE 12–13

AREA OF ASSESSMENT

	Attention	Executive Functioning	Mental Status	Memory	Orientation
Allen Cognitive Level Test—Original		X			
Allen Cognitive Level Test—Problem Solving		X			
Large Allen Cognitive Level Test		X			
Cognitive Performance Test		X			
Routine Task Inventory		X			
Autobiographical Memory Interview				X	
Bay Area Functional Performance Evaluation	X	X			
Cognitive Assessment of Minnesota	X	X		X	X
Cognitive Behavior Rating Scales		X	X	X	X
Contextual Memory Test				X	
Continuous Visual Memory Test				X	
Dementia Rating Scale	X			X	
Doors and People Test				X	
Loewenstein Occupational Therapy Cognitive Assessment		X			X
Mini-Mental State Exam	X	X	X	X	X
Middlesex Elderly Assessment of Mental State			X		
Neurobehavioral Cognitive Status Examination	X	X	X	X	X
Raven's Progressive Matrices		X			
Rey Complex Figure Test		X		X	
Rivermead Behavioral Memory Test				X	
Severe Impairment Battery	X	X	X	X	X
Short Category Test		X			
Short Portable Mental Status Questionnaire			X		X
Stroop Color and Word Test	X				
Symbol Digit Modalities Test	X				
Test of Orientation of Rehabilitation Patients	X				
Wisconsin Card Sorting Test		X			

parts of the BaFPE and the ABS. The authors believed that the BaFPE was helpful in learning about the patients and how they approached tasks. Houston and colleagues (1989) found that therapists working in psychiatry liked the BaFPE but found it too long. A training course has been available to teach clinicians how to administer and score the BaFPE, which the authors found beneficial. The BaFPE is available from Consulting Psychologists Press, 3830 E. Bayshore Road, Palo Alto, CA 94303, (415) 969–8901.

COGNITIVE ASSESSMENT OF MINNESOTA

The Cognitive Assessment of Minnesota (CAM) was developed by occupational therapists to assess a broad range of cognitive abilities in persons with brain damage (Rustad et al., 1993). The CAM was developed as a screening tool from a rehabilitation framework rather than as a diagnostic tool for patients with psychiatric diagnoses. Its authors designed the test to quantify the presence of cognitive deficits for intervention. The test consists of the manual, score sheet, and some common objects, such as paper, a pencil, blocks, and a toothbrush. It takes approximately 40 minutes to administer. Subtests of the CAM include attention, memory, visual neglect, following directions, orientation, temporal awareness, matching, object identification, visual and auditory memory and sequencing, recall and recognition, money skills, math skills, foresight and planning, safety and judgment, concrete problem solving, and abstract reasoning. The authors considered the test appropriate for patients at Rancho Level IV and higher and for patients who have had a CVA. The CAM is not appropriate for patients with severe perceptual deficits, visual acuity deficits, and aphasia. Scoring varies based on the subtest. Scores for each area are plotted on a graph with a breakdown of no impairment to severe impairment rankings.

Norms were developed on administration of the CAM to 200 normal subjects, aged 18 to 70. There were no effects from age or level of education. Interrater reliability was demonstrated. Test-retest reliability was demonstrated with retesting in 1 week. Validity was established with 200 normal patients and 39 patients with brain injury and right CVA. The CAM correctly identified over 95 percent of the patients with cognitive impairment. Significant correlations have been demonstrated for the CAM with the Porteus Maze Test and the Mini-Mental State Exam. For more information, contact Therapy Skill Builders, 3830 East Bellevue, P.O. Box 42050-4SW, Tucson, AZ 85733.

COGNITIVE BEHAVIOR RATING SCALES

The Cognitive Behavior Rating Scales (CBRS) were developed to formalize observation of cognitive abilities in patients who are not testable by other test batteries (Williams, 1987). The CBRS comprise 116 items in the areas of language deficit, apraxia, disorientation, agitation, need for routine, depression, higher cognitive deficits (memory, abstract reasoning, language, and motor execu-

tion), memory disorder, and dementia. Scores are obtained from observation by a reliable person, in some instances a family member. The patient is rated on a five-point scale from 1 ("not at all like this person" or "this person's ability is very low") to 5 ("very much like this person" or "this person's ability is very high"). The CBRS can be completed in 15 to 20 minutes. Raw scores are transformed into T-scores and percentiles. A profile of the patient's functioning in all areas is graphed so that strengths and weaknesses may be identified.

Williams (1987) states that the CBRS are best utilized with patients with dementia. The test was developed by creating items from interviews with families and from the literature that is pertinent to patients with dementia and depression. The original number of items was scaled down by a group of 10 neuropsychologists. Some of the initial research of the CBRS suggests that the tool may discriminate between patients with dementia and patients with depression. Family members were found to be reliable raters. Norms are based on a sample of 688 people. Research has been proposed on patients with TBI and CVA. For more information, contact Psychological Assessment Resources, Inc., P.O. Box 998, Odessa, FL 33556.

CONTEXTUAL MEMORY TEST

The Contextual Memory Test (CMT) was developed by an occupational therapist to assess awareness of memory deficits (Toglia, 1993b). It was designed to be used with a range of diagnoses, including CVA, TBI, dementia, depression, schizophrenia, and other neurologic disorders. The CMT assesses a patient's metamemory, or awareness of his or her memory capabilities, as well as a patient's memory capacity, recall, and strategy use. The CMT is intended as an adjunct to other, more conventional memory tests. The test consists of the manual, two large presentation cards, 40 recognition cards, and a scoring booklet. Two versions of the test, the restaurant version and the morning version, allow for reassessment. In the first part of the test, the patient is presented with a card on which are 20 line drawings (Fig. 12–26). The patient is not told that the items on the card relate to a theme or context. The patient is asked to study the card and try to remember as many items as possible. In the second part of the test, the patient is provided with the context in which the pictures are related. This is done to determine if providing contextual cues improves the patient's performance and his or her awareness of his or her performance. The patient is asked to recall items from each part of the test. If on part two the patient continues to be unable to recall, then the recognition cards may be used. Delayed recall may also be assessed after approximately 20 minutes. Prior to the presentation of the stimulus card and after the recall, the patient is asked a series of questions about his or her perception of his or her memory and awareness of strategies utilized to remember.

Several scores are obtained: recall, recognition, aware-

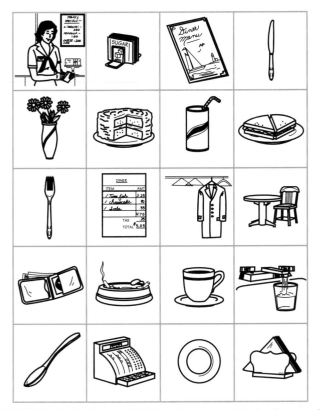

FIGURE 12–26. A card of 20 line drawings used in the Contextual Memory Test. (Approximation of test item.) (Courtesy of Therapy Skill Builders, Tucson, AZ.)

ness, and strategy use. Several recall scores are broken down into immediate, delayed, and total. The scores can be converted to standard scores and compared with normals. Three measures are used under the awareness score. These include prediction, or the ability to predict amount of information to be recalled; estimation, or the difference between the amount of data the person said he or she remembered and that which was actually remembered; and a response to general questioning in which point values are assigned to some of the responses. Strategy use is utilized in three ways: the effect of context, the total strategy score, and the order of recall. This is helpful in determining what strategies the patient utilized. Several patterns of performance are addressed in the manual, with treatment implications provided.

An initial study of 112 patients with brain injury did not demonstrate differences in the context and noncontext versions of the test. Concurrent validity was established in 33 patients with brain injury with the CMT and the Rivermead Behavioral Memory Test (RBMT). The CMT correctly discriminated 332 of 375 nondisabled subjects and 134 of 159 patients with brain injury, using the immediate and delayed scores. A few less were identified when the total strategy and discrepancy score was factored in. Significant differences have been noted between controls and patients with brain injury in relation to their ability to predict their memory capabilities. The patients who performed the poorest on estimation had the largest

discrepancy in their recall versus predicted recall. Patients with brain injury also demonstrated lower strategy scores. For more information on the CMT, contact Therapy Skill Builders, 3830 East Bellevue, P.O. Box 42050-4SW, Tucson, AZ 85733.

CONTINUOUS VISUAL MEMORY TEST

The Continuous Visual Memory Test (CVMT) is an assessment of visual memory (Trahan & Larrabee, 1983). It comprises three subtests: an Acquisition Task, a Delayed Recognition Task, and a Visual Discrimination Task. The Acquisition Task assesses recognition memory by asking the patient to discriminate between new and repeated stimuli of complex designs. The designs are presented rapidly. This is repeated in the Delayed Recognition Task. In the Visual Discrimination Task, the patient is asked to perceive and discriminate among stimuli so that visual discrimination deficits can be distinguished from visual memory deficits. The test may assist in distinguishing between acquisition and retrieval deficits. The test consists of 137 stimulus cards and a scoring form. For the CVMT to be administered, the patient must be able to understand the nature of the test, have adequate visual acuity, and be capable of providing a response. Impaired performance on the CVMT may reflect impaired visual perception in some patients, which is why the Visual Discrimination Task was included. The test takes 45 to 50 minutes to perform. Scores are obtained from performance on the Acquisition Task and the Delayed Recognition Task. Norms are available on persons from 18 to 91 years but are most reliable up to 60 years of age. No differences were found due to sex and education. Percentile scores, in addition to normal means and normal standard deviations, are available.

Some validity studies have been performed on the CVMT in patients with TBI, Alzheimer's type dementia, and amnesiac syndrome. All of these groups scored significantly lower than normals matched for age. Patients with right hemisphere lesions scored significantly lower than normals, as compared with the patients with left hemisphere damage (receptive aphasics excluded) who scored the same as the controls. For more information, contact Psychological Assessment Resources, Inc., P.O. Box 998, Odessa, FL 33556.

DEMENTIA RATING SCALE

The Dementia Rating Scale (DRS) was developed to measure the differences between demented patients and normals. It was designed to measure decline in neurologic, behavioral, and cognitive functions (Mattis, 1973). The scale is composed of 36 tasks with five subscales: attention, initiation and perseveration, construction, conceptualization, and memory. Stimulus items are familiar to most patients. The test is designed in a hierarchic manner, in that patients passing the first item in each subscale are given credit for the remainder tasks in the subscale and therefore

Heaton, R., Chelune, G., Talley, J., Kay, G., & Curtiss, G. (1981). *Wisconsin Card Sorting Test Manual: Revised and Expanded*. Odessa, FL: Psychological Assessment Resources.

Heaton, R., & Pendleton, M. (1981). Use of neuropsychological tests to predict adult patient's everyday functioning. *Journal of Consulting and Clinical Psychology, 6*, 807–821.

Hecaen, H., & Albert, M. (1978). Disorders of memory. In *Human neuropsychology*. New York: John Wiley and Sons.

Heimann, N., Allen, C., & Yerxa, E. (1989). The Routine Task Inventory: A tool for describing the functional behavior of the cognitively disabled. *Occupational Therapy Practice, 1*, 67–74.

Houston, D., Williams, S., Bloomer, J., & Mann, W. (1989). The Bay Area Functional Performance Evaluation: Development and standardization. *American Journal of Occupational Therapy, 44*, 170–183.

Itzkovich, M., Elazor, B., Aberbuch, S. (1990). *Loewenstein Occupational Therapy Cognitive Assessment (LOTCA) Manual*. Pequannock, NJ: Maddox, Inc.

Josman, N., & Katz, N. (1991). A Problem-solving version of the Allen Cognitive Level Test. *American Journal of Occupational Therapy, 45*, 331–338.

Katz, N., & Heimann, N. (1990). Review of research conducted in Israel on cognitive disability instrumentation. *Occupational Therapy in Mental Health, 10*, 1–15.

Kiernan, R., Mueller, J., Langston, J. W., & Van Dyke, C. (1987). The Neurobehavioral Cognitive Status Examination: A brief but differentiated approach to cognitive assessment. *Annals of Internal Medicine, 107*, 481–485.

Klyczek, J., & Mann, W. (1990). Concurrent validity of the Task-Oriented Assessment Component of the Bay Area Functional Performance Evaluation with the American Association on Mental Deficiency Adaptive Behavior Scale. *American Journal of Occupational Therapy, 44*, 907–912.

Kopelman, M., Wilson, B., & Baddeley, A. (1990). The Autobiographical Memory Interview: A new assessment of autobiographical and personal semantic memory in amnesic patients. *Journal of Clinical Experimental Neuropsychology, 11*, 724–744.

Levin, H., O'Donnell, V., & Grossman, R. (1979). The Galveston Orientation and Amnesia Test: A practical scale to assess cognition after head injury. *Journal of Nervous and Mental Disease, 11*, 675–684.

Lezak, M. (Ed.). (1983). *Neuropsychological assessment*. New York: Oxford University Press.

Lezak, M. (1985). Neuropsychological assessment. In P. Vinken, G. Bruyne, & H. Klawans (Eds.), *Handbook of Clinical Neurology. Vol. 1* (pp. 515–530). New York: Elsevier.

Lindenmuth, J., Breu, C., & Malooney, J. (1980). Sensory overload. *American Journal of Nursing, 80*, 1456–1458.

Loring, D., Lee, G., & Meador, K. (1989). Issues of assessment of the elderly. *Clinics in Geriatric Medicine, 5*, 565–581.

Mattis, S. (1973). *Dementia Rating Scale, Professional Manual*. Odessa, FL: Psychological Assessment Resources, Inc.

Meyer, J., & Meyer, K. (1995). *Rey Complex Figure Test and Recognition Trial*. Odessa, FL: Psychological Assessment Resources, Inc.

Montgomery, K., & Costa, L. (1983). Concurrent validity of the Mattis Dementia Rating Scale.

Morse, A. (1986). Neuropsychological tools and techniques of cognitive assessment. In *Brain injury: Cognitive and prevocational approaches to rehabilitation* (pp. 51–88). New York: The Tiresias Press.

Naugle, R., & Kawczak, K. (1989). Limitations of the Mini-Mental State Examination. *Cleveland Clinic Journal of Medicine, 56*, 277–284.

Newcombe, F. (1985). Rehabilitation in clinical neurology. In J.A.M. Frederiks (Ed.), *Handbook of clinical neurology. Vol. 46* (pp. 609–642). Amsterdam and New York: Elsevier Science Publishers.

Nissen (1986). Neuropsychology of attention and memory. *Journal of Head Injury Rehabilitation, 1*, 13–21.

Panisset, M., Roudier, M., Saxton, J., & Boller, F. (1994). Severe Impairment Battery: A neuropsychological test for severely demented patients. *Archives of Neurology, 51*, 41–45.

Pfeiffer, E. (1974). A Short Portable Mental Status Questionnaire for the assessment of organic brain deficit in elderly patients. *Journal of the American Geriatrics Society, 23*, 433–441.

Raven, J. C., Court, J. H., & Raven, J. (1988). *Manual for Raven's Progressive Matrices and Vocabulary Scales* (1988 Edition). London: Oxford Psychologists Press.

Raven, J., Raven, J. C., & Court, J. (1991). *Manual for Raven's Progressive Matrices and Vocabulary Scales. General overview* (1991 Edition). London: Oxford Psychologists Press.

Rustad, R., DeGroot, T., Jungkunz, M., Freeberg, K., Borowick, L., & Wanttie, A. (1993). *The Cognitive Assessment of Minnesota*. Tucson, AZ: Therapy Skill Builders.

Saxton, J., McGonigle, K., Swihart, A., Boller, F. (1993). *The Severe Impairment Battery*. Suffolk, England: Thames Valley Test Company.

Saxton, J., & Swihart, A. (1989). Neuropsychological assessment of the severely impaired elderly patient. *Clinics in Geriatric Medicine, 5*, 531–543.

Schmitt, F., Ranseen, J., & DeKosky, S. (1989). Cognitive mental status examinations. *Clinics in Geriatric Medicine, 5*, 545–564.

Schwamm, L., VanDyke, C., Kiernan, R., Merrin, E., Mueller, J. (1987). The Neurobehavioral Cognitive Status Examination: Comparison with the Mini-Mental State Examination in the neurosurgical population. *Annals of Internal Medicine, 107*, 486–491.

Smith, A. (1982). *Symbol Digit Modalities Test, manual*. Los Angeles: Western Psychological Services.

Spreen, O., & Strauss, E. (1991). *A compendium of neuropsychological tests*. New York: Oxford University Press.

Squire, L., & Cohen, N. (1984). Human memory and amnesia. In G. Lynch, J. McGaugh, & N. Weinberger (Eds.), *Neurobiology of learning and memory*. New York: Guilford Press.

Strub, R., & Black, F. W. (1977). *The Mental Status Examination in Neurology*. Philadelphia: F. A. Davis Company.

Toglia, J. (1993a). Attention and memory. In C. B. Royeen (Ed.), *American Occupational Therapy Association self-study series: Cognitive rehabilitation*. Rockville, MD: American Occupational Therapy Association.

Toglia, J. (1993b). *Contextual Memory Test*. Tucson, AZ: Therapy Skill Builders.

Trahan, D., & Larrabee, G. (1983). *Continuous Visual Memory Test*. Odessa, FL: Psychological Assessment Resources.

Veltman, R., VanDongen, S., Jones, S., & Blostein, P. (1993). Cognitive screening in mild head injury. *Journal of Neuroscience Nursing, 25*, 367–371.

Warren, M. (1993). A hierarchical model for evaluation and treatment of adult acquired brain injury, Part 1. *American Journal of Occupational Therapy, 47*, 42–54.

Wetzel, L., & Boll, T. (1987). *Short Category Test, booklet format manual*. Los Angeles: Western Psychological Services.

Williams, J. M. (1987). *Cognitive Behavior Rating Scales manual*. Odessa, FL: Psychological Assessment Resources.

Wilson, B., Baddeley, A., Cockburn, J., & Hiorns, R. (No date). *The Rivermead Behavioural Memory Test. Supplement 2: Validation study*. Titchfield, Hants, England: Thames Valley Test Company.

Wilson, B., Cockburn, J., & Baddeley, A. (1991). *The Rivermead Behavioural Memory Test*. Edmunds, England: Thames Valley Test Company.

Winograd, C. H. (1984). Mental status tests and the capacity for self care. *Journal of the American Geriatrics Society, 32*, 49–55.

Zemke, R. (1994). Task skills, problem solving, and social interaction. In C. B. Royeen (Ed.), *American Occupational Therapy Association self-study series: Cognitive rehabilitation*. Rockville, MD: American Occupational Therapy Association.

Zoltan, B. (1990). Evaluation and treatment of cognitive dysfunction. In L. Pedretti & B. Zoltan (Eds.), *Occupational therapy practice skills for physical dysfunction*, third edition. St. Louis, MO: C. V. Mosby Company.

Age-Related Assessment

about the child's performance may be influenced by constraints of time, space, equipment, and skill or preparation.

Evaluation of the Young Child

Assessing young children can be challenging in ways that are different than the assessment of adults. Issues such as the separation of the child from his or her parents during the evaluation process and the developmentally typical reactions children have to new and different situations can affect the process. Young children are often resistive to the testing protocol and procedures and therefore may make the use of highly standardized devices difficult. They often resist moving from one activity to the other and are difficult to motivate, as they fail to grasp the meaning of the activities. These challenges may affect the child's performance on test items and try the skills of even the most experienced examiner.

DEVELOPMENTAL ASSESSMENTS

A therapist may wish to have an overview of the child's developmental progress to determine if the child is delayed developmentally. Developmental delay is determined by a delay in the achievement of recognized developmental milestones, regardless of the primary diagnostic reason. Children who are the most severely affected are often identified at birth. Others who are referred or later determined to need developmental assessment appear to have varying levels of "slowness" achieving developmental milestones (Clancy & Clark, 1990).

Children that appear to have developmental delays are most often assessed by a team of health professionals that may include an occupational, physical, and speech therapist, and a psychologist, among others. It is essential that the team members understand that in pediatrics we are dealing with a developing and emerging child. As the central nervous system develops over time, functional skills and developmental milestones change as perception, motor coordination, cognition, language, emotional, and social development occur. As intervention will be remedial and compensatory in varying degrees, general guidelines for assessment of developmental delay include identifying the child's current developmental level of function and some prediction of the progression of the child's progress. These goals cannot be reached, and effective decisions cannot be made based on one evaluation. Assessment in pediatrics is a process or collection of data from several sources and several viewpoints representing the many spheres of influence on children's development (Meisils & Provence, 1989).

A variety of developmental instruments are available to therapists working with children suspected of having or being at risk for developmental delay. Several have been selected for review and discussion here, and others are included in Table 13–1.

The Early Intervention Developmental Profile

The Early Intervention Developmental Profile (EIDP) (Brown et al., 1981; Rogers & D'Eugenio, 1981) is part of a comprehensive developmental assessment and systematic intervention system for young children from newborn to 6 years old. The assessment instrument was designed to provide a general overview of developmental milestones based on specific age-related skills for children with all types of disabilities. The initial assessment, originally developed in 1977, is designed to test skills between 0 and 36 months. The second part, developed in 1981, includes skills from 3 to 6 years. The test's developers combined tasks and normative data developed in the literature and on standardized tests of developmental functioning. Areas evaluated include perceptual and fine motor, cognition, language, social and emotional, self-care, and gross motor skills. No composite scores are figured, but age levels for each of the six areas are determined.

The profile is designed to be administered by a team of evaluators, each area being assessed by the team member most highly trained to do so. The profile can be administered in approximately 1 hour. After completion, the team has a profile of the child's current level of functioning in each area with basal and ceiling levels of performance. This gives those involved with the child a baseline of information to plan intervention strategies.

This instrument is not standardized and should not be used as a diagnostic tool. However, used in combination with other evaluations, it does provide an intervention team with a baseline of performance. The test booklet can be used several times to document a change in skill levels over time. Scores can be charted out on a composite profile to illustrate areas of strengths and concerns.

Studies of both age sections of this tool have been conducted with small samples. However, it has been found in studies conducted by the developers that interrater and test-retest studies have been excellent (89 and 90 percent). In correlation studies using the Bayley Motor Scales, the Slossen Intelligence Test for Children and Adults, and the Vineland Social Maturity Scale, the EIDP showed strong criterion-related validity.

The Denver II

The Denver II (Frankenberg et al., 1990; Frankenberg et al., 1992) is a screening instrument that was originally published in 1967 as the Denver Developmental Screening Test (DDST). Since that time it has undergone a major revision and restandardization. It is now titled the Denver II,

Table continued on following page

TABLE 13-1

ASSESSMENTS FOR CHILDREN SUSPECTED OF HAVING OR BEING AT RISK FOR DEVELOPMENTAL DELAY

Developmental Screens	Target Population	Purpose	Time	Comments	Psychometric Properties	References
Movement Assessment of Infants Screening Test (MAI-ST)	2–18 mo	Identify movement patterns that interfere with normal development	10–15 minutes	Individually administered; domains: muscle tone, primitive reflexes, volitional movement	Reliability: TR = 0.87 to 0.97; IR = 0.81 to 0.95 No validity information	Chandler, 1986; Chandler et al., 1988
Denver II	0–6 y	Initial screen of well children suspected of having or being at risk for developmental delay	20–35 minutes	Individually administered, norm-referenced test; domains: personal-social, fine-motor adaptive, language, and gross motor. Test form can be used several times to document progress; child's behavior during testing recorded on form	Original version (DDST) standardized on over 2000 normal children Reliability: IR & TR = 0.90 to 0.99. No correlation studies available Validity: content validity shown through wide use of DDST and expert review	Frankenberg et al., 1992; Frankenberg et al., 1990
Miller Assessment for Preschoolers (MAP)	2 yr, 9 mo–5 yr, 8 mo	Assist in the identification of preschoolers with mild to severe developmental delays	30–40 minutes	Individually administered, norm-referenced test; domains: sensory and motor abilities, cognitive functioning, and combined abilities. Total, composite battery scores can be calculated, as well as percentile scores on each index	Standardization sample: 1200 normal children Reliability: IR = 0.84 (coordination index) to 0.99 on individual index scores, 0.978 for battery score. TR = 72% (coordination index) to 94% Validity: Content validity by review of experts and literature, also by a pilot or research edition	Miller, 1988; Miller & Schouten, 1988; Miller & Sprong, 1987
Battelle Developmental Inventory Screening Test (BDI-ST)	0–8 yr	Identify children that are at risk for developmental delays	10–30 minutes	Individually administered; domains: personal-social, adaptive, motor, communication, cognition	No reliability information Validity: Scores correlated to full BDI (0.92 or above)	Newborg et al., 1988
Battelle Developmental Inventory (BDI)	0–8 yr	Identify developmental strengths and weaknesses of both children with disabilities and nondisabled children	1–2 h	Individually administered standardized test; domains: personal-social, adaptive, motor, communication, cognition. Basal and ceiling levels are established; training is encouraged	SEM for total BDI was 20.02, range of 2.12–9.05. TR for total BDI was 0.99, range of 0.90–0.99. IR for total BDI was 0.99, range of 0.88–0.99 (1984 version) Validity: Content established by expert review, construct correlations generally above 0.80 with muscle control lowest at 0.56, total BDI correlation of 0.97	Newborg et al., 1988

TABLE 13-1

ASSESSMENTS FOR CHILDREN SUSPECTED OF HAVING OR BEING AT RISK FOR DEVELOPMENTAL DELAY *Continued*

Developmental Screens	Target Population	Purpose	Time	Comments	Psychometric Properties	References
Early Intervention Developmental Profile (EIDP)	0–6 y	Provide a general overview of developmental milestones based on specific age-related skills of children with all types of disabilities	1 h	Individually administered norm-referenced test; domains: perceptual/fine motor, cognition, language, social/emotional, self-care, and gross motor skills. Provides a profile of the child's current performance with basal and ceiling levels established; test form can be used several times to document progress	Criterion-related validity to Vineland, Developmental Activities Screening Inventory, and Stanford Binet Reliability: IR = 0.89, TR = 0.90 Validity: Content correlates strongly with Bayley Motor Scales, Slossen Intelligence Test, and Vineland Social Maturity Scale	Brown et al., 1981; Rogers & D'Eugenio, 1981
Bayley Scales of Infant Development II (BSID-II)	1–42 mo	Assess current developmental function, diagnose developmental delay, plan intervention strategies	30–60 min	Individually administered standardized test; subscales: Motor Scale; Mental Scale; Behavior Rating Scale. Basal and ceiling levels are established. Scores are converted to a Mental Development Index, Psychomotor Development Index, and percentiles; training is encouraged	Normative data: Nationally stratified random sample of 1700 children Reliability: IC = 0.88 for Mental Scale, 0.84 for Motor Scale, 0.88 for Behavior Rating Scale SEM = 5.21 for Mental Scale, 6.01 for Motor Scale. TR = 0.87 for Mental Scale, 0.78 for Motor Scale. IR = 0.96 for Mental Scale, 0.75 for Motor Scale Validity: Content, construct and criterion related described in manual	Bayley, 1993

IC = Internal consistency reliability; IR = interrater reliability; SEM = standard error of measurement; TR = test-retest reliability.

and its normative data have been updated, individual test items have been eliminated or revised, and new language items and a behavioral rating scale that records subjective behavioral observations have been added. The developers were also concerned about training in test administration and interpretation, so they have made available a video training program and a technical manual to aid in proficiency.

The Denver II was developed for use with well children or children that have no symptoms of overt problems. It is used as an initial screening or to monitor the developmental progress of children suspected of having or being at risk for developmental delays. As a screening test, it is designed not for diagnosis but to assist in planning or identifying the need for diagnostic evaluation. As such, the test does not provide a composite score, nor is it a predictor of future developmental progression; rather, it gives an overall picture of a child's developmental progress over several developmental domains.

The test can be used on more than one occasion to screen children from birth to 6 years old. Consisting of 125 task items, the test is arranged by area of development and by the growth curves used to assess normal performance of developmental skills. Areas screened are personal and social, fine motor and adaptive, language, and gross motor skills. Test behavior is recorded after completion of the items, providing a record of the behaviors and how they affected performance. Taking between 20 and 35 minutes to administer, individual test items are scored based on the average percentage of children that have achieved that skill by the determined age range. Each developmental task has been further delineated by when 25, 50, 75, and 90 percent of children in the standardization sample achieved the specific task. The child's performance receives a score based on these designations: a "caution" when between 75 and 90 percent of children have achieved the task, or a "delay" when 90 percent have achieved it. The overall number of items on which a child receives a "caution" or "delayed" score determines the need for further testing or observation.

When the Denver II was assessed for two types of reliability, examiner-observer and test-retest stability, the average scores were higher than the original version and were in the 90 to 99 percent range. Correlational studies have not been done.

The individual test items of the original version (DDST) were standardized on more than 2000 children in 1988. The age at which children passed each item and the determination of the percentage designations were determined from this sample.

Content validity relies on the wide acceptance of the utility of the original DDST, as well as the fact that the items were written and selected by professionals in the field of pediatric development and screening (Frankenburg et al., 1990). Other types of validity studies have not been conducted.

The Miller Assessment of Preschoolers

The Miller Assessment of Preschoolers (MAP) (Miller, 1988; Miller & Schouten, 1988; Miller & Sprong, 1987) is a preschool screening test designed to assist in the identification of developmentally delayed preschoolers. Areas of preacademic skills are assessed. Preacademic skills are those prerequisite skills and behaviors that appear to predict successful performance in school. The test is designed to assess children who exhibit mild to severe problems that affect one or more developmental areas and are between the ages of 2 years 9 months and 5 years 8 months. The MAP assesses sensory and motor abilities, cognitive functioning, and the combined abilities or skills that require the use of sensorimotor and cognitive abilities together. The 27 test items and structured observations are arranged in five indexes: foundations, coordination, verbal, nonverbal, and complex tasks. Humphrey and King-Thomas (1993) suggest that the best use of the MAP might be to assist in identifying the child's current strengths and intervention needs. They also suggest that the data obtained from the administration of this test are particularly useful for planning treatment and documenting changes in performance.

The test items, manual, and score sheets are notable for their simplicity and ease in use. A score reflecting the total or composite performance on the battery can be calculated. Also, individual scores on each index compare the child's performance to the norm and can be used to determine specific areas that need more in-depth testing. The developers have found scores on this assessment to be predictive of school-rated behaviors. However, poor performance on the MAP should not be used as a means to diagnose intellectual or medical problems, but the information obtained through the use of the test should be combined with more detailed diagnostic assessment. Percentile scores are interpreted as indicating that the child a) is at risk and in need of a referral for further testing, b) has some areas of concern and is in need of a follow-up assessment, or c) exhibited normal performance. The MAP can be administered to document developmental progress and intervention efficacy after a suitable time lapse of 6 months to 1 year.

The assessment takes approximately 30 to 40 minutes to administer by a trained evaluator. Although the test is designed for use by professionals with varied backgrounds and training, the evaluator should have experience in psychological and developmental assessment, experience with preschool-aged populations, and familiarity with standardized testing procedures. Along with practice administering the assessment, a prospective evaluator should obtain a learning videotape or attend a continuing education workshop to ensure that he or she is administering the test and observational items in a standardized manner. The manual contains clear and specific instructions for the administration of each test item, scoring instructions, and interpretation.

Reliability. The use of the MAP has been found to be a reliable and consistent method of screening preschool sensorimotor performance. The interrater reliability, conducted by two examiners and 40 normal children on the MAP, ranged from 0.84 to 0.99 on individual test indexes and was 0.978 for the total test. The performance index of coordination (0.84) was the only score that was below 0.97. Test-retest reliability was conducted by three examiners on 80 normal children. The reliability was calculated on the stability of the child's total score. The scores expressed as percentages in the MAP manual ranged from a low of 72 percent (coordination index) to a high of 94 percent (nonverbal index) agreement after retest. Internal reliability for the MAP was calculated to be near 0.80 for both item raw scores and the average item-to-test correlations.

Validity. The MAP has been found to be a valid measure of sensorimotor performance in preschool. Content validity was established by review by content experts and a review of the literature. Content validity of test items was also determined by a pilot field test of a "try-out" or research edition of the MAP.

Standardization. The MAP was standardized on 1200 normal children using a random, stratified sampling procedure. Variables considered were age, geographic region, race, sex, community size, and socioeconomic status.

Although the MAP is one of the better instruments available for use by pediatric occupational and physical therapists, it does have a number of problems (Schouten & Kirkpatrick, 1993). Considerable dialogue about this tool has taken place in the OT research literature (Short-Degraff, 1993).

The Battelle Developmental Inventory

The Battelle Developmental Inventory (BDI) (Newborg et al., 1988) is nationally standardized and administered individually over a 1- to 2-hour period. The primary purpose of the BDI is identification of developmental strengths and weaknesses of children both with and without disabilities. Two versions have been published, the first in 1984 and the revised edition in 1988. The BDI also assists with developing and implementing individual education plans (IEPs). The full BDI battery includes five domains: (a) personal and social, with subdomains of adult interaction, expression of feelings and affect, self-concept, peer interaction, coping, and social roles; (b) adaptive, with subdomains of attention, eating, dressing, personal responsibility, and toileting; (c) motor, with subdomains of muscle control, body coordination, locomotion, fine muscle control, and perceptual motor; (d) communication, with subdomains of receptive and expressive; and (e)

cognitive, with subdomains of perceptual discrimination, memory, reasoning and academic skills, and conceptual development. Each domain may be administered individually, or the entire battery can be administered. Information can be obtained through structured administration of items, observation, and interviews.

Basal and ceiling levels are established in administered subdomains. Scores range from 0 (incorrect response) to 1 (attempt that does not meet the full criteria), to 2 (response meets the full criteria). Ten age levels have been established. Raw scores are converted to percentile ranks, standard scores, and age equivalency. The scores allow the examiner to compare (a) the total score with each domain, (b) domains with one another, (c) subdomains with the domains, and (d) subdomains with one another.

The BDI was designed for use by teachers and others interested in measuring a child's functional abilities. The developers recommend that the examiner familiarize himself or herself with the items and practice administering the test. The BDI is for children from birth to 8 years of age who have a single disability or any combination of disabilities. Some test items include specific adaptations for children with specific impairments.

Normative Sample. Stratified random sampling of the four major geographic regions from the U.S. census was used for the norming sample. Forty-two test administrators at 28 test sites in 24 states participated. A total of 800 children were tested, with equal numbers across 10 age ranges. The sampling method is outlined in the manual.

Reliability and validity information were recalculated in the 1988 version. The standard error of measurement for the total BDI was 20.02, with a range of 2.12 to 9.05, depending on the age range. Test-retest reliability was 0.99 for the total test and ranged from 0.90 to 0.99 for the age ranges. No interrater reliability is reported in the 1988 revision.

Validity. Content validity was established by having content experts review the BDI. Construct validity was demonstrated through the correlation of the subdomains to each other and to the domains in a logical way. The correlations were generally above 0.80, with a BDI total correlation of 0.97. The lowest area was muscle control (0.56). The authors suggested that this was low due to the ceiling effect of the test. A factoral analysis indicated that each subdomain was located in the correct domain. In comparing BDI scores for children with a variety of disabling conditions with those for nondisabled children, the BDI accurately identified children with developmental problems across the five domains. Criterion-related validity was established by comparing the BDI with the Vineland Social Maturity Scale (Vineland), Developmental Activities Screening Inventory (DASI), Stanford-Binet Intelligence Scale, Wechsler Intelligence Scale for Child—Revised, and Peabody Picture Vocabulary Test scores. Overall, the BDI total score correlated best with the Vineland (0.94), and DASI (0.91).

The BDI is a widely used inventory (Goodman & Pollak, 1993). A problem that has been identified with this test is that for children whose chronologic age falls at a cut-off point between age categories, extremely different scores can be obtained, depending on how the child's birthdate is compared with the age category (Boyd, 1989). One problem found with the literature is that the authors do not indicate which version of the BDI was used, making comparisons difficult.

NEONATAL ASSESSMENT

Low–birth weight infants and those with high-risk factors are surviving in increasing numbers because of advances in neonatology. Therapists providing services in the neonatal intensive care unit (NICU) must be aware of medical as well as developmental issues in the neonate. The therapist must be sensitive to a variety of physiologic state, motor, attention, and interactive behaviors. These behaviors are constantly interacting and changing, which alters the ways in which the neonate responds to the sensory input from the environment. Most neonatal assessments address the infant's neurobehavioral organization. The neurobehavioral assessment allows the therapist to assess the stability of the physiologic state, self-regulation behaviors, and attention and interaction systems during handling. Other components of development that may be included in neonatal assessment would be reflexive development, muscle tone, motor activity, and postural development.

The assessment process provides the therapist with baseline information and allows the therapist to document progress (Miller & Quinn-Hurst, 1994). During the assessment, the therapist's focus is on the neonate's reactions to specific types of stimuli. Careful attention is given to the amount of environmental support necessary to achieve the neonates' responses (Als et al., 1982). A variety of instruments are available to therapists working with neonates suspected of having or being at risk for developmental delay. Several have been selected for review and discussion here, and others are included in Table 13–2.

Some of the neonatal neurobehavioral assessments require certification for the examiner, and others do not. The Neonatal Neurobehavioral Evaluation (NNE) (Morgan et al., 1988), the Neurological Assessment of the Preterm and Full-Term Infant (NAPFI) (Dubowitz & Dubowitz, 1981), and the Neurologic Evaluation of the Newborn and the Infant (Amiel-Tison & Grenier, 1983) do not require certification. The Neonatal Behavioral Assessment Scale (NBAS) (Brazelton, 1973, 1984), the Assessment of Premature Infant Behavior (APIB) (Als et al., 1982), and the Naturalistic Observation of Newborn Behavior (NONB) (Als, 1984) all require certification. The trainee should have a strong background in normal and abnormal infant development. Training occurs via workshops or videotapes. The trainee then practices the assessment prior to concluding reliability training. Specific centers that provide certification are listed in the back of each individual manual.

Other areas of assessment that may be performed based on specific problems that the infants may exhibit include assessment of feeding and pulmonary ability and biomechanical problems, such as limitations in range of motion and splinting needs.

The Neurological Assessment of the Preterm and Full-Term Infant

The NAPFI (Dubowitz & Dubowitz, 1981) was designed to provide a developmental profile of full-term and preterm infants. This test can be administered shortly after birth and is designed for sequential uses. It has been developed to provide information concerning the current functional state of the infant's nervous system.

The test items were selected from other recognized tests of preterm and full-term infant behavior (Brazelton, 1984; Prechtl, 1977; Saint-Anne Dargassies, 1977). The testing items include those that assess aspects of higher-order neurologic function, as well as more traditional neurologic testing items. The areas of infant behavior assessed are habituation, movement and tone, reflexes, and neurobehavioral responses (orientation, alertness and excitability, irritability and consolability, defensive reactions, and crying).

The NAPFI can be administered quite quickly and is very easy to score. Organized through the use of illustrations, the test requires no specific training to administer; however, it is recommended that users should have practice administering the test to healthy infants before using it for clinical purposes. The test manual contains detailed instructions for administration of test items and procedures. The testing form is easy to use and is arranged in a recommended sequential order; however, this order can be varied according to the infant's state and needs. An experienced examiner can administer this test in approximately 15 to 20 minutes.

Reliability. The NAPFI is reported to have good interrater reliability, but no other measures of statistical soundness have been reported.

The Assessment of Preterm Infant Behavior

The APIB (Als et al., 1982) is one of the most comprehensive standardized evaluations available for the assessment of the neurobehavioral functioning in preterm infants. The AIPB is based on the NBAS (Brazelton, 1973, 1984), extending the types and amounts of data collected and refining the use of the test for premature infants. The scoring and interpretation of this assessment is quite complex, requiring a certification process that requires approximately 1 year to complete. Therapists who seek to become certified in the use of this instrument should have excellent evaluation skills and experience, extensive expe-

TABLE 13–2

ASSESSMENTS FOR INFANTS WITH LOW BIRTH WEIGHT AND THOSE INFANTS AT HIGH RISK FOR DEVELOPMENTAL DIFFICULTIES

Neonatal	Target Population	Purpose	Time	Comments	Psychometric Properties	Reference
Assessment of Premature Infant Behavior (APIB)	Premature infants	Provide a comprehensive neurobehavioral assessment	45–60 min	Standardized assessment of subsystem stability before, during, and after administration of 27 items and 19 reflexes arranged according to amount of stimulation provided; scoring and interpretation are complex and require in-depth training	Reliability: IR = examiners must be trained in administration and in scoring at 0.90 level prior to using the assessment Validity: Content validity based on NBAS; construct validity discriminates at-risk, high-risk, and normal infants	Als et al., 1982; Als et al., 1988a, 1988b
Naturalistic Observation of Newborn Behavior (NONB) (also referred to as Neonatal Individualized Developmental and Care Assessment Plan [NIDCAP])	Premature infants	Identify infant's stability and self-regulation abilities during medical procedures; treatment plans are directed to support and develop self-regulation abilities	50–60 min	Observation and time samples of physiologic, motor, and state behaviors; approach and withdrawal signs immediately prior to, during, and after a procedure; individualized care and follow-up plans are developed based on the assessment	Reliability: IR = examiners must be trained in observations and in scoring at 0.90 level prior to using the assessment Content validity: Based on APIB	Als, 1984
Neonatal Behavioral Assessment Scale (NBAS)	Neonates 37–44 w gestational age	Assess the infant's current behavior capabilities in response to environmental stimuli and handling; the examination is a "snapshot" of the infant	20–30 min	Designed to show parents their infant's capabilities with emphasis on eliciting the best response; 37 items scored on a 9-point scale and 19 reflexes (based on Prechtl, 1977) scored on a 3-point scale. Manual describes administration, scoring, and interpretation; frequently used in research	Reliability: IR = examiners must be trained in observations and in scoring at 0.90 level prior to using the assessment Content validity: Based on wide test use	Brazelton, 1973, 1984
Neonatal Neurobehavioral Examination (NNE)	32–42 w gestational age	Describe neurobehavioral characteristics at specific conceptual ages in quantitative terms	15 min	Standardized battery; domains: tone and motor patterns, primitive reflexes, and behavioral responses. Scored on a three-point scale and summed for all sections; behavioral responses section also included cluster scores. Mean and standard deviations for both groups are given	Sample: 54 normal, full-term infants and 298 randomly selected infants in the NICU Reliability: IR = 0.88 on individual test items and 0.95 on section scores Validity: Content established by review of research on infant assessment; construct validity discriminates between high-risk and normal infants	Morgan et al., 1988

Test	Age Range	Purpose	Time	Description	Psychometric Information	Reference
Neurologic Evaluation of the Newborn and Infant	0–12 mo	Identify abnormal neuromotor development and provide sequential follow-up during the first year; designed for neonatologists but can supplement the neurodevelopmental examination	10–15 min	Critical ages are birth, 2, 7, and 12 months; domains: physical examination; historical data about state behaviors, posture, and spontaneous motor behaviors; and passive and active muscle tone. Scores are on a continuum with pictures and descriptions of items; the same form can be used for repeated administration to track progress. No total score obtained	Correlations among test sections were 0.498 to 0.630 indicating overlap of constructs between sections Reliability: IR = (individual items) 0.50 to 0.90. TR = 0.90 (Wetzel & Wetzel, 1984). Construct validity: The test discriminates between normal and abnormally developing infants	Amiel-Tison & Grenier, 1983; Amiel-Tison, 1973
Neurological Evaluation of the Preterm and Full-term Newborn (Dubowitz)	Premature infants	Assess neurologic stability and identify abnormalities as they occur	10–15 min	Quick screen including habituation, movement and tone, reflexes, visual and auditory responses, state, and irritability; scores are on a continuum with pictures and brief descriptions. The same form can be used for repeated administration to track progress; no interpretation	Construct validity: Test discriminates those neonates that have an interventricular hemorrhage from normal neonates No other psychometric information available	Dubowitz & Dubowitz, 1981
Neurological Screening Examination of the Newborn Infant	Newborns	Assess reflexes, provide comprehensive neurologic assessment	30 min	Manual provides specific information administration of neonatal reflexes; includes the infant's state, motor activity, and responsiveness during the examination	No psychometric information	Prechtl, 1977
Reflex Evaluation	Any age	Assess primitive reflexes and postural reactions	20–30 min	Programmed text provides overview and discussion of all reflexes and reactions assessed by therapists (includes obligatory and pathologic) Evaluation form includes pictures of reflexes and reactions	No psychometric information	Barnes et al, 1978

rience working with newborns, and good memory and judgment (Vergara, 1991). The APIB provides information concerning the infant's response to stress, interactive abilities, and the physiologic "cost" of stress and interaction, among other data. The data are collected in six areas or "packages," which are arranged sequentially, placing increasing demands on the response abilities of the infant. The examiner identifies which tasks or handling procedures to which the infant responds well without intervention, the tasks the infant needs environmental support to handle well, and the tasks the infant is not capable of handling with or without support (Als et al., 1988).

The infant must have the physiologic stability to tolerate a number of handling procedures. The APIB takes between 45 and 60 minutes to administer. As it also takes about the same amount of time to score and interpret, it can be quite costly and time consuming. However, this can be balanced by the comprehensive nature of the data collected on completion.

As the APIB requires very comprehensive training and certification, the interrater reliability can be perceived as high. Each certified examiner must administer and score the test at $r = 0.90$ or higher before using the instrument.

The validity of the APIB is based on its original version, the NBAS. The construct validity has been determined as adequate in discriminating between at-risk, high-risk, and normal children.

The Neonatal Behavioral Assessment Scale

The NBAS (Brazelton, 1973, 1984) was developed to measure the neurobehavioral responses of infants between 36 weeks and 44 weeks gestation. The test addresses neurobehavioral organization in the context of the infant's interactive abilities. Originally intended for use with full-term infants as a parental training tool, it is often used with premature infants as well. However, as performance on the test items requires greater physiologic stability than some of other instruments assessing infant behavior (e.g., the NONB, which does not require the handling of the infant), it is recommended that the NBAS be used as the preterm infant approaches full-term gestational age (Miller & Quinn-Hurst, 1994).

The NBAS has 28 behavioral items and 18 elicited responses (reflexes). The test items are grouped into clusters of behaviors, providing a description of the infant's overall behavior. The clusters include habituation, orientation, motor behaviors (including tone, response to sensory information, and reflexes), range and regulation of state behaviors, and autonomic stability. The Kansas Supplementary items are for the evaluation of high-risk infants (Brazelton, 1984).

Certification and training in the administration of this assessment are needed. Information concerning the requirements for this process are available from The Brazel-

ton Neonatal Assessment Center in Boston, Massachusetts.

The Bayley Scales of Infant Development–Second Edition

The Bayley Scales of Infant Development–Second Edition (BSID-II) (Bayley, 1993) are based on the original Bayley Scales of Infant Development (BSID) (Bayley, 1969). Much of the original content has been retained, and new materials created. The purpose of the BSID-II is to assess the current developmental function of infants and children. The BSID diagnoses developmental delay and assists in planning intervention strategies. The BSID-II is a nationally standardized, individually administered assessment. Three scales are included: 1) the Mental Scale, which includes memory, habituation, problem solving, early number concepts, generalization, classification, vocalizations, language, and social skills; (2) the Motor Scale, which includes control of gross and fine muscle groups; and (3) the Behavior Rating Scale (BRS) (formerly the Infant Behavior Record), which encompasses qualitative aspects of behavior, including attention and arousal, orientation and engagement, emotional regulation, and motor quality. The BRS provides supplemental information for the Mental and Motor Scales.

The child receives credit or no credit on administered items. Basal and ceiling levels are established in the Mental and Motor Scales. Raw scores, based on the number of items receiving credit, are calculated for all three scales. The BRS raw scores are converted to percentiles. The raw scores are converted into Mental Development Index (MDI) and Psychomotor Development Index (PDI) scores, with a 90 or 95 percent confidence interval based on one of the 17 age levels. Based on the MDI, PDI, and percentiles, the child's performance can be classified as within normal limits or mildly, moderately, or significantly delayed.

Examiners using the BSID-II should have extensive experience in administration and interpretation of assessments of young children. The instructions should be followed exactly. When testing a child with a physical or perceptual deficit, the examiner may choose to adapt the test items. However, the authors state that if the instructions are changed, the results cannot be compared with those of the normative sample. Interpretation should be completed as suggested by the Standards for Educational and Psychological Testing (American Psychological Association, 1992). All test materials and forms are provided in the BSID-II kit. The BSID-II is intended for children between the ages of 1 and 42 months.

Standardization. Several pilot studies were conducted. Based on the pilot studies, changes were made to test materials, scoring, or the manual. Try-out testing was then done with a stratified sample of 643 children. Stratification was on the basis of race or ethnicity, parent education level, gender, and age. Examiners used selected items from the

BSID Mental and Motor Scale, as well as the new items for the BSID-II. After try-out testing, the BSID-II was evaluated for racial and gender bias. In addition, an expert panel reviewed the test items for bias. The norms for the BSID-II came from a national, stratified (age, gender, race or ethnicity, geographic region, and parent education) random sample that was representative of the U.S. population for children from 1 to 42 months of age. A total of 1700 children participated, with 100 children in each of the 17 age groups.

Reliability. The reliability for each scale at each of the age levels was calculated using coefficient alpha. The average coefficient for the Mental Scale is 0.88, for the Motor Scale is 0.84, and for the total behavior rating scale is 0.88. Standard error of measurements averaged 5.21 for the Mental Scale and 6.01 for the Motor Scale.

Test-retest reliability was computed for four age levels (1, 12, 24, and 36 months). The interval between testing ranged from 1 to 16 days, with an average of 4 days. The Mental and Motor Scale coefficients for 1 and 12 months were 0.83 and 0.77, respectively. At 1 month, coefficients ranged from 0.48 to 0.70 for the behavior rating scale; at 12 months, they ranged from 0.57 to 0.90. At 24 and 36 months, Mental and Motor Scale coefficients were 0.91 for the Mental Scale, 0.79 for the Motor Scale, and 0.60 to 0.71 for the behavior rating scale. The total coefficients for the combined ages were 0.87 for the Mental Scale and 0.78 for the Motor Scale.

Interrater reliability was completed by having a second rater discretely observe the administration of the BSID-II. Each rater independently scored the child. The MDI and PDI scores were compared. Coefficients were 0.96 for the Mental Scale and 0.75 for the Motor Scale. The authors believe that the Motor Scale requires physical manipulation of the child, which may have contributed to the lower coefficients. Coefficients were also calculated for the BRS for the youngest (0.70) and oldest (0.88) age groups.

Validity. Content validity for the three scales was established by having experts review both domains to be tested and the individual items. Construct validity for the Mental and Motor Scales was established by correlating each item with the total score for each age for which the item was included. Items were placed in the scale where they had the highest correlation. Correlations between the MDI and PDI tended to be low to moderate. This supports interpreting the two scales independently. Construct validity for the BRS was established by a factor analytic study. The reason for this was that the authors wanted to assure that all aspects of behavior were included. For children from 1 to 5 months of age, two factors were identified, which accounted for 44 percent of the variance. Factor one was motor quality, and factor two was attention or arousal. Three factors were identified for the 6- to 12-month age group, which accounted for 46 percent of the variance. Factor one was orientation or engagement, factor two was motor quality, and factor three was emotional regulation. Three factors were identified for the 13- to 42-month age

group, which accounted for 53 percent of the variance. Factor one was emotional regulation, factor 2 was orientation or engagement, and factor 3 was motor quality.

The BSID-II scores were compared with scores on the original BSID for 200 children. Moderate correlations were found between the MDI ($r = 0.62$) and PDI ($r = 0.63$). This was expected due to the changes in the BSID-II. The mean score on the BSID-II was lower for both the MDI and the PDI. The BSID-II was also correlated with other tests. Details are in the manual. Thompson and colleagues (1994) and Wasserman and coworkers (1993) examined the validity of the BSID-II. Both studies confirmed that the BSID-II had adequate construct validity.

CONCLUSIONS

The areas included and the type of instrument selected for developmental and neonatal assessment depend primarily on the purpose of the evaluation. Some referrals clearly specify the reasons for referral and the areas or components of function that should be assessed, but in the majority of cases, these decisions are left to the therapist. Assessment in the areas of developmental and neonatal assessment is most often a team process to provide the best overall view of the child's strengths and problems.

This chapter has presented an overview of just some of the variety of instruments available for evaluation of children with developmental issues. Therapists should be cautious about interpreting the results of those evaluations in which they do not have the appropriate training or expertise.

GLOSSARY

Consolability—The ability of a child to be consoled or comforted after a disruption of state.

Developmental milestones—A progressive continuum of recognized developmental skills and abilities.

Full term—An infant born between 37 and 41 weeks after conception.

Gestation—The length of time between conception and birth.

Habituation—A sensory processing ability that allows a child to inhibit irrelevant stimuli; when exposed to numerous repetitions of the same stimulus, the intensity of the response diminishes and often the child stops responding altogether.

Individual educational plan (IEP)—A process federally mandated by the Education for Handicapped Children Act (Public Law 94-142) and Handicapped Act Amendments of 1986 (Public Law 99-457) for children preschool through secondary educational level who are the

TABLE 14-1

PEDIATRIC ASSESSMENTS *Continued*

Sensorimotor—Gross and Fine Motor Tests	Target Population	Purpose	Time	Comments	Psychometric Properties	Reference
Sensorimotor Performance Analysis (SPA)	5–21 y	Screening tool that analyzes the underlying sensorimotor components of performance during fine and gross motor tasks; information assists in program planning	20–30 min	Criterion-referenced, individually administered observation of postural mechanisms, sensory processing, developmental lags, postural tone, and bilateral integration. Seven tasks are involved. Each task includes performance components. Scoring is on a continuum. Raw scores are transferred to a scoring profile. The profile groups related sensorimotor components to a performance component.	Normative sample: Not available. Reliability: IR ranged from 0.5–0.91; TR ranged from 0.89–0.97. Concurrent validity was unable to be determined; construct validity established through theoretical basis for test; SPA could differentiate children with mental retardation	Richter & Montgomery, 1989
Toddler and Infant Motor Evaluation (TIME)	4 mo–3.5 y	Comprehensive, diagnostic assessment for children with suspected motor delays that assists with appropriate program planning	45–60 min	Individually administered, standardized test. Administration is in partnership with parents. Eight subtests: five are primary subtests (mandatory): mobility, stability, motor organization (child is evaluated in only one of four levels), functional performance, social/emotional abilities. Three are clinical subtests (optional): component analysis, quality rating, and atypical positions. Examiners must be familiar with motor development; some training in neuro-developmental treatment will help. Clinical subtests require advanced training. Can complete subtests over several sessions. Raw scores from each subtests form the total score. Raw scores are converted to standard scaled scores and percentiles.	Normative sample: 75 trained testers participated; tester's sample was selected randomly, stratified by race or ethnicity, gender; socioeconomic status, and age; 875 children participated. Reliability—All coefficients are by subtest; IC coefficients ranged from 0.72–0.97; TR = 0.96 and up; IR = 0.89 and up; SEM = 0.52–1.59. Validity: Content—expert review; construct validity—theoretical constructs underlying test given; there is age differentiation; factor analysis completed; criterion-related—discriminates between normal children and children with delays; classification analysis shows low false negative (less than 3.2%) and low false positive (less than 11.8%)	Miller & Roid, 1994

BSID = Bayley Scales of Infant Development; IR = interrater reliability; SEM = standard error of the mean; TR = test-retest reliability.

those of other motor development tests (Bayley Scales of Infant Development [BSID] and the West Haverstraw). The correlation coefficient for the BSID Mental Scale with the PDMS total Fine Motor Scale was 0.78, with skill categories ranging from 0.26 to 0.80. The coefficient for the BSID Motor Scale with the PDMS total Gross Motor Scale was 0.37, with skill categories ranging from 0.05 to 0.64. Correlation to the West Haverstraw was similar. This range of coefficients was what the authors expected.

The Erhardt Developmental Prehension Assessment

The Erhardt Developmental Prehension Assessment (EDPA) (Erhardt, 1982) is designed to assess the development of hand function in children. This test measures qualitative change in hand function and was designed to aid in the treatment planning process. The EDPA is widely used by pediatric therapists (Henderson, 1991). This criterion-referenced test assesses the development of prehension patterns from gross upper extremity movements to fine fingertip prehension. Based on the sequential progressions and age levels of the development of prehension from the work of Gesell and Halverson, the test is designed to be used with children who have developmental delays by comparing performance with the normal developmental progression of hand function.

The instrument is divided into three sections. The first two sections evaluate involuntary positional and reflexive patterns and voluntary cognitively directed patterns from birth to 15 months of age. The third section addresses pencil grasp and prewriting skills from 1 to 6 years of age. The first two sections of the test are useful for evaluating the postural prerequisites of prehension for children who have not yet developed independent hand function. Erhardt (1982) states that the 15-month-old skills as described in this scale represent mature prehension and present an approximate norm for assessing the prehension skills of older children.

Each developmental pattern is depicted in a drawing, and the child is scored on the age-appropriate skill, as well as on the sequential prerequisite components needed for each pattern. The assessment is scored using a four-level hierarchic rating of a plus (+) or minus (–) scale. From highest to lowest, each pattern is scored as well integrated and normal (+), not present (–), emerging or not well integrated (±), or transitional (++).

The EDPA, originally published and distributed nationally in 1979, has undergone two revisions by Erhardt. The current version now in use was revised in 1982. In its current form, this instrument continues to lack the psychometric requirements necessary as a standardized, objective measure. The administrative and scoring instructions are not clearly presented, and the testing environment is not specified (Pollock et al., 1991). In a critique of this test, Dunn (1983) has stated that research studies are needed to

study its reliability and validity. Although some studies have been conducted, many questions remain concerning the test-retest reliability, internal consistency, and validity of this test. An interrater reliability study was conducted using an earlier version, but is not reflective of the current EDPA (Erhardt, Beatty, & Hertsgaard, 1981). In a study of intrarater and interrater objective reliability in trained and untrained examiners, examiners rated children's performance by use of videotape (Scheer et al., 1994). The study demonstrated high levels of intrarater objectivity among trained examiners (with median correlation coefficients of 0.91 and 0.88) and interrater reliability in the moderate to high range (with a median correlation of 0.77). In their analysis, the authors showed that the interrater reliability was improved by training. In two recent studies of interrater reliability, altered versions of the test have been used (Pollock et al., 1991; Tomacelli & Palisano, 1990). Both of these studies have shown promising results, but the alterations of the items and the scoring procedures make it difficult to apply the results to the assessment available and to clinical use.

The Bruininks-Oseretsky Motor Development Scale

The Bruininks-Oseretsky Motor Development Scale (BOTMP) (Bruininks, 1978) is a standardized test of developmental gross and fine motor skills. It is administered to individual children from 4.5 to 14.5 years old who appear to have motor problems not related to obvious neurologic dysfunction. Forty-six test items are divided into eight subtests. The fine motor subtests are upper limb coordination, speed and dexterity, response speed, and visual-motor control. The gross motor subtests are: running speed and agility, balance, bilateral coordination, and strength. The test takes approximately 45 minutes to administer and requires a large room to accommodate the balance beam, running, and other gross motor items. This standardized assessment appears to be widely used by pediatric therapists. The BOTMP is easy to learn to use and has a clearly detailed manual with administration and scoring instructions.

On each item the child is scored on how long it takes to complete the task, the number of repetitions performed, the number of errors made, or by passing or failing according to set criteria. The child's raw score on each item is converted to a point score, the point scores are totaled, and each subtest is computed to a gross motor, fine motor, and total battery composite score. Subtest scores can be converted to standard scores, percentile ranks, or age-equivalent scores. Separate norms for boys and girls are provide for the total battery score. Directions and scoring instructions are included for a short screening form of the battery, which takes approximately 15 to 20 minutes to administer and score.

Reviews of the psychometric properties of this testing

instrument are mixed, and although it is recommended as a good evaluative tool, the therapist needs to be aware of its limitations. A test-retest study on nondisabled children found fair to good test-retest reliability for second and sixth grade nondisabled children (DeGangi, 1987). The reliability coefficients for the total battery and for the short form version of the test were above 0.80 for both grades. The coefficients for grade two were 0.77 for the gross motor composite, 0.88 for the fine motor composite, and 0.85 and 0.68, respectively, for the sixth grade children. Coefficients for individual subtests ranged from 0.58 to 0.89 for second grade and from 0.29 to 0.89 for sixth grade. They were above 0.80 for all subtests except for Balance and Response Speed. Interrater reliabilty has only been evaluated for one of the eight subtests. The interrater reliability was determined for the Visual-Motor subtest only and was reported by Bruininks (1978) to be 0.77 to 0.97 on individual test items in the subtest.

To measure construct validity, Bruininks (1978) cited three studies in the manual contrasting the performance of children with and without mental and learning disabilities; only the Response Speed subtest did not discriminate among the groups of children. In studying the relationship of subtest scores to chronologic age, correlations ranged from 0.57 to 0.86, indicating a strong relationship. In measuring internal consistency, correlating individual test items with subtest scores and the total test scores, Bruininks (1978) reported moderate to high correlations, indicating that the functions in each subtest were related and that the subtests are measuring overall fine and gross motor development.

The standard error of measurement (SEM) for this instrument is rather large, complicating the scoring process for examiners. As reported by Bruininks in the test manual (1978), the SEM for subtests, which have a mean of 15 and a standard deviation of 2, is 2 or 3 standard score points. For the composite scores, which have a mean of 50 and a standard deviation of 10, an SEM of 4 or 5 standard points is applied.

Wilson and colleagues (1995) make several suggestions in light of their analysis of the BOTMP. Because of the lack of interrater reliability studies, they caution that the test, when used to show improvement, should be administered by the same examiner. They also make other suggestions as a result of their examination of the use of the BOTMP in reevaluation and as documentation of the efficacy of treatment. The authors note that the normative standard and composite scores that were based on a population of nondisabled children may not show change if the progress is slower than normal developmental maturation. As a result, they suggest that therapists use the subtest point scores rather than the composite and standard scores for comparison. From their analysis, they also report that the subtests Running Speed and Agility, Balance, Visual Motor Control, Upper Limb Speed and Dexterity appear to provide the greatest degree of discrimination between children with and without motor problems. Therefore, the

point scores on these subtests will be the best indicators of the child's strengths and deficits in motor function. The low test-retest reliability on the Response Speed and Balance subtests is problematic as well, with the Response Speed subtest having the least value (see Table 14–1).

SENSORY INTEGRATION

Sensory integration addresses the integration and organization of the information from the different sensory modalities. This input is received from the environment and from ones's body and is used in dealing effectively with the environment (Ayres, 1991). Sensory integrative theory and practice is based on the work of A. Jean Ayres. The theory of sensory integration continues to be modified and revised through the research that continues in neurobiologic processing and treatment efficacy studies being conducted by therapists. The goal of Ayres' research was to describe the relationships between behaviors, such as sensorimotor and academic learning, and neural functioning. Ayres felt that in studying these relationships, it was important to look not only at the visual system but also at the vestibular, proprioceptive, and tactile systems (Walker, 1993).

Children with sensory integrative problems exhibit problems integrating and processing sensory and motor behavior. They display deficits in cognition, language, perception, and motor skills, and they often have difficulties with emotional stability (Ayres, 1972; DeGangi et al., 1993). Often, the problems of children with these difficulties go unrecognized until they enter school and begin the process of learning reading, writing, and mathematics. Most often these children are identified as being learning disabled; however, it has become increasingly recognized that similar problems are apparent in children with developmental delays.

Several instruments measuring sensory integrative functioning are presented here and in Table 14–2. The tools were selected as a representative sample of those available to test areas of sensory processing and function.

The DeGangi-Berk Test of Sensory Integration

The DeGangi-Berk Test of Sensory Integration (TSI) (Berk & DeGangi, 1987) is a standardized, criterion-referenced assessment that measures sensory integrative abilities. The purpose of the test is to detect sensory integrative dysfunction in the early years. The test results can be used for screening or diagnosis, depending on the needs of the child. The TSI is intended for children from ages 3 to 5 with suspected sensory integration problems and should not be used alone to determine the diagnosis. The TSI includes 36 items that are divided into three

TABLE 14-2

PEDIATRIC ASSESSMENTS

Sensory Integration	Target Population	Purpose	Time	Comments	Psychometric Properties	Reference
A Guide to Testing Clinical Observations in Kindergarten	5–6 y	Clinical observation of children's performance on variety of tasks; provides a foundation for further study	30–45 min	Nineteen subtests, with focus on postural mechanisms and reflex integration, including eye dominance and eye movements. Administration and scoring described in manual. No overall interpretation. Evaluators should be familiar with sensory integration theory.	No psychometric information; does provide standard z scores for some items	Dunn, 1981
DeGangi-Berk Test of Sensory Integration (TSI)	3–5 y	Detects sensory integrative dysfunction	30 min	Thirty-six items on three subtests: postural control, bilateral motor integration, and reflex integration. Scores are interpreted as normal, at-risk, or deficient. Some equipment comes in the kit. Evaluators should be familiar with sensory integration theory.	Normative sample: 101 normal children and 30 delayed children in the Washington DC area and 8 delayed children in Indiana. Reliability: IR = 0.67–0.79 for postural control; 0.74–0.76 for bilateral motor integration; 0.14–0.49 for reflex integration, and 0.73–0.79 for the total test. Decision reliability = 0.79–0.93; TR = 0.85–0.96. Validity: Content—panel of experts reviewed; construct—items demonstrated a significant discrimination index; classification accuracy for test = 81%; least effective subtest was reflex integration; intercorrelation matrix showed moderately low subtest coefficients (0.39–0.65)	Berk & DeGangi, 1983, 1987

Table continued on following page

TABLE 14–2

PEDIATRIC ASSESSMENTS *Continued*

Sensory Integration	Target Population	Purpose	Time	Comments	Psychometric Properties	Reference
Pediatric Clinical Test of Sensory Integration for Balance (P-CTSIB)	4–9 y	Assessment of a child's ability to use sensory cues to adapt motor response for the maintenance of balance	30 min	Child is tested in two standing positions (heels together and heel to toe) under six sensory conditions. Three (eyes open, eyes closed, and visual sway) on normal surface and the same on a foam surface. Administration outlined in article. Requires two therapists to administer—one to record data and to measure sway, the other to give directions, position child, and time durations. No overall interpretation available.	Normative data collected in two studies (Dietz et al., 1991; Richardson et al., 1992); no established norms. Reliability: IR (Spearman's rank order correlation coefficient) = 0.69 (feet together, visual sway) and 0.92 (heel-toe eyes open); TR (Spearman's rank order correlation coefficient) for duration = 0.29 (heel-toe, eyes closed, normal surface) to 0.83 (heel-toe, eyes closed, normal surface); for sway = 0.05 (heel-toe, visual sway, foam surface) to 0.75 (heel-toe, visual sway, normal surface); for combined sensory conditions = 0.44 (heel-toe, vision absent) to 0.83 (heel-toe, somatosensory inaccurate). Validity: Content—established through review of the literature	Dietz et al., 1991
Sensory Assessment	5–18 y	Standardized sensory assessment	20 min	Five sensory modalities: pressure sensitivity, moving two-point discrimination, stereognosis, proprioception, and directionality	Normative sample: 41 children. Reliability: All were reported in percentage of agreement; IR (nondominant hand) = 87.5%–100%; (dominant) = 81.25%–100%; TR (nondominant) = 94%–100% (dominant) = 88%–100%. Validity: Content presents a review of the literature	Cooper et al., 1993
Sensory Integration and Praxis Tests (SIPT)	4 y–8 y, 11 mo	Clinical assessment of several practice abilities, the status of sensory processing, and the behavioral manifestations of deficits in sensory integration	1.5–2 h	Domains of sensory integration and praxis: tactile and vestibular processing, form and space perception and visuomotor coordination, praxis, and bilateral integration and sequencing. Standardization, administration, and scoring procedures complex. Certification in SI theory and test administration required through Sensory Integration International.	Standardization sample: 2000 normal children nationwide. See manual and attend coursework for comprehensive coverage of current reliability and validity information	Ayres, 1991

Sensory Profile	3–10 y	Profile reveals a child's typical and atypical sensory responses, as reported by the parent	20 min	Parent checklist of 99 statements, divided into auditory, visual, taste/smell, movement, body position, and touch/sensory categories, and emotional/social and activity level behavioral categories. Items scored on Likert scale. No overall interpretation. Assists in program planning.	Normative sample: Convenience sample of 64 children. Reliability: Not available. Validity: Content—items selected based on a review of the literature	Dunn, 1994
Sensory Rating Scale	0–3 y	Identifies and quantifies sensory responses	20 min	Domains divided into six sections: touch; movement and gravity; hearing; vision; taste and smell; temperament; and general sensitivity. Two forms: 0–8 mo and 9 mo–3 y. Items are scored on a Likert scale. No overall interpretation. Assists in program planning.	Normative sample: Parents of 120 normal children. Reliability: Internal consistency (total score) = 0.83 for 0–8 mo (range 0.46–0.81) and 0.90 for 9 mo–3 y (range 0.52–0.82); TR (interrater) $r = 0.889$ for mothers and $r = 0.95$ for fathers (Pearson product-moment correlation); IR $r = 0.43$. Validity: Content by review of literature	Provost & Oetter, 1993
Knickerbocker Sensorimotor History Questionnaire (KSHQ)	Parents of children	Can focus attention on problem behaviors during assessment and treatment; evaluators should be familiar with sensory integration theory	30 min	Seven subscales: gross motor organization, olfactory system, tactile system, auditory system, visual system, academically related questions, and social adjustments. Key organizes concerns into groupings.	Normative data: Not available. Reliability: IC = 0.59 (Social Adjustment) to 0.77 (Tactile System) (Carrasco, 1990). Validity: Not available	Knickerbocker, 1983
Teacher Questionnaire on Sensorimotor Behavior (TQSB)	Teachers of children in preschool and school	Gives teachers a basis for referral of atypical children: children with learning or emotional problems or minimal dysfunction; evaluators should be familiar with sensory integration theory	30 min	Adapted from KSHQ. Six subscales: motor organization, somatosensory system, visual system, auditory system, olfactory system, and social adjustment. "Yes" answers are totaled and converted to high, suspect, or no risk scores. Contact first author for more information.	Normative data: Not available. Reliability: IC = 0.64–0.89, or 0.76–0.90 if items with low or negative alpha reliability were deleted; supports homogeneity. Validity: Not available	Carrasco & Lee, 1993

Table continued on following page

TABLE 14–2

PEDIATRIC ASSESSMENTS Continued

Sensory Integration	Target Population	Purpose	Time	Comments	Psychometric Properties	Reference
Touch Inventory for Elementary-School-Aged Children (TIE)	6–12 y	Screening test for tactile defensiveness	10 min	Language competency of 6 years old; IQ of 80; no physical disabilities. Items can be repeated until the child understands. Equipment easy to make. Some training required. TIE included in appendix.	Normative data: 415 children included. Reliability: IC = 0.79 (Royeen, 1986); TR = 0.59 (Royeen, 1987a); IR = 1.00. Validity: Content through panel of experts (Royeen, 1985); discriminates between normal and children with tactile defensiveness (85% accuracy) (Royeen, 1986)	Royeen, 1985, 1990
Touch Inventory for Preschoolers (TIP)	Teachers of children 2.5–4.5 y	Screening test for tactile defensiveness	60 min	Teachers of the children were interviewed about a child's behaviors	Normative data: Not available—patterns of scores presented. Reliability: IC = 0.90. Validity: Content through review by experts	Royeen, 1987b

IC = Internal consistency; IR = interrater reliability; TR = test-retest reliability.

subtests. These subtests represent three subdomains of sensory integration. The subtests are (a) postural control, which includes antigravity postures and muscle cocontraction; (b) bilateral motor integration, which includes bilateral motor coordination, trunk rotation, crossing the midline, rapid unilateral and bilateral hand movements, stability of the upper and lower extremities in bilateral symmetrical postures, and dissociation of the head and trunk; and (c) reflex integration, which includes the asymmetric and symmetric tonic neck reflexes. Specific training is not required to use this test, but examiners should be familiar with sensory integration principles.

The test is individually administered in about 30 minutes. Some test items are included in the test kit. A protocol booklet includes criteria for all scores. The scores are arranged in columns that correspond to the three subtests. A score is obtained for each subtest. The three are added together to arrive at the total test score. In addition, a profile score is obtained for the postural control and bilateral motor integration subtests. Scores from each of the three sections are totaled, then are added together to get the total test score. The reflex integration score is not looked at individually, but it does contribute to the total score. Scores are interpreted as normal, at-risk, or deficient.

Normative data were collected on 101 normal children and 30 delayed children from the Washington DC area and 8 delayed children from Indiana. Interrater reliability ranged from 0.67 to 0.79 for postural control, 0.74 to 0.76 for bilateral motor integration, 0.14 to 0.49 for reflex integration, and 0.73 to 0.79 for the total test. Decision reliability (placing the student in the correct functioning level) was 0.79 to 0.93. Test-retest reliability was 0.85 to 0.96 (DeGangi & Berk, 1983).

Content validity was established by a panel of experts. Construct validity was established at three levels of performance: item, subtest, and total test. The test items demonstrated a significant discrimination index. Classification accuracy for the total test was 81%. Overall, the least effective subtest was reflex integration. These scores are included in the total test score. An intercorrelation matrix showed moderately low subtest coefficients (0.39–0.65) (DeGangi & Berk, 1983).

The authors of the TSI state in the theoretic background that the test is based on "vestibular based functions" because it is the easiest feature of sensory integration to measure. These functions form the basis for the three subtests. Royeen (1988) expressed concern that calling these functions vestibular based may not be entirely accurate. She believed that a more accurate description of the subtests was "a test of three areas of brain stem and spinal cord level motor functions which are related to sensory processing generally, and vestibular system processing specifically" (p. 74). In addition, Royeen stated that the test is probably more valid for 3- and 4-year-old children because of the number of children in the normative sample from that age range.

The Sensory Integration and Praxis Tests

The Sensory Integration and Praxis Tests (SIPT) (Ayres, 1991) assist in the clinical assessment of the ability of the child to process sensory input from the body and the environment and the organization of that input into behaviors. The SIPT is designed to clinically evaluate children 4 through 8 years old who exhibit mild to moderate learning, behavioral, or developmental difficulties (Ayres & Marr, 1991). The 17 subtests of the SIPT are individually administered. The subtests are arranged into four groups: 1) tactile and vestibular sensory processing, 2) form and space perception and visuomotor coordination, 3) praxis, and 4) bilateral integration and sequencing. This well-standardized instrument takes the experienced examiner approximately 1.5 hours to administer.

The tests of sensory integration (SI) have been revised several times and evolved through the work of Ayres. Several individual tests were initially published and then combined to form the Southern California Sensory Integration Tests (SCIPT) and the Southern California Postrotary Nystagmus Test; the current version, the SIPT, was published in 1989. This version includes the Postrotary Nystagmus Test, and 12 of the original subtests of the SCIPT were revised and also included. Four new tests of praxis were added to the SIPT. The publisher of the test, Western Psychological Services (WPS), computer scores the revised scoring system to aid in more precise and complex statistical comparisons. This WPS report includes descriptive information about the child's performance on each subtest and a graph comparing the child's scoring patterns to six diagnostic clusters. Factor and cluster analysis has resulted in the identification of groups of children who score in a similar pattern on the SIPT; these clusters identify children that have bilateral integration and sequencing deficits, visuo- or somatodyspraxia, verbal dyspraxia, or normal function.

Therapists who would like to administer the SIPT need to be specially trained, have substantial pediatric experience, and have knowledge of statistics and measurement. The three courses required in SI theory and the SIPT Competency Examination required for SI certification are offered by Sensory Integration International.

The SIPT (Ayres, 1991) was standardized on a nationwide sample of about 2000 children, and the normative sample was taken from children 4 years to 8 years, 11 months. This analysis determined sex and age differences for subtests of the SIPT; therefore separate norms have been developed for boys and girls in 12 age groups.

Extensive reliability and validity information has been published in the literature, and it continues to be added to as a result of the accumulation of current studies concerning sensory integration evaluation and treatment efficacy. The therapist is referred to the coursework and literature by WPS, Sensory Integration International, and others for the more extensive information needed to use this test battery in the clinic competently.

PSYCHOSOCIAL ASSESSMENT

Psychosocial assessment in pediatrics addresses a variety of behaviors, ranging from the normal stresses and transitions of childhood to the persistent maladaptive problems that result in a label of psychopathology. Most children being treated by therapists are at risk for difficulties in psychosocial and emotional development no matter what their primary diagnosis. Often in looking for the sensorimotor deficits underlying behaviors, therapists often overlook these domains and their effect on self-care, play, communication, and school performance (Cronin, 1996).

In choosing an appropriate evaluation tool, it is important to remember that a child's performance on assessments of psychosocial functions can be influenced by the stimulation level of the test environment and the effects of the medications often prescribed to influence behavior. Therefore, information and data collected should be confirmed through skilled observations of the child in the natural settings and environments in which the child is expected to perform, such as the classroom, community, and home. It is also valuable to obtain information through direct interviews with the child, teachers, and caregivers.

Several of the instruments available for the assessment of pediatric psychosocial function and dysfunction are discussed both in the text and in Table 14–3. Tests of cognition and intelligence are not covered here, as the assessment of these domains of psychological functioning are most often conducted by other professionals. The tools selected for discussion here are meant to be a representative sample of the types instruments available to assess the areas of psychosocial performance as both a primary and secondary diagnosis.

The Adolescent Role Assessment

The Adolescent Role Assessment (Black, 1976) is an instrument designed to identify adolescents at risk for making poor occupational choices. Occupational choices are those decisions that culminate in the selection of an occupational role. This assessment is based on the premise that occupational choice is a developmental decision-making process (Ginzberg, 1972). The Adolescent Role Assessment explores the teenager's past and present performance through the use of a semistructured interview. Intervention decisions can then be based on the hypothesis that the skills needed to make occupational choice decisions have not been developed as part of the childhood developmental process (Black, 1982).

Through the use of a guided dialogue, the examiner asks questions related to the adolescent's childhood play experiences and functions within the family, at school, and with peers. The willingness of the teenager to cooperate appears critical to the establishment of a rapport early in the interview process. The interview takes approximately 1 hour. The questions are divided into six sections representing the developmental stages of the occupational choice process. Rating criteria are predetermined for each individual question; as the criteria are based on evidence of normative behaviors rather than on the behavior itself, the author feels subjective value judgments can be eliminated from influencing the scoring of the items. Using a plus and minus system of scoring, the appropriate behaviors (+), marginal or borderline behaviors (0), and inappropriate behaviors (–) are identified.

The content of this assessment was developed by a review of the literature on child and adolescent role behaviors. A test-retest study was conducted on a sample of 12 adolescents diagnosed with psychiatric dysfunctions and 28 normal subjects. The median coefficient was 0.91, indicating high reliablity in this small sample (Black, 1982).

The Preschool Play Scale

The purpose of the Preschool Play Scale (PPS) (Knox, 1974) is to provide a descriptive measure of free play. The PPS is designed to measure play behaviors in children from birth to 6 years of age. Play behaviors are described in yearly increments across four dimensions: space management, material management, imitation, and participation. The dimensions include 16 categories of play behavior. Through observation, the child's level of play is recorded for each dimension. Descriptions of the play behaviors are on the score sheet. The examiner records the presence or absence of each of the 16 behaviors. The examiner then looks at each dimension's behaviors and decides on an age level that most of the descriptors are in. The play age is determined by averaging the dimensional scores. A play quotient can be calculated by dividing the play age by the child's chronologic age and multiplying by 100. The play observer needs a general understanding of the four dimensions of the scale and adequate knowledge of early childhood development. The observation period may last from 15 to 30 minutes. Longer periods may increase reliability (Harrison & Kielhofner, 1986).

Interrater reliability was examined with 90 subjects between the ages of 4 months and 6 years. Correlation coefficients were 0.996 for the overall play age, with ranges of 0.98 to 0.99 for the four dimensions. Test-retest reliability was completed after a 1-week interval, with coefficients of 0.96 for the play age and 0.86 to 0.96 for the four dimensions (Bledsoe & Shepherd, 1982).

Content validity was established because the items were based on play theory literature (Knox, 1974). Concurrent validity was established by comparing play ages with chronologic ages, with a correlation of 0.89 to 0.95 for the four dimensions and 0.96 for the total score. Scores on the

TABLE 14–3

PEDIATRIC ASSESSMENTS

Visual Perception	Target Population	Purpose	Time	Comments	Psychometric Properties	Reference
Developmental Test of Visual Perception II (DTVP-2)	4–10 y	Identifies presence and degree of visual perception deficits to refer those children for services, to evaluate effectiveness of intervention, and to serve as research tool	30–60 min	Eight subtests: Four require eye-hand coordination (eye-hand coordination, copying, spatial relations, visual-motor speed), and four are motor reduced (position in space, figure-ground, visual closure, form constancy). Kit includes all materials	Normative sample: 1972 children in 12 states representing four major U.S. Census districts; sites selected from PRO-ED's customer files; 14 data collectors represented 16 schools and tested all children in the school (demographic information in manual) Reliability: IC = 0.96 for total test, 0.93 or above for subtests; TR = 0.95 for total test, 0.80–0.92 for subtests; IR = 0.98 for total test, 0.87–0.98 for subtests Validity: Content and concurrent established with literature review; construct—age differentiation occurs; intercorrelation coefficients were all significant; factor analysis revealed one factor	Hammill et al., 1993
Motor-Free Visual Perception Test (MVPT)	4–8 y	Provides a quick screening of visual perceptual abilities without requiring the child to have motor skills	10 min	Domains of visual perceptual function: spatial relationships, visual discrimination, figure ground, visual closure, and visual memory. Scores converted to a perceptual age and a perceptual quotient.	Sample: 881 normal children Reliability:TR = 0.81 and inter-item = 0.71–0.82 with total value 0.86 for 4–8 y Validity: Content based on literature review; construct based on comparison with test of visual perception (r = 0.49), intelligence (r = 0.31), and school performance and readiness (r = 0.36)	Hammill et al., 1993
Test of Visual Motor Skills (TVMS)	2–13 y	Measures eye-hand coordination through copying figures	3–6 min	Test may be administered individually or in groups. Child copies 26 shapes on provided booklet. Scoring is completed after the child is done. Raw scores are converted into motor age, standard scores, and percentiles from 1 of 11 age levels.	Normative sample: 1009 children from the San Francisco Bay area participated, with an age range of 2 y, 3 mo–12 y, 11 mo; testing was conducted at 13 schools; item difficulty ranged from 0.37–0.98 Reliability: IC = 0.31–0.90 SEMs ranged from 0.88–2.99 Validity: Content established by experts; item—correlated with another test; no correlations given; criterion-related—established by comparing two tests	Gardner, 1986

Table continued on following page

Perception. The purpose of the DTVP-2 is fourfold: (a) to identify the presence and degree of visual perceptual or visual-motor difficulties in a child, (b) to identify children who should be referred for services, (c) to evaluate the effectiveness of intervention programs, and (d) to function as a research tool. The DTVP-2 is a battery of eight subtests, each measuring a different part of visual perception and visual-motor abilities. All eight subtests are interrelated. Four of the subtests are motor enhanced, meaning that they require eye-hand coordination: (a) eye-hand coordination, (b) copying, (c) spatial relations, and (d) visual-motor speed. The other four subtests are motor reduced, meaning that the child may point to a correct answer: (a) position in space, (b) figure-ground, (c) visual closure, and (d) form constancy.

The DTVP-2 is appropriate for children between 4 and 10 years of age. The directions can be adapted for children who are non–English speaking or hearing impaired. The test can also be used for children with motor impairments. In these instances, the examiner should determine the appropriateness of administering the motor-enhanced subtests.

The equipment includes the examiner's manual, a picture book, a response booklet, and a profile/examiner form. Standardized instructions and scoring criteria are included in the manual. Some subtests have ceilings; others do not. Raw scores are obtained for each subtest. These are converted to age equivalencies, percentile rankings, and standard scores according to the child's chronologic age. Composite quotients, percentiles, and age equivalencies are also obtained for the overall test, the motor-reduced subtests, and the motor-enhanced subtests. Standard scores can be placed on a graph. Space is also available to record administration conditions.

The battery can be administered by anyone interested in looking at visual perceptual skills in children. The authors recommend that examiners receive formal training in assessment. The test takes approximately 30 to 60 minutes to administer. It can be administered in as many sessions as needed.

Normative information was collected on 1972 children. Data collection sites were selected from PRO-ED's (Austin, TX) customer files. Fourteen data collectors representing 16 schools participated. The data collectors represented the four major U.S. census districts. All collectors tested all appropriate children in the school (unless the parent had not given permission). Complete demographic information on the children is in the manual.

Internal consistency reliability coefficients for the DTVP-2 were 0.96 or above for the total test and 0.93 or above in the motor-enhanced and motor-reduced subtests. Individual subtests are 0.80 or higher. The average SEM values for each subtest were 1, 2 for the motor-reduced subtests, 2.5 for the motor-enhanced subtests, and 2 for the total test. Test-retest reliability, with a 2-week interval between tests, ranged from 0.80 to 0.92 for the subtests

and 0.95 for the total test. Interrater reliability was established by having two people independently score 88 protocols. The coefficients ranged from 0.87 to 0.98 for the subtests and 0.98 for the total test.

Content validity was established through the rationale for the content of the subtests and demonstrated by the results of the item analysis procedures that were used during the test construction. Concurrent validity was established by comparing the DTVP-2 with the MVPT (Colarusso & Hammill, 1972) and the Developmental Test of Visual-Motor Integration (VMI) (Beery, 1989). The coefficients comparing the DTVP-2 with the MVPT range from 0.27 to 0.82 for the subtests and 0.78 for the total test. The coefficients for the DTVP-2 and the VMI range from 0.41 to 0.95 for the subtests and 0.87 for the total test. These indicate that the DTVP-2 has concurrent validity. Construct validity was supported through age differentiation because children's performance increases with age. The DTVP-2 scores were intercorrelated. The coefficients were all significant ($P < 0.01$). The median coefficient was 0.36. This indicates that a low degree of relationship exists between the subtests. The DTVP-2 was compared with the National Teacher Assessment and Referral Scales (NTARS) (Hammill & Hresko, 1993). The coefficients indicated that perceptual skills were different from cognitive skills. Factor analytic studies of the DTVP-2 yielded one factor. This supported its validity as an assessment of visual perception.

Because this is a new test no other research studies are available.

FUNCTIONAL ASSESSMENTS

Comprehensive pediatric assessment should always include the evaluation of age-appropriate functional abilities. Developing independence in the daily functional skills of self-care and environmental competence, such as feeding, mobility, dressing, and grooming, are critical components of the developmental processes. Assessment of the child's performance in these areas provides information concerning the child's ability to apply the discrete developmental milestones to mastery and independence in his or her environment. Treatment goals in pediatric intervention include enhancing the quality of life of children with disabilities by aiding in the inclusion of such children in the home, school, and community at large; to do so means that therapists and caregivers must include daily functional skills in treatment and assessment activities. This section of the chapter and Table 14–5 provide an overview of a sample of the assessment tools available for the evaluation of functional skills and abilities in children. The value of including the assessment of functional skills is that it provides valuable information concerning the application of discrete developmental milestones to the child's home, community, and educational intervention goals.

TABLE 14-5

PEDIATRIC ASSESSMENTS

Functional Assessments	Target Population	Purpose	Time	Comments	Psychometric Properties	Reference
Behavioral Assessment Scale of Oral Functions in Feeding	Children with feeding problems	Provides an objective and graded method of documenting the major aspects of oral function in relation to feeding difficulties	15–30 min	Assesses feeding functions: jaw closure, lip closure, tongue control, swallowing, chewing, and drinking. Criterion-based scoring; descriptions of scoring are on the test form. Scores range from 0 (nonfunctional) to 5 (normal). Results are documented as percentage of occurrence of scores.	Reliability: Internal consistency of the scale ranged from 0.67–0.78; IR was computed using intraclass correlation coefficients of agreement ranged from 0.72–0.84; TR intraclass correlation coefficients was 0.67–0.79; both IR and TR are marginally acceptable (Ottenbacher et al., 1985)	Stratton, 1981
Evaluation of Oral Structures	Neonates	Provides a description of oral-motor behaviors that are based on understanding the infant's medical problems and maturity level	10–15 min	Descriptive information about tongue, jaw, lips, checks, and palate function during feeding, with emphasis on the infant's resting position and components of movement needed for feeding. Includes multisensory observation prior to and during feeding. Information presented is specific to the neonate.	No psychometric information available	Glass & Wolf, 1994
Pediatric Evaluation of Disability Inventory (PEDI)	6 mo–7.5 y	Measures the child's daily functional capabilities and skills performance; identifies skills child performs independently and with assistance	Varies	Assesses self-care mobility, and social functioning through three scales; Functional Skills, Caregiver Assistance, and Modification Scales. Data collected through observation or interview.	Normative sample: 412 children Reliability: Internal consistency—ICC = 0.95–0.99, IR was ICC = 0.96–0.99 on Assistance Scale and .91 and 1.00 on Modification Scale (social function = 0.79) Validity: Construct—score changes in normative sample consistent with progression of normal developmental change concurrent; PEI and BDIST were 0.73 and 0.71	Haley et al., 1992
Pre-Feeding Scale	Children with feeding problems	Provides an objective assessment of oral motor abilities and other issues related to feeding	30–60 min	Descriptive information only—readers referred to text chapter on normal acquisition of feeding skills. Includes parent questionnaire to obtain feeding history. Information includes family issues and concerns; the learning, communicative, physical, and sensory environment; normal oral-motor skills; limiting oral motor skills; treatment explorations; and a feeding plan.	No psychometric information available	Morris & Klein, 1987

Table continued on following page

TABLE 14-5

PEDIATRIC ASSESSMENTS *Continued*

Functional Assessments	Target Population	Purpose	Time	Comments	Psychometric Properties	Reference
Neonatal Oral-Motor Assessment Scale (NOMAS)	34 w gestational age and up	"Differentiate tongue and jaw movements during both nonnutritive and nutritive sucking; identify normal and deviant oral-motor patterns; and quantify oral-motor skills" (p. 14)	10–15 min	Evaluates components of rate; rhythmicity; consistency of degree of jaw excursion; and direction, range, and timing of tongue movement during nutritive and nonnutritive sucking. Scores are criterion referenced and descriptions are on the score sheet. All scores are totaled. Scores are classified as normal, disorganized, or dysfunctional.	No psychometric information available	Braun & Palmer, 1985
Vineland Adaptive Behavior Scales	Birth–18 y, 11 mo	Evaluates daily living scales necessary to independently perform personally and socially	Varies	Measures four domains: communication, daily living skills, socialization, and motor skills. Three scales: interview survey, comprehensive interview, and classroom edition. Test manuals are clear, but scoring and administration are quite complex, requiring familiarity.	Reliability and validity conducted on each individual scale Information available in the manual of each version of the Scales	Sparrow et al., 1984

IC = Internal consistency; IR = interrater reliability; TR = test-retest reliability.

The Vineland Adaptive Behavior Scales

The Vineland Adaptive Behavior Scales (Sparrow et al., 1984) use a semistructured interview or a questionnaire format for the evaluation of the daily living skills that are necessary to independently perform personally and socially. The instrument measures behavior in four domains: communication, daily living skills, socialization, and motor skills. The original testing instrument, the Vineland Social Maturity Scale (Doll, 1936), has been revised several times, and this work has resulted in three versions of the scales. The interview survey form edition requires approximately 20 to 40 minutes to complete, while the more comprehensive interview edition requires 60 to 90 minutes. This expanded edition was developed to provide more specific information for use in treatment planning. These scales are scored according to the answers of a parent or caregiver. The third version, the classroom edition, is a questionnaire that is completed by the classroom teacher in approximately 20 minutes. Scores for each domain are calculated, along with an adaptive behavior composite score, age-equivalent score, and national percentile rank.

The survey and expanded interview forms of the test scales were developed and normed with a large national sample of individuals from birth to 18 years, 11 months old and a supplementary sample of children with disabilities. The classroom version was developed and standardized for children between the ages of 3 years and 12 years, 11 months. Supplementary data for all three scales were collected with a sample of individuals with various cognitive and sensory disabilities.

Administration and scoring of the scales is complex, requiring the examiner to be very familiar with the format, scoring, and procedures. The test manuals are clear and comprehensive, making standardization procedures easy to adhere to with practice. As the test items are not administered directly to the subject, it is important that the person being interviewed correctly understands what is being asked. The examiner is able to ask additional "probes" for clarification or for additional information. Also, because the examiner does not directly observe the performance of the subject, it is possible that the information gathered by this instrument might be biased by the parent's, caretaker's, or teacher's perception of the child's performance.

Information on reliability has been conducted on individual scales and summarized in the respective manuals. Construct, content, and criterion validity is summarized in individual version manuals.

The Pediatric Disability Index

The Pediatric Disability Index (PEDI) (Haley et al., 1992) is a judgment-based, standardized instrument that assesses the functional capabilities and performance of children. A software program is available that enables the examiner to enter performance data, calculate scores, and develop a profile of the child, based on the normative sample. Normative standard scores are available for 14 age levels between the ages of 6 months and 7 years, 6 months. The three content domains addressed by the PEDI through three measurement scales are self-care, mobility, and social functioning. The hierarchic levels of the items allow for the test to also be used with older children if their functional skill level is lower than that of a nondisabled 7.5-year-old child.

The child's functional capability is measured on a Functional Skills Scale identifying the daily functional skills that the child has mastered and performs without assistance. For this scale of 197 items, the parent indicates the specific tasks the child performs competently and independently. Each functional task is criterion referenced, and the format is arranged along the normal developmental continuum. The level of assistance that the child needs to perform these activities is recorded by use of a Caregiver Assistance Scale. The amount of the assistance is measured on a five-point scale ranked "total assistance" to "independence." Added to the information provided by these two skills is a third scale, the Modification Scale, that measures the extent of the environmental modifications and the adaptive equipment the child needs to perform key daily functional tasks. This scale does not yield a normative score but provides information concerning the frequency and degree of the adaptations necessary to the child's performance. The PEDI is designed to be administered by occupational or physical therapists, nurses, teachers, or other pediatric health care practitioners. The data can be collected by various methods, such as structured caregiver interview, observations of the child by caregiver or practitioner, or clinical and professional judgment. Experienced examiners can complete this assessment with a child in 20 to 30 minutes, while completion of the PEDI by interview requires approximately 45 to 60 minutes. The authors report that these times may vary with the age and level of disability of the child.

Standardization and the collection of normative data were conducted with a sample of 412 nondisabled children from the New England region of the United States. The reliability of the PEDI was evaluated for the internal consistency of each of the individual scales, the interinterviewer reliability of the Caregivers Scales, and the reliability of two different respondents on the Caregiver Scales. The reliabilities of the scales were calculated, and the intraclass correlation coefficients ranged between 0.95 and 0.99, indicating excellent internal consistency within the scales. The interinterviewer reliability on the normative sample with the assistance scales was also quite high (ICC = 0.96 to 0.99), while the scores on the modifications were high (ICC = 0.91 and 1.00), except for the Social Functions component (0.79), which was still acceptable. Reliability with a clinical sample of children with various disabilities was also studied using the assistance scales; the intraclass correlation coefficients ranged from 0.84 to 1.00, indicating a high level of agreement between the two scales. A study of a sample of children with disabilities was conducted to address the question of reliability among respondents on functional status. When comparing the responses of the child's parents and the child's rehabilitation team members, almost all scales had a high level of reliability. However, the Social Function component of the Modifications Scale proved to be problematic again (ICC = 0.30), leading to some changes in the methods for scoring these items. The authors indicate in the manual that studies are being conducted into the interrater reliability and test-retest reliability among rehabilitation team members.

Validity studies of the PEDI have studied construct, concurrent, discriminative, and evaluative validity. The authors (Haley et al., 1992) studied construct validity by comparing the scores of children in the normative sample at three different age levels (infant, preschool, and school age). The curves or changes in scores among the age levels were consistent with the authors' expectations of the changes during the normal developmental process. Feldman and associates (1990) further addressed construct and discriminative validity when comparing the scores of children with and without disabilities on the PEDI and the Battelle Developmental Inventory Screening Test (BDIST). In this study, the disabled sample scored significantly lower on the PEDI than did the nondisabled sample. The Modifications and the Functional Skill Scales of the PEDI were found to be the best discriminators between groups, correctly identifying over 70% of the children.

The PEDI manual cites the previously mentioned study and others addressing concurrent validity. Scores on the PEDI Functional Skills and Caregiver Assistance Scales summary scores have been compared with scores on the BDIST and the children's version of the Functional Independence Measure (Wee-FIN). Correlations between the scores on the BDIST and PEDI for the total sample of disabled and nondisabled children were moderately high (r = 0.73 and 0.71). The Social Function Scales again proved problematic; however, this study was conducted with the developmental version of the test before the scoring procedures for this scale were changed. The concurrent validity studies with the Wee-FIN also provided high correlations (r = 0.80–0.97).

Another area of validity would be the ability of this instrument to identify change in functional status over time or evaluative validity. Two clinical studies were conducted with children with minor to moderate injuries and with severe disabilities. According to the authors, the results of these studies indicate that the PEDI is responsive selectively to specific clinical populations (Haley et al., 1992). Further research is currently being conducted to assess the responsiveness of the instrument to changes in child's functional performance (Haley & Coster, 1993). Also currently under development is a classroom functional assessment instrument for use with children 5 through 12 years of age.

In their critique of the PEDI, Reid and colleagues (1993) state that the PEDI provides promise as a comprehensive and unique instrument for the evaluation of a wide range of clinically significant functional behaviors and also as a research tool. However, they continue with criticisms of some of the scoring and administration procedures. They also address the issue of how to reflect the quality of the child's performance. Other issues that Reid and coworkers discuss include the lack of information from this tool to address cognitive function, and those behaviors that can influence performance, such as attention and motivation.

CONCLUSIONS

This chapter has focused on a sampling of the assessment instruments available to evaluate specific areas of function and dysfunction in the pediatric population. When assessing a child, it is often necessary to evaluate discrete skills and areas of performance. These specific areas might include prerequisite capacities such as visual-perceptual, sensorimotor, sensory integrative, psychosocial, and functional performance.

Assessing specific areas of function often helps the therapist to understand the effects these specific components have on the child's overall functioning. Assessment of more specific areas of performance can be accomplished through the use of standardized instruments, as well as through activity analysis and clinical observation. It is important for the assessment process, however, that the therapist maintain an overview of the child's total functioning within his or her environment and not reduce the child's difficulties to these areas of discrete function.

GLOSSARY

Adaptive behaviors—The ability to alter behavioral responses to changes in input from the environment.

Caregiver(s)—The person or people who provide various types of care needed by the child.

Integration—The organization of information from several sources into a unifying whole.

Occupational choice—The developmental decision process by which adult independence of occupation is achieved; recognition of personal strengths and liabilities.

Praxis—The ability to plan and execute a coordinated movement.

Visual-motor skills—Abilities related to the coordination of visual sensory information with motor responses.

REFERENCES

Ayres, A. J. (1972). Improving academic scores through sensory integration. *Journal of Learning Disabilities, 5*, 338–343.

Ayres, A. J. (1991). *Sensory Integration and Praxis Test*. Los Angeles: Western Psychological Services.

Ayres, A. J., & Marr, D. B. (1991). Sensory integration & praxis tests. In A. G. Fisher, E. A. Murray, & A. C. Bundy (Eds.), *Sensory integration and practice*. Philadelphia: F. A. Davis Company.

Beery, K. (1989). *Developmental Test of Visual-Motor Integration*. Los Angeles: Western Psychological Services.

Behnke, C. J., & Fetkovich, M. M. (1984). Examing the reliability and validity of the play history. *The American Journal of Occupational Therapy, 38*, 94–100.

Berk, R. A., & DeGangi, G. (1987). *DeGangi-Berk Test of Sensory Integration*. Los Angeles: Western Psychological Services.

Black, M. M. (1976). Adolescent role assessment. *The American Journal of Occupational Therapy, 30*, 73–79.

Black, M. M. (1982). Adolescent role assessment. In B. Hemphill (Ed.), *The evaluative process in psychiatric occupational therapy*. Thorofare, NJ: Slack, Inc.

Bledsoe, N. P., & Shepherd, J. T. (1982). A study of reliability and validity of a pre-school play scale. *The American Journal of Occupational Therapy, 36*, 783–788.

Braun, M. A., & Palmer, M. M. (1985). A pilot study of oral motor dysfunction in "at-risk" infants. *Physical and Occupational Therapy in Pediatrics, 5*(4), 13–25.

Bruininks, R. H. (1978). *Bruininks-Oseretsky Test of Motor Proficiency: Examiner's manual*. Circle Pines, MN: American Guidance Service.

Carrasco, R. C. (1990). Reliability of the Knickerbocher Sensorimotor History Questionnaire. *Occupational Therapy Journal of Research, 10*(5), 280–282.

Carrasco, R. C., & Lee, C. E. (1993). Development of a teacher questionnaire on sensorimotor behavior. *Sensory Integration Special Interest Section Newsletter, 16*(3), 5, 6.

Case-Smith, J. (1993). Postural and fine motor control in preterm infants in the first six months. *Physical and Occupational Therapy in Pediatrics, 13*(1), 1–17.

Case-Smith, J. (1988). *Posture and Fine Motor Assessment of Infants*. Bethesda, MD: American Occupational Therapy Foundation.

Case-Smith, J. (1989). Reliability and validity of the Posture and Fine Motor Assessment of Infants. *Occupational Therapy Journal of Research 9*(5), 259–272.

Case-Smith, J. (1992). A validity study of the Posture and Fine Motor Assessment in Infants. *The American Journal of Occupational Therapy, 46*, 597–605.

Chandler, L. S., Andrews, M. S., & Swanson, M. W. (1980). *Movement Assessment of Infants: A manual*. Rolling Bay, WA: Movement Assessment of Infants.

Colarusso, R., & Hammill, D. (1972). *Motor-Free Visual Perception Test manual*. Novato, CA: Academic Therapy Publications.

Cooper, J., Majnerner, A., Rosenblatt, B., & Birnbaum, R. (1993). A standardized sensory assessment for children of school-age. *Physical and Occupational Therapy in Pediatrics, 13*(1), 61–80.

Coster, W. J., Haley, S., & Baryza, M. J. (1994). Functional performance of young children after traumatic brain injury: A 6-month follow up study. *The American Journal of Occupational Therapy, 48*(3), 211–218.

Cronin, A. F. (1996). Psychosocial/emotional domains of behavior. In P. N. Pratt & A. S. Allen (Eds.), *Occupational therapy for children* (3rd ed.). St. Louis, MO: C. V. Mosby Company.

Crowe, T. K., Dietz, J. C., Richardson, P. K., & Atwater, S. W. (1990). Interrater reliability of the Pediatric Clinical Test of Sensory Interaction for Balance. *Physical and Occupational Therapy for Pediatrics, 48*(4), 1–27.

DeGangi, G. (1987) Sensorimotor tests. In L. King-Thomas & B.J. Hacker (Eds.), *A therapist's guide to pediatric assessment*. Boston: Little, Brown & Company.

DeGangi, G. A., & Berk, R. A. (1987). *The DeGangi-Berk Test of Sensory Integration (TSI)*. Los Angeles: Western Psychological Services.

DeGangi, G. A., & Berk, R. A. (1983). Psychometric analysis of the Test of Sensory Integration. *Physical and Occupational Therapy in Pediatrics, 3*(2), 43–60.

DeGangi, G. A., Wietlisbach, S., Goodin, M., & Scheiner, N. (1993). A comparison of structured sensorimotor therapy and child-centered activity in the treatment of preschool children with sensorimotor problems. *The American Journal of Occupational Therapy, 47*, 777–786.

DeMatteo, C., Law, M., Russell, D., Pollack, N., Rosenbaum, P., & Walter, S. (1993). The reliability and validity of the Quality of Upper Extremity Skills Test. *Physical and Occupational Therapy in Pediatrics, 13*(2), 1–18.

Dietz, J. C., Richardson, P., Atwater, S. W., Crowe, T. K., & Odiorne, M. (1991). Performance of normal children on the Pediatric Clinical Test of Sensory Interaction for Balance. *Occupational Therapy Journal for Research, 11*(6), 336–356.

Doll, E. (1936). Vineland Social Maturity Scale. Vineland, NJ: The Training School at Vineland, New Jersey.

Dunn, W. (1983). Critique of the Erhardt Developmental Prehension Assessment. *Physical and Occupational Therapy in Pediatrics, 3*(4), 59–68.

Dunn, W. (1981). *A guide to testing clinical observations in kindergarteners*. Bethesda, MD: American Occupational Therapy Association.

Dunn, W. (1994). Performance of typical children on the Sensory Profile: An item analysis. *The American Journal of Occupational Therapy, 48*, 967–974.

Ellison, P. H. (1986). Scoring sheet for the Infant Neurological International Battery (INFANIB). *Physical Therapy, 66*, 548–550.

Ellison, P. H., Horn, J. L., & Browning, C. A. (1985). Construction of an Infant Neurological International Battery (INFANIB) for the assessment of neurological integrity in infancy. *Physical Therapy, 65*, 1326–1331.

Erhardt, R. P. (1982). *Developmental hand dysfunction: Theory, assessment, treatment*. Laurel, MD: Ramsco Publishing Company.

Erhardt, R. P., Betty, P. A., & Hirtsgaard, D. M. (1981). A developmental prehension assessment for handicapped children. *The American Journal of Occupational Therapy, 35*, 287–242.

Feldman, A. B., Haley, S. M., & Coryell, J. (1990) Concurrent and construct validity of the Pediatric Evaluation of Disability Inventory. *Physical Therapy, 70*(10), 602–610.

Folio, M. R., & Fewell, R. R. (1983). *Peabody Developmental Motor Scales and activity card*. Chicago: Riverside.

Frostig, M. (1964). *Frostig Visual Perceptual Program*. Chicago: Follett Publishing Co.

Gardner, M. F. (1986). *TVMS: Test of Visual-Motor Skills*. San Francisco: Health.

Gardner, M. F. (1982). *TVPS: Test of Visual-Perceptual Skills (Non-motor)*. San Francisco: Health.

Ginzberg, E. (1972). Toward a theory of occupational choice: A restatement. *Vocational Guidance, 20*, 169–172.

Glass, R. P., & Wolf, L. S. (1994). A global perspective on feeding assessment in the neonatal intensive care unit. *The American Journal of Occuaptional Therapy, 48*, 514–526.

Haley, S. M., & Coster, W. J. (1993). Response to Reid, D.T. et al.'s critique of the Pediatric Evaluation of Disability Inventory. *Physical and Occupational Therapy in Pediatrics, 13*(4), 89–92.

Haley, S. M., Coster, W. J., Ludlow, L. H., Haltiwanger, J. T., & Andrellos, P. J. (1992). *Pediatric Evaluation of Disability Inventory: Development, standardization, and administration manual*. Version 1.0. Boston: New England Medical Center Hospitals, Inc.

Hammill, D. D., & Hresko, W. (1993). *National Teacher Assessment and Referral Scales*. Austin, TX: PRO-ED.

Hammill, D. D., Pearson, N. A., & Voress, J. K. (1993). *Developmental Test of Visual Perception* (2nd ed.). Austin, TX: PRO-ED.

Harrison, H., & Kielhofner, G. (1986). Examining reliability and validity of the Preschool Play Scale with handicapped children. *The American Journal of Occupational Therapy, 40*, 167–173.

Henderson, A. (1991). Memorandum to all occupational therapist program directors from the chairman of the pediatric core curriculum committee. Rockville, MD: The American Occupational Therapy Association, September 3.

Hinderer, K. A., Richardson, P. K., & Atwater, S. W. (1989). Clinical implications of the Peabody Developmental Motor Scales: A constructive review. *Physical and Occupational Therapy in Pediatrics, 9*(2), 81–105.

King-Thomas L. (1987) Responsibilities of the examiner. In L. King-Thomas & B. J. Hacker (Eds.), *A therapist's guide to pediatric assessment*. Boston: Little, Brown & Company.

Knickerbocker, B. M. (1983). *A holistic approach to the treatment of learning disorders*. Thorofare, NJ: Slack.

Knox, S. H. (1974). A play scale. In M. Reilly (Ed.), *Play as exploratory learning* (pp. 247–266). Beverly Hills, CA: Sage.

Miller, L. J., & Roid, G. H. (1994). *The T.I.M.E. Toddler and Infant Motor Evaluation: A standardized assessment*. Tucson, AZ: Therapy Skill Builders.

physical function, perceptual-motor training, prosthetic and orthotic training, prevocational exploration, homemaking, and supportive therapy.

Since these early beginnings, both OT and PT assessment and treatment have evolved with societal changes to include the independent living movement, with the emphasis on utilizing the strengths of the individual and peer support groups. In 1989, Hasselkus suggested that the evolving attitudes toward health care in general and care of the elderly in particular have resulted in assessment and treatment along a continuum from the traditional rehabilitation to independent living. In actuality, assessment and treatment of the elderly is unique because of an element that is often overlooked in health care literature regarding the elderly; i.e., the perceptions of the elderly regarding functional assessment and intervention may be affected by their valuing of such activities in relation to the effects on their total life at this stage of their lives. This may be why many elderly individuals are resistive to turning their home into a hospital-type environment. Their primary goal may be to keep their environment as normal, aesthetically pleasing, and as comforting as possible, even if this means compromising some functional independence. However, the health professionals' primary goals are to advocate any modifications to behavior or the physical environment that will increase the autonomy or independence of the elderly person. To be effective, assessment and treatment must be shaped by the particular elderly population and the setting of the intervention.

For purposes of this discussion, OT assessment is organized under the two categories of functional ability and the environment. Both functional ability and the environment are organized around the theory of human occupation. The assessment of functional ability is grouped around the three categories of 1) the patient's perception of competence and interests in choosing daily living activities (volition), 2) the patient's recurrent patterns of behavior in daily living (habituation), and 3) the patient's organization and capacity for occupational performance in daily life (performance); the fourth category includes factors that facilitate or hinder occupational performance (environment).

Assessment of functional ability in this context is multiphasic and includes the person's volitional areas, such as interests, values, and ability to be autonomous, plus his or her habits and roles, as well as the more traditionally emphasized skill components and the ability to perform various activities. The environment includes both physical and social components, including physical resources and social supports, particularly the caretaker. The physical and social environments are intermeshed to compose occupational behavior settings that constitute a meaningful context for performance (Kielhofner, 1995a). Looking at the occupation of elderly individuals from this perspective accommodates the unique needs of individuals shaped by their personal profiles, including their personal perceptions, roles, habits, and performance abilities within their environmental context.

Physical therapy assessment has been organized around the "SOAP" framework (Subjective, Objective, Assessment, Plan) for assessment of performance. Both occupational therapy and physical therapy assess the environment from their unique perspective.

FUNCTIONAL ASSESSMENT

Relationship Between Function and Disease

In addition to the frequent functional presentations of disease in old age that may be characterized by the absence of classic or typical clinical findings, another phenomenon common with the elderly is the poor correlation between type and severity of functional disability and the number of diagnoses. Since illness and functional loss both increase with age, it is often assumed that the frequency of diseases or conditions of older persons correlates with the kind and intensity of functional disability. However, this is not the case. A long list of problems or illnesses accumulated by an old person does not necessarily result in serious loss of function. Many elderly persons with very long lists of serious problems still maintain independence. Another common error is to assume that the specific functional impairment is related to the organ or system with the disease. For example, mobility problems would be attributed to musculoskeletal or neurologic disorders and incontinence to the bladder. This causality principle does not necessarily apply with the elderly. Certain vulnerable tissues and organ systems may be likely to decompensate as a result of systemic disease anywhere in the body, which may compromise the functional integrity of an elderly individual (Besdine, 1988). The systems that are most vulnerable to impairment vary with each individual; therefore, the areas of functional ability that may be compromised in each individual will also vary. Two important implications for these noncorrelations between functional ability and diagnoses are pivotal for good care of the elderly. First, functional impairment should be assessed independent of the medical diagnoses. Secondly, although specific pathology may exist in a particular organ system, it does not mean that the primary pathology exists in that specific organ system or that any functional loss due to disease is attributed to that particular system. Health professionals can manage this phenomenon specific to the elderly by enumerating functional impairments parallel with the clinical findings of impairment when developing therapeutic goals to increase independence (Besdine, 1988).

A study by Baron and others (1987) of hand function of the elderly in relation to osteoarthritis (OA) supported this notion of noncorrelations. Osteoarthritic patients assessed with The Smith Hand Function Test (Smith, 1973) showed correlations to age, coordination, and hand strength but not to the degree of OA. However, results of subjective hand disability measured by the Stanford Health Assessment Questionnaire (HAQ) (Fries et al., 1982) correlated with radiographic OA manifestations and joint tenderness, as well as sex and hand strength. The authors concluded that OA does not seem to contribute significantly to the objective decline in hand function but may contribute to a subjective sense of functional limitation.

As the elderly person becomes more frail, small changes in the individual's ability to perform daily activities or the ability of a caregiver to provide support can have a major impact on the person's style and quality of life. Chances are much greater that such small changes will have more of an impact on the lifestyles of elderly individuals than on those of younger persons.

Functional Decrease as a Sign of Illness

In addition to impact on lifestyle, a decrease of functional ability in the elderly can be the first sign of new illness or exacerbation of a chronic disease. Unlike younger persons, the elderly often do not exhibit a single, specific complaint that helps to determine a differential diagnosis, but rather they exhibit one or more nonspecific problems indicated by functional impairment. Functional presentation of illness might include any of the following: cessation of eating or drinking, falling, urinary incontinence, dizziness, acute confusion, new onset or worsening of previously mild dementia, loss of weight, and generalized failure to thrive (Besdine, 1988). If we accept that the onset of problems is not easily recognized by many health professionals, family members, and the elderly themselves, then this apparent age difference in manifestation of illness is very important to the case management of the elderly. It is important that elderly individuals and the people who compose their formal and informal support systems be aware that disruption of homeostasis by any pathology is likely to be expressed in the most vulnerable or delicately balance systems. Therefore the weakest links are likely to fail, and the results may be ADL or instrumental activities of daily living (IADL) problems rather than the usual classic symptoms seen in the younger population (Besdine, 1988). The implication for the elderly and everyone involved with their care is that deterioration of functional independence in previously unimpaired active elders may be an early, subtle sign of an unidentified illness. Rapid and thorough clinical evaluation of the presenting functional impairments may be the only way that independence and the quality of life can be maintained (Besdine, 1988). Leaders in the field have recommended that health care providers routinely carry out a functional assessment that is complementary to the traditional diagnostic work-ups that precede treatment recommendations. This combined process has been called Comprehensive Functional Assessment (CFA) (Champlin, 1985).

The ultimate functional disability is death. In the update of the Massachusetts Health Care Panel Study (Branch, 1980), four variables were associated with a greater likelihood of the elderly dying within 15 months. Two of these were related to functional ability: 1) if the person is no longer self-sufficient in personal care (ADL), and 2) if the person is no longer able to do heavy work around the house without help (IADL).

Central Indicator for Treatment Planning

Functional assessment is important for all persons with loss of independence, but it is especially important for the elderly for whom independent abilities are more easily affected by the broad array of illnesses and problems common in old age (Besdine, 1988). As people age, the possibility that they will have difficulty with functional activities increases, particularly past the age of 85 years. The report of the Health and Public Policy Committee of the American College of Physicians recognized that decreased functional ability of the elderly is an increasingly major issue as the population ages. "Although most elderly noninstitutionalized adults are functionally competent, the percentage who need help doing everyday activities doubles with each successive decade up to age 84, and triples between ages 85 and 94" (Almy, 1988, p. 70). Kane and Kane (1981) supported the concept that functional ability, rather than the absence or presence of disease, is the central issue with the elderly. "Measures of functional status that examine the ability to function independently despite disease, physical and mental disability, and social deprivation are the most useful overall indicators to assist those who care for the elderly" (p. 1).

Even though there is general agreement that independence is the key issue of health care for the elderly and assessment of functional ability is of prime importance, trends in reimbursement for maintenance of function are directly counter to this need. Home health care is limited to only about 12 to 15 percent of those who actually need such services. Branch and others (1988) found that requirements for assistance in ADL and functional dependency are factors placing the elderly at high risk for needing home care. Assistance required with ADL or IADL is not covered by Medicare, so the elderly must often seek assistance from family or friends. This lack of funding for personal care grew out of the movement away from the medical model and the belief that intervention when the elderly person is medically stable could lead to perpetuation of the sick role and unnecessary dependency. "Management of medically stabilized disability is primarily a personal matter and only secondarily a medical matter" (DeJong, 1979, p. 440). However, this lack of support for maintenance of the frail elderly when needed may increase the strain on family caregivers until they can no longer cope and thus actually hasten institutionalization of the elderly.

Assessment Methods

Assessment of the elderly usually includes one or more of the following forms: 1) self-reports by the patient, 2) ratings based on observations of the patient's performance by a rater or attendants, and 3) direct examination by a trained professional, such as the occupational or physical therapist (Maguire, 1995a).

Self-Report. In initial data collection, information is usually obtained through some type of self-report if the elderly person or an informant is capable of giving accurate information. Self-report information is usually in the form of interviewing or surveying the elderly individual. Self-report supplies information about peoples' perceptions of their competence and their situations and not necessarily objective data. However, self-report is very important as part of the total picture. Research with the elderly indicates that self-report may be more indicative of the way the elderly function rather than of the number of measurable medical conditions. In addition to learning how a person perceives his or her functional ability, research on the elderly has suggested that self-ratings of health are more closely related to attitudes and behaviors of the elderly than clinical evaluations of health by others (Graney & Zimmerman, 1981). Skrastins and others (1982) have suggested that older people are often slow to bring problems to medical attention because their symptoms are vague or because they accept their disability as part of old age. Self-reports often include information about the person's performance and habits in ADL and IADL. Activities of daily living include the self-care activities of eating, hygiene, grooming, and dressing. Depending on the assessments used, information is not always obtained on the resources available and needed to continue to be as independent as possible. The Assessment of Living Skills and Resources (ALSAR) (Williams et al., 1991) does combine both (performance and resources) and is easy to use. In any multidimensional assessment of the elderly, information concerning the balance of functional ability with available resources is essential. It is this balance that often determines if a person is able to remain living in the community rather than in an institutional setting. For example, an elderly person may need assistance with getting in and out of the bathtub, general housecleaning, transportation to medical appointments and social activities, shopping, cooking, and planning nutritious meals. This person needs assistance with only one self-care activity—bathing. Assistance is needed with five IADL activities, but only cooking is needed daily. Even food can be prepared for several days at one time if the person is able to reheat the food. Assistance is needed for a number of activities, but the person could still remain in his or her own home if a consistent combination of personal or physical resources were available to meet these needs. In this example, a constant companion is not necessary, but consistent assistance is. Often this assistance is supplied by a family caregiver, such as a spouse or adult daughter.

When a family caregiver is not available, a combination of neighbors, friends, and paid help may be utilized, but this is precarious and leaves the older person more vulnerable to a breakdown in the system. (See a more extensive discussion regarding caregivers in this chapter under Caregivers in Environmental Assessment.) It is usually more successful in the long term if the older person can manage temporarily without help if his or her social support system breaks down. When regular support is no longer available, the person often has to enter some type of institutional setting. In the restrictive environment of an institution, the amount of assistance given is often more than is needed, which leads to decreased autonomy and eventual loss of independence.

Observations of Behavior. Assessment using observation of behavior is based on observations of the elderly person's performance by a rater. An example of this type of assessment is The Parachek Geriatric Behavior Rating Scale (Miller & Parachek, 1974). The authors report that a hospital technician who is well acquainted with the patient can do the ratings within 3 to 5 minutes without the patient being present (Maguire, 1995a).

Assessment by Direct Examination. Most occupational and physical therapists use direct examinations to rate performance of the elderly to give the detailed information that is usually needed for treatment planning. However, ratings of performance are often difficult to standardize, particularly for complex activities such as homemaking (Maguire, 1995a). Examples of assessments utilizing direct examination are the Katz Index of ADL (Katz et al., 1963), the Barthel Index (Mahoney & Barthel, 1965), and The Klein-Bell Activities of Daily Living Scale (Klein & Bell, 1982).

OCCUPATIONAL THERAPY ASSESSMENT

Volitional Level

The volitional level, as the highest system in human occupation, directs the habituation and performance systems and affects the elderly person's choice of occupation. The volitional process involves the procedures of attending, choosing, interpreting, and experiencing occupational behavior (Kielhofner et al., 1995).

Values. Values assign significance, personal conviction, and commitment to occupations (Kielhofner et al., 1995). Values determine the elderly person's perception of what is valuable in life. It is expected that with consistency of personality, values will also be somewhat consistent throughout the life span. At the same time, the adaptation that individuals must go through in response to normal aging and disease or trauma necessitates reappraisal of values to adapt to role and performance changes. Rogers and Snow (1985) have suggested that successful aging requires agreement between elderly individuals' values, capabilities, and activities.

The need to determine patients' values and health beliefs to incorporate these beliefs into their therapeutic programs is important for all patients but is more central for the elderly than for younger persons. At a stage in life when the elderly are more susceptible to having their autonomy eroded, care must be taken to ensure that the therapist tailors assessment and treatment interventions to elderly individuals' personal values and beliefs rather than emphasizing how they need to conform to the health care system, no matter how good are the therapist's intentions.

Personal Causation. The need for personal control and the drive to master the environment continues to be important throughout the life cycle, including in old age. The potential multiple losses in roles, performance ability, and resources make the elderly person more vulnerable to experiencing a diminished sense of competence and personal control. Elderly persons may become more externally oriented due to their perception that they have little control over many of these changes (Rogers & Snow, 1985). Some evidence exists that an internal rather than external control orientation is associated with more successful aging (Kuypers, 1972). Autonomy, or the right of self-determination, is the volitional area that is most vulnerable to erosion for elderly individuals. Increased dependence in the performance area is often associated with elderly individuals and their professional and informal caregivers equating loss of autonomy with loss of independence. As roles and performance decrease, individuals can feel a lack of efficacy and personal control over their lives.

Management of Self-Care. Assessment of the management of self-care is part of the overall assessment of self-care but not synonymous with assessment of the performance components of ADL and IADL. It is a somewhat artificial distinction to separate the two, but it is being done here to emphasize this facet of the concept. Hasselkus (1989) points out that the concept of self-care puts non–health care workers, including the elderly consumer, in a position of dominance and the health care provider in the position of consultant. She suggests that even though the patient in the position of dominance may not be an appropriate power balance for acute or crisis medical situations, it may be the appropriate power balance for long-term chronic care, which is a large proportion of the medical care for the elderly. Assessment strategies for the management aspect of self-care must determine if the elderly need to move from the dependency of the acute-care role and to reestablish control and self-directedness in their lives. Part of this assessment process is to determine elderly people's values and beliefs concerning their health needs so that these factors can be incorporated into an appropriate educational program. Patient education includes those learning activities designed to assist people in making changes in their behavior conducive to health while affirming the role of patients in a partnership-type arrangement. Occupational therapy

assessments may include questions regarding who makes decisions around IADL, such as scheduling appointments and arranging business matters.

Interests. Interests serve to partially structure the choice, frequency, and valuing of occupation throughout the life span. In the postretirement years, people usually have a greater proportion of unobligated time as compared with earlier stages of life. Although interests may stay somewhat constant throughout peoples' lives, the opportunity for participation in both type and frequency of activities is influenced by their roles at particular stages of life. Therefore, peoples' participation in activities at any point in their lives may not necessarily be representative of their interests. Pursuing particular interests is further mediated by how people value the activities that are a result of certain interests. For example, a woman may have always been interested in volunteering in her religious institution but never had sufficient time before she retired. During her young and middle adult years, her energy and resources were directed to job related activities, raising children, and then caring for elderly parents. Her value system dictated that she take care of "her own" before using her energy to care for others. Once retired, she may give a lot of time to church activities and receive more satisfaction from this volunteer activity than she did from her job. However, this is a very personal reaction; others may miss their work interests and find no comparable alternate interests associated with their retirement roles. In addition, roles and activities may have to be modified as a person ages owing to personal and social changes, even if the associated interests remain strong. Performance deficits may make former interests not viable. Rogers and Snow (1985) have suggested that although the frail elderly may participate more in sedentary and solitary pursuits, they may still desire to be involved in more active and social pursuits.

Measures of Volition. In addition to tests designed specifically to measure the volitional area, related measurements such as values clarification, life satisfaction surveys, inventories of interests, measures of internal versus external locus of control, and perceptions of competence may be helpful. (See the Appendix at the end of this chapter for listings of specific instruments.)

Habituation

The habituation process guides the structure of behavior in daily life and the change in roles and habits over time (Kielhofner, 1995b). The habituation level is very important because a good part of our daily activities are performed in a routine manner, without needing a lot of conscious thought. This is generally very helpful and efficient.

Habits. Most of the time we only become aware of how much habits help conserve our energy when the routine way we do things does not work. An example of the importance of habituation is when family members or close long-term memory, orientation, expressive and receptive speech, apraxias, and higher cognitive functions (Skrastins et al., 1982). A study of 40 institutionalized elderly women was undertaken to determine if changes occurred in mental status and functional abilities over the course of 1 year. Findings indicated a decline in mental status and an increase in functional dependency (Hamilton & Creason, 1992). However, the authors suggest that cognitive impairment did not always result in a self-care deficit.

Many of the assessment instruments commonly used with the elderly combine one or more performance components or functional activities. In addition to having to be concerned about assessing the components and actual functional activities, the health care professional must be concerned about the validity and reliability of the actual instruments. In a longitudinal study of the functional status among community elders, Branch and others (1984) found that the choice of operational ADL measures is important in trying to interpret assessment data. There was a great difference in the rate of loss of independence recorded, depending on the measure. For example, adding two items to a four-item ADL scale greatly increased the scale's sensitivity to changes in functional status.

Because most of the assessments of skill in occupational performance are covered in other areas of this text, just a few types of assessments that may be useful for the elderly population are mentioned.

Measures of Performance. Measures of performance might include a history of falls and screening for mental status, depression, ADL and IADL, sensory deficits, functional range of motion, and functional muscle strength. If serious deficits are noted, more detailed testing can be administered. See the Appendix at the end of this chapter for a listing of specific tests.

PHYSICAL THERAPY ASSESSMENT

The PT assessment is challenging owing to the uniqueness and variety of the physical and mental attributes of the geriatric patient, which have been previously discussed. This section relates these unique issues specifically to PT assessment of the elderly.

Recent literature suggests that a move is occurring toward computerized rehabilitation assessment to improve the efficiency of documentation and communication (Koch et al., 1994). A standardized geriatric functional assessment is not a new idea and has been supported by many (Besdine, 1988). However, one standardized geriatric assessment form has not been universally accepted in the clinical or academic community (O'Sullivan & Schmitz, 1994). This is partly due to the uniqueness of the geriatric patient. Haley and colleagues (1994) gave the example that persons with the same level of physical impairment may or may not have the same physical problems using a toilet. One obvious difference might include the physical location

and distance that the toilet is from the individual (environment). Variables like this and many others need consideration before one functional assessment form can eventually be adopted. However, the goal of equivalent and well-documented data for research and functional instruments will continually be supported (Besdine, 1988; Kutner et al., 1992; Mellette, 1993). Because no one perfect evaluation exists for every type of clinical situation, therapists must be trained to develop their own descriptive assessments or to utilize several existing standardized formats (O'Sullivan & Schmitz, 1994). A combination of using both is a good idea. Some of the more standardized formats are the Tufts Assessment of Motor Performance (TAMP) (Gans et al., 1988), the Katz Index of Activities of Daily Living (Katz et al., 1963), the Functional Independence Measure (FIM) (Uniform Data System for Medical Rehabilitation, 1990), the Barthel Index (Mahoney & Barthel, 1965), and the Functional Status Index (Cech & Martin, 1995). The following section reviews some of the more important aspects of developing your own age-related assessment tools.

The Assessment

A good assessment relates to all types of patients. It must be adaptable to different situations. It must address the hospitalized geriatric nonambulatory patient as well as the elderly patient who has an active lifestyle but developed a shoulder problem during a golf game. Because of the varied possibilities that are present in this age group, physical therapists must prepare themselves with a different assessment philosophy. This philosophy might best be explained as having an awareness of the age-related conditions that need consideration when performing the evaluation. These considerations will be addressed from the traditional SOAP note format which describes the *Problem* first, and then the *Subjective, Objective, Assessment,* and *Plan* (Kettenbach, 1995). In planning the assessment, the physical therapist must not forget normal developmental changes as well as the presenting pathology. The age-related data are needed to formulate a logical conceptual framework applicable to the individual assessment (Haley et al., 1994).

PROBLEM LIST

Problem lists of the elderly are different when compared with those of younger patients. Persons over age 65 demonstrate increased functional impairment. In fact, 75 percent have at least one chronic illness. More than a third can not perform their major activity independently, and 5 percent are confined to home. In the over-75 age group, 15 percent are confined to home, and even more debilitation exists in the over-80 age group, of which 25 percent cannot go outdoors. When ill, the elderly and younger patients differ; the younger patients usually have specific singular complaints. The elderly generally report more than one complaint, and many times it is nonspecific. The multiple problems of the elderly also affect many mobility functions and ADL. The good news is that the problems are usually successfully treated if detected by assessment (Besdine, 1988).

SUBJECTIVE INFORMATION

Subjective information can be the most important part of the assessment. When first meeting the patient, physical therapists immediately begin gathering subjective information from comments, observations, as well as from others associated with the elderly, particularly their caregivers. (See Assessment Methods.) At this point, the therapist must immediately decide how much assessment time is practical for the initial session. The patient's medical status may only allow 15 minutes or less. This time-limiting factor is obviously more important in evaluating the elderly than when assessing younger patients. Subjective information involves patients' orientation, cognitive level, pain, shortness of breath, communication abilities, and family relationships. While gathering this subjective information, the physical therapist will be assessing many sensory functions. It is well known that normal developmental aging results in decreasing sensory functions. One noted change is decreased visual function, resulting in decreased depth perception and contrast recognition. The contrast deficits are commonly associated with lack of light. Other diminished sensory changes are hearing loss, diminished touch, and less acute taste and smell abilities (Maguire, 1995b). It is interesting to note in animal studies that pain thresholds may increase. This phenomenon may possibly explain why the elderly report difficulty localizing pain (Hall & Perlmutter, 1985). During assessment it should be kept in mind that the elderly need more time for information processing and also for learning new motor tasks. Reaction times are longer, and memory skills diminish (Haywood, 1993). The therapist must keep in mind the variability among elderly individuals. Disease may result in more serious physical and mental declines in function. During the subjective assessment, the therapist will easily identify the more serious pathologic problems such as advanced Alzheimer's disease, speech deficits, and severe depression (Cherney, 1995).

This subjective assessment can be influenced by attitudes of the therapist as well as of the patient. Your assessment should not be biased by ageism or discriminatory influences. Studies have shown that therapists sometimes think older patients are less worthy of rehabilitation. If patients detect this "internal ageism," the therapist may interpret patient reactions to this ageism as poor motivation (Bonder & Wagner, 1994).

It is at this point that the physical therapist must determine the most important objective data to collect. The therapist must be practical and consider the available time and the mental and physical status of the patient. The therapist decides whether to use an informal tool, a standardized form, or a combination of both.

OBJECTIVE DATA

The assessment also depends on collecting key point objective data. The ultimate assessment includes a musculoskeletal, neurologic, cardiorespiratory, vascular, dermatology, and endocrine system evaluation. All of these assessments are lengthy and important but not always practical with the elderly. As previously mentioned, the patient's condition is the restricting factor. Difficult decisions must be made immediately as to what the assessment will include. Minimally, it should be based on your knowledge of normal and pathologic disease of elders. One physical therapist suggests assessing only the three areas of dressing, feeding, and walking (Bottomley, 1989). Although this tri-area classification seems overly simplified, it does impress one with the reality of basic functional needs.

When planning objective data collection, normal aging changes that are musculoskeletal in nature must be considered, including decreased strength, flexibility, endurance, and coordination. As a result of these changes, the elderly have decreased postural stability, impaired balance when walking, a slower gait, increased episodes of falling, and less ability to carry out their ADL.

Kutner and others (1992) emphasize this further and report that these musculoskeletal areas are the major key points in preventing injury and reducing loss of function. The physical therapist must also be cognizant of declining cardiovascular efficiency and endocrine functions, thus alerting the evaluator to precautions involving patients' cardiac status, shortness of breath, and osteoporosis (Kutner et al., 1992; Lewis, 1995). Strength assessment is a very important aspect of the elderly assessment. It is generally agreed that atrophy is associated with aging. Strength is maximal during the 20s and 30s. Decreases are noted thereafter but are not functionally significant until around 75 years of age. The most commonly affected muscle groups are the antigravity muscles. These muscle groups are needed for many ADL, such as getting up out of a chair, sitting down, climbing stairs, and standing. In people 75 to 84 years of age, Kutner and others (1992) found that 15 percent were unable to climb stairs and 24 percent were unable to lift a 10-lb weight. The causes are sometimes due to sedentary living, but there are normal physiologic explanations related to changes in muscle fiber types and neuronal motor unit degeneration (Haywood, 1993). However, studies now show that the elderly can significantly decrease the loss of strength from disuse or a sedentary life through exercise (Cech & Martin, 1995; Lewis, 1995).

Range of motion and joint mobility or flexibility also decrease with age as a result of both normal development and pathologic conditions. Age-associated losses of flexibility may be the result of increased collagen formation and sedentary lifestyle. Common postural changes include a

APPENDIX

Assessments Useful with the Elderly

Activities of Daily Living (From OARS) (George & Fillenbaum, 1985)

Assessment of Communication & Interaction Skills (MOHO Clearing House, 1995)

Assessment of Living Skills and Resources (Williams et al., 1991)

Assessment of Motor and Process Skills (AMPS Project, 1995)

Assessment of Occupational Functioning (Watts et al, 1989)

BaFPE Social Interaction Scale (Williams & Bloomer, 1987)

BaFPE Task Oriented Assessment (Williams & Bloomer, 1987)

Barth Time Configuration (Barth, 1985)

Caregiver Reaction Assessment (Given et al., 1992)

Caregiver Strain Index (Robinson, 1983)

Cognitive Capacity Screening Examination (Jacobs et al., 1977)

Comprehensive Assessment and Referral Evaluation (Gurland et al., 1977–1978)

Environment Assessment Scale (Kannegieter, 1986)

Environmental Questionnaire (Dunning, 1972)

Family Burden Interview (Zarit et al., 1980)

Family Environment Scale (Moos, 1976)

Functional Activities Questionnaire (Pfeiffer et al., 1982)

Functional Assessment Inventory (Pfeiffer et al., 1981)

Functional Independence Measure (FIMS) (Uniform Data System for Medical Rehabilitation, 1990)

Health Assessment Questionnaire (Fries et al., 1982)

Home Hazard Checklists (Tideiksaar, 1986)

Instrumental Activities of Daily Living (From OARS) (George & Fillenbaum, 1985)

Interpersonal Support Evaluation List (Cohen et al., 1985)

Klein-Bell Activities of Daily Living Scale (Klein & Bell, 1982)

Kohlman Evaluation of Living Skills (Kohlman-Thompson, 1992)

London Psychogeriatric Rating Scale (Hersch et al., 1978)

Mini-Mental Status Examination (Anthony et al., 1982)

Modified Interest Checklist (Occupational Therapy Department, 1995)

Multidimensional Functional Assessment Questionnaire (From OARS) (George & Fillenbaum, 1985)

Multidimensional Observation Scale for Elderly Subjects (Helmes, 1988)

NIH Activity Record (Furst, 1995)

Occupational Case Analysis Interview and Rating Scale (Slack Book Order Dept, 1995)

Occupational Performance History Interview (American Occupational Therapy Association, 1995)

Occupational Questionnaire (MOHO Clearing House, 1995)

Older Americans Resources and Services (George & Fillenbaum, 1985)

Role Checklist (Oakley, 1995)

Scorable Self Care Evaluation (Clark & Peters, 1992)

Screen for Caregiver Burden (Vitaliano et al., 1991)

Self Assessment of Occupational Functioning (MOHO Clearing House, 1995)

Self-Efficacy Scale (Scherer & Maddux, 1982)

Services Assessment Questionnaire (From OARS) (George & Fillenbaum, 1985)

Short Portable Mental Status Questionnaire (Pfeiffer, 1975)

Volitional Questionnaire (MOHO Clearing House, 1995)

Worker Role Interview (MOHO Clearing House, 1995)

Zarit Burden Scale (Zarit et al., 1985)

REFERENCES

Almy, T. P. (1988). Comprehensive functional assessment for elderly patients. *Annals of Internal Medicine, 1,* July.

American Occupational Therapy Association, 4720 Montgomery Lane, PO Box 31220, Bethesda, MD 20824-1220, Phone: (301) 652-2682, Fax: (301) 652-7711, Order # 1690.

AMPS Project, Occupational Therapy Building, Colorado State University, Fort Collins, Colorado 80523, Information on Required Training.

Anthony, J. C., LeResche, L., Niaz, U., VonKorff, M. R., & Folstein, M. F. (1982). Limits of the "Mini Mental State" as a screening test for dementia and delirium among hospital patients. *Psychological Medicine, 12,* 397–408.

Atchley, R. C. (1972). *Social forces in later life: An introduction to social gerontology.* Belmont, CA: Wadsworth.

Baron, M., Dutil, E., Berkson, L., Lander, P., & Becker, R. (1987). Hand function in the elderly: Relation to osteoarthritis. *Journal of Rheumatology, 14,* 815–819.

Barth, T. (1985). *Barth time construction.* New York: Health Related Consulting Services.

Besdine, R. W. (1988). Functional assessment as a model for clinical evaluation of geriatric patients. *Public Health Report, 103* (pp. 530–536). Washington, DC: U.S. Department of Health and Human Services.

Bidabe, D. L., & Lollar, J. M. (1988). *Mobility opportunities via education.* Report of the Kern County Superintendent of Schools, Bakersfield, CA.

Birren, J. E. (1964). *The psychology of aging.* Englewood Cliffs, NJ: Prentice-Hall.

Blau, Z. S. (1973). *Old age in a changing society.* New York: New Viewpoints.

Bonder, B. R., & Wagner, M. B. (1994). *Functional performance across the life span.* Philadelphia: W. B. Saunders Company.

Bottomley, J. (1989). *Geriatric assessment: Functional assessment in the elderly.* Baltimore: Video Press, University of Maryland at Baltimore.

Botwinick, J. (1973). *Aging and behavior: A comprehensive integration of research findings.* New York: Springer.

Branch, L. G. (1980). Functional abilities of the elderly: An update on the Massachusetts health care panel study. In S. G. Haynes & M. Feinleib (Eds.), *Second conference on the epidemiology of aging* (pp. 237–265). Washington DC: U.S. Department of Health and Human Services. NIH publication No. 800969.

Branch, L. G., Katz, S., Kniepmann, K., & Papsidero, J. (1984). A prospective study of functional status among community elders. *American Journal of Public Health, 74,* 266–268.

Branch, L. G., Wetle, T. T., Scherr, P. A., Cook, N. R., Evan, D. A., Hebert, L. E., Masland, E. N., Keough, M. E., & Taylor, J. O. (1988). A prospective study of incident comprehensive medical home care use among the elderly. *American Journal of Public Health, 78,* 255–259.

Brody, H., & Vijayashanker, N. (1977). Anatomical changes in the nervous system. In C. Finch & L. Hayflick (Eds.), *Handbook of the biology of aging.* New York: Van Nostrand Reinhold.

Brown, L., Potter, J., & Foster, B. (1990). Caregiver burden should be evaluated during geriatric assessment. *Journal of the American Geriatrics Society, 38,* 455–460.

Cech, D., & Martin, S. (1995). *Functional movement development across the life span.* Philadelphia: W. B. Saunders Company.

Champlin, L. (1985). Functional assessment: A new tool to improve geriatric care. *Geriatrics, 40*(2), 120–125.

Cherney, L. R. (1995). The effects of aging on communication. In C. L. Bernstein (Ed.), *Aging: The health care challenge.* Philadelphia: F. A. Davis Company.

Clark, E. N., & Peters, M. (1992). *Scorable self-care evaluation.* Thorofare, NJ: Slack.

Cohen, S., Mermelstein, R., Kamrack, T., & Hobermad, H. M. (1985). Measuring the functional components of social support. *In* I. G. Sarason & B. R. Sarason (Eds.), *Social Support: Theory, research and applications* (pp. 73–94), Boston: Martinus Nijhioff.

Corbin, J., & Strauss, A. (1988). *Unending work and care: Managing illness at home.* San Francisco: Jossey-Bass Publishers.

Corso, J. F. (1971). Sensory processes and effects in normal adults. *Journal of Gerontology, 26,* 90–105.

Crutchfield, C. A., & Barnes, M. R. (1993). *Motor control and motor learning in rehabilitation.* Atlanta: Stokesville Publishing Co.

Culler, K. (1993). Home and family management. In H. Hopkins & H. Smith (Eds.), *Willard and Spackman's occupational therapy* (8th ed.) (pp. 207–226). Philadelphia: J. B. Lippincott.

Daleiden, S., & Lewis, C. B. (1990). Clinical implications of neurologic changes in the aging process. In C. B. Lewis (Ed.), *Aging: The health care challenge* (2nd. ed.). Philadelphia: F. A. Davis Company.

DeJong, G. (1979). Independent living: From social movement to analytic paradigm. *Archives of Physical Medicine and Rehabilitation, 60,* 435–446.

Drinka, T., Smith, J., & Drinka, P. (1987). Correlates of depression and burden for informal caregivers of patients in a geriatrics referral clinic. *Journal of the American Geriatrics Society, 35*(6), 522–525.

Duke University Center for the Study of Aging and Human Development. (1978). *Multidimensional functional assessment: The OARS methodology.* Durham, NC: Duke University Center for the Study of Aging and Human Development.

Dunning, H. D. (1972). Environmental occupational therapy. *American Journal of Occupational Therapy, 26,* 292–298.

Fisher, A., & Kielhofner, G. (1995a). Mind-brain-body performance subsystem. In G. Kielhofner (Ed.), *Model of human occupation: Theory and application.* Baltimore: Williams & Wilkins.

Fisher, A., & Kielhofner, G. (1995b). Skill in occupational performance. In G. Kielhofner, (Ed.), *A model of human occupation: Theory and application.* Baltimore: Williams & Wilkins.

Fries, J. F., Spitz, P. W., & Young, D. Y. (1982). The dimensions of health outcomes: The health assessment questionnaire, disability and pain scales. *Journal of Rheumatology, 9,* 789–793.

Furst, G., MPH, OTR, Department of Rehabilitation Medicine, National Institutes of Health, 9000 Rockville Pike, 10/6S235, Bethesda, MD 20892.

Gans, B. M., Haley, S. M., Hallenborg, S. C., Mann, N., Inacia, C. A., & Fass, R. M. (1988). Description and interobserver reliability of the Tufts Assessment of Motor Performance. *Physical Medicine and Rehabilitation, 67,* 202–210.

George, L. K., & Fillenbaum, G. G. (1985). OARS methodology: A decade of experience in geriatric assessment. *Journal of the American Geriatrics Society, 33*(9), 607–615.

Given, C., Given, B., Stommel, M., Collins, C., King, S., & Franklin, S. (1992). The caregiver reaction assessment (CRA) for caregivers to persons with chronic physical and mental impairments. *Research in Nursing and Health, 15,* 271–283.

Graney, M. J., & Zimmerman, R. M. (1981). Causes and consequences of health self-report variations among older people. *International Journal of Aging and Human Development, 12*(4), 291–300.

Gurland, B., Kuriansky, J., Sharpe, L., Simon, R., Stiller, P., & Birkett, P. (1977–1978). The comprehensive assessment and referral evaluation (CARE)—Rationale, development and reliability. *International Journal of Aging and Human Development, 8*(1), 9–41.

Haley, S. M., Coster, W. J., & Bindea-Sundberg, K. (1994). Measuring physical disablement: The contexual challenge. *Physical Therapy, 74*(5), 443–451.

Hall, M., & Perlmutter, E. (1985). *Adult development and aging.* New York: John Wiley & Sons.

Hamilton, L. W., & Creason, N. S. (1992). Mental status and functional abilities: Change in institutionalized elderly women. *Nursing Diagnosis, 3*(2), 81–86.

Hasselkus, B. R. (1974). Aging and the human nervous system. *American Journal of Occupational Therapy, 28,* 16–21.

Hasselkus, B. R. (1991). Ethical dilemmas in family caregiving for the elderly: Implications for occupational therapy. *American Journal of Occupational Therapy, 45*(3), 206–212.

Hasselkus, B. R. (1989). Occupational and physical therapy in geriatric rehabilitation. *Physical and Occupational Therapy in Geriatrics, 7*(3), 3–20.

Haywood, K. M. (1993). *Life span motor development* (2nd ed.). Champaign, IL: Human Kinetics Publishers.

Helmes, E. (1988). Multidimensional observation scale for elderly subjects (MOSES). *Psychopharmacology Bulletin, 24*(4), 733–745.

Hersch, E. L., Kral, V. A., & Palmer, R. B. (1978). Clinical value of the London psychogeriatric rating scale. *Journal of the American Geriatrics Society, 26*(8), 348–354.

Hislop, H. J. (1975). The not-so-impossible dream. *Physical Therapy, 55,* 1069–1081. *Home care for persons 55 and over, U.S., July 1966–June 1968.* (1972). National Center for Health Statistics, Series No. 10, No. 73, DHEW publication HSM72-1062.

Huston, P. (1990). Family care of the elderly and caregiver stress. *American Family Physician, 42*(3), 671–676.

Jacobs, J. W., Bernhard, M. R., Delgado, A., & Strain, J. J. (1977). Screening for organic mental syndromes in the medically ill. *Annals of Internal Medicine, 86,* 40–45.

Kane, R. A., & Kane, R. L. (1981). *Assessing the elderly.* Lexington, MA: D.C. Heath Company.

Kannegieter, R. B. (1986). The development of the environment assessment scale. *Occupational Therapy in Mental Health, 6,* 67–83.

Katz, S., Ford, A. B., Moskowitz, R. W., Jackson, B. A., & Jaffe, M. W. (1963). The index of ADL. *Journal of the American Medical Association, 185,* 914–919.

Kettenbach, G. (1995). *Writing soap notes* (2nd ed.). Philadelphia: F. A. Davis.

Kielhofner, G. (1995a). Environmental influences on occupational behavior. In G. Kielhofner (Ed.), *A model of human occupation: Theory and application* (2nd ed.) Baltimore: Williams & Wilkins.

Kielhofner, G. (1995b). Habituation subsystem. In G. Kielhofner (Ed.), *A model of human occupation: Theory and application* (2nd ed.). Baltimore: Williams & Wilkins.

Kielhofner, G. (1982). *Health through occupation.* Philadelphia: F. A. Davis Company.

Kielhofner, G. (Ed.). (1985). *A model of human occupation: Theory and application.* Baltimore: Williams & Wilkins.

Kielhofner, G., Borell, L., Burke, J., Helfrich, C., & Nygard, L. (1995). Volitional subsystem. In G. Kielhofner (Ed.), *A model of human occupation: Theory and application* (2nd ed.). Baltimore: Williams & Wilkins.

Kiernat, J. (1991). The rewards and challenges of working with older adults. In J. Kiernat (Ed.), *Occupational therapy and the older adult: A clinical manual* (pp. 2–10). Gaithersburg, MD: Aspen Publishers.

Kim, M. J., McFarland, G. K., & McLand, A. M. (Eds.). (1984). Classification of nursing diagnoses: Proceedings of the fifth national conference. St. Louis, MO: Mosby-Year Book.

Kisner, C., & Colby, L. A. (1990). *Therapeutic exercise foundations and techniques* (2nd ed.). Philadelphia: F. A. Davis Company.

Klein, R. H., & Bell, R. (1982). Self-care skills with the Klein-Bell ADL scale. *Archives of Physical Medicine and Rehabilitation, 63,* 335–338.

Koch, M., Gottschalk, M., Baker, D. I., Palumbo, S., & Tinetti, M. E. (1994). An impairment and disability assessment and treatment protocol for community-living elderly persons. *Physical Therapy, 74*(4), 286–291.

Kohlman-Thompson, L. (1992). *The Kohlman evaluation of living skills.* Rockville, MD: American Occupational Therapy Association.

Kutner, N. G., Ory, M. G., Baker, D. I., Schechtmen, K. B., Hornbrook, M. C., & Mulrow, C. D. (1992). Measuring the quality of life of the elderly in health promotion intervention clinical trials. *Public Health Report, 107* (pp. 530–539). Washington DC: U.S. Department of Health and Human Services.

Kuypers, J. A. (1972). Internal-external locus of control, ego functioning, and personality characteristics in old age. *Gerontologist, 12,* 168–173.

Lewis, C. B. (1995). Musculoskeletal changes with age: Clinical implications. In C. B. Lewis (Ed.), *Aging: The health care challenge* (3rd ed.). Philadelphia: F. A. Davis Company.

Maguire, G. H. (1995a). Activities of daily living. In C. B. Lewis (Ed.), *Aging: The health care challenge* (3rd ed.). Philadelphia: F. A. Davis Company.

Maguire, G. H. (1990). Occupational therapy. In W. Abrams & R. Berkow (Eds.), *The Merck manual of geriatrics.* New Jersey: Merck & Co., Inc.

Maguire, G. H. (1995b). Sensory changes in the elderly. In C. B. Lewis (Ed.), *Aging: The health care challenge* (3rd ed.). Philadelphia: F. A. Davis Company.

Mahoney, F. L., & Barthel, D. W. (1965). Functional evaluation: Barthel index. *Maryland State Medical Journal, 14,* 61–65.

Mellette, S. J. (1993). Cancer rehabilitation. *Journal of the National Cancer Institute, 85,* 781–784.

Miller, E. R., & Parachek, J. F. (1974). Validation and standardization of a goal-oriented, quick screening geriatric scale. *Journal of the American Geriatrics Society, 22,* 278–283.

MOHO Clearing House, Department of Occupational Therapy M/C 811, University of Illinois at Chicago, 1919 West Taylor Street, Chicago, Illinois 60612. Fax: (312) 413-0256.

Moos, R. H. (1976). *Family environmental scale.* Palo Alto, CA: Consulting Psychologist Press.

North American Nursing Diagnosis Association. (1990). *Taxonomy I—Revised.* St. Louis, MO: NANDA.

Oakley, F., MS, OTR/L. Occupational Therapy Department, Rehabilitation Medicine, NIH, Bldg. 10, Rm. 65235, 9000 Rockville Pike, Bethesda, MD 20892.

Orem, D. (1985). *Nursing concepts of practice* (3rd ed.). New York: McGraw-Hill.

O'Sullivan, S. B., & Schmitz, T. J. (1994). *Physical rehabilitation: Assessment and treatment* (3rd ed.). Philadelphia: F. A. Davis Company.

Payton, O., Nelson, C., & Ozer, M. (1990). *Patient participation in program planning: A manual for therapists.* Philadelphia: F. A. Davis Company.

Peloquin, S. M. (1990). The patient-therapist relationship in occupational therapy: Understanding visions and images. *American Journal of Occupational Therapy, 44*(1), 13–21.

Perry, G. R., & de Meneses, M. R. (1989). Cancer patients at home: Needs and coping styles of primary caregivers. *Home Healthcare Nurse, 7*(6), 27–31.

Pfeiffer, E., Johnson, T. M., & Chiofolo, R. C. (1981). Functional assessment of elderly subjects in four service settings. *Journal of the Americans Geriatrics Society, 29*(10), 488–437.

Pfeiffer, R. I. (1975). A short portable mental status questionnaire for the assessment of organic brain deficit in elderly patients. *Journal of the American Gerontology Society, 23*(10), 433–441.

Pfeiffer, R. I., Kurosake, T. T., Harrah Jr., C. H., Chance, J. M., & Filos, S. (1982). Measurement of functional activities in older adults in the community. *Journal of Gerontology, 37*(3), 323–329.

Robinson, B. (1983). Validation of a caregiver strain index. *Journal of Gerontology, 38*(3), 344–348.

Rogers, J. C. (1987). Occupational therapy assessment for older adults with depression: Asking the right questions. *Physical and Occupational Therapy in Geriatrics, 5*(2), 13–33.

Rogers, J. C., & Snow, T. L. (1985). Later adulthood. In G. Kielhofner (Ed.), *A model of human occupation: Theory and application.* Baltimore: Williams & Wilkins.

Rusk, H. A. (1977). *Rehabilitation medicine* (4th ed.). St. Louis: C. V. Mosby Company.

Rzetelny, H., & Mellor, J. (1981). *Support groups for caregivers of the aged.* New York: Community Service Society.

Sasano, E. M., Shepard, K. F., Bell, J. E., Davies, N. H., Hansen, E. M., & Stanford, T. L. (1977). The family in physical therapy. *Physical Therapy, 57,* 153–159.

Saxon, S. V., & Etten, M. J. (1978). *Physical changes and aging: A guide for the helping professions.* New York: Tiresias Press.

Scherer, M., & Maddux, J. E. (1982). Self efficacy scale: Construction and validation. *Psychological Reports, 51,* 663–671.

Schirm, V. (1989). Functionally impaired elderly: Their need for home nursing care. *Journal of Community Health Nursing, 6*(4), 199–207.

Sheppard, H. L. (1976). Work and retirement. In R. H. Binstock & E. Shanas (Eds.), *Handbook of aging and the social sciences.* New York: Van Nostrand Reinhold.

Shestack, R. (1977). *Handbook of physical therapy.* New York: Springer.

Skrastins, R., Merry, G. M., Rosenberg, G. M., & Schuman, J. E. (1982) Clinical assessment of the elderly patient. *Canadian Medical Association Journal, 127*(3), 203–206.

Slack Book Order Department, 6900 Grove Road, Thorofare, NJ 08086-9447, Phone: 1-800-257-8290, Fax: (609) 853-5991, Order # 30543.

Smith, H. B. (1973). Smith hand function evaluation. *American Journal of Occupational Therapy, 27,* 244–251.

Stone, R., Cafferata, G., & Sangl, J. (1987). Caregivers of the frail elderly: A national profile. *The Gerontologist, 27*(5), 616–626.

Tideiksaar, R. (1986). Preventing falls: Home hazard checklists to help older patients protect themselves. *Geriatrics, 41,* 26–29.

Tracey, C. A. (1989). Etiologies of the nursing diagnosis of self-care deficit. In R. Carroll-Johnson (Ed.), *Classification of nursing diagnoses: Proceedings of the eighth national conference* (pp. 349–351). Philadelphia: J. B. Lippincott Company.

Uniform Data System for Medical Rehabilitation. (1990). *Guide to the Uniform Data Set.* New York: State University of New York at Buffalo.

Vitaliano, P., Russo, J., Young, H., Becker, J., & Maiuro, R. (1991). The screen for caregiver burden. *The Gerontologist, 31*(1), 76–83.

Watson, P. G. (1987). Family participation in the rehabilitation process: The rehabilitators' perspective. *Rehabilitation Nursing, 13,* 70–73.

Watts, J. H., Brollier, C., Bauer, D., & Schmidt, W. (1989). The assessment of occupational functioning: The second revision. *Occupational Therapy in Mental Health, 8*(4), 61–67.

Williams, J. H., Drinka, T. J., Greenberg, J. R., Farrell-Holtan, J., Euhardy, R., & Schram, M. (1991). Development and testing of the assessment of living skills and resources (ALSAR) in elderly community-dwelling veterans. *The Gerontologist, 31*(1), 84–91.

Williams, S., & Bloomer, J. (1987). *Bay area functional performance evaluation* (2nd ed.). Palo Alto, CA: Consulting Psychologist Press.

Zarit, S. H., Orr, N. K., & Zarit, J. M. (1985). *The hidden victims of Alzheimer's disease: Families under stress.* New York: New York University Press.

Zarit, S. H., Reever, K., & Bach-Peterson, J. (1980). Relatives of the impaired elderly: Correlates of feelings of burden. *The Gerontologist, 20*(6), 649–655.

Assessment of Activities of Daily Living

evaluating the construct validity of the FIM have been completed. These include studies of patterns of difficulty with the motor and cognitive FIM items (Granger et al., 1993), prediction of burden of care (Granger et al., 1990), ability of the FIM to measure changes in motor and cognitive function during rehabilitation (Heinemann et al., 1993), patterns of results of items on the FIM when subjected to Rasch analysis (Heinemann et al., 1993), and prediction of rehabilitation outcome after stroke (Oczkowski & Barreca, 1993).

OVERALL UTILITY

The FIM is a clear and concise self-care assessment whose primary purpose is to evaluate change over time in rehabilitation programs. Its observer reliability and validity for program evaluation use have been well established. Therapists should be cautioned not to use the FIM for evaluation of change in individual clients, as it is less responsive in this situation.

Functional Status Index

The Functional Status Index (FSI) was developed as part of a Pilot Geriatric Arthritis Program and is designed for use in a program evaluation for clients with arthritis. It is available from Allen M. Jette, PT, MGH Institute of Health Professions, 15 River Street, Boston, MA 02108-3402.

CLINICAL UTILITY

The FSI is a self-report tool in which clients are asked to rate their performance as well as the degree of pain and difficulty in accomplishing tasks. The FSI includes 18 items in the areas of gross mobility, hand activities, personal care, home chores, and social activities. It has four personal care items. Clients are asked to rate degree of assistance for each activity on a scale of 0 to 4, with 0 indicating independent and 4, unable or unsafe to do the activity. Clients are then asked to rate the degree of pain and the degree of difficulty on a scale of 1 to 4 with 1 meaning no pain or no difficulty and 3, severe pain or severe difficulty. Completion time is approximately 20 to 30 minutes.

STANDARDIZATION AND RELIABILITY

The FSI is a standardized instrument, and a manual is available. Using coefficient alpha, the internal consistency of the FSI categories ranged from 0.23 for hand activities to 0.81 for social and role activities. Internal consistency of personal care was 0.67. Using interclass correlation coefficients, interrater reliability ranges from 0.64 for hand activities to 0.89 for social and role activities (Jette, 1987). Test-retest reliability ranges from 0.40 for social and role activities to 0.87 for home chores. Personal care is 0.82.

Reliability for the pain and difficulty indices are also in the acceptable range.

VALIDITY

The FSI was developed using extensive information from previous self-care measures and from the literature followed by factor analysis to reduce the number of items from 45 to 18. Correlations of the FSI with health professional assessments, including Arthritis and Rheumatism Association (ARA) functional classification, ARA stage of disease, and professional global assessment of function and disease activity, ranged from 0.25 to 0.49 (Jette, 1987). Rates of agreement between the FSI and observation of performance in self-care and IADL tasks ranged from 0.77 to 0.95.

OVERALL UTILITY

The FSI is a well-developed assessment that covers a number of domains applicable to clients with arthritis. Its reliability and validity have been well tested.

Goal Attainment Scaling

Goal attainment scaling (GAS) is a method of evaluating the effectiveness of the therapy intervention. Through this process, goals are set in collaboration with clients, and changes over time are documented and scored. It is applicable to all clients. GAS is a methodology that is available at no cost from Stolee and associates (1992), Cot & Finch (1991), or Ottenbacher & Cusick (1990).

CLINICAL UTILITY

Goal attainment scaling assesses change in performance on specific goals in self-care. The goals are set by rehabilitation professionals, usually in collaboration with clients.

There is a standard procedure for GAS. A specific problem area in self-care is identified. The expected level of performance is then set. Levels of performance attainment that are less than expected and better than expected are then set. The expected level of performance is rated 0, and other levels are rated from +2 to −2. After intervention, the achieved level of performance is scored according to the five attainment levels that had been preset. Change scores for single or multiple goals can be calculated using a standard score expressed as a T score. T scores have a mean equal to 50 and a standard deviation of 10. Completion time ranges from 15 to 45 minutes for each client.

STANDARDIZATION AND RELIABILITY

Standard procedures have been established and outlined in the literature for using GAS. The mathematic calculations of GAS are complex. For reliability, internal consistency has not been reported. Interclass correlation scores of 0.87 to 0.88 were obtained between physician and primary care nurses with 15 seniors in a geriatric program (Stolee et al., 1992). Substantial training of rehabilitation personnel is required to ensure consistency in goal setting across individuals. Test-retest reliability has not been reported.

VALIDITY

Content validity is ensured because GAS is an individualized measure and the content is determined individually by each client. In the study by Stolee and colleagues (1992), the correlation of GAS scores with global outcome rating was 0.82. The authors also found that the correlation of change in GAS score to change in Barthel was 0.86. The average change in GAS score was a gain of 23.9 points (standard deviation was 7.4), compared with a gain on the Barthel index of 18.3 points (standard deviation was 19.8).

OVERALL UTILITY

Goal attainment scaling represents a useful method to measure change in individualized goals in clients. It is useful in multidisciplinary settings and can apply to all clients. It is more suitable as a clinical rather than a research tool. The training to ensure consistency of GAS application has been found to be extensive. Also, mathematic calculation of the GAS is complex and controversial.

Katz Index of Activities of Daily Living

The Katz Index is a short ADL index designed to classify individuals in rehabilitation who have self-care problems and to predict need for later attendant requirements. It is available in the article by Katz and coworkers (1970).

CLINICAL UTILITY

The Index of ADL is scored by a rehabilitation professional after observation of client behavior. The Index of ADL includes six items, one each for bathing, dressing, toileting, transfers, continence, and feeding. Each item is scored on a nominal scale of independence or dependence. Completion time is 30 minutes.

STANDARDIZATION AND RELIABILITY

No instruction administration manual is available for the Katz Index of ADL. Some of the administration instructions, particularly related to intermediate descriptions of function, may be confusing. Internal consistency has not been reported. Interrater reliability, measured using observer agreement, is adequate. Test-retest has not been reported.

VALIDITY

In developing the Katz Index of ADL, the authors used items from the literature. Guttman scaling was used to confirm the hierarchic nature of the index. The Katz has been compared to the Barthel Index and the Kenny Self-Care Evaluation (Gresham, Phillips & Labi, 1980) and was found to be less responsive than either measure. In a study of 194 nursing home residents, correlation between the Katz and the Sickness Impact profile was found to be 0.39 (Mulrow et al., 1994).

OVERALL UTILITY

The Katz Index of ADL is a quick, simple, basic self-care assessment. Its most clinically useful purpose is as a descriptive or predictive assessment to gather information efficiently about self-care.

Kenny Self-Care Evaluation

The Kenny Self-Care Evaluation (Iverson et al., 1973) describes self-care abilities and evaluates changes in self-care over time in adults involved in rehabilitation. It is available from the Kenny Rehabilitation Institute, 1800 Chicago Avenue, Minneapolis MN 55404. Cost is limited to the cost of printing the measure.

CLINICAL UTILITY

Items on the Kenny are scored by therapists after observation. The evaluation contains 17 items rated from 0 to 4, with 0 indicating dependent and 4, independent. Items evaluated include bed activities, transfers, locomotion, dressing, personal hygiene, and feeding. Instructions and format are concise and easy to follow. Each of the seven categories of self-care is broken down into specific tasks for that activity. The activities are scored 0 to 4, and a category score is calculated that is the average of the activities scores. Completion time is usually less than 1 hour.

STANDARDIZATION AND RELIABILITY

An administration manual with instructions is available. Internal consistency has not been reported. Interrater reliability is good (0.74), except for locomotor items (0.42) (Kerner & Alexander, 1981). Test-retest reliability has not been reported.

VALIDITY

The Kenny Evaluation appears to adequately cover the domain of self-care assessment. Its ability to detect change in self-care assessment is greater than the Barthel or the Katz (Donaldson et al., 1973). Studies of its construct validity have not been reported.

OVERALL UTILITY

The Kenny Self-Care Evaluation provides a clear and concise reading form to assess physical self-care tasks. It appears to adequately cover the domain of self-care activities. A limited number of reliability and validity studies are available for this measure.

Klein-Bell Activities of Daily Living Scale

The Klein-Bell ADL Scale was developed specifically to evaluate change in self-care abilities over time for adults in rehabilitation and children encountering problems in self-care. It is available from HSCER Distribution, HSBT 281 SB 56, University of Washington, Seattle, WA 98195. The cost of a manual, which includes scoresheets, is $10, plus $5 for shipping.

CLINICAL UTILITY

The Klein-Bell is administered by a therapist, and scoring is based on direct observation of task performance. This scale documents basic ADL in the areas of dressing, elimination, mobility, bathing, hygiene, eating, and emergency telephone communication. Each area has been broken down into specific tasks so that there are 170 items on the scale. Tasks are scored as achieved or not achieved. Individuals who use adapted equipment to complete a task also receive an achievement score. Scores are totaled and can be profiled on a graph for interpretation to clients and others. The assessment takes approximately 1 hour to complete.

STANDARDIZATION AND RELIABILITY

The Klein-Bell is a standardized assessment, and a manual with instruction forms is available. Internal consistency reliability has not been reported. Interrater agreement of 92% was reported (Klein & Bell, 1982). In using the Klein-Bell assessment with children, interrater reliability was 0.96 (Law & Usher, 1987). Test-retest reliability has not been reported.

VALIDITY

The Klein-Bell ADL Scale was developed using specific criteria to yield a measure that would be sensitive to small changes in functioning. The authors used information from previous scales and from the literature to develop the items. Criterion validity has not been reported. A correlation of

−0.86 was found between Klein-Bell score discharge and amount of personal care assistance required, indicating that assistance increases as Klein-Bell score decreases (Klein & Bell, 1982). Scores on the Klein-Bell Scale were able to indicate children who had self-care problems due to disability (Law & Usher, 1987). Law & Usher also found that the Klein-Bell Scale was responsive to changes over time, as indicated by therapist and parent judgmental change. Unruh and others (1993) found that parent reports of children's function on the Klein-Bell Scale agreed with therapist ratings more that 85% of the time.

OVERALL UTILITY

The Klein-Bell ADL Scale was developed to be sensitive to small changes in function over time. It has been shown to be reliable and valid in measuring change in ADL. The Klein-Bell is most suitable to use in clinical situations when therapists want very specific information about a client's self-care function and wish to have a measure that is sensitive to small changes in self-care ability over the course of rehabilitation.

Patient Evaluations Conference System

The PECS was developed to help set goals for adult rehabilitation clients and to evaluate progress toward meeting these goals. It is available from Dr. R. Harvey, Marianjoy Hospital, P.O. Box 795, Wheaton, IL 60189.

CLINICAL UTILITY

The PECS includes 79 items covering domains of self-care, mobility, travel, home management, medical condition, mental capacity, work resources, social interaction, and communication. Only eight items on the PECS address self-care directly. Each item is scored on an ordinal scale of 1 to 7, with 1 being total dependence and 7 being total independence. A goal score is also identified. The PECS is completed by rehabilitation professionals based on their observation of client performance. Each section of the PECS is completed by the service provider most appropriate for that section. Completion time has not been reported.

STANDARDIZATION AND RELIABILITY

The PECS has undergone many standardization studies. A complete manual is available. Much of the standardization work for the PECS has been the completion of Rasch analysis to ensure that the PECS can provide interval level measurement. Internal consistency has not been reported. Interrater reliability ranges from 0.68 to 0.80, while test-retest reliability has not been reported.

VALIDITY

Studies on the PECS have indicated four factors: cognitive competence, motoric competence, applied self-care, and impairment severity (Silverstein et al., 1991). The results of the studies using Rasch analysis have indicated that the self-care tasks increase in difficulty, with the easiest task being performance in a bladder program and the most difficult task, knowledge of medications (Kilgore et al., 1993). Moderate correlations between PECS and Brief Symptom Inventory have been found (Jellinek et al., 1982). Change on the PECS during rehabilitation after head injury has been shown to relate to severity of brain lesion, as measured by computerized tomographic scan (Rao et al., 1984).

OVERALL UTILITY

The PECS appears to be a very comprehensive measure for use in setting rehabilitation goals and evaluating progress. Development of the PECS continues, with the primary recent focus being Rasch analysis to ensure the interval nature of the assessment. Further studies regarding the validity of the measure are required.

Physical Self-Maintenance Scale

The Physical Self-Maintenance Scale was developed as a measure to describe problems in the independent living status of elderly people in the hospital. It is available from the article by Lawton and Brody (1969).

CLINICAL UTILITY

The Physical Self-Maintenance Scale includes six items in the areas of bathing, dressing, grooming, eating, toileting, and mobility. These items are scaled using a Guttman scale so that they are hierarchic. Clients are rated by the amount of assistance required for each task. The scale can be completed using a self-report format or by scoring based on direct observation of client performance. Completion time for scoring takes about 30 minutes. Extra time is necessary for observation of tasks.

STANDARDIZATION AND RELIABILITY

The Physical Self-Maintenance Scale has clear and concise instructions, and an administration manual is available. Internal consistency has not been reported. Initial studies by Lawton and Brody (1969) indicated an interrater reliability coefficient of 0.96. Edwards (1990) also found interrater reliability of 0.96. Test-retest reliability, as measured by Edwards (1990), was $r = 0.59$.

VALIDITY

The Physical Self-Maintenance Scale was adapted from the Langley-Porter scale, so its content validity may be limited. A study by Rubenstein and coworkers (1984) found that self-report scores on the Physical Self-Maintenance Scale were significantly higher than scores on the Katz ADL. Studies by Edwards (1990) and Rubenstein and colleagues (1984) confirmed that the self-report format of the Physical Self-Maintenance Scale overestimates functional abilities. Scores on the Physical Self-Maintenance Scale were significantly higher for clients able to be discharged home (Edwards, 1990).

OVERALL UTILITY

The Physical Self-Maintenance Scale is a quick assessment of self-care abilities and provides useful information to describe the extent of self-care problems. In its observational format, it appears to be both reliable and valid. In the self-report format, it may overestimate functional abilities.

PULSES Profile

The PULSES profile is designed to provide a descriptive measure of severity of disability and to evaluate change over time in adults with physical impairments. It is available from the article by Moskowitz and McCann (1957).

CLINICAL UTILITY

Items on the PULSES profile are scored after observation of client performance by a rehabilitation professional. Scores are assigned using a four-point scale for items in areas of physical, upper extremity, lower extremity, abilities, sensory components, continence, and supports. In total, the PULSES profile includes 14 items in six areas. The PULSES takes 15 to 20 minutes to score. Clinical observation is independent of this time.

STANDARDIZATION AND RELIABILITY

Instructions for the PULSES profile are easy to follow. However, no administration manual is readily available. Internal consistency reliability has not been reported. Interrater and test-retest reliability over 0.87 has been found.

VALIDITY

The PULSES profile contains only 14 items to cover six self-care areas. Therefore, it does not fully sample the potential content for each area. A study comparing the Index of Independence in Activities of Daily Living, the

PULSES profile, and the Physical Self-Maintenance Scale (Settle & Holm, 1993) found that the PULSES profile did not provide enough information to plan rehabilitation intervention. Scores on the PULSES profile were higher for those who returned to an independent living situation after rehabilitation (Granger et al., 1979).

OVERALL UTILITY

The PULSES profile provides a comprehensive overview of self-care function but is not likely to be responsive to change because it is limited to a few items.

The Safety Assessment of Function and the Environment for Rehabilitation

The Safety Assessment of Function and the Environment for Rehabilitation (SAFER) tool is designed to evaluate seniors' abilities to function safely within their living environment (Oliver et al., 1993). Its primary purpose is to describe safety problems present within a living situation. Safety and self-care tasks are included in the measure. It is available from Community Occupational Therapy Associates (COTA), 3101 Bathurst Street, Suite 200, Toronto, Ontario M6A 2A6, Canada. Guidelines for administration and scoring, along with the SAFER measure, cost $75.00.

CLINICAL UTILITY

The SAFER is completed by the occupational therapist after observation of client performance in his or her living environment. The SAFER tool includes 97 items, which are scored on a dichotomous (problem/not a problem) scale. Items are scored after performance of self-care and other ADL and IADL tasks are observed in the living environment. Scores are calculated as the percentage of applicable items that are considered to be a safety problem. Completion time takes 20 minutes to 2 hours, depending on the nature of the living environment.

STANDARDIZATION AND RELIABILITY

The SAFER is a standardized measure, and guidelines for the administration and scoring of the tool are available. In a study with 56 community-dwelling seniors, the Kuder Richardson-20 internal consistency coefficient was 0.83. Observer and test-retest reliability are currently being tested.

VALIDITY

Content validity of the SAFER tool was established initially by searching for items within the literature and was followed by a review by a panel of occupational therapists and seniors. Items were defined and reviewed using a consensus procedure. Criterion and construct validity are currently being tested.

OVERALL UTILITY

The SAFER is a clinically useful assessment to evaluate safety. Reliability and validity testing is currently being completed.

Structured Assessment of Independent Living Skills

The Structured Assessment of Independent Living Skills (SAILS) was developed to assess everyday activities in clients with dementia to document or describe problems and potentially evaluate change over time. It is available from the article by Mahurin and colleagues (1991).

CLINICAL UTILITY

The SAILS is a criterion-based measure in which a number of test items are administered to a client and scored based on his or her performance at that time. It includes items in the areas of fine motor skills, gross motor skills, dressing skills, eating skills, cognitive tasks, receptive language, expressive language, time and orientation, money-related skills, instrumental activities, and social interaction. Most items are scored on a four-point scale, with 0 indicating no performance and 3, correct response to all items. Some items are also timed. Completion time ranges from 1 to 1.5 hours.

STANDARDIZATION AND RELIABILITY

The SAILS is a relatively new measure. A short manual with instructions is available from the authors. Standardization to date has involved preliminary studies using 36 individuals. An internal consistency study found an alpha coefficient of 0.90 for the SAILS. Interrater reliability between two raters was $r = 0.99$. In a study using 10 clients, test-retest reliability was 0.81 for total score and 0.97 for motor time (Mahurin et al., 1991).

VALIDITY

Items for the SAILS were selected after a review of current assessment techniques. Inclusion of items was based on three criteria: theoretic relevance, practicality, and gradation of task difficulty (Mahurin et al., 1991). Correlations of the SAILS were as follows: with the Geriatric Depression Scale, 0.39; with the Mini-Mental State Exam, 0.60; with the Weschler Adult Intelligence Scale, 0.73 to 0.79; and with the Global Deterioration Scale, 0.69. Scores on the SAILS for a group of clients with Alzheimer's disease were significantly lower than those of a control group of elderly clients who were the same age and had similar years of education.

OVERALL UTILITY

The SAILS is a new measure and has received limited psychometric testing. It appears to provide clinically useful information in a number of self-care areas. Initial testing for reliability and validity demonstrated acceptable reliability and construct validity.

The Structured Observational Test of Function

The Structured Observation Test of Function (SOTOF) is designed as a simultaneous descriptive assessment of self-care abilities of older adults and underlying neuropsychological function contributing to these abilities. It is available from NFER-Nelson Publishing Company, Darville House, 2 Oxford Road East, Windsor Brookshire, England SL4 1DF. The cost for a complete set, including the manual, five instruction cards, 50 record forms, and 25 ADL neuropsychological record forms is $59.95.

CLINICAL UTILITY

In the SOTOF, abilities for self-care tasks are rated by a clinician after direct observation of performance in these tasks. The SOTOF includes a brief screening assessment to describe sight, hearing, balance, comprehension, and limb function. Clients are then observed doing four self-care tasks: eating from a bowl, washing hands, pouring and drinking liquid, and putting on a long-sleeved shirt. A number of items are listed under each task, and the client's ability to do or not to do each task is recorded. Also included is room for information about further problems or assessments and what neuropsychological functions may be contributing to performance difficulties with each task. The SOTOF does not give an overall score because its main purpose is to enable the clinician to describe difficulties that the client is encountering and to use that information to plan intervention. Each of the four ADL tasks takes 10 minutes to complete.

STANDARDIZATION AND RELIABILITY

The SOTOF is a standardized assessment, and manual rating forms and complete instructions are available. Internal consistency was examined by testing consistency between performance on the four SOTOF ADL tasks and the deficit items for each task on the neuropsychological checklist. Results indicated high levels of consistency on the neuropsychological checklist but some variability across the four self-care tasks. The authors have recommended that all four tasks be given. Kappa statistics for interrater reliability were 0.92 for the screening assessment, 0.37 to

0.67 for the four self-care tasks, and 0.54 for the neuropsychological checklist. Test-retest reliability using Kappa statistics were 0.92 for the screening assessment, 0.5 to 0.77 for the four self-care tasks, and 0.55 for the neuropsychological assessment.

VALIDITY

The SOTOF was developed using a framework from the National Council of Medical Rehabilitation Research, which outlines an assessment model ranging from pathophysiology to impairment to functional limitation to disability. The four tasks that are evaluated cover important self-care tasks and can be used to identify major neuropsychological problems leading to difficulties in self-care. Correlations above 0.05 level of statistical significance were found between the SOTOF and other measures such as the River-Mead Perceptual Reception Battery, National Adult Reading Test, Chesington OT Neurological Assessment Battery, and River-Mead ADL Assessment for Stroke Patients. Deficits of ADL performance and a neuropsychological on the SOTOF were found to be very similar to those deficits identified on other measures used in the criteria validity study.

OVERALL UTILITY

The SOTOF is a very new measure that combines direct observation of self-care tasks with an analysis of the neuropsychological functions underlying performance or difficulties in performances with these tasks. For a new measure, the SOTOF has had considerable standardization and research. A clinical utility study was used to ensure that the SOTOF was easily understood and quick to administer. The SOTOF currently has evidence of adequate observer and test-retest reliability and initial evidence of criterion and construct validity. Further use by clinicians and more research will contribute to our knowledge of the utility of this measure.

GLOSSARY

Clinical utility—The overall usefulness of an assessment in a clinical situation, including its ease of administration and interpretation of scores, reasonable cost, and time to complete.

Construct validity—The ability of an assessment to perform as hypothesized (e.g., individuals discharged to an independent living situation should score higher on a self-care assessment than individuals discharged to a long-term care living situation).

Content validity—The comprehensiveness of an assessment and its inclusion of items that fully represent the attribute being measured.

Criterion validity—The ability of an assessment to truly measure a certain attribute when compared with an external standard (e.g., another assessment of the same attribute).

Reliability—The consistency of an assessment score under different administration conditions, such as at different times (test-retest reliability) or with different therapists (observer reliability).

Responsiveness—The ability of an assessment to measure change in performance over time in situations where change truly occurs. Responsiveness is a type of construct validity for assessments used to measure change over time.

REFERENCES

Buchwald, E. (1949). Functional training. *Physical Therapy Review, 29,* 491–496.

Canadian Association of Occupational Therapists. (1991). *Occupational therapy guidelines for client-centered practice.* Toronto, Ontario: CAOT Publications ACE.

Cot, C., & Finch, E. (1991). Goal setting in physical therapy practise. *Physiotherapy Canada, 43,* 19–22.

DeHaan, R. D., Horn, J., Limburg, M., Van Der Meulen, J., & Bossuyt, P. (1993). Comparison of five stroke scales with measures of disability handicap and quality of life. *Stroke, 24,* 1178–1181.

Donaldson, S. W., Wagner, C. C., & Gresham, G. E. (1973). A unified ADL evaluation form. *Archives of Physical Medicine and Rehabilitation, 54,* 175–179.

Edwards, M. M. (1990). The reliability and validity of self-report activities of daily living skills. *Canadian Journal of Occupational Therapy, 57,* 273–278.

Feinstein, A. R., Josephy, M. S., & Wells, C. K. (1986). Scientific and clinical problems in indexes of functional disability. *Annals of Internal Medicine, 105,* 413–420.

Fisher, A. G. (1994). *Assessment of motor and process skills manual.* Fort Collins, CO: Colorado State University.

Fortinsky, R. H., Granger, C. V., & Seltzer, G. B. (1981). The use of functional assessment in understanding home-care needs. *Medical Care, 19,* 489–497.

Gowland, C., Torresin, W., Stratford, P., Ward, M., VanHullenaar, S., Moreland, J., & Sanford, J. (1992). Chedoke-McMaster Stroke Assessment: A comprehensive clinical measure. *Physiotherapy Canada, 44,* 13–19.

Granger, C. V., Albrecht, G. L., & Hamilton, B. B. (1979). Outcome of comprehensive medical rehabilitation measurement by Pulses Profile and the Barthel index. *Archives of Physical Medicine and Rehabilitation, 60,* 145–154.

Granger, C. V., Cotter, A. C., Hamilton, B. B., Fiedler, R. C., & Hens, M. M. (1990). Functional assessment skills: A study of persons with multiple sclerosis. *Archives of Physical Medicine and Rehabilitation, 71,* 870–875.

Granger, C. V., Hamilton, B. B., Linacre, J. M., Heinemann, A. W., & Wright, B. D. (1993). Performance profiles of the Functional Independence Measure. *American Journal of Physical Medicine and Rehabilitation, 72,* 84–89.

Granger, C. V., Hamilton, B. B., & Sherwin, F. S. (1986). *Guide for use of the Uniform Data Set for medical rehabilitation.* Buffalo, NY: Buffalo General Hospital.

Gresham, G. E., Phillips, T. F., & Labi, M. L. C. (1980). ADL status in stroke: Relative merits of three standard indexes. *Archives of Physical Medicine and Rehabilitation, 61*(8), 355–358.

Harvey, R. F., & Jellinek, H. M. (1981). Functional performance assessment: A program approach. *Archives of Physical Medicine and Rehabilitation, 62,* 456–461.

Hebert, R., Carier, R., & Bilodeau, A. (1988). The functional autonomy measurement system (SMAF): Description and validation of an instrument for the measurement of handicaps. *Age and Aging, 17,* 293–302.

Heinemann, A. W., Linacre, J. M., Wright, B. D., Hamilton, B. B., & Granger, C. V. (1993). Relationships between impairment and physical disability as measured by the functional independence measure. *Archives of Physical Medicine and Rehabilitation, 74,* 566–573.

Iversen, I. A., Silberberg, N. E., Stever, R. C., & Schoening, H. A. (1973). *The revised Kenny Self-Care Evaluation: A numerical measure of independence in activities of daily living.* Minneapolis, MN: Sister Kenny Institute.

Jellinek, H. M., Torkelson, R. M., & Harvey, R. F. (1982). Functional abilities and distress levels in brain injured patients at long-term follow-up. *Archives of Physical Medicine and Rehabilitation, 63,* 160–162.

Jette, A. M. (1980). Functional Status Index: Reliability of the chronic disease evaluation instrument. *Archives of Physical Medicine and Rehabilitation, 61,* 395–401.

Jette, A. M. (1987). The Functional Status Index: Reliability and validity of the self-report functional disability measure. *Journal of Rheumatology, 14,* 15–19.

Katz, S., Downs, T. D., Cash, H. R., & Grotz, R. C. (1970). Progress in the development of ADL. *The Gerontologist, 10,* 20–30.

Keith, R. A. (1984). Functional assessment measures in medical rehabilitation: Current status. *Archives of Physical Medicine and Rehabilitation, 65,* 74–78.

Kerner, J. F., & Alexander, J. (1981). Activities of Daily Living: Reliability and validity of gross vs. specific ratings. *Archives of Physical Medicine and Rehabilitation, 62,* 161–166.

Kilgore, K. M., Fisher, W. P., Silverstein, B., Harley, P., & Harvey, R. F. (1993). Application of Rasch analysis to the patient evaluation conference system. *Physical Medicine Rehabilitation Clinics of North America, 4,* 493–515.

Kivela, S. L. (1984). Measuring disability—Do self-ratings and service provider ratings compare? *Journal of Chronic Disease, 37,* 27–36.

Klein, R. M., & Bell, B. (1982). Self-care skills: Behavioral measurement with the Klein-Bell ADL scale. *Archives of Physical Medicine and Rehabilitation, 63,* 335–338.

Klein-Paris, C., Clermont-Michel, T., & O'Neill, J. (1986). Effectiveness and efficiency of criterion testing versus interviewing for collecting functional assessment information. *American Journal of Occupational Therapy, 40,* 486–491.

Laver, A., & Powell, G. (1995). *The Structured Observational Test of Function.* Windsor Brookshire, England: NFER-Nelson Publishing Company.

Law, M. (1993). Measuring activities of daily living: Directions for the future. *American Journal of Occupational Therapy, 47,* 233–237.

Law, M., Baptiste, S., Carswell, A., McColl, M., Polatajko, H., & Pollock, N. (1991). *The Canadian Occupational Performance Measure.* Toronto: CAOT Publications.

Law, M., Baptiste, S., Carswell, A., McColl, M., Polatajko, H., & Pollock, N. (1994a). *Canadian Occupational Performance Measure, second edition.* Toronto: CAOT Publications.

Law, M., & Letts, L. (1989). A critical review of scales of activities of daily living. *American Journal of Occupational Therapy, 43,* 522–528.

Law, M., Polatajko, H., Pollock, N., McColl, M. A., Carswell, A., & Baptiste, S. (1994b). Pilot Testing of the Canadian Occupational Performance Measure: Clinical and measurement issues. *Canadian Journal of Occupational Therapy, 61,* 191–197.

Law, M., & Usher, P. (1987). Validation of the Klein-Bell ADL scale for pediatric occupational therapy. *Canadian Journal of Occupational Therapy, 55,* 63–68.

Lawton, M. P., & Brody, E. M. (1969). Assessment of older people: Self-maintaining in instrumental activities of daily living. *Gerontologist, 9,* 179–186.

Letts, L., & Marshall, L. (1995). *Evaluating the validity and consistency of the Safer tool.* Toronto, Ontario: Community Occupational Therapy Associates. Unpublished manuscript.

Long, W. B., Sacco, W. J., Coombes, S. S., Copes, W. S., Bullock, A., & Melville, J. K. (1994). Determining normative standards for Functional Independence Measure, transitions in rehabilitation. *Archives of Physical Medicine and Rehabilitation, 75,* 144–148.

Mahoney, S. I., & Barthel, D. W. (1965). Functional evaluation: The Barthel Index. *Maryland State Medical Journal, 14,* 61–65.

Mahurin, R. K., DeBettignies, B. H., & Pirozzolo, F. J. (1991). Structured Assessment of Independent Living Skills: Preliminary report of performance measure of functional abilities in dementia. *Journal of Gerontology, 46,* 58–66.

Merbitz, C., Morris, J., & Grip, C. (1989). Ordinal scales and foundations of misinference. *Archives of Physical Medicine and Rehabilitation, 70,* 308–312.

Moskowitz, E., & McCann, C. B. (1957). Classification of disability in the chronically ill and aging. *Journal of Chronic Disease, 5,* 342–346.

Mulrow, C. D., Gerety, M. B., Cornell, J. E., Lawrence, B. A., & Canten, D. N. (1994). The relationship between disease and function and perceived health in very frail elders. *Journal of the American Geriatrics Society, 42,* 374–380.

Nakayama, H., Jorgensen, H. S., Raaschou, H. O., & Olsen, T. S. (1994). The influence of age on stroke outcome: A Copenhagen stroke study. *Stroke, 25,* 808–813.

Nygard, L., Bernspang, B., Fisher, A. G., & Winblad, B. (1993). Comparing motor and process ability in home versus clinical settings with persons with suspected dementia. *American Journal of Occupational Therapy, 48,* 689–696.

Oczkowski, W. J., & Barreca, S. (1993). The Functional Indepence Measure: Its use to identify rehabilitation needs in stroke survivors. *Archives of Physical Medicine and Rehabilitation, 74,* 1291–1294.

Oliver, R., Blathwayt, J., Brackley, C., & Tamaki, T. (1993). Development of the safety assessment of function in the environment for rehabilitation (Safer tool). *Canadian Journal of Occupational Therapy, 60,* 78–82.

Ottenbacher, K. J., & Cusick, A. (1990). Goal attainment scaling as a method of clinical service evaluation. *American Journal of Occupational Therapy, 44,* 519–525.

Park, S., Fisher, A. G., & Velozo, C. A. (1993). Using the Assessment of Motor and Process Skills to compare performance between home and clinical settings. *American Journal of Occupational Therapy, 48,* 697–709.

Ranhoff, A. H., & Laake, K. (1993). The Barthel ADL Index: Scoring by the physician from patient interview is not reliable. *Age and Aging, 22,* 171–174.

Rao, N., Jellinek, H. M., Harvey, R. F., & Flynn, M. M. (1984). Computerized tomography head scans as predictors of rehabilitation outcome. *Archives of Physical Medicine and Rehabilitation, 65,* 18–20.

Rubenstein, L. Z., Schairer, C., Wieland, G. D., & Kane, R. (1984). Systematic bases in functional status assessment of elderly adults: Effects of different data sources. *Journal of Gerontology, 39,* 686–691.

Settle, C., & Holm, M. B. (1993). Program planning: The clinical utility of three activities of daily living assessment tools. *American Journal of Occupational Therapy, 487,* 911–918.

Shah, S., & Cooper, B. (1991). Documentation for measuring stroke rehabilitation outcomes. *Australian Medical Record Journal, 21,* 88–95.

Shiner, D., Gross, C. R., Bronstein, K. S., Licata-Gehr, A. E., Eden, D. T., Cabrera, A. R., Fishman, I. G., Roth, A. A., Barwick, J. A., & Kunitz, S. C. (1987). Reliability of the activities of daily living scale and its use in telephone interview. *Archives of Physical Medicine and Rehabilitation, 68,* 723–728.

Silverstein, B., Kilgore, K. M., Fisher, W. P., Harley, J. P., & Harvey, R. F. (1991). Applying psychometric criteria to functional assessment in medical rehabilitation: 1. Exploring unidimensionality. *Archives of Physical Medicine and Rehabilitation, 72,* 631–637.

Stolee, P., Rockwood, K., Fox, R. A., & Streiner, D. L. (1992). The use of goal attainment scaling in a geriatric care setting. *Journal of the American Geriatrics Society, 40,* 574–578.

Streiner, D. L., & Norman, G. R. (1989). *Health Measurement Scales: A practical guide to their development and use.* New York: Oxford Medical Publications.

Unruh, A. M., Fairchild, S., & Versnel, J. (1993). Parent's and therapist's rating of self-care skills in children with spina bifida. *Canadian Journal of Occupational Therapy, 60,* 145–148.

Wilcox, A. (1994). *A study of verbal guidance for children with developmental coordination disorder.* London, Ontario: University of Western Ontario. Unpublished Masters thesis.

Wylie, C. M. (1967). Measuring end results of rehabilitation of patients with stroke. *Public Health Report, 82,* 893–898.

OBSERVATIONAL GAIT ANALYSIS

The clinician typically divides gait into a stance and a swing phase. Within each of these phases it is possible to describe observed deviations from the expected normal gait pattern. To do this the therapist must either be very familiar with normal parameters of gait or at times may be able to make comparison to the contralateral and less involved limb. However, these observations are subjective and somewhat vague. For example, range of motion of a specific joint may be simply described as normal, excessive, or decreased. It may be that a clinician will attempt to indicate the motions at a joint through the gait cycle. Thus, for a patient whose motion at the ankle is limited to minus 5 degrees of dorsiflexion, the clinician will probably observe initial contact with the flat foot, an early heel rise during mid-stance and possibly a weak push-off. In swing the clinician notes increased knee flexion to ensure toe clearance. Although there appears to be limited push-off, the clinician thinks that the contralateral step length is shorter owing to the shortened ipsilateral stance time. Clearly, other inferences could be made about joint motions or timing and distance data but the information would be subjective, making it very difficult to eventually document specific changes after treatment.

Patla and colleagues (1987) developed a questionnaire to determine the need and usefulness of live visual observation of gait. The questionnaire was given to 24 physical therapists in a multidisciplinary rehabilitation center. The results of the questionnaire indicated that gait analysis was a necessary clinical tool especially for amputees, neurologic patients, and patients with a pathologic process in the lower extremity. Most clinicians expressed confidence in their ability to identify gait deviations but that recording methods (e.g., video) could be helpful, although there was some apprehension in using complex equipment. It appeared that most clinicians performed a comprehensive analysis of a patient's gait where time and distance parameters of stride length and cadence were determined to be extremely important, especially in the sagittal plane. Unfortunately, the final report from the therapist was a simple and brief narrative with no apparent evidence that these comments were determined by those gait parameters observed. The authors concluded that a more automated recording system is needed and that reliability and validity data are required for visual observation of gait.

Goodkin and Diller (1973) reported on the reliability of live visual analysis of gait. There was a high percentage of agreement between therapists on such gait deviations as trunk bending, knee flexion and extension, and vaulting. Less agreement was noted for deviations such as adduction, circumduction, and hip rotation. The therapists were simply asked to rate these motions as being either acceptable, needs to be minimized, or needs to be encouraged. However, little agreement was reported when therapists were asked to name the patient's two major deviations.

These authors also recommended the development of recording devices to more objectively assess a patient's gait performance.

It is not surprising, therefore, that many advocate video recording as a preferred method of gait observation as opposed to live visual observation. A video recording of a patient's gait pattern has many advantages for the patient as well as the therapist when compared with visual analysis (Turnbull & Wall, 1985). The recording would clearly provide a record that could be used as the basis for comparison against other patients or normal subjects or between visits by the same patient. The patient would need to walk far less because the recording could be played over and over as the therapist observed and made notes of the gait, thus avoiding possible fatigue. The recording could be slowed down to better see rapid movements and even stopped on a given frame to better assess a given event or body configuration. It is not only amusing to speed up the video recording but also enlightening because it may exaggerate, and therefore highlight, a gait deviation such as a lateral lurch filmed in the frontal plane. Those of you who have seen the Charlie Chaplin silent black and white movies will appreciate this point. Thus the subjective assessment of gait would be greatly enhanced by the use of video.

However, do the enhancements achieved through the use of video make gait assessment more reliable? Krebs and associates (1985) videotaped the gait of children with a lower limb disability that required the use of bilateral knee-ankle-foot orthoses. Experienced physical therapists were "well" trained to use an observational gait analysis form, as outlined in Figure 17–1, on which joint deviations were rated as noticeable, just noticeable, or very noticeable. Joint motion of children's gait was observed with and without their orthoses during stance phase only. Stance phase was further divided into early-, mid-, and late-stance. There were four rating sessions. Average full within-rater agreement (between observation sessions) was only 69 percent while the average between-rater agreement (within observation sessions) was 67.5 percent. The average within-rater Pearson product-moment correlation was $r = 0.60$. The average intraclass coefficient (ICC) for between-rater observations was 0.73. The authors concluded that even well-trained clinicians are only moderately reliable in recording gait deviations from videotape but, nevertheless, probably more reliable than live recording. We have only reported correlations across joints, phases of stance, and rating sessions. Krebs and colleagues (1985) appropriately indicate, however, that the observation of certain joints within certain planes (e.g., sagittal vs. frontal) for different phases of stance are more reliable than others. For example, the ICCs for observation of the hip in the frontal plane were higher than that in the transverse plane and the ICCs for observation of foot valgus and varus were comparatively low for all stance phases.

Eastlack and coworkers (1991) used a number of raters to record gait deviations from videotape of three patients with rheumatoid arthritis. They were specifically interested

Child Prosthetic-Orthotic Studies
New York University

KAPO Comparison Study
Form 1

OBSERVATIONAL GAIT ANALYSIS

Subject _____ Date _____ Examiner _____

Ambulator Aids: None   (1 or 2)   Axillary Crutches   (1 or 2)   Forearm Crutches   Cane   Walker   Rollator

Orthoses worn during this trial: Leather/Metal   Plastic/Metal   Hip Strap   Knees Locked

Key: 0:   Not Noticeable   +:   Just Noticeable   ++:   Very Noticeable

GAIT DEVIATIONS	HS-FF Early	LEFT FF-HO Mid	HO-TO Late	HS-FF Early	RIGHT FF-HO Mid	HO-TO Late	COMMENTS
Knee flexion							
Knee extension							
Hip flexion							
Hip extension							
Genu varum							
Genu valgum							
Hip adduction							
Hip abduction							
Hip internal rotation							
Hip external rotation							
Pes varus							
Pes valgus							

Step Length: L > > R   L = R   L < < R

FIGURE 17–1. Observational gait analysis rating form. Each cell was completed by all raters for all subjects. Raters noted 0 for normal gait, + for just noticeably abnormal gait, or ++ for very noticeably abnormal gait. (From Krebs, D. E., Edelstein, J. E., & Fishman, S. [1985]. Reliability of observational gait: Kinematic gait analysis. *Physical Therapy, 65,* 1027–1033, with the permission of the APTA.)

in motion at the knee at initial ground contact, mid-stance, heel-rise, and toe-off as well as genu valgum. The raters also monitored temporal and distance factors. The evaluation form is shown in Figure 17–2. However, to improve the reliability of gait observation they used slow and stop-action techniques, a strategy recommended by Krebs and colleagues (1985) after their study. Raters recorded knee flexion as being either inadequate, normal, or excessive and temporospatial factors (see Fig. 17–2) as decreased, normal, or increased. There was only slight to moderate agreement between raters. For knee motion the assessment of genu valgum received the highest agreement followed by knee flexion at mid-stance. For temporal and distance factors the raters showed moderate agreement on stride length. Genu valgum (ICC = 0.69) and stride length (ICC = 0.49) showed the highest ICC (2,1). The raters not being knowledgeable of the normal values of the variables being observed could explain the low-to-moderate values

reported in this study. The authors, however, made two interesting observations. First, although the reliability of gait observation was moderate at best in this study it probably is higher than the normal clinical assessment in which therapists do not use videotape analysis. Second, if raters were able to view a videotape of normal gait, then this would clearly facilitate observation techniques given the descriptive variables used to define joint motion in this study.

The previously mentioned studies only considered reliability (i.e., how reproduceable were the results obtained). Hughes and Bell (1994) measured both the reliability and validity of visual gait analysis of patients with hemiplegia. Validity measures how well the clinician's assessments agreed with those obtained from an objective measurement system. Patients were filmed and a split-screen technique was used to simultaneously show lateral and anteroposterior views of gait. The raters were experienced physical

TABLE 17-1

CHARACTERISTICS OF HEMIPLEGIC GAIT ACCORDING TO STAGE OF MOTOR RECOVERY

Variable	Stage of Motor Recovery				Total Patients n = 23	Normal n = 5
	3	*4*	*5*	*6*		
Walking speed (m/s)	0.16 ± 0.07	0.17 ± 0.08	0.40 ± 0.15	0.65 ± 0.11	0.31 ± 0.21	1.14 ± 0.10
Stride period (sec)	2.8 ± 0.7	2.8 ± 0.7	2.0 ± 0.4	1.4 ± 0.1	2.3 ± 0.8	1.2 ± 0.1
Cadence (steps/min)	45 ± 9	45 ± 9	63 ± 11	85 ± 9	57 ± 18	104 ± 9
Stride length (m)	0.41 ± 0.12	0.44 ± 0.16	0.73 ± 0.20	0.91 ± 0.09	0.60 ± 0.25	1.32 ± 0.12
Stance period (sec)						
Affected side	1.9 ± 0.7	1.9 ± 0.8	1.2 ± 0.3	0.89 ± 0.11	1.6 ± 0.7	0.68 ± 0.07
Unaffected side	2.5 ± 0.7	2.3 ± 0.8	1.5 ± 0.3	0.95 ± 0.13	1.9 ± 0.8	0.68 ± 0.08
Swing period (sec)						
Affected side	0.89 ± 0.21	0.88 ± 0.33	0.74 ± 0.12	0.53 ± 0.07	0.78 ± 0.25	0.48 ± 0.03
Unaffected side	0.34 ± 0.11	0.44 ± 0.11	0.52 ± 0.12	0.47 ± 0.06	0.44 ± 0.12	0.48 ± 0.03
Stance/swing ratio						
Affected side	2.4 ± 1.3	2.6 ± 1.7	1.7 ± 0.5	1.7 ± 0.3	2.1 ± 1.2	1.4 ± 0.1
Unaffected side	8.1 ± 3.2	6.0 ± 3.1	2.9 ± 0.7	2.1 ± 0.4	5.0 ± 3.2	1.4 ± 0.1
Double support (percent of stride)	54 ± 14	50 ± 15	34 ± 9	29 ± 5	43 ± 15	17 ± 2
Stance symmetry (affected/unaffected)	0.77 ± 0.11	0.82 ± 0.14	0.83 ± 0.09	0.94 ± 0.17	0.83 ± 0.12	1.00 ± 0.03
Swing symmetry (unaffected/affected)	0.41 ± 0.16	0.55 ± 0.21	0.70 ± 0.13	0.91 ± 0.19	0.62 ± 0.23	0.99 ± 0.02
Stance/swing ratio symmetry (affected/ unaffected)	0.33 ± 0.18	0.47 ± 0.22	0.59 ± 0.19	0.88 ± 0.30	0.53 ± 0.27	1.01 ± 0.06

From Brandstater, M. E., deBruin, H., Gowland, C., & Clark, B. (1983). Analysis of temporal variables. *Archives of Physical Medicine and Rehabilitation, 64,* 583–587.

(1994), gait velocity would have to either decrease by at least 4.54 m/min or increase by at least 9.30 m/min for the clinician to say with confidence that a real change due to therapeutic intervention actually took place. Respective limits for cadence were 14.89 and 18.29 steps/min and for stride length, 0.05 and 0.14 m. According to Hill and associates (1994), these broad confidence intervals are due to between-patient variability, whereas the strong correlation coefficients are the result of within-patient consistency between individual trials. The authors discuss potential strategies for reducing measurement error. If reduction of error can be achieved then clearly, such electrical contact systems could provide the clinician with an appropriate measuring device that is simple to use, that is relatively inexpensive when compared with motion analysis systems, and that provides objective data on time and distance parameters of gait that can be used to detect change in patient performance.

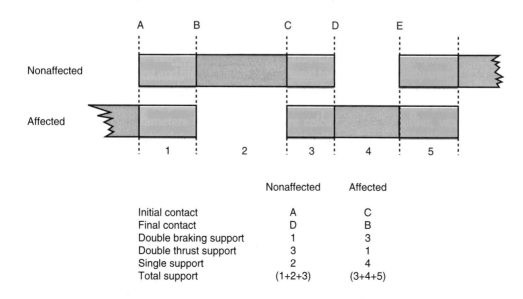

FIGURE 17-6. Temporal phases of gait cycle. A complete stride includes support and swing phases and is commonly regarded as starting with initial contact of one foot with ground and terminating with same foot again making contact (from A–E). Swing phase is equivalent to single support on contralateral side. (From Wall, J. C., & Turnbull, G. I. [1986]. Gait asymmetries in residual hemiplegia. *Archives of Physical Medicine and Rehabilitation, 67,* 550–553.)

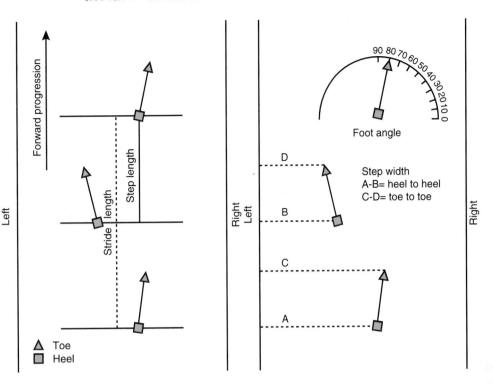

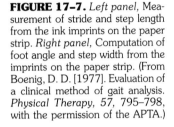

FIGURE 17–7. *Left panel,* Measurement of stride and step length from the ink imprints on the paper strip. *Right panel,* Computation of foot angle and step width from the imprints on the paper strip. (From Boenig, D. D. [1977]. Evaluation of a clinical method of gait analysis. *Physical Therapy, 57,* 795–798, with the permission of the APTA.)

ANALYSIS OF TEMPORAL AND DISTANCE PARAMETERS—SIMPLE CLINICAL ASSESSMENTS

There is a defined need for objective measurement of gait because without it the quality of treatment decisions is reduced because of the subjective and often unreliable nature of the assessment. Objective measures must also be employed if one is to demonstrate the efficacy of a treatment protocol, a function that will become increasingly important as health care resources become more strained and health care providers are held more accountable.

From the previous paragraphs it should now be evident that temporal and distance parameters of gait can provide meaningful measures of performance if measurement error is controlled. Other less expensive methods of obtaining temporal and distance gait parameters have been reported. Various attempts have been made to obtain footprint impressions. Boenig (1977) placed moleskin on the heel and toe of the shoe of healthy subjects. When the moleskin was saturated with ink then imprints of heel-strike and toe-off were left on a paper walkway. Measures of stride length, step width, step length, foot angle, and cadence were obtained. How these measures were recorded are shown in Figure 17–7. A stopwatch was used to determine the time taken to walk a predetermined length from which cadence (steps/min) was derived. Strong test-retest correlation coefficients were reported for stride length ($r = 0.925$), step length ($r = 0.972$), and cadence ($r = 0.905$). Obviously symmetry data could not be obtained because of the failure to measure the time of bilateral

heel-strike and toe-off during the walk. Shores (1980) actually had subjects stand in paint before walking, only to obtain similar data as Boenig (1977), although no reliability data were reported. Absorbent paper laid over a water-soaked material has also been recommended as a possible mechanism of obtaining footprint data (Clarkson, 1983).

In somewhat more comprehensive studies, Holden and coworkers (1984, 1986) used ink patches placed on patients' shoes and a digital stopwatch to derive timing and distance parameters of gait. They provided data on both interrater and test-retest reliability. Both patients with hemiparesis and multiple sclerosis were tested. Extremely high correlation coefficients were noted for gait velocity, cadence, step length, and stride length for interrater reliability for hemiplegic ($r = 0.99$ to 1.00) and multiple sclerosis patients ($r = 0.90$ to 1.00) and for test-retest reliability for the same patient groups ($r = 0.94$ to 0.97 and $r = 0.92$ to 0.98). Similar strong correlations were noted for test-retest reliability for patients placed in groups based on functional ambulation (Table 17–2). The ability of temporal and distance gait parameters to predict levels of ambulation was shown by r^2 values of 0.45 for gait velocity, 0.38 for cadence, 0.39 and 0.31 for step length, and 0.47 and 0.43 for stride length. The authors considered these values to be meaningful when the potential of variance within ambulation levels can be explained by a number of other different variables, such as age, gender, duration of disability, nature of clinical symptoms, and type of walking aid or orthosis. In a later paper (Holden et al., 1986) the temporal and distance parameters of gait were compared with selected clinical characteristics, ambulation category, and type of ambulation aid of the same group of patients. Their mean data for temporal distance parameters are

TABLE 17–2

TEST-RETEST RELIABILITY* OF TEMPORAL-DISTANCE MEASURES IN SUBJECTS WITH NEUROLOGIC IMPAIRMENTS BY FUNCTIONAL CATEGORY

Temporal-Distance Measure	Functional Ambulation Category				
	1 **Physical Assistance Level II** **(n = 10)**	**2** **Physical Assistance Level I** **(n = 15)**	**3** **Supervision** **(n = 6)**	**4** **Independent on Level** **(n = 8)**	**5** **Independent** **(n = 22)**
Velocity	0.97	0.94	0.94	0.99	0.95
Cadence	0.92	0.94	1.00	1.00	0.97
Left step length	0.95	0.98	0.53	0.94	0.93
Right step length	0.96	0.95	0.80	0.99	0.96
Left stride length	0.98	0.96	0.66	0.98	0.96
Right stride length	0.97	0.96	0.70	0.99	0.96
Left step length: stride length	0.97	0.95	0.68	0.98	0.95
Right step length: stride length	0.97	0.96	0.70	0.99	0.96
Step-time differential	0.91	0.99	0.72	0.94	0.98
Stride-time differential	0.18	0.57	0.23	0.97	0.19

*Pearson correlation coefficients.
From Holden, M. K., Gill, K. M., Magliozzi, M. R., Nathan, J., & Piehl-Baker, L. (1984). Clinical gait assessment in the neurologically impaired. *Physical Therapy, 64,* 35–40, with the permission of the APTA.

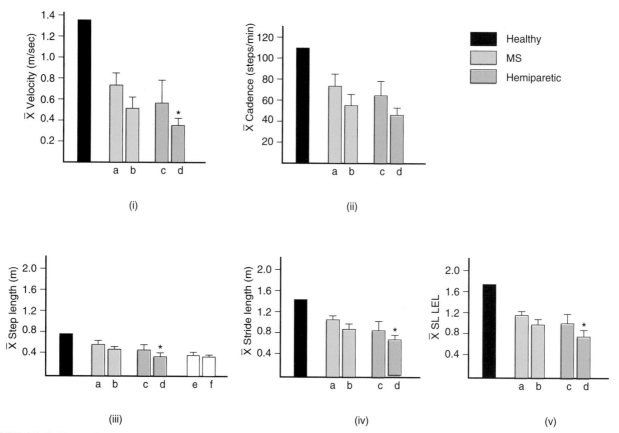

FIGURE 17–8. Mean values and 95 percent confidence intervals for five temporal-distance measures in neurologically impaired subjects (MS, n = 24; hemiparetic, n = 37). a, Functionally independent MS subjects (n = 12); b, all MS subjects; c, functionally independent hemiparetic subjects (n = 10); d, all hemiparetic subjects; e, hemiparetic involved lower extremity; and f, hemiparetic uninvolved lower extremity. Healthy values are weighted averages compiled from published values. *Asterisk* indicates significant difference from MS group (*P* < 0.03). (From Holden, M. K., et al. [1986]. Gait assessment for neurologically impaired patients. *Physical Therapy, 66,* 1530–1539, with the permission of the APTA.)

TABLE 17–3

RELATIONSHIP* OF AMBULATION AID USED AND FUNCTIONAL AMBULATION CATEGORY TO TEMPORAL-DISTANCE MEASURES

Temporal-Distance Measure	Ambulation Aid Category		Functional Ambulation Category	
	Hemiparesis†	*Multiple Sclerosis†*	*Hemiparesis†*	*Multiple Sclerosis†*
Velocity	−0.63	−0.85	0.59	0.80
Cadence	−0.69	−0.89	0.53	0.74
Step length	−0.47‡	−0.68	0.53	0.73
Stride length	−0.47‡	−0.69	0.54	0.73
Stride length: lower extremity length	−0.49‡	−0.72	0.52	0.71
Involved extremity step length	−0.31		0.55†	
Uninvolved extremity step length	−0.43		0.38	

*Spearman rank-order correlation coefficient.
†$P < 0.001$.
‡$P < 0.005$.
  Modified from Holden, M. K., Gill, K. M., & Magliozzi, M. R. (1986). Gait assessment for neurologically impaired patients. *Physical Therapy, 66,* 1530–1539, with the permission of the APTA.

shown in Figure 17–8. The data for healthy subjects were extrapolated from the literature. The differences between gait of healthy individuals and the sample of hemiparetic and multiple sclerosis patients is apparent. For hemiparetic patients, strong correlations were not noted between the temporal distance parameters of gait (see Fig. 17–8) and the clinical characteristics of age, duration of disability, number of clinical symptoms, and number of gait deviations ($r = 0.40$ to 0.28). Similar data were reported for the multiple sclerosis patients ($r = -0.35$ to $r = -0.19$). For both groups of patients more impressive correlations, however, were noted between time and distance parameters of gait and functional ambulation category and type of ambulation aid used. These correlations are shown in Table 17–3. Functional ambulation was categorized as the patient being able to ambulate independently on all surfaces, independently on level surfaces only, dependent for supervision, dependent for physical assistance (light touch), or dependent for physical assistance (support body weight). Type of ambulation aid was categorized as one cane or crutch, two canes or crutches, or a walker. As can be seen from Table 17–3, the stronger correlations were noted for the patients with multiple sclerosis. The relationship between velocity and cadence and the categories of ambulation aid and functional ambulation appear to be the most impressive for both groups of patients.

RECENT ADVANCES

Video technology has vastly improved in recent years, and features are available on modern videocassette recorders and camcorders produced for the home market that were only available to industrial users previously. Some of these features have allowed for the development of a number of techniques for objectively measuring the temporal and distance gait parameters from video. Gaudet and coworkers (1990) showed how step widths and step lengths could be accurately and reliably measured from video. They suggested that the technique could be improved if a camcorder had an automatic focus, a feature common to most camcorders currently available. Wall (1991) showed how the ability to advance a video through one field at a time and identify each field could be used to determine the temporal phases of the gait cycle. The validity and reliability of this technique has been reported on by Wall and Crosbie (1996a). Footswitches were placed on the heel and great toe of each foot and were connected to light-emitting diodes. The subjects were filmed by a video camera as they walked across a force plate ("gold standard"). The camera also filmed the image of the light-emitting diodes. A signal from a time code generator was added to the videotape. The timing data from the force plate and footswitches allowed the determination of right and left total support time, right step time, and right braking double support. For barefoot walking these values for data from the force plate were 0.76, 0.74, 0.59, and 0.15 second, respectively. Corresponding data from the footswitches were 0.75, 0.73, 0.59, and 0.16 second. Similar differences were noted for heel contact and toe-off where the switches tended to close after heel strike on the force plate and open before toe-off from the force plate. The data from the force plate and footswitches are indeed remarkably similar. However, the authors determined that their modified video-based system was more accurate for determining the times of heel contact and toe-off than the use of footswitches. Interrater reliability (ICC [2, 1]) for observation from the video of both right and left total support time was 0.94, for right step time, 0.95, and for right braking double-support, 0.46. The superb slow-motion capability afforded by videocassette recorders with four heads is the basis for a number of techniques to measure the durations of the temporal phases of the gait cycle. Timing can even be achieved with a multimemory stopwatch (Wall & Scarborough, 1996) or a personal computer (Wall & Crosbie, 1996b). Given the advantages of using video to enhance subjective assessment, the ability to obtain objective measurements from the recording should make these techniques very applicable to use in the clinical environment.

CONCLUSION

Gait assessment is an everyday responsibility for the practicing therapist. Visual assessment, which is almost universally used for this purpose, has been shown to be unreliable at best. Measurement of the temporal and distance factors of gait have been found to be clinically useful. It has been suggested that the use of video might be a helpful adjunct to visual assessment. Techniques that now allow for these measurements to be made objectively from a video recording have been developed and should prove useful for clinical use.

GLOSSARY

Cadence—Steps per minute.

Double support—Period of time during gait when both feet are in contact with the ground.

Electromyography—Provides information as to what muscles are active during gait.

Force platform—The output of the force platform is the ground reaction force.

Ground reaction force—Forces at the ground that react to the forces generated while walking.

Heel contact—Contact on the ground by the heel, which in normal gait signifies the beginning of stance.

Kinematics—Measures of movement without reference to the forces that cause the movement.

Stance phase—Period of time the foot is in contact with the ground during gait.

Step length—Heel contact of one foot to heel contact of the other foot, measured along the line of progression.

Stride—Heel contact of one foot to heel contact of the same foot (two steps).

Time code generator—Equipment that adds information on time to a video tape, allowing field identification.

Toe off—Foot leaving contact with the ground, which signifies the end of stance and the beginning of swing.

REFERENCES

Bajd, T., & Kralj, A. (1980). Simple kinematic gait measurements. *Journal of Biomedical Engineering, 2,* 129–132.

Boenig, D. D. (1977). Evaluation of a clinical method of gait analysis. *Physical Therapy, 57,* 795–798.

Brandstater, M. E., de Bruin, H., Gowland, C., & Clark, B. (1983). Hemiplegic gait: Analysis of temporal variables. *Archives of Physical Medicine and Rehabilitation, 64,* 583–587.

Cerny, K. (1983). A clinical method of quantitative gait analysis. *Physical Therapy, 63,* 1125–1126.

Cheung, C., Wall, J. C. & Zelin, S. (1983). A microcomputer based system for measuring the temporal phases of amputee gait. *Prosthetics and Orthotics International, 7,* 131–140.

Clarkson, B. H. (1983). Absorbent paper method for recording foot placement during gait. *Physical Therapy, 63,* 345–346.

Crouse, J. G., Wall, J. C., & Marble, A. L. (1987). Measurement of the temporal and spatial parameters of gait using a microcomputer based system. *Journal of Biomedical Engineering, 9,* 64–68.

Eastlack, M. E., Arvidson, J., Snyder-Mackler, L., Danoff, J. V., & McGarvey, C. L. (1991). Interrater reliability of videotaped observational gait-analysis assessments. *Physical Therapy, 71,* 465–472.

Gaudet, G., Goodman, R., Landry, M., Russell, G., & Wall, J. C. (1990). Measurement of step length and step width: A comparison of videotape and direct measurement. *Physiotherapy Canada, 42,* 12–15.

Gifford, G., & Hughes, J. (1983). A gait analysis system in clinical practice. *Journal of Biomedical Engineering, 5,* 297–301.

Goodkin, R., & Diller, L. (1973). Reliability among physical therapists in diagnosis and treatment of gait deviations in hemiplegics. *Perceptual and Motor Skills, 37,* 727–734.

Grieve, D. W., & Gear, R. (1966). The relationship between length of stride, step frequency, time of swing and speed of walking for children and adults. *Ergonomics, 5,* 379–399.

Harris, G. F., & Wertsch, J. J. (1994). Procedures for gait analysis. *Archives of Physical Medicine and Rehabilitation, 75,* 216–225.

Hill, K. D., Goldie, P. A., Baker, P. A., & Greenwood, K. M. (1994). Retest reliability of the temporal and distance characteristics of hemiplegic gait using a footswitch system. *Archives of Physical Medicine and Rehabilitation, 75,* 577–583.

Holden, M. K., Gill, K. M., & Magliozzi, M. R. (1986). Gait assessment for neurologically impaired patients. *Physical Therapy, 66,* 1530–1539.

Holden, M. K., Gill, K. M., Magliozzi, M. R., Nathan, J., & Piehl-Baker, L. (1984). Clinical gait assessment in the neurologically impaired. *Physical Therapy, 64,* 35–40.

Hughes, K. A., & Bell, F. (1994). Visual assessment of hemiplegic gait following stroke: Pilot study. *Archives of Physical Medicine and Rehabilitation, 75,* 1100–1107.

Klenerman, L., Dobbs, R. J., Weller, C., Leeman, A. L., & Nicholson, P. W. (1988). Bringing gait analysis out of the laboratory and into the clinic. *Age and Aging, 17,* 397–400.

Krebs, D. E., Edelstein, J. E., & Fishman, S. (1985). Reliability of observational gait kinematic gait analysis. *Physical Therapy, 65,* 1027–1033.

Mizrahi, J., Susak, Z., Heller, L., & Najenson, T. (1982a). Objective expression of gait improvement of hemiplegics during rehabilitation by time-distance parameters of the stride. *Medical and Biological Engineering and Computing, 20,* 628–634.

Mizrahi, J., Susak, Z., Heller, L., & Najenson, T. (1982b). Variation of time-distance parameters of the stride as related to clinical gait improvement in hemiplegics. *Scandinavian Journal of Rehabilitation Medicine, 14,* 133–140.

Nichols, P. J. R. (1979). Rehabilitation of the stroke patient. *Age and Aging, 8,* Suppl., 67–75.

Patla, A. E., Proctor, J., & Morson, B. (1987). Observations on aspects of visual gait assessment: a questionnaire study. *Physiotherapy Canada, 39,* 311–316.

Pinzur, M. S., DiMonte-Levine, P., Trimble, J., Haag, K., & Sherman, R. (1986). Temporal gait monitoring: A new device. *Archives of Physical Medicine and Rehabilitation, 67,* 344–345.

Robinson, J. L., & Smidt, G. L. (1981). Quantitative gait evaluation in the clinic. *Physical Therapy, 61,* 351–353.

Rosenrot, P., Wall, J. C., & Charteris, J. (1980). The relationship between velocity, stride time, support time and swing time during normal walking. *Journal of Human Movement Studies, 6,* 325–335.

Shores, M. (1980). Footprint analysis in gait documentation. *Physical Therapy, 60,* 1163–1167.

Stern, G. M., Franklyn, S. E., Imms, F. J., & Prestidge, S. P. (1983). Quantitative assessments of gait and mobility in Parkinson's disease. *Journal of Neural Transmission, Suppl. 19,* 201–214.

Turnbull, G. I., & Wall, J. C. (1985). The development of a system for the clinical assessment of gait following a stroke. *Physiotherapy, 71,* 294–298.

Wall, J. C. (1991). Measurement of the temporal gait parameters from videotape using a field counting technique. *International Journal of Rehabilitation Research, 14,* 344–347.

Wall, J. C., & Ashburn, A. (1979). Assessment of gait disability in hemiplegics. *Scandinavian Journal of Rehabilitation Medicine, 11,* 95–103.

Wall, J. C., Charteris, J., & Turnbull, G. I. (1987). Two steps equals one stride equals what?: The applicability of normal gait nomenclature to abnormal walking patterns. *Clinical Biomechanics, 2,* 119–125.

Wall, J. C., & Crosbie, J. (1996a). Accuracy and reliability of gait measurement. *Gait & Posture.*

Wall, J. C., & Crosbie, J. (1996b). Temporal gait analysis using slow motion video and a personal computer: accuracy and reliability. *Physiotherapy.*

Wall, J. C., & Scarbrough, J. (1996). The use of a multimemory stopwatch to measure the temporal gait parameters. *Journal of Orthopedic and Sports Physical Therapy.*

Wall, J. C., & Turnbull, G. I. (1986). Gait asymmetries in residual hemiplegia. *Archives of Physical Medicine and Rehabilitation, 67,* 550–553.

CHAPTER 18

Home Management

Shirley J. Jackson, MS, OTR/L

Felecia Moore Banks, MEd, OTR/L

SUMMARY Assessments in home management are rarely standardized and are fraught with methodologic, philosophical, and theoretic differences. Therefore, therapists must exercise skilled judgment in comparing and selecting home assessment tools based on disability populations, task demands, aging process, physical functioning, and cognitive abilities. Few instruments address culture, patient goals, lifestyle, or values that may determine the need for a home assessment and impact performance. This section examines the assessment issues related to the performance roles and tasks of the homemaker as reflected in the various assessment scales typically used by therapists.

HISTORICAL PERSPECTIVE

Assessment and instruction in home management skills can be dated as far back as the early 1900s. Assessment and training in skills such as learning how to plan and prepare a meal in the home; use the telephone; manipulate furniture items or gadgets such as drawers, faucets, or keys; and to provide locomotion and traveling training have been among a few of the areas addressed by therapists in preparation for discharge to the home (Buchwald, 1949). However, it was only after World War II, as the demand for services for people with disabilities increased, that subsequent growth in assessment procedures occurred. The Architecture Barrier Act of 1968 (Public Law 90-480) and Section 504 of the Rehabilitation Act of 1973 (Public Law 93-112) required programs and buildings that received federal funds to be accessible to people with disabilities.

The Rehabilitation Act of 1973 and the Social Services Act of 1974 particularly emphasized the pertinence and urgency of developing comprehensive programs for individuals who were homebound to promote independent living. Homemaking became a viable occupation and was considered for governmental funding.

Amendments in 1978 to the Rehabilitation Act of 1973 established Title VII, called "Comprehensive Services for Independent Living." The Comprehensive Services for Independent Living, under the jurisdiction of the state, provided grants for independent living centers, independent living programs for the older blind person, and protection and advocacy programs to guard the rights of persons with severe disabilities (Walker, 1979).

The Fair Housing Act, as amended in 1988 (Public Law 100-420), played a significant role in establishing accessibility requirements for all buildings with four or more housing units. Under this law, landlords were prevented from screening out people with disabilities. As a result of the many legislative acts regarding the rights of people with disabilities, the independent living movement emphasized making the community more accessible for persons with disabilities. This movement not only acknowledged the rights of people with disabilities but also offered persons with special needs greater consumer control, creating new assessment tools and markets of technology.

Current trends in health care and advancements in technology have influenced the development of standardized clinical assessments and realistic clinical simulations of home and community, where therapists can directly evaluate the performance of home management skills. For example, Easy Street (HSM Group, 1992), recently renamed Independence Square, an advanced technologic simulation, creates a realistic community and home environment in the clinic setting. This allows the patient and therapist to discuss structural differences that may adversely affect in-home performance.

Assessment tools of home management skills have expanded in various directions over the past 50 years. While some rehabilitation programs continue to allow therapists to complete at-home evaluations with their patients, most have adopted more cost-effective measures. Such measures include component skills assessment using the Assessment of Motor and Process Skills (AMPS), the Bay Area Functional Performance Evaluation (BaFPE), the Milwaukee Evaluation of Daily Living Skills (MEDLS), or a simulated home environment, which allows direct observation of performance (see Table 18–2).

Currently, the particular challenge continues to be the creation of assessments that provide functional outcome measures that are norm referenced and reliable and that have good predictive validity but are useful to a clinician when time constraints are of utmost importance. Since many new markets have emerged, including home economists, biomechanical engineers, and architects, together with occupational and physical therapists, more statistically sound and efficient home assessment tools are anticipated. Additionally, with third-party payors demanding functional outcomes and rehabilitation's continued emphasis on discharge to home, greater efforts will yield better instrumentation.

THEORETIC APPROACHES

Theoretic approaches that undergird home management are highly dependent on and embedded in notions about physical functioning and task performance. These notions are advanced in postulates such as developmental hierarchies, dysfunctional-functional continuums, and the process of task analysis. Home management can easily be addressed under several theoretic treatment approaches because of its multidimensional nature. However, the occupational performance model is considered one unified, task-oriented, conceptual framework that addresses the functional elements of performance of the homemaker role. This framework embodies treatment approaches consistent with rehabilitation and the model of human occupation.

A person's ability to maintain a home environment is

ADL HIERARCHY

Management
COMPLEX ADLs
- Care of others
- Money management
- Household maintenance
- Shopping
- Cleaning
- Meal preparation and clean-up
- Clothing care
- Safety precautions

SIMPLEX ADLs
Self-care
- Feeding
- Hygiene
- Bathing
- Basic communication

Mobility
- Ambulation
- Wheelchair propulsion
- Transfers
- Bed mobility

FIGURE 18–1. ADL hierarchy. (Adapted from Functional Performance in Older Adults. Bonder, B., & Wagner, M. B. [1994]. *Functional performance in older adults.* Philadelphia: F.A. Davis Company.)

probably one of the most important roles he or she will experience during a lifetime (Culler, 1993). Oakley (1981) defined a home maintainer as a person who has responsibility at least one day a week for the upkeep of the home, e.g., for tasks such as house cleaning or yard work. Home management not only includes cleaning and yard work but also consists of clothing care, meal preparation and clean-up, shopping, money management, household maintenance, and safety procedures. According to Rogers and Holm (1994), there are three categories of daily living tasks, which are generally perceived to be hierarchically arranged from simple to complex and include mobility, self-care, and complex activities of daily living (ADL). Home management tasks are among the most complex ADLs and are identified at the highest end of the hierarchy. Mobility is placed at the lowest end of the hierarchy, and self-care is identified at midpoint (Fig. 18–1).

Conceptually, home assessments are multidimensional. At least two hierarchy systems are used to classify home management skills: the ADL hierarchy and the dysfunctional hierarchy.

Activities of Daily Living Hierarchy

The ADL hierarchy basically separates foundational self-care skills and mobility from home management tasks. The hierarchy is ordered by increased levels of performance difficulty and recognizes the increased demand for cognitive abilities required to accomplish the higher-order tasks. The term *Instrumental Activities of Daily Living* (IADL), or *complex ADL,* is commonly used to identify high-level activities such as in the area of home management.

Dysfunctional Hierarchy

The concept of a dysfunctional hierarchy in rehabilitation is an outgrowth of the traditional medical model's influence on terminology related to disrupted performance. For years, the words chosen to reflect the impact of disease on daily life were interchangeable, with no distinction between how the terms "impairment," "disability," or "handicap" were used (Christiansen, 1991). In 1980, the World Health Organization (World Health Organization, 1980; Wood, 1980) classified these terms in a level of dysfunctional hierarchy (Fig. 18–2), according to the International Classification of Diseases (ICD), which was later incorporated into a document called the *International Classification of Impairment, Disability, and Handicap* (ICIDH) (Wood, 1980).

This dysfunctional hierarchy, according to Christiansen (1991), was among the first used as a means of classifying assessment tools in rehabilitation. Explanations are provided from a systems approach. The hierarchy assigns meaning to the impact of a condition on daily living. For example, "impairment" is viewed as permanent or temporary loss or abnormality affecting psychological, physiologic, or anatomic structures or function. The term *disability* is defined as the result of an impairment that restricts one's ability to perform one's life activities or to fulfill one's life role. The term *handicap* was described as a disadvantage resulting from an impairment or disability that limits or prevents normal role fulfillment, as viewed by the patient. Attention is given to age, sex, social, cultural, environmental, and economic consequences of the individual. Degrees of restriction by severity or disability groups are not provided with this hierarchy, making it difficult to use effectively for assessment purposes.

Task Approach

The traditional task-oriented approach continues to be the most popular approach among therapists. This approach requires direct observation of the patient performing a task and the therapist's analyzing the skill performance and level of performance. This type of assessment yields three measures: level of independence, degree of safety while performing the task, and length of time it takes to complete the task. The time frame yields a reality check. For example, if a patient takes 20 minutes to make a cup of coffee and serve it, one might determine that this is an unrealistic task for this patient to perform. The task-oriented approach provides valuable data about the individual's potential level of performance. Consistent observation and analysis are concepts unique to this approach and are essential for use of any good home evaluation instrument. Task-oriented approaches can be viewed in theoretical models of practice such as the occupational performance model.

Occupational Performance Model

The occupational performance approach (American Occupational Therapy Association, 1974) focuses on the "doing process" of an activity or occupational task to be accomplished. In this occupational performance taxonomy, the role of the task performer is clearly defined, and the activities and tasks required for successful role performance are closely examined. For example, if a primary role of a patient is that of a mother, wife, and home maintainer, the tasks that she might be required to perform (based on distinct social expectations) would be tasks such as preparing a meal, cleaning the house, and shopping (see Appendix D). The performance skills needed to perform such tasks would involve decision making, problem solving, and the ability to handle objects. The process of assessing home management should provide the best possible picture of an individual's level of functional performance in the role that he or she is expected to resume. For this reason, this task-oriented performance-based model appropriately assesses the characteristic behaviors or performance demonstrated by the person in a natural context.

Kielhofner (1985) proposed a continuum of occupational function and dysfunction that would incorporate concepts of competence, efficacy, and helplessness. The optimum level of occupational functioning would include achievement, competence, and exploration based on McClelland's (1961) progress in the continuum of normal development from exploration to achievement. Occupational function (exploration to achievement), depicts a progressive development of skills and habits into satisfactory role performance. Models of practice that incorporate function-dysfunction hierarchies are shown in Table 18–1. Although the use of hierarchies is valuable, more research is needed before their full potential for use can be actualized.

HANDICAP

DISABILITY

IMPAIRMENT

FIGURE 18–2. World Health Organization dysfunctional hierarchy.

ASSESSMENT FACTORS

Many factors must be considered when assessing home management skills. The cultural values of the patients and

TABLE 18-1

EXAMPLES OF HOW FUNCTION-DYSFUNCTION ACROSS THREE MODELS IS DETERMINED

Role: Homemaker

World Health Organization Hierarchy	Occupational Performance Dysfunction-Function Hierarchy		Functional Assessment
Handicap: A disadvantage for a given individual resulting from an impairment or disability that limits or prevents the fulfillment of a role (Wood, 1980)	Occupational role (American Occupational Therapy Association, 1974): Task-oriented approach to performance		Role performance: Self-report questionnaire Interview Direct observation of role performance
	Function: Able to fulfill role as a homemaker	Dysfunction: Unable to perform duties or skills as a homemaker	
Disability: Restriction or inability to perform a task or activity within a normal range or function without assistance	Occupational performance task: Function: Able to judge distance of cup and pour hot coffee into the cup	Dysfunction: Unable to judge distance of cup while pouring hot coffee	Task performance: Self-report Interview Direct observation and analysis
Impairment: Loss or abnormality of psychological, physiologic, or anatomic structures or function	Occupational performance components: Function: Normal muscle tone; normal visual processing	Dysfunction: Abnormal muscle tone; deficits in spatial relations	Performance component enablers: Specific tests in the area of range of motion, tone, sensation, strength, cognition, and perception
Pathology: Disruption of blood flow to the brain	Pathology: RCVA	Pathology: RCVA	Pathology: RCVA

RCVA = Right cerebrovascular accident.

Adapted from American Occupational Therapy Association (1993). Self-Study Series: Assessing function. Bethesda, MD: American Occupational Therapy Association.

their families, the living situation, finances and other resources, and the patient's medical status, as well as task demands, must be considered.

Cultural Values

A patient's family and cultural values are critical to successful management in the home. Client-provider collaboration on treatment goals can result in shorter hospital stays (Shendell-Falik, 1990) and better goal attainment (Czar, 1987). Patients and families often lack consistent, comprehensive information to enable them to effectively adjust and cope with family members returning to the home. Studies indicate that a family's ability to cope with chronic illnesses can make a significant impact on adaptation and rehabilitation. Thus, it is important to determine whether the patient's and family's cultural values and beliefs support the need for independence in home management. For example, a patient's husband found it difficult to allow her to perform a task independently because the task appeared to be difficult. Other family members may find it necessary to perform home management duties for their loved one because it is traditional and customary to do so.

Living Situation

Living situation influences recommendations for further assessment in the area of home management, home

modifications, and adaptations. For example, a patient who lives in a private home will have different equipment needs than a person who lives in a rental apartment. Also, the "home" for a patient could be a homeless shelter that sleeps six people in a room.

Finances and Other Resources

A patient's financial situation and available resources can significantly affect decisions that are made when assessing the home and management skills. Although cost-effective recommendations are routinely the goal of most therapists, a person who does not have the financial resources to make the suggested modifications in the home might have to consider modifications that are even less costly. Information gathered by the therapist about insurance coverage, community and family foundations, and other local support, can help therapists and their clients make tough decisions that might make the difference between whether a patient can return home or must be placed in a nursing facility.

Medical Status and Performance Components

Because home management tasks require a significant amount of physical and cognitive skills, it is important that a therapist consider the patient's most recent medical status and level of performance components such as range of motion, muscle strength, cognition, and emotional factors (see Appendix C). If a patient has underlying factors that prevent him or her from performing basic self-care skills and requires significant assistance from others, a home management assessment might not be appropriate. As a patient's functional status improves, a home management assessment would be recommended. Nonetheless, an assessment of the home environment can be initiated if discharge is imminent. Today, early discharge from acute care settings requires therapists to assess the home for architectural barriers and to provide home programs for the patient, family, or caregiver, when the patient is acutely ill. These patients often return home with follow-up home therapy and other home supports. Home management assessments are completed by the home therapist when appropriate.

Task Demands

It also is important to understand what is required to perform a particular task that is to be considered. A home management task could involve primarily physical characteristics, such as the use of weight-bearing joints with lifting and shifting of weight from one point to another (e.g., moving a hot coffee pot off the stove to the table). It is also important to consider the cognitive and emotional skills required for performing a given task. This is why it is important to complete a task analysis as part of the assessment process. This analysis will give a clearer picture of the task demands. Shopping requires a person to be able to problem-solve to get the items purchased from the store to home. Carrying a grocery bag is a task demand that should be considered when shopping. Therapists and patients should also be familiar with the options available when considering the task demands of shopping. For example, a person could use a shopping cart or have groceries delivered to the home. However, until physical, cognitive or perceptual, and psychosocial demands of this task have been considered closely, proposing solutions, such as delivering groceries to the home, is not very useful. Task demands also are perceived by each patient differently. A therapist's perception of task demands and a patient's perceptions could differ considerably. This is a likely reason why many standardized home management assessments are not available and why it is important to find out from the patient or family how tasks are usually performed. A therapist's skill and judgment in considering all factors, including the demands of the task, can often have a greater impact on the assessment of complex ADL than on basic self-care assessments (Hopkins & Smith, 1993). Since few standardized instruments on complex ADL exist, professional skill and judgment are required for performing home management assessments.

In summary, the role of the therapist in assessing home management skills is a challenging one. High-level ADL assessment requires considerable complex problem solving

on the part of the patient and therapist; therefore, a more detailed analysis of task performance is required. The problem-solving process involved in home management assessment is illustrated with a specific case study in Appendices A and B.

SELECTING A HOME ASSESSMENT TOOL

One of the most critical responsibilities a therapist has is the selection of an appropriate assessment instrument. The therapist must understand the statistical concepts and philosophic and theoretic bases behind the development of the instrument. Knowing these essentials makes it easier to analyze available instruments to determine their value and utility for a given situation or for a particular client.

In reviewing the statistical characteristics of an assessment, the therapist should, at a minimum, select an instrument with validity and reliability data.

The *validity* of an instrument is of utmost concern to the researcher and the therapist. Validity is the statistical descriptor that indicates how accurately the instrument measures what it claims to measure. Among home management instruments, validity is fairly easy to achieve since it measures certain concrete physical properties and common attributes well agreed on by most therapists.

The primary types of validity critical to the selection of home assessment scales are *content validity, construct validity,* and *predictive validity* (see Chapter 1 for an in-depth description of validity and reliability.)

Content validity refers to the items selected to be included in a test as representative of the universe of possible items. Without making an assessment too long or too short, one must determine if the assessment is inclusive enough to adequately represent the many homemaking tasks and situations a patient may commonly encounter. Second, one must consider whether the measure is reflective of the way each task is commonly accomplished in the patient's home.

Construct validity unites psychometric notions with theoretic notions. What does performance on this measure really mean? Other factors that may influence the performance outcome (e.g., whether the patient is too tired or too weak and whether it is the optimum time of day) must be teased out to determine if the instrument validly measures the construct it claims to measure, i.e., the construct of home management ability.

Predictive validity (Kerlinger, 1973) compares the test measure with the actual measure of performance of the attribute in the home situation. In other words, a client's performance on a clinical assessment of homemaking tasks should adequately predict performance of the client in the real home situation. Predictive validity is the most important type of validity to consider when dealing with practical problems and outcomes. Therefore, all home assessment scales must have acceptable predictive validity to make them useful assessment tools.

To be interpretable, a test must be reliable. Unless one can depend on the results of the measurement instrument, one cannot make accurate predictions. *Reliability* is essential to dependability in measurement. Furthermore, reliability is reflected in an instrument as stability or consistency of a measure across time. For example, when an infinite number of therapists uses a measuring tape to determine the height of a countertop or the width of a door sill, they should each record the same tape measurement. The tape measure calibrations are consistent no matter what shape, distance, or object it measures.

Many of the ADL assessments report *test-retest reliability*. This type of reliability indicates whether the test measures the construct in the same way each time the assessment measure is used. Specifically, *test-retest* refers to the client being retested using the same instrument, usually by the same therapist. If the test is reliable, the score will be essentially the same unless a change occurs in the patient.

The majority of the standardized home assessments report *interrater reliability,* which may be determined by having two therapists simultaneously observe the same client perform a given assessment task. Each rater assigns a score based on preestablished criteria. The two therapists' ratings on each performance item are compared for interrater agreement.

Whether the author has reported reliability and validity is noted for assessments recorded in this section (Table 18–2). Since for almost all assessments listed in the table, the coefficient was at least 0.80, an acceptable coefficient, only an "X" is recorded, indicating that these data were reported.

HOME MANAGEMENT ASSESSMENT FOR SPECIAL NEEDS

To assess a patient's ability to perform tasks in the home, the previous assessment factors should be considered. In addition, a therapist must know the patient's age, diagnosis, and pertinent precautions that might have an impact on function.

The Postsurgical Patient

To assess a patient with surgical diagnoses, therapists should anticipate that the patient will need to adhere to certain precautions. For this reason, therapists often intervene early during the assessment process by providing the patient and family the restrictions and precautions and guiding the use of adaptive equipment and methods of compensation.

Surgical procedures such as total hip replacement involve the placement of a prosthesis and, like many surgical procedures, require a period of immobilization or restrictions that might prevent a patient from performing certain types of activities. For a total hip replacement, a patient is not allowed to flex the hip beyond 90 degrees. Therefore, activities that involve reaching, placing, and bending need to be carefully assessed. Because surgical procedures are often temporary by nature, a patient might decide to have someone perform home management tasks until the recovery period has ended. The need for equipment also is assessed for temporary use. With an expected level of recovery, approaches that focus on restoring performance components such as range of motion, muscle strength, and endurance (biomechanical approaches) might be paired with performance-oriented approaches that examine tasks related to role performance.

The Older Adult

For the older adult, factors such as changes in neuromuscular status, impaired vision, and cognitive changes need to be considered. Because some of these changes result in problems such as loss of balance, falls, and memory impairment, a variety of assessment areas should be closely considered.

A common problem in assessing older adults emerges because of fluctuation in capability and performance. Most established assessment instruments assume that stability is present; however, performance stability is less likely in elders than in younger persons. For example, older persons may choose not to or may be unable to clean the front yard on a very hot day or a cold and snowy day. Regardless of rating criteria used, frequency in performance can vary. It is also important to take a complete history of the older adult; some older adults have never learned to perform home management duties that are not gender specific (Rogers and Holm, 1994). For example, an older male might not be accustomed to cooking and would not have a problem relying on a family member to cook, whereas, an older woman may not have learned to make repairs to the house or mow the lawn. With the older adult, expectations need to be considered closely. With home management tasks being optional in nature, the older adult might choose to have assistance rather than learn a new task or perform an old task that might require a lot of time and energy. Also, cost is often a concern with the older adult who lives on a fixed income.

The Person with Brain Damage

Following a brain injury, a patient might be unable to focus on relevant internal or external stimuli. As a result, he or she might not be able to exert the cognitive influences

TABLE 18–2

HOME MANAGEMENT ASSESSMENTS

Name of Test	Authors	Special Population	Descriptive Summary	Assessment Method	Reliability/ Validity*
Assessment of Motor and Process Skills (AMPS)	Fisher (1994)	General	Assesses IADL (e.g., meal preparation, home management) as the client would normally perform them. Person chooses to perform two or three familiar tasks from among 50 possibilities. Person's performance is rated in two skill areas: IADL motor and IADL process.	Observation	X/X
Bay Area Functional Performance Evaluation (BaFPE)	Asher & Williams (1989)	Psychiatric clients	Assesses functional performance of ADL, motor skills, sensation endurance, cognition, sensory motor functioning, and appearance. Two subtest: Task Oriented Assessment (TOA) and Social Interaction Scale (SIS).	Task observation and interview	X/X
Comprehensive Evaluation of Basic Living Skills	Casanova & Gerber (1976)	Chronic adult psychiatric inpatients	Rates client's performance in personal care and hygiene across seven basic living skills; meal planning, use of telephone, transportation, shopping and meal preparation, service, and clean-up.	Observation	
Functional Activities Questionnaire (FAQ)	McDowell & Newell (1987)	Normal and older adults and those with senile dementia	Screening tool for assessing activities necessary for higher-level independent skills including personal finances, managing forms, e.g., taxes and Social Security Insurance, shopping, making coffee, playing a game, tracking current events, and mobility.	Paper/pencil completed by spouse or significant others	Predictive
Maguire's Tri-Level ADL Assessment	Maguire (1985)	Geriatric clients	Assesses ADL across six categories: communications, food needs, dressing, hygiene, organization, and mobility across three environmental levels: personal home, or sheltered environment.	Observation	None

Table continued on following page

*X indicates that reliability or validity is present. X/X indicates both are present.

TABLE 18-2

HOME MANAGEMENT ASSESSMENTS *Continued*

Name of Test	Authors	Special Population	Descriptive Summary	Assessment Method	Reliability/ Validity*
Milwaukee Evaluation of Daily Living Skills (MEDLS)	Leonardelli (1988)	Long-term psychiatric clients (chronic schizophrenics)	Behavioral assessment of basic ADL skills in money handling, safety awareness, use of public transportation and telephone, medication management, clothing care, use of community resources, ability to read and write, meal planning and preparation and other household care are not included.	Observation	Interrater reliability/ criterion
Older Americans Resources and Services Instruments (OARS)	Kane & Kane (1981)	Geriatric clients	Assesses ability to use telephone and higher level ADL, e.g., financial management, shopping, housekeeping, and meal preparation.	Interview clients or significant others	None
Philadelphia Geriatric Center (PGC) Scale	Lawton (1980)	Geriatric clients	Assesses higher-level ADL, including shopping, food preparation, housekeeping, laundry, use of public transportation, financial and medication management.	Interview client or responsible other	None
The Rabideau Kitchen Evaluation-Revised: An Assessment of Meal Preparation Skill (RKE-R)	Neistadt (1992)	Adults with traumatic brain injury (TBI) or subtle cognitive perceptual deficits	Assessment of skill performance in simple meal preparation of a sandwich and hot beverage. Scored from dependent (1) to independent (7).	Observation	Test-retest/ none
Independent Living Skills Evaluation (ILSE)	Johnson et al. (1980)	Chronically emotionally disturbed clients living in apartments	Rated functional levels using behavioral descriptors across 10 categories, including money management (banking and budgeting), meal preparation and storage, clothing care, and use of transportation		None
Index of ADL	Katz (1983)		Assesses functional independence in self-care activities using a ranking score		X/X
Barthel Index (The Maryland Disability Index)	Mahoney & Barthel (1965)	Neuromuscular and musculoskeletal disorders	Adapted version scores the functional level of the client across 10 self-care tasks and mobility, using weighted ranges from 0 to 100 (independent in all tasks).	Observation of task performance	Test/retest 0.89/ predictive validity

Klein-Bell ADL Scale	Klein & Bell (1982)	Well individuals and persons with mental and physical dysfunctions	Using scaled scores, assesses basic self-care and higher-level ADL across five categories (170 items), including self-care, safety and money management, transportation and telephone, work, and leisure.	Observation	X/X
Kohlman Evaluation of Living Skills (KELS)	Kohlman-Thompson (1979)	Multiple populations	Assesses minimum standards for independent living across 18 daily living skills areas: self-care, safety and health, money management, transportation, telephone, work, and leisure. Provisions also to assess cognition, memory, attention span, comprehension, reality-testing, and sound judgment.	Interview and observation of task	Interrater reliability/predictive validity
The Role Checklist: Parts I and II	Oakley (1981); Barris et al. (1987)	Adolescents, adults, and elderly with physical and psychological dysfunction	A written inventory along a temporal continuum, where Part I is designed to assess one's major life role(s) based on occupational components, and Part II measures the degree to which the individual values each life role.	Paper/pencil self-report inventory	Interrater/content
Satisfaction with Performance Scaled Questionnaire (SPSQ)	Yerxa et al. (1982)	Normal and physically challenged persons	Using a five-point frequency scale score across two subscales: home management (24 items) and social community problem solving (22 items). Score indicates percentage of time (25%–100%) client is satisfied with his or her performance in these independent living areas.	Interview (self-report)	X/X
Scorable Self-Care Evaluation	Clark & Peters (1984)	Adults with psychosocial disabilities	Assess areas of personal self-care housekeeping tasks, money management, work, and leisure.	Observation	X/X

necessary to bring stability, structure, and organization to the environment in which home tasks are to be completed. Behavioral characteristics of cognitive and perceptual disruptions can prevent the brain-damaged patient from performing tasks safely in the home. For example, a patient is considered unsafe during the performance of a home management task such as cooking. Given further intervention, this patient may become safe with this task, but at present requires too much cuing for the therapist to suggest that this patient can perform this task safely in the home. Behavioral characteristics include such disruptions as incompleteness of thought and action, reduced learning potential, and reduced initiation and inhibition. Major problems identified with the brain-damaged population are the inability to handle time and the inability to function socially and emotionally within the family and community.

For assessment of the brain-damaged patient in the area of home management to be practical, it is recommended that a patient reach the following functional status: a) independence in mobility with or without equipment; b) functional use of one upper extremity with or without adaptive equipment; and c) independence in self-care (i.e., dressing, hygiene, grooming, bathing, and toileting) or have an attendant assist with these needs (Malkmus et al., 1980).

The Person with Cardiopulmonary Problems

Before a patient is assessed for management of home activities, it is important that the patient's condition is stable and that he or she has no medical complications that will interfere with his or her ability to perform high-level tasks in the home. Assessing a patient's ability to perform high-level ADL should be viewed very much like a form of exercise testing. Baseline measures such as heart rate and rhythm, breathing frequency, systolic and diastolic blood pressure, rate pressure product, and perceived exertion should be included since they provide valuable information about a patient's ability to perform ADL (Dean, 1994). The therapist should have a clear picture of the physiologic demands of the task that a person will be performing. High-level ADL can require changes in body position, which could cause a change metabolically. The metabolic demand of activities is measured in metabolic equivalents (METs). One MET is equal to 3.5 ml of oxygen per kilogram of body weight per minute. Charts identifying the metabolic demands of activities can be used to help assess patients with cardiopulmonary disorders by providing the therapist with baseline activities. An important point to remember is that functional performance and functional capacity are assessments both needed for a patient diagnosed with a cardiopulmonary disorder.

FUNCTIONAL GOAL-SETTING

A major reason for assessment of home maintenance tasks is to determine if functional goals have been met. Functional goals need to state specifically what tasks the patient will perform related to the task demands. For example, if a task requires a patient to judge the distance to a cup and pour coffee into the cup, the functional goal could simply read as follows:

Patient will reach forward and pick up the coffee pot and pour the hot water into the cup with two verbal prompts.

Long-term goals are written with the intent that a patient will achieve a certain level of function by the termination of therapy. To achieve long-term goals, the therapist plans a series of short-term goals that are building blocks leading to one or more long-term goals (Trombly, 1995). When treatment is focused on performance components, such as visual processing, cognition, range of motion, or muscle tone, it is important to include such components as a part of the treatment goal. For example, functional goals with performance components might be written in the following terms:

Patient will demonstrate 90 degrees of volitional movement of right shoulder flexion to pick up the coffee pot from the stove.

It is not required that performance components be identified in the goal that is written. However, factors that interfere with performance should be considered and reported in the initial evaluation and progress note (American Occupational Therapy Association, 1992). It is important to indicate the level of function in the goal writing. Expected level of function should be based on criteria that are established by the therapist in collaboration with the patient and the caregiver. The expected level of function should be established at a point where mastery should be achieved. For example, success in two of five trials, or 50 percent accuracy, does not indicate mastery of a task. On the other hand, success in five of five trials, or 100 percent accuracy, is a better indicator of mastery and is more likely to ensure safe task performance. Moreover, goals should be prioritized and should address issues that concern the client and affect safety first. Today, most reviewers of documentation are looking for functional progress with measurable outcomes. Such expected functional goals should delineate criteria that are needed to move the patient from an at-risk to a safe, functional, and healthy status (Rogers & Holm, 1994). Other samples of home management functional goals follow:

- Given two verbal cues, patient will generate a list of items from a menu with 100 percent accuracy
- Patient will dial 911 and give requested information accurately in three of three practice trials
- Patient will independently sweep a floor the size

of her room at home while using good body mechanics

HOME VISITS

Kielhofner and colleagues (1980) define the environment as the physical, social, and cultural setting in which a person operates. A person cannot exist without interaction with the environment, which includes external objects, people, and events that influence the person's actions. Lawton (1980) indicates that person-environment congruence is important. To achieve this congruence, the following important environmental attributes have been identified by Bonder and Wagner (1994):

1. Safety—The degree to which an environment minimizes accidents and hazards and affords assistance should the need occur
2. Security—The degree to which the environment provides psychological reassurance and meets other personal needs
3. Accessibility—The degree to which the environment affords entry, transport, and the use of its resources; most functional health, time use, and social behaviors are facilitated by accessibility
4. Legibility—The degree to which the environment can be comprehended

A home visit is usually performed by an occupational and physical therapist to assure functional independence and safety in the home. Important items to take on a home visit include a measuring tape, a flashlight, a transfer belt, a screwdriver, ambulatory equipment, and a home assessment check list (see Appendix E). Following is a format that therapists can use to prepare the patient and family to return home:

1. Evaluate the family's level of understanding and willingness to adjust to the disabled family member.
   a. Where will the patient live? What room?
   b. What kind of adjustments does the family anticipate?
   c. What kind of adjustment is the family willing to accept?
2. Evaluate the usefulness of the rehabilitation.
   a. Will the methods used in rehabilitation be useful in home situations?
   b. Is the equipment functional in the home?
3. Assess for architectural barriers and other potential barriers.
4. Identify problems that the patient and family will need to resolve prior to discharge.
5. Offer problem-solving strategies to the patient and family or caregiver.

Finally, the following is a list of basic principles we believe should be considered when assessing home management skills:

1. Home management is viewed as a complex ADL. Such activities include cooking, cleaning, shopping, and financial management. Therefore, it is considered the highest level of ADL function from a hierarchic perspective, with mobility at the lower end of the hierarchy and self-care at the midpoint.
2. Task-oriented, performance-based models of function-dysfunction provide a framework for assessing home management and can serve as helpful guides to functional performance in the home.
3. Every patient does not require an assessment in home management. The role of the home maintainer should be determined based on the patient's lifestyle, culture, level of function (cognitive, physical, emotional), and personal goals and desires.
4. To determine functional performance in the home, a considerable amount of judgment and skill is required by the therapist.
5. Performance of home management tasks also requires a higher level of problem-solving and proficiency on the part of the patient.
6. Clinical assessment tools should have good reliability and predictive validity for in-home task performance; i.e., the direct observations of tasks in the clinic should have similar characteristics to the tasks completed at home.
7. Task demands should be considered. A detailed activity analysis should be performed to determine the level of skill needed for successful in-home task performance.
8. Goals should have functional implications based on the patient's level of functional abilities.

CONCLUSIONS

Since current health care trends lead us to believe that more and more patients will need to be discharged early and directly to their homes, it is vital that occupational and physical therapists provide careful assessments if patients are to function safely in their home environment. This chapter has dealt with the major issues in this important area of assessment.

GLOSSARY

Assistive technology—Any item, piece of equipment, or product system, whether acquired commercially, off the shelf, customized, or modified, that is used to increase, maintain, or improve functional capacities of individuals with disabilities.

Disability—Limitation of a person's ability to carry out personal, social, and familial responsibilities caused by health problems.

Home assessment—A process by which therapists evaluate an individual's living environment and identify measurable factors that might interfere with functioning in the home.

Home management—Higher-level ADL that individuals perform in the home environment. Such activities include organization of the home, housekeeping routines, shopping, budgeting, and money management.

Independence—Having adequate resources to accomplish everyday tasks.

Instrumental activities of daily living (IADL)—Higher-order activities that support independence, including housekeeping duties, shopping, budgeting, and money management.

Mobility tasks—Those tasks that involve moving the body from one position or place to another.

Occupational performance—Task accomplishment in everyday living within a desirable role.

Occupational performance component—Any subsystem that contributes to the performance of tasks in every day living; underlying factors such as motivation, range of motion, cognition.

Performance—Routine task behavior, in contrast to capacity, which is the ability to perform a task.

Personal self-care tasks—Those tasks that involve taking care of body-oriented, fundamental, personal needs like feeding and toileting.

Roles—Set of expectations governing the behavior of persons holding a particular position in society.

Tasks—Work assigned to, selected by, or required of a person related to a skill. A collection of activities related to accomplishment of a goal.

REFERENCES

American Occupational Therapy Association. (1992). *Effective documentation for occupational therapy: On target guidelines (or notewriting that works)*. Bethesda, MD: American Occupational Therapy Association.

American Occupational Therapy Association. (1974). *The performance frame of reference: A curriculum guide for occupational therapy educators*. Bethesda, MD: American Occupational Therapy Association.

American Occupational Therapy Association. (1994). Uniform terminology, third edition. *American Journal of Occupational Therapy, 4*(11), 1074.

Asher, B., & Williams, C. (1989). *Bay Area Functional Evaluation Test*. Palo Alto, CA: Psychologist Press.

Barris, R. (1982). Environmental interactions: An extension of the Model of Human Occupation. *American Journal of Occupational Therapy, 36*, 637–644.

Barris, R., Oakley, F., & Keilhofner, G. (1987). The Role Checklist: Parts 1 and 2.

Bonder, B., & Wagner, M. (1994). *Functional performance in older adults*. Philadelphia: FA Davis Co.

Buchwald, E. (1949). Functional training. *The Physical Therapy Review, 29*(1), 491–496.

Casanova, J., & Gerber, J. (1976). Comprehensive evaluation of basic living skills. *American Journal of Occupational Therapy, 30, 2*.

Christiansen, C., & Baum, C. (Eds.) (1991). *Occupational therapy: Overcoming performance deficits*. Thorofare, NJ: Slack.

Clark, E. N., & Peters, M. (1984). *Scorable self care evaluation*. Thorofare, NJ: Slack.

Culler, K. (1993). Home and family management. In H. Hopkins & H. Smith (Eds.), *Willard and Spackman's occupational therapy* (8th ed.) (pp. 207–226). Philadelphia: J. B. Lippincott Company.

Czar, M. (1987). Two methods of goal setting in middle-age adults facing critical life changes. *Clinical Nurse Specialist, 1*, 171–177.

Dean, E. (1994). *Cardiopulmonary development in functional performance in older adults*. Philadelphia: F. A. Davis Company.

Devaney, J. (1994). Tracking the American dream: Fifty years of housing history from the Census Bureau: 1940 to 1990. *U.S. Census Housing Reports*. Washington DC: U.S. Department of Commerce Economics and Statistics Administration; U.S. Government Printing Office.

Fillenbaum, G. (Ed.). (1987). Development of a brief, internationally usable screening instrument. In G. Maddox & E. Buse (Eds.), *Aging: The universal human experience*. New York: Springer.

Fisher, A. (1994). Assessment of motor and process skills (AMPS) [Unpublished manual]. Dept. of Occupational Therapy, University of Illinois at Chicago.

Frey, N. (1989). Functional Outcome: Assessment and Evaluation. In DeLisa, J. A. (ed): Rehabilitation Medicine. Philadelphia: J. B. Lippincott.

Hemphill, B. (1988). *Mental health assessment in occupational therapy*. Thorofare, NJ: Slack.

Hopkins, H., & Smith, H. (Eds.). (1993). *Willard and Spackman's occupational therapy* (8th ed.). Philadelphia: J. B. Lippincott Company.

HSM Group, Ltd. (1992). *Easy street*. Scottsdale, AZ: HSM Group, Ltd.

Hunt, L. (1994). *Functional performance in older adults* (pp. 284–294). Philadelphia: F. A. Davis Company.

Johnson, J., Johnson-Vinnicombe, B., & Merril, G. (1980). The independent living skills evaluation. *Occupational Therapy in Mental Health, 2*, 5–18.

Kane, R. E., & Kane, R. L. (1981). Older Americans Resources and Services Instrument (OARS). In *Assessing the elderly*. Lexington, MA: Lexington Books.

Katz, S. (1983). Assessing self-maintenance: Activities of daily living, mobility, and instrumental activities of daily living. *Journal of American Geriatric Society, 31*.

Kerlinger, F. (1973). *Foundations of behavioral research* (2nd ed.). New York: Holt, Rinehart, & Winston, Inc.

Kielhofner, G. (1985). *A model of human occupation: Theory and application*. Baltimore: Williams & Wilkins.

Kielhofner, G., Burke, J., & Igi, C. (1980). A model of human occupation, Part IV. Assessment and intervention. *American Journal of Occupational Therapy, 34*.

Klein, R. M., & Bell, B. (1982). Self-care skills: Behavioral management with Klein-Bell ADL scale. *Archives of Physical Medicine & Rehabilitation, 63*, 335–338.

Kohlman-Thompson, L. (1979). Kohlman evaluation of living skills (KELS). In L. K. McGourty (Ed.), *KELS research*. Bethesda, MD: American Occupational Therapy Association.

Law, M., & Letts, L. (1989). A critical review of scales of activities of daily living. *American Journal of Occupational Therapy, 43*(8).

Lawton, E. (1980). Activities of daily living test: Geriatric consideration. *Physical and Occupational Therapy in Geriatrics, 1*, 11–20.

Leonardelli, C. (1988). *Milwaukee Evaluation of Daily Living Skills* (MEDLS). Thorofare, NJ: Slack, Inc.

Llorens, L. A. (1984). Changing balance: Environment and individual. *American Journal of Occupational Therapy, 38*.

Maguire, G. H. (1985). Activities of daily living. In C. Lewis (Ed.). *Aging: The health care challenge*. Philadelphia: F. A. Davis Company.

Mahoney, F., & Barthel, D. (1965). Functional Evaluation Index. *Maryland State Medical Journal, 14*.

Malkmus, D., Booth, B.J., & Kodimer, C. (1980). *Rehabilitation of the head injured adult: Comprehensive management*. Downey, CA: Professional Staff Association of Rancho Los Amigos Hospital, Inc.

McClelland, C. (1961). *The achieving society*. Princeton, NJ: Van Nostrand.

McDowell, I., & Newell, C. (1987). *Measuring health: A guide to Rating Scale Questionnaire*. New York: Oxford Press.

Neistadt, M. E. (1992). The Rabideau Kitchen Evaluation Revised. Durham, NH: University of New Hampshire Department of Occupational Therapy, School of Health and Human Services.

Oakley, F. (1981). *Role checklist presented at workshop on enhancing clinical effectiveness: Practical application of the model of human occupation*. Chicago: University of Illinois at Chicago, July 24-25, 1989.

Pedretti, L., & Zoltan, B. (1990). Occupational therapy: Practice skills for physical dysfunction (3rd ed.). St. Louis: C. V. Mosby Company.

Rogers, J., & Holm, M. (1994). *Functional performance in older adults* (pp. 181–200). Philadelphia: F. A. Davis Company.

Rogers, J., & Holm, M. AOTA Self-Study Series 1. The therapist's thinking behind functional assessment I. Bethesda, MD: American Occupational Therapy Association.

Rowles, G. (1987). A place to call home. In L. Carstensen & B. Edelstein (Eds.), *Handbook of clinical gerontology.* Riverside, NJ: Pergamon Press.

Shendell-Falik, W. (1990). Creating self-care units in the acute care setting: A case study. *Patient Education and Counseling, 15,* 39–45.

Trombly, C. (1995). *Occupational therapy for physical dysfunction* (4th ed.). Baltimore: Williams & Wilkins.

Trombly, C., & Scott, A. (1983). *Occupational therapy for physical dysfunction.* Baltimore: Williams & Wilkins.

Walker, J. M. (1979). A guide to organizations, agencies, and federal programs for handicapped Americans. Washington, DC: Handicapped American Reports.

Wood, P. H. N. (1980). Appreciating the consequences of disease: The international classification of impairments. *Disabilities and handicap. World Health Organization Chronicle, 34* 376–380.

World Health Organization (1980). International classification of impairments, disabilities, and handicaps (ICIDH). Geneva: World Health Organization.

Yerxa, E. J., Burnett-Beaulieu, S., Stocking, S., & Azen, S. (1982). Development of the Satisfaction with Performance Scaled Questionnaire (SPSQ). *The American Journal of Occupational Therapy, 36*(10).

APPENDIX A

Case Study

Sherry is a 41-year-old woman who lives with her husband and 7-year-old son. She loves to jog and explore new and innovative cooking ideas. Many of Sherry's friends consider her to be an expert in ethnic cooking. Two weeks ago, Sherry was found conscious on the bathroom floor, unable to move the left side of her body. She was rushed to the emergency department, where a complete work-up revealed an occlusion to the right middle cerebral artery. Sherry was diagnosed with a right cerebrovascular accident, with residual left-sided weakness and was hospitalized for continued follow-up care and rehabilitation. At present, Sherry has shown significant improvement since her admission to the hospital. She has increased muscle tone in the left upper extremity and is able to perform volitional movement patterns and use her arm to assist with simple ADLs, such as eating or hygiene, with supervision. Sherry is very anxious to return home, and discharge is planned for within the next 2 days. She looks forward to seeing her family and cooking again. Although Sherry is able to perform her simple ADLs with supervision, the therapist has concerns about her ability to perform more complex ADLs (IADLs) such as cooking, house cleaning, and shopping.

Sherry ambulates with a cane on the unit; however, in a busy clinic, she often misjudges the distance of some items from others and has difficulty lifting weighted items in her room. Today, Sherry's therapist will have her prepare a meal. Before Sherry completes such a task, the therapist asks her questions based on her distinct role as a home maintainer that provide a clear picture of the task demands in the area of cooking. This enables simulation of this activity, as much as possible, in a natural context. For example, Sherry's therapist wants to know how often she cooks meals, what type of meals she prepares, and what kinds of kitchen equipment are commonly used.

Activities of Daily Living and Home Management Clinical Problem

To assess a person's ability to perform tasks in the home, complex problem solving on the part of the therapist is required. Listed below are a series of questions that should be used to identify and solve problems in the area of home management. This approach involves a two-stage process that consists of problem identification and problem resolution. Examples given refer to Sherry, the patient introduced in the case study in Appendix A.

PROBLEM IDENTIFICATION

1. What is the etiology and nature of the diagnosis?

   EXAMPLE: Mild right cerebrovascular accident with residual left-sided weakness

2. What are the implications of the diagnosis?

   EXAMPLE: Unable to accurately judge distance of objects; unable to perform normal volitional movement patterns

3. How do these implications impact function?

   EXAMPLE: Unable to judge distance of cup; difficulty lifting objects such as a coffee pot

4. With what functional problems does the patient present?

   EXAMPLE: Unable to safely perform a cooking task

5. Will these functional problems prevent the patient from performing tasks required for role performance in the home?

   EXAMPLE: Yes, unable to complete the task of cooking required for role as home maintainer

6. Does the patient have the desire and interest to resolve such functional problems?

   EXAMPLE: Yes, very anxious for recovery. Would especially like to cook.

7. Is the family supportive of the patient's desire to resolve the functional problems?

   EXAMPLE: Very supportive; husband is willing to assist with chores at home

8. How do these functional problems affect safety?

   EXAMPLE: Unsafe in kitchen handling hot water; potential safety problems in other areas of ADL

9. Is the patient's functional problem in the area of simple or complex ADL?

   EXAMPLE: Prominent deficits in complex ADL

PROBLEM RESOLUTION

1. Among all of the functional problems identified, which are amenable to rehabilitation?

   EXAMPLE: Inability to judge distance of cup and lift hot coffee pot

2. Which approach would best resolve the problem (remedial, compensation/adaptation, or both)?

   EXAMPLE: Based on time frame for discharge, functional task-oriented approach of compensation/adaptation would be selected

3. What specific methods of treatment would correspond to the patient's individual needs?

ENDURANCE LIMITATIONS

Difficulty in completing any home activity that requires sustained effort or movement over a specified period of time, such as the following:
- Preparing large meals for family
- Unpacking clothes
- Performing yard work

COGNITIVE OR PERCEPTUAL DIFFICULTY

- Recognizing self-limitations
- Recognizing signs of fatigue
- Knowing when a meal is finished cooking
- Following a menu

- Writing a menu
- Following appropriate emergency procedures
- Finding items in a cluttered kitchen or shopping mall
- Keeping track of schedules, such as which day to put out the trash
- Finding his/her way to the store
- Juggling more than one task at a time such as answering the telephone and washing

SOCIAL AND EMOTIONAL DIFFICULTY

- Selecting appropriate dress for the occasion and/or what to say when guests arrive
- Using appropriate social graces
- Tolerating standing in crowded line to pay a bill
- Handling criticism from others

Home Management Terminology

1. **Home management:** Obtaining and maintaining personal and household possessions and environment
   a. **Clothing care:** Obtaining and using supplies, sorting, laundering (hand, machine, and dry clean), folding, ironing, storing, and mending
   b. **Cleaning:** Obtaining and using supplies, picking up and puting away, vacuuming or sweeping and mopping floors, dusting, polishing, scrubbing, washing windows, cleaning mirrors, making beds, and removing trash and recyclables
   c. **Meal preparation and clean-up:** Planning nutritious meals, preparing and serving food, opening and closing containers and cabinets and drawers, using kitchen utensils and appliances, cleaning up, and storing food safely
   d. **Shopping:** Preparing shopping lists (grocery and other), selecting and purchasing items, selecting method of payment, and completing money transactions
   e. **Money management:** Budgeting, paying bills, and using bank systems
   f. **Household maintenance:** Maintaining home, yard, garden, and appliances
   g. **Safety procedures:** Knowing and performing preventive and emergency procedures to maintain a safe environment and to prevent injuries

2. **Care of others:** Providing for children, spouse, parents, pets, or others, such as giving physical care, nurturing, communicating, and using age-appropriate activities

From the American Occupational Therapy Association. (1994). Uniform terminology, third edition. *American Journal of Occupational Therapy, 4*(11), 1074.

A P P E N D I X   E

Occupational Therapy Home Evaluation

Patient's Name: _____

Diagnosis: _____

Date of Birth: _____

Hosp. No.: _____

Inpatient or Outpatient   (Circle One)

Unit: _____   (If Applicable)

Home Address:

_____

Home Telephone:

_____

Number of Persons in the Home: _____

Patient's Primary Role in the Home:

_____

1. **OFF-STREET PARKING**
   a. Is an off-street parking area available to building?
      YES   NO
   b. If adjacent off-street parking is not available, identify and give location of nearest and most convenient parking area: _____
      _____
   c. Is the surface of the parking area paved (no sand, gravel, etc.)?
      YES   NO

2. **PASSENGER LOADING ZONE**
   a. Is there a passenger loading zone?
      YES   NO
   b. If yes, where is it located in relation to selected entrance? _____

3. **TYPE OF RESIDENCE**
   a. Is this a private home?
      YES   NO

   b. If yes, is it multilevel?
      YES   NO
   c. If no, is it single level?
      YES   NO
   d. Is this an apartment:
      YES   NO
   e. On what floor does patient reside? _____

4. **APPROACH TO SELECTED ENTRANCE**
   a. Which entrance was selected as most accessible?
      _____
   b. Is the approach to the entrance door ground level?
      YES   NO
   c. Is there a ramp at the entrance?
      YES   NO
   d. If there are any steps in the approach to the entrance, give total number of steps: _____
   e. If there are steps, is there a sturdy handrail in the center, on at least one side?
      YES   NO

468

5. **ENTRANCE DOOR**
   a. With door open, what is the width of the entrance doorway? _____
   b. Is the door automatic?
      YES   NO
   c. Are there steps between entrance and main areas?
      YES   NO
   d. If yes, what is the total number of steps? _____
   e. If there are steps, is there a sturdy handrail in the center, or at least one side?
      YES   NO
   f. What is the width of the interior door (if applicable)? _____

6. **ELEVATOR**
   a. Is there a passenger elevator?
      YES   NO
   b. Does it serve all essential areas?
      YES   NO

7. **ENVIRONMENTAL AND ECOLOGY SAFETY**
   a. Are floors free of rough places, and are tile or rugs free of holes?
      YES   NO
   b. Are all areas such as basement or attic stairs well lit?
      YES   NO
   c. Are electric cords run under rugs, furniture, or doors, or across the floor? _____
   d. Are stairs, halls, and exits free from clutter?
      YES   NO
   e. Are throw rugs eliminated or fastened down?
      YES   NO
   f. Are strong banisters or railings placed along each stairway?
      YES   NO
   g. Is furniture arranged to allow free movement in heavy traffic areas?
      YES   NO
   h. Is heavy furniture equipped with casters?
      YES   NO
   i. Is storage space easy to reach in areas where often-used items are stored?
      YES   NO
   j. Is there adequate ventilation in the home?
      YES   NO
   k. Does the home have a regulated cooling and heating system?
      YES   NO
   l. Are there signs of leakage from appliances or other areas of the home?
      YES   NO
   m. Is running hot water present?
      YES   NO
   n. Is there an adequate waste disposal system?
      YES   NO

8. **BEDROOM**
   a. Where is the bedroom located? _____
   b. Is it accessible?
      YES   NO
   c. If no, give doorway width and any other reasons: _____
   d. What kind of bed does patient use? _____
   e. Is there any adaptive equipment present?
      YES   NO
   f. If yes, please list: _____
   g. If yes, is it being used?
      YES   NO
   h. If no, why not? _____
   i. Is there space for a wheelchair to turn?
      YES   NO

9. **BATHROOM**
   a. Where is the bathroom located? _____
   b. Is it accessible?
      YES   NO
   c. If not, give doorway width and any other reasons: _____
   d. Is there space for a wheelchair to turn?
      YES   NO
   e. Is there a tub?
      YES   NO
   f. If yes, state type and give height from floor: _____
   g. Are there fixtures?
      YES   NO
   h. If yes, put a check beside the appropriate fixtures:
      rail mounted next to commode _____
      rail mounted on tub wall _____
      one faucet _____
      two faucets _____
   i. Is there a shower?
      YES   NO
   j. Is there any adaptive equipment present?
      YES   NO
   k. If yes, please list: _____
   l. If yes, is it being used?
      YES   NO
   m. If no, why not? _____
   n. Are there nonskid surfaces on tub or shower?
      YES   NO
   o. Is a first-aid kit available at all times?
      YES   NO
   p. What type of toilet is present, and give height from floor: _____

10. **KITCHEN**
   a. Where is the kitchen located? _____
   b. Is it accessible?
      YES   NO
   c. Is there space for a wheelchair to turn?
      YES   NO
   d. If not, give doorway width or any other reasons: _____
   e. Are corners on cabinets, counters, and furniture rounded and protected?
      YES   NO

f. Are work surfaces accessible?
    YES   NO
g. Are pots and pans too large and heavy?
    YES   NO
h. Is there any adaptive equipment present?
    YES   NO
i. If yes, please list: _____
j. If yes, is it being used?
    YES   NO
k. If no, why not? _____
l. Are there any safety hazards?
    YES   NO
m. If yes, please list: _____

11. **TELEPHONE**
    a. Where is the most accessible phone located?
        _____
    b. What type (wall, desk, booth)?_____
    c. If phone is in a booth, what is the width of the booth door with door open? _____
    d. Is the handset 48 inches or less from the floor?
        YES   NO
    e. Are there any adaptations to the phone?
        YES   NO
    f. If yes, please list: _____
    g. Is there an attendant who will take calls?
        YES   NO

12. **ASSISTANCE AND AIDS AVAILABLE**
    a. Is there help available for those needing assistance in entering (doorman, etc.)?
        YES   NO

EQUIPMENT LIST
Please list all items patient currently has:

b. If not, is help available for those needing assistance, if arranged for in advance?
    YES   NO
c. Who should be called in advance for assistance?
    _____
d. What is the above person's telephone number?
    _____
e. Is there anyone in the household to provide assistance?
    YES   NO
f. If yes, who? _____
g. Is there any one living outside the household who regularly assists the patient? _____
h. If yes, please give name and telephone number of that person: _____
i. List any other assistance patient receives: ___
    _____
j. Are there members in your household who are not in good health?
    YES   NO
k. Is there any one in the household who is non-English speaking?
    YES   NO

13. **ACCESS TO PUBLIC TRANSPORTATION**
    a. Give location of nearest bus stop: _____
        _____
    b. Is it accessible?
        YES   NO
    c. Is subway accessible?
        YES   NO

RECOMMENDATIONS

_____
Evaluator

Data from Shirley J. Jackson and Felecia M. Banks, Howard University Occupational Therapy Department, 1995.

CHAPTER 19

Community Activities

Carolyn Schmidt Hanson, PhD, OTR

SUMMARY   Integrating the individual with an illness or injury into the community is important for therapists to consider. Within the community, public areas need to be accessible for individuals with disabilities. Legislation such as the Americans with Disabilities Act of 1990 has facilitated barrier removal and modification of structures in the public sector. Informal and formal community integration assessments used by clinicians are discussed in this chapter. In addition, a special section on driving is presented.

After being hospitalized owing to trauma or illness, an individual typically engages in basic activities of daily living while recovering in an institution. As therapists, we need to consider methods of integrating the individual back into the community, whether the person is in an acute care facility or a rehabilitation program. Once discharged home, this individual may begin to perform more activities independently and eventually venture into the community. However, tasks may be more difficult and take longer to perform after hospitalization. Whereas driving to the bank and withdrawing money used to take 10 minutes, it may now require more than twice that time and require a family member to drive the newly recuperating individual to the bank. A 10-minute task for one has just become a 30-minute task for two people. This chapter focuses on assessments used to integrate individuals with physical disabilities back into the community.

According to Law and colleagues (1995), three major factors help explain why physical and occupational therapy goals are currently more community based:

1. The independent living movement
2. The increased number of elderly living in our society
3. Legislation such as the Americans with Disabilities Act (ADA) of 1990

The combination of these factors has led to more emphasis being placed on making the environment accessible to all. Although physical and, particularly, attitudinal barriers remain, people with disabilities are finding it easier to participate in community activities than in the past (Reynolds, 1993).

LEGISLATION

The intention of the ADA has been likened to the philosophy of occupational therapy: engaging in purposeful activity is essential to humans (Bachelder & Hilton, 1994). Owing to its legal ramifications, the ADA is having an impact on our society. The ADA is not new legislation but a direct outgrowth of Section 504 of the Rehabilitation Act of 1973, otherwise known as the Handicapped Bill of Rights. Although it extends the scope of Section 504 to encompass all public facilities and is not just limited to federal agencies, the intent of the ADA is no different than this passage from the Rehabilitation Act of 1973:

No otherwise qualified handicapped individual in the United States shall, solely by reason of his

471

handicap, be excluded from participation in, be denied the benefits of or be subjected to discrimination under any program or activity receiving federal financial assistance.

(FEDERAL REGISTER, P. 163)

The ADA mandates accessibility of public accommodations (Title III) and federal and state government entities (Title II). Title I applies to employment opportunities for individuals with a disability, and Title IV pertains to telecommunications. Title V is a miscellaneous category. As can be seen by the five titles, individuals with all types of disabilities are covered by this legislation. No longer will stairs to a courthouse or restrooms with small, heavy doors prevent an individual using a wheelchair from entering these areas. Structured modifications will be needed to provide access to all people. Compliance with the ADA is expected, but it is not being monitored per se. If a violation is reported, the case will be reviewed by the court and action taken.

Public accommodation guidelines meeting ADA specifications are available through regional Disability and Business Technical Assistance Centers (see Appendix at the end of this chapter). To evaluate the accessibility of a particular building, therapists can use *The ADA Checklist for Readily Achievable Barrier Removal* (Adaptive Environments Center, 1992). This checklist reviews entranceways, parking, accessibility of goods and services, usability of restrooms, and miscellaneous items, such as telephone and drinking fountain heights. The checklist enables a therapist or any other interested person to evaluate whether a building is accessible or not and additionally provides possible solutions for inaccessible areas. The checklist was designed for buildings already in existence.

COMMUNITY REINTEGRATION

Informal Assessments

An ideal time to work on community activities is when the individual is first hospitalized. Individuals in some facilities may have the opportunity to eat in a public dining room, attend a religious service, and even get a haircut while being treated by health professionals (Goggins et al., 1990). In addition to these common activities, individuals may be able to visit the post office and bank and to pick up a few items from the grocery store—all under one roof. A wide variety of facilities across the country have used Independence Square™ (developed by the creator of "Easy Street") to bridge the gap from hospital to home (Henderson, 1994). Independence Square™ consists of realistic modules, each being a replica of places of business and leisure, such as a bank, grocery store, restaurant, and beach. Numerous modules are available, but custom ordering is possible for a specific location. For example, since

Miami is on the coast, the beach is a familiar place to visit; therefore, a hospital in south Florida might request a beach module. The modules known as "enhanced care environments" are motivating and fun for people. Dix (1992) stated that individuals involved in Independence Square™ activities viewed their therapy as being more beneficial when they were rehearsing skills in a more realistic environment. Not always is it possible to observe individuals in their own communities. With Independence Square™, the community can be brought to the individual. In this manner, skills can be assessed in a structured and controlled environment.

Gradually extending rehabilitation efforts into the community allows the practicing of necessary functional skills in more meaningful and unpredictable situations. Observing individuals during a planned community outing is one method of determining physical and psychological competence. For example, a comprehensive program focusing on reintegrating the postgrafted burned individual into the community (Goggins et al., 1990) consisted of the following phases: **preparation** (financial considerations of institutional reimbursement for the community activity; roles of the team members, individual, and family; individualized goal setting), **performance** (preparing the person mentally, physically, and emotionally for the activity; coaching and prompting the individual during the activity; considering the particular situation—noting the individual's interactions with the environment), and **evaluation** (the individual with burns plays an active role in discussing how goals were met and how the outing was viewed, along with feedback from team members). Individuals benefit from these structured outings, but cost effectiveness needs to be documented.

El-Ghatit and coworkers (1980) mentioned that standard evaluation of individuals with spinal cord injuries entailed residing in an apartment 7 miles away from the hospital before discharge was planned. The apartment complex was located near stores, churches, and public transportation to facilitate the transition of the individual into community activities. The hospital was just far enough away from the apartment complex to encourage independent functioning.

An outpatient intensive group-oriented program has been found to assist individuals with mild to moderate brain injury to find employment and be more active in the community (Smigielski et al., 1992). To be considered for this program, an individual must undergo a 2-day interdisciplinary assessment conducted by a physiatrist, clinical neuropsychologist, physical therapist, occupational therapist, speech pathologist, medical social worker, and nurse. A team conference is held after the assessment to determine if the individual with a brain injury is capable of full participation. The patient and interested family members then meet with the interdisciplinary team to discuss treatment. This assessment has proved to be a valuable resource owing to its comprehensive nature. Whether the individual is accepted into the outpatient program or not, recommendations are made for medical treatment, residential placement, and vocational planning, as appropriate.

Formal Assessments

The Community Integration Questionnaire (CIQ), originally designed for persons with traumatic brain injury (TBI), consists of 15 questions in three domains: home integration, social integration, and productive activities (Willer et al., 1994). This questionnaire is to be completed by the individual with the brain injury or the person most familiar with the individual. Alternate forms of the CIQ include telephone and computerized versions. The CIQ takes approximately 15 minutes to answer questions relating to the use of transportation, social, employment, and school-related activities, in addition to household responsibilities.

Willer and others (1994) have reported high test-retest reliability (greater than 0.90) and good validity of the CIQ. Formalized interrater reliability studies have not been conducted, but comparisons have been made between responses made by family members and the individuals themselves. Significant differences on all sections of the CIQ and the total CIQ score were found between able-bodied individuals (control group) and individuals with TBI. Also, significant differences were found between those with TBI who lived independently as opposed to in a supported living situation (Willer et al., 1994). In a sample of 352 individuals with TBI and 237 nondisabled people, Willer and colleagues (1993) discovered that individuals with TBI were significantly less integrated on every subscale of the CIQ than the nondisabled, except for one area: Females with TBI were integrated into home activities to the same extent as nondisabled females. Further research is needed to evaluate reliability over time and for different methods of administering the CIQ. Other areas for exploration include comparison of the CIQ with related assessments and using this instrument with different populations.

The Craig Handicap Assessment and Reporting Technique (CHART) was developed to determine rehabilitation outcomes in relation to activities that society views as being productive (Whiteneck et al., 1992). Handicap in this assessment is defined in the same fashion as the World Health Organization (WHO) definition: An impairment or disability that interferes with the fulfillment of roles considered appropriate for an individual's age, gender, and culture. While constructing the items in this inventory, Whiteneck and associates (1992) paid attention to the variety of ways in which social roles were fulfilled. Designed for the spinal cord population, CHART is a survey consisting of the following components: physical independence, mobility, occupation, social integration, and economic self-sufficiency. A maximum score of 500 points is possible, with 100 points allotted for each of the five components. CHART was calibrated on the able-bodied population. Good test-retest reliability has been documented on 135 individuals with spinal cord injury (SCI) who

were tested by an examiner on two separate occasions a week apart (Whiteneck et al., 1992). For interrater reliability, the ratings of the individual with SCI were compared with those of a spouse or close relative (Table 19–1). Content validity was found to be adequate when rehabilitation professionals rated individuals with various levels of SCI. In a pilot sample, a high correlation was found on the subscale of productive activity for the CIQ and occupation on the CHART but not for the social integration subscales (Willer et al., 1994). Across all five dimensions, the more severe the impairment, the more significant the handicap. However, considerable variability in handicap was evident in those with similar impairments (see Table 19–1).

The Reintegration to Normal Living (RNL) Index was developed to evaluate how successfully individuals were integrated into their communities after sustaining an injury or managing a chronic condition. According to RNL authors Wood-Dauphinee and colleagues (1988), reintegration was defined by the following domains: indoor, community, distant mobility, self-care, daily activity, recreational activity, social activity, general coping skills, family roles, personal relationships, and presentation of self to others. "I spend most of my days occupied in a work activity that is necessary or important to me" is an example of one of the statements used in the RNL questionnaire. The aforementioned items are rated according to a scale of 1 to 10, ranging from "this statement does not describe my situation" (1) to "this statement fully describes my situation" (10). A second version of the questionnaire was developed for people who require adaptive devices, motor aids, or human assistance. The RNL is available in both French and English.

Preliminary studies have shown high internal consistency of the RNL (0.90 and higher). In determining interrater reliability, Wood-Dauphinee and associates (1988) found higher correlations when the responses of cancer patients were compared with those of their significant others (0.63) as opposed to those of the health professionals caring for them (0.40). With this in mind, the researchers excluded the ratings of health professionals from future studies. Authors of the RNL Index recommended that populations other than cancer patients be studied and monitored for longer periods of time (Wood-

TABLE 19–1

RELIABILITY OF THE CRAIG HANDICAP ASSESSMENT AND REPORTING TECHNIQUE

	Test-Retest	Interrater
Physical independence	0.92	0.80
Mobility	0.95	0.84
Occupation	0.89	0.81
Economic self-sufficiency	0.80	0.69
Social integration	0.81	0.57
Overall	0.93	0.83

Dauphinee et al., 1988). Regarding construct validity, a moderately strong correlation was found between the RNL and the Quality of Life (QL) Index. The QL was designed for physicians to use with individuals with cancer and other chronic diseases. Requiring only several minutes to administer, the domains measured include activity, daily living, health, support, and outlook on life. High internal consistency and interrater reliability of the QL have been reported (Spitzer et al., 1981).

DRIVING

Driving is an important activity to a great number of people, as it represents independence. When unable to drive, one has to rely on others to engage in activities outside of the home. No particular driving assessment is considered standard, as individuals with disabilities vary, as do driving evaluators. Currently, professionals involved in disabled driving have the opportunity to become recognized as driver rehabilitation specialists by taking a certification examination.

Driving assessments mentioned in the literature include computerized and standardized psychometric tests, visual tests, and on-the-road driver evaluations (Brooke et al., 1992; Engrum et al., 1989; Korner-Bitensky et al., 1994). Many of the same perceptual tests were found in these different assessments, such as the Trail Making test of the Halstead-Reitan Neuropsychological Battery and portions of the Wechsler Adult Intelligence Scale (WAIS-R) (Lezak, 1983). The Cognitive Behavioral Driver's Index (CBDI) is one such instrument that combines the aforementioned tests and the Driver Performance Test. The CBDI was designed for the neurologically involved individual and has shown high internal consistency and reliability and good validity (Engrum et al., 1989).

Gouvier and others (1988) mentioned five components that were essential in determining driving ability: gross sensory and motor function; cognitive and perceptual ability; knowledge of rules of the road and judgment regarding driving situations (as measured by the Driver Performance Test [DPT]); computerized driving simulator and small vehicle (e.g., golf cart) maneuvering competence on a closed course; and full-size vehicle maneuvering competence on a closed course and public highways. If at any point during the evaluation process a person does not adequately master one of the components, the test is ended. Training may then be implemented to correct the specific deficit. This assessment was designed for the population with TBI and for other severely disabled individuals. Further validation of the five components is needed. However, the DPT used in component three has been standardized on 8000 automobile and light truck drivers and has good predictive validity (Weaver, 1982); i.e., significantly higher automobile accident rates occur in people who score below the average classification rating on the DPT.

In 1990, Galski and associates reported that a typical driver evaluation consisting of predriver components (perceptual and cognitive tasks) and on-the-road components had no predictive validity or criterion validity with individuals who had had a stroke or TBI. The evaluator's decision to pass or fail an individual with a neurologic impairment was based not on any of the subtests but more on subjective information. Components of the predriver evaluation did not correlate with on-the-road tests. Galski and others (1990) emphasized the necessity of clearly identifying skills necessary for driving. Galski and colleagues (1992) proposed a particular model of driving (the cybernetic model), which they tested on 35 individuals with TBI. Individuals were given a predriver evaluation (various neuropsychological tests), simulator evaluation (two-dimensional driving exercise), and behind-the-wheel evaluation (on a protected course, as well as in usual traffic). Results indicated that 93% of the variability of the driving outcome was explained cumulatively by the predriver and simulator evaluations in addition to behavioral measures (e.g., inattention, distractibility). In fact, the seven neuropsychological tests alone primarily accounted for driving outcome. Following up on their past recommendations, Galski and coworkers (1993) evaluated 58 individuals with TBI and 48 with cerebrovascular accident (CVA) on behind-the-wheel driving performance. They again found that the predriver evaluation, along with the simulator evaluation and behavioral measures, was the best method of determining driving ability because of its high sensitivity and the safety it provides the patient and driving evaluator.

Sprigle and colleagues (1995) surveyed driving evaluators across the country regarding their driving assessments and satisfaction with their evaluations and equipment. The 21-question survey was returned by 138 evaluators from 44 states and consisted of occupational therapists (62% of the evaluators), with the main location of driver training being a medical facility (80%) for all evaluators. The most commonly measured physical characteristics were range of motion, manual muscle testing, sensation, grip and pinch strength, fine motor dexterity, and eye-hand coordination. Driving characteristics most commonly measured included gas, brake, and steering force and brake and steering reaction time. Sprigle and others (1995) commented on the lack of standardized methods for identifying driving ability and the reliance on subjective functional tests. Despite this, they noted that 66% of the survey respondents were satisfied with their evaluations and equipment (e.g., simulators). Further research to be conducted should identify assistive driving equipment and essential driving characteristics that predict driving ability.

After passing the various components of a driver assessment, individuals may require adaptations to their vehicles. Sabo and Shipp (1989) have identified equipment and strategies for a variety of disabilities. Since each person with a disability presents a unique challenge, generalizations concerning any diagnosis and its relation to driving are difficult to make. For more information regarding driving and the disabled, refer to the Appendix that follows.

APPENDIX

Resources

ASSOCIATION OF DRIVER EDUCATORS FOR THE DISABLED (ADED): An international organization providing service in the field of driver education for the disabled. Responsible for the development of the Certified Driver Rehabilitation Specialist (CDRS) examination. A list of driver training evaluators in each state is available on request. For more information, call Ric Cerna at (608) 884-8833.

LOUISIANA TECH UNIVERSITY CENTER FOR REHABILITATION SCIENCE AND BIOMEDICAL ENGINEERING: Several booklets written by experienced driving evaluators are available regarding motor vehicle selection, adaptive driving devices, and vehicle modifications. Workshops on driver assessment and training of staff are conducted by the professionals at the Center. For more information, contact Mike Shipp at (318) 257-4562 or 711 S. Vienna, P.O. Box 3185, Ruston, Louisiana 71272.

GUYNES DESIGN INC. (GDI): Creator of Independence Square™ Rehabilitation Centers enhanced care environments (creator of the original "Easy Street"). For more information, contact Patricia Moore at (602) 254-6690.

ADA CHECKLIST FOR READILY ACHIEVABLE BARRIER REMOVAL: To obtain a copy, ask for the Disability and Business Technical Assistance Center in your geographic region by calling 1-800-949-4ADA.

GLOSSARY

Accessibility—Pertaining to the physical arrangement of a building, outside facility, or other structure and the ease with which people with disabilities can enter the structure and benefit from its services and products.

Americans with Disabilities Act (ADA)—Legislation enacted in 1990 mandating that people with disabilities have the same opportunities as the nondisabled in finding employment and accessing public accommodations and public transportation.

Cognitive Behavioral Driver's Inventory (CBDI)—Test battery that measures cognitive and behavioral skills applicable to driving; is available in software form. The CBDI was developed and researched in a clinical rehabilitation setting of brain-injured individuals.

Community integration—Refers to getting people with an injury or disease back into regular activities within the community, such as working, socializing, engaging in leisure skills, performing activities of daily living, and driving.

Community Integration Questionnaire (CIQ)—Assesses the degree of community integration of individuals with a disability. Originally designed for the population with TBI.

Craig Handicap Assessment and Reporting Technique (CHART)—Community assessment designed originally for individuals with an SCI.

Driver Performance Test (DPT)—Tests knowledge of rules of the road and judgment regarding driving situations.

Handicap—An impairment or disability that interferes with the fulfillment of roles considered appropriate for an individual's age, gender, and culture.

Independence Square™—Realistic modules of businesses and leisure areas in which people with disabilities can bridge the gap from hospital to home by practicing various activities.

Quality of Life Index (QL)—Designed for physician use, this concise questionnaire measures how well individuals with chronic problems are performing at home.

Reintegration to Normal Living Index (RNL)—Designed originally for chronic populations, this questionnaire assesses how well an individual is faring within the community and home.

REFERENCES

Adaptive Environments Center. (1992). *The Americans with Disabilities Act checklist for readily achievable barrier removal.* Washington DC: National Institute on Disability and Rehabilitation Research.

Bachelder, J. M., & Hilton, C. L. (1994). Implications of the Americans with Disabilities Act of 1990 for elderly persons. *American Journal of Occupational Therapy, 48,* 73–81.

Brooke, M. M., Questad, K. A., Patterson, D. R., & Valois, T. A. (1992). Driving evaluation after traumatic brain injury. *American Journal of Physical Medicine and Rehabilitation, 71,* 177–182.

Dix, A. (1992). Life on Easy Street . . . Using simulated streets to rehabilitate patients to the real world outside. *Nursing Times, 88,* 26–29.

El-Ghatit, A. Z., Melvin, J. L., & Poole, M. A. (1980). Training apartment in the community for spinal cord injured patients: A model. *Archives of Physical Medicine and Rehabilitation, 61,* 90–92.

Engrum, E. S., Lambert, E. W., Scott, K., Pendergrass, T., & Womac, J. (1989). Criterion-related validity of the Cognitive Behavioral Driver's Index. *Cognitive Rehabilitation, 7,* 22–31.

Federal Register. (1973). Rehabilitation Act of 1973. Federal Register, 41(August 23), 163.

Galski, T., Bruno, R. L., & Ehle, H. T. (1992). Driving after cerebral damage: A model with implications for evaluation. *American Journal of Occupational Therapy, 46,* 324–332.

Galski, T., Bruno, R. L., & Ehle, H. T. (1993). Prediction of behind-the-wheel driving performance in patients with cerebral brain damage: A discriminant function analysis. *American Journal of Occupational Therapy, 47,* 391–396.

Galski, T., Ehle, H. T., & Bruno, R. L. (1990). An assessment of measures to predict the outcome of driving evaluations in patients with cerebral damage. *American Journal of Occupational Therapy, 44,* 709–713.

Goggins, M., Hall, N., Nack, K., & Shuart, B. (1990). Community reintegration program. *Journal of Burn Care Rehabilitation, 11,* 343–346.

Gouvier, W. D., Schweitzer, J. R., Horton, C., Maxfield, M., Shipp, M., Seaman, R. L., & Hale, P. N. (1988). A systems approach to assessing driving skills among TBI and other severely disabled individuals. *Rehabilitation Education, 2,* 197–204.

Henderson, J. (1994). Humanity by design. *Interiors, 8,* 58, 59.

Korner-Bitensky, N., Sofer, S., Kaizer, F., Gelinas, I., & Talbot, L. (1994). Assessing ability to drive following an acute neurological event: Are we on the right road? *Canadian Journal of Occupational Therapy, 61,* 141–148.

Law, M., Stewart, D., & Strong, S. (1995). Achieving access to home, community, and workplace. In C. Trombly (Ed.), *Occupational therapy for physical dysfunction* (pp. 361–375). Baltimore MD: Williams & Wilkins.

Lezak, M. D. (1983). *Neuropsychological assessment.* New York: Oxford Press.

Reynolds, R. (1993). Recreation and leisure lifestyle changes. In Paul Wehman (Ed.), *The ADA mandate for social change.* Baltimore, Maryland: Paul H. Brookes Publishing Co.

Sabo, S., & Shipp, M. (1989). Disabilities and their implications for driving. Washington DC: National Institute on Disability and Rehabilitation Research.

Smigielski, J. S. Malec, J. F., Thompson, J. M., & DePompolo, R. W. (1992). Mayo Medical Center brain injury outpatient program: Treatment procedures and early outcome data. *Mayo Clinic Proceedings, 67,* 767–774.

Spitzer, W. O., Dobson, A. J., Hall, J., Chesterman, E., Levi, J., Shepherd, R., Battista, R. N., & Catchlove, B. R. (1981). Measuring quality of life of cancer patients: Concise QL-Index for use by physicians. *Journal of Chronic Disease, 34,* 585–597.

Sprigle, S., Morris, B. O., Nowachek, G., & Karg, P. E. (1995). Assessment of the evaluation procedures of drivers with disabilities. *Occupational Therapy Journal of Research, 15,* 147–164.

Weaver, J. K. (1982). *Driver Performance Test.* Dunwoody, GA: SPA Productions.

Whiteneck, G. G., Charlifue, S. W., Gerhart, K. A., Overholser, J., & Richardson, G. N. (1992). Quantifying handicap: A new measure of long-term rehabilitation outcomes. *Archives of Physical Medicine and Rehabilitation, 73,* 519–526.

Willer, B., Ottenbacher, K. J., & Coad, M. L. (1994). The community integration questionnaire. A comparative examination. *American Journal of Physical Medicine and Rehabilitation, 73,* 103–111.

Willer, B., Rosenthal, M., Kreutzer, J. S., Gordon, W. A., & Rempel, R. (1993). Assessment of community integration following rehabilitation for traumatic brain injury. *Journal of Head Trauma Rehabilitation, 8,* 75–87.

Wood-Dauphinee, S. L., Opzoomer, A., Williams, J. I., Marchand, B., & Spitzer, W. O. (1988). Assessment of global function: The reintegration to normal living index. *Archives of Physical Medicine and Rehabilitation, 69,* 583–590.

CHAPTER 20

Work Activities

Bruce A. Mueller, OTR/L, CHT

Ellen D. Adams, MA, CRC, CCM

Carol A. Isaac, PT, BS

SUMMARY   Work evaluation includes evaluation of the injured or the potential worker, type of work to be performed, and how that work is performed. In this chapter we explore the history of work evaluation and the interrelationship of the workers' attitudes and temperaments and the job. Evaluation systems are explored, as well as the role of the evaluators. Musculoskeletal evaluations, standardized testing, and computerized testing are also examined. Maximum voluntary effort, abnormal illness behavior, and functional testing are explored in light of the ever-changing medicolegal milieu. A case study (see Appendix A at the end of this chapter) is presented to illustrate the interactions of an interdisciplinary functional capacity evaluation, work hardening, and eventual return to work. It is recommended that documentation of the assessment be concise, devoid of overly technical language, well-supported by current research, and readable by the major players in the work-injured person's rehabilitation. Those individuals are the injured worker and his or her family members, occupational and physical therapists, the insurance adjustor, the rehabilitation or vocational counselor, the physician, the attorney, the psychologist, and the judge of workers' compensation claims. A sample Functional Capacity Evaluation (see Appendix B at the end of this chapter) is presented, emphasizing the interaction of the assessment of the evaluee's physical abilities by either an occupational therapist or a physical therapist and the psychosocial and vocational history by a rehabilitation counselor. Physician and attorney statements (see Appendix C at the end of this chapter) also are presented.

HISTORY

In the past, "occupational therapy took root in a rich soil of work activities for the mentally ill. In the early 1920s, the first occupational therapists documented steps for a uniform program of curative activity" (Marshall, 1985, p. 297). Currently, physical therapists such as Keith Blankenship, Glenda Key, and Duane Saunders have taken a major step forward in the development of work assessment systems and industrial medicine. However, most of the early work programs and work assessments were done from the field of occupational therapy. In contrast to the current theory, in the early 1900s, work was a modality of treatment—not the goal of treatment. "Despite recent technological advances, physical disability work programs of the 1990s are distinctly similar to those of the early 1900s" (Hanson & Walker, 1992, p. 56). Hanson and Walker have cited numerous references that document that moral treatment stemmed from the use of recreation, employment, and self-care as a mode of treatment for mental illness. The mentally ill were no longer treated as subhuman. Work was prescribed to increase self-esteem and to meet unconscious needs.

In the early years, the pioneers of occupational therapy used the environment around them as a mode of treatment, a situation not unlike today when a work hardening facility has a group lunch prepared by a primary school food service worker. In the 30s "some considered the entire hospital to be an occupational therapy department" (Marshall, 1985, p. 297). As Edwina Marshall points out, the occupational therapist had "clearly defined" responsibilities and "industrial therapy or employment therapy was born." She further notes that "the occupational therapists initiated and supervised the program using activities necessary for the normal function of patients and employees as in treatment modalities. Work assignments were matched with experience, aptitude, and interests of the patient" (Marshall, 1985, p. 297). One would have to search the literature to its depths to find a description of the goals of work assessment and work hardening that is better written, more on target, and more simply stated yet complex.

In the 1930s and 1940s, workshops were beginning to become respected modes of treatment. However, occupational therapy's role and work evaluation changed in the 1950s due to the burgeoning field of vocational rehabilitation and through occupational therapy volitional distancing from this field. During an occupational therapy conference in the late 1950s, only 2 of 34 curriculum directors defended work evaluation as a necessary component of all occupational therapy treatment for all age and disability groups. Opponents placed work evaluation in a back room with vocational counselors and would not consider it occupational therapy (Marshall, 1985, p. 298). Some occupational therapists did not follow this consensus. In the early 1950s "the paradigm of occupation was attacked by both members of the medical profession and occupational therapy" (Harvey-Krefting, 1985, p. 304). A paradigm, by definition, is an example serving as a pattern. As Kuhn (1970) suggests, a paradigm explains what the profession does and how it is done. As Harvey-Krefting (1985) notes, the occupational therapy paradigm indicated "the health-restoring effect of occupation in the extensive use of crafts as work projects" (p. 303). She notes that Kielhoffer and Burke (cited in Harvey-Krefting, 1985) describe the occupational paradigm period as one when therapists treated problems stemming from interruptions in work or lack of occupation. Idleness, poor work habit formation, and lack of social skills were seen as demoralizing and as fostering a sick or invalid role. Work was introduced to break this cycle (Harvey-Krefting, 1985). Again, work was the treatment

modality, not the goal. Barton (cited in Hanson & Walker, 1992) indicates that therapeutic work was preliminary to and dovetailed with real vocational education, which was beyond the scope of occupational therapy.

As Harvey-Krefting (1985) points out, "therapists began to feel uncomfortable with the simple operating principle that it was good for disabled people to keep busy. This discomfort eventually led to the borrowing and adopting of knowledge from other disciplines and hence, the development of the 'inner-mechanism paradigm'" (p. 304). In the inner-mechanisms paradigm, therapists began to establish work evaluation programs and to develop work samples that reflected specific jobs. This new scientific approach that therapists should not be just observers; they should take a more scientific, objective, and professional approach, was emphasized. Harvey-Krefting (1985) further notes that "holistic principles accepted during the occupational paradigm were sacrificed to narrow, more precise concepts such as defense mechanisms and sensory integration" (p. 304). During this new way of looking at the therapeutic use of work, new definitions of work assessment and work therapy were developed. Work as an end in gainful employment became the crux of the program. Harvey-Krefting (1985) notes that "evaluation in the occupational paradigm was mainly prevocational in nature and used crafts or daily living skills to assess readiness for work therapy" (p. 303).

In the 1950s, structured prevocational programs became popular. The TOWER (Testing Orientation Work Evaluation and Rehabilitation) System drew therapists from around the country. As Ogden-Niemeyer and Jacobs (1989) indicate in their book *Work Hardening, State of the Art*, prevocational evaluation and vocational evaluation were originally part of the same service that provided both primary and secondary vocational assessment, which then became specialized. Primary vocational assessment deals with the general trainability, or potential for further intensive testing or training for employment. Secondary vocational assessment deals with potential for specific training areas, i.e., work evaluation, in what was then (in the late 1950s and early 1960s) part of the already mentioned growing field of vocational evaluation. "Results from the evaluations yielded production features of neatness, safety, work habits, intellectual and attitudinal factors" (Hanson & Walker, 1992, p. 60). Hanson and Walker further note that other programs included prevocational assessment geared for the person who did not have a work history or who had not worked for many years. Although the TOWER System was preeminent during this time, it was not without drawbacks. While being comprehensive (it was used for 2 weeks to 6 months minimum, 5 to 6 hours per day graduated to 8 hours per day), it needed a large city population base and was expensive.

Other tests produced in the 1950s were done in association with *The Dictionary of Occupational Titles* (Field & Field, 1988; described later in this chapter), as indicated by Wegg (1960). Wegg further indicates that norms involving production and proficiency ratings were available for each testing kit. These early work samples led the way for the Jewish Evaluation Vocational System (JEVS) and Valpar Work Samples. The McCarron-Dyal Work Evaluation System was also established primarily for the mentally retarded and the chronically mentally ill. Singer was an evaluation system for unspecified target groups and had 20 work samples for skilled trades. In Velozo's (1993) article, he states "vocational evaluations (work evaluations developed by vocational evaluators) generally provide testing in one or more of the following areas: A) vocational interests; B) aptitudes and achievements; C) motor skills; D) work samples" (p. 204). Since vocational evaluations emerged from the Carl Perkins Vocational Act, most of these have been designed to assess the potential worker, e.g., the disabled student. These types of tests do not readily transfer to the injured worker attempting to return to work. The vocational evaluation would be the evaluation of choice (as long as the physical abilities and limitations are known) for the injured worker who has a desire to return to work but is unable to return to his or her usual and customary job and has no transferrable skills. As Velozo (1993) further points out, "unlike traditional vocational assessments, no single discipline can lay claim to developing evaluations for the injured worker" (p. 204). We agree since it is our intent to recommend that evaluation of the injured worker not be done by a single discipline. Evaluation of the injured worker is best done within the scope of an interdisciplinary program. Issues addressed include prior and current work history, the individual's current psychosocial and vocational milieu, abnormal illness behaviors, medical history, diagnosis and biomechanical issues, physical abilities and limitations, current litigation, and funding sources. No one therapist can adequately address all of these areas, even when the issues to be assessed are clear. We recommend a continuum of care from a focused 1- to 2-hour evaluation for the simple release to work parameters to a full-blown interdisciplinary functional capacity evaluation utilizing a physical or occupational therapist (depending on diagnosis) and a vocational rehabilitation counselor.

In summary, work assessment has evolved over a number of years and has its roots in the pioneers of occupational therapy. No one discipline of occupational or physical therapy or vocational evaluation can claim to be the full developer of work assessment. It is our contention that work assessment is best done in an interdisciplinary program that is specifically geared to deal with the workers' compensation system and that deals specifically with the injured worker population's needs.

KINDS OF PATHOLOGY

During the initial stages of work assessment (work as a therapeutic medium), the diagnoses assessed were psychi-

atric disorders. Now the majority of work assessment is done within the scope of physical dysfunction.

Low back pain is the most commonly assessed disorder for return-to-work functional capacity evaluations (FCEs). Mayer and Gatchel (1988) indicate "low back pain is the most expensive, benign condition in industrialized countries. It is also the number one cause of disabilities in persons under the age of 45" (p. 93). They further note that more than 1 percent of the working-age population is totally and permanently disabled by the problem. Our own research indicates the following statistics regarding percentages of FCEs by diagnosis:

- Low back problems (strains and sprains, herniated discs, and fusions), 39 percent
- Upper extremities or hand injuries, 36 percent
- Cervical injuries, 14 percent
- Other (lower extremities and multiple injuries), 11 percent

The physical demand levels of the injured workers' jobs who presented for FCEs were broken down as follows:

- Sedentary work (lifting less than 10 lb, infrequent standing and walking), 8 percent
- Light work (lifting 10 to 20 lb occasionally, frequent standing and walking), 43 percent
- Medium work (occasional lifting 20 to 50 lb, frequent lifting 10 to 20 lb), 46 percent
- Heavy work (lifting 100 lb maximum with frequent lifting or carrying of objects up to 50 lb) or very heavy work (lifting objects in excess of 100 lb with lifting or carrying of objects 50 lb or more), 3 percent

These categories of work are further clarified in the section on *The Dictionary of Occupational Titles* (Field & Field, 1988).

INTRODUCTION TO FUNCTIONAL CAPACITY EVALUATION

The FCE is an interdisciplinary evaluation that is used to assess the physical, functional, vocational, and psychosocial status of an injured worker. The importance of the FCE has been made clear by the comments of a physician and an attorney who usually represent the insurance company in workers' compensation litigation (see Appendix C at the end of this chapter). Musculoskeletal testing, computerized and standardized testing, vocational and psychosocial history (see Appendix D at the end of this chapter), and abnormal illness behavior are addressed. These areas are described in detail in the following sections.

Identifying Data

Prior to the actual performance and administration of an FCE, many details require the assistance of support staff and professional staff. The referral for the FCE most often comes from the treating physician. Other referral sources include the insurance adjustor (also known as the carrier), rehabilitation providers, plaintiff or defense attorneys, and employers. In some instances, the referring physician is not actually treating the injured worker but is seeing the individual for an independent medical evaluation. Some states require a prescription from a doctor to perform a FCE. This is a good practice whether or not it is required by law, as it allows the injured worker and the evaluators to have the confidence that the physician supports this type of testing and agrees that the client is able to participate in the testing.

At the time of the referral, the referral source is asked for certain identifying data on the client, including the client's name, address, age, phone number, date of injury, diagnosis, surgeries, employer, insurance carrier, rehabilitation provider, and attorney and physician information. This information becomes part of the permanent record. At this time it is also important to request medical records for the evaluators to review prior to the injured worker's arrival for their evaluation.

Once the referral is received, verbal authorization to perform the FCE is obtained from the insurance adjustor, and the price for the FCE is established. It is a good idea at that point to follow up the conversation with a letter confirming the date and time of the appointment and the charge that was agreed on. Some states regulate the fees and the professionals required to perform the evaluations.

After authorization for the service is obtained, the injured worker should be notified by phone and in writing of his or her appointment time. The injured worker should be encouraged to call with any questions he or she may have to help alleviate any fears regarding the purpose and nature of the testing. Making phone contact with the person to be evaluated increases compliance in attending the scheduled appointment. The letter sent to the client should include the date and time of testing, who requested and authorized the FCE, what to wear, directions to the facility, and encouragement for the client to inform the therapist in advance of medical problems that are not related to the injury but could interfere with testing. The letter should direct the client to call to confirm the appointment and to clarify any questions he or she may have. Other persons involved in the care of the injured worker, i.e., the rehabilitation provider, medical doctor, and adjustor, should always be kept informed of appointment dates, times, and changes if they occur to promote ongoing and open communication and to prevent the injured worker from "falling through the cracks," or getting lost in the system, thereby increasing the overall cost by delaying the return to work. Additionally, keeping everyone informed eases the process of coordinating return medical appointments.

When the injured worker arrives for his or her appointment, he or she is initially oriented to the facility, which includes introduction of the staff with whom he or she will work and locating restrooms, rest areas, and fire plan and exits. Release forms (Figs. 20–1 and 20–2) to request additional medical, vocational, or psychological reports and to release the results of the FCE to the appropriate persons are signed by the client and witnessed by the staff. Additional medical history is assessed, and a general health screen is administered. The client's blood pressure and pulse are taken to make sure they are within safe, testable limits.

The client is asked to sign an FCE Participation Agreement (Fig. 20–3), which is explained to the injured worker by the therapist who will be performing the FCE. This form tells the client what is expected in terms of exertion. The client is instructed to stop an activity if abnormal discomfort (i.e., discomfort other than what he or she usually feels) is experienced. The client is told verbally and in writing that consistency of effort and maximum voluntary effort is being assessed throughout the testing. The client and the therapist both sign this form.

The client's past medical history is secured by means of a questionnaire that is filled out by the client and reviewed for pertinent information that may affect or limit aspects of the evaluation. The client is asked to report on any surgery ever had, medications currently being taken, and all doctors currently treating him or her for any condition. The client is asked to report to the therapist the diagnosis as he or she understands it, and it is compared with the diagnosis given to the therapist by the physician. At times the client may have more current information on his or her condition than was relayed at referral. The client is also asked to describe his or her symptoms verbally, to answer questions on several pain assessment questionnaires, and to complete a pain drawing and rating diagram. Facilities and FCE systems vary widely on pain and behavioral questionnaires administered and the degree of health screening.

As part of the evaluation, a psychosocial and vocational history questionnaire (see Appendix D at the end of this chapter) is mailed to the client to fill out prior to coming to the evaluation, or it is given to the client on arrival to the facility. The purpose of this questionnaire is to obtain information regarding the injured worker's perception of his or her social, vocational, educational, financial, family, and recreational activities prior to and since the injury. It is recommended that a certified rehabilitation counselor further explore this information with the injured worker to assess the impact of the injury on the client's life. This information is also used to assist the client in developing realistic vocational goals as he or she begins the return-to-work process and to identify other potential, non–injury-related barriers to successfully returning to work. It is important to note that no current assessment tool can establish motivation or lack thereof. The professionals involved in the FCE process have a responsibility to report objective data and professional observations.

PHYSICAL RESTORATION CENTERS
of Florida

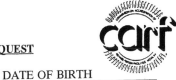

<u>INFORMATION RELEASE/REQUEST</u>

REGARDING _____ DATE OF BIRTH_____

(State full name and date of birth of person to whom disclosure refers)

INFORMATION SOURCE ___The Physical Restoration Center_____

___3601 SW 2nd Ave, Suite S, Gainesville, FL 32607_____

INFORMATION RECIPIENT (Specify individual, title, program, agency, address, any or all as appropriate)

       DOCTOR:_____

       INSURANCE CARRIER:_____

       REHABILITATION:_____

       CLIENT ATTORNEY:_____

       OTHER:_____

PURPOSE _____

FORM: WRITTEN, VERBAL, AUDIO, ELECTRONIC

I consent to the release of information described above. I may revoke my consent at any time by delivery of a written notice to the source of information specified above. It will be effective upon the date notice is received by them, but excluding information already furnished by them before that date. In the absence of my formal written notice, this consent is revoked automatically on the date indicated below.

_____

Signature of person to whom disclosure refers/Signature of parent or other authorized person (If person to whom disclosure refers is a minor or incompetent)

_____

Date of consent

_____

Date automatically revoked

_____

Signature of Witness

_____

Date witnessed

<u>To the recipient of this information:</u> This information is being disclosed to you from records whose confidentiality is protected by Federal Law. Federal regulations prohibit you from making any further disclosure of it without the specific written consent of the person to whom it pertains, or as otherwise permitted by such regulations (42 CRF Part 2). A general authorization for the release of medical or other information is NOT sufficient for this purpose.

PRC Rev 6/95

3601 S.W. 2ND AVENUE, SUITE S GAINESVILLE, FLORIDA 32607-2802 • PHONE (904) 336-6830 FAX (904) 336-6910

FIGURE 20–1. Permission form for releasing results of the evaluation to stated persons.

Musculoskeletal Examination

An orthopedic assessment of the spine is covered elsewhere in this book. Patients coming to the clinic for an FCE usually have had a complete musculoskeletal examination elsewhere. Insurance companies are more and more reluctant to pay for duplicate services, and the real goal of an FCE is to test function specific to a client's ability to work. However, some tests specific for the industrial rehabilitation client should be included, especially if the patient has never been evaluated by a physical or occupa-

tional therapist. Numeric data can be obtained, and certain abnormal illness behavior tests can be easily performed at this time. Occasionally, a secondary injury from another area will be found, which may be what is restricting the patient's ability to work rather than the primary area of complaint; this situation should be well documented.

There are many ways to measure range of motion of the spine. General flexibility should be observed, but it has been shown that visual assessment of spinal flexibility is unreliable. An inexpensive way of assessing lumbar range of

and is appropriate for the person who reports that he or she is able to return to the same job and does not have overt behavioral or psychosocial problems.

This type of evaluation generally takes an hour or less to perform by one therapist, it does not have a validity component, and it does not address specific job duties. This evaluation should not be used for the person who has not progressed appropriately in physical therapy, for the person who reports that he or she is unable to return to work, for the person who has no job to return to, or for the person with overt pain behaviors. Appendix E at the end of this chapter is an example of a format for a physical abilities assessment.

Maximum Voluntary Effort

What is the state of the art, state of the science, state of the "guess" when evaluating maximum voluntary effort? As clinicians who work in the field of FCEs and return-to-work programs, we are deluged with physicians, insurance adjustors, and attorneys who want to know "Is this person for real?" "Is he or she exaggerating the symptoms?" "Does he or she have real problems?" Knowing if the injured worker produces a maximum voluntary effort (MVE) is imperative to the outcome validity of the FCE. The therapist needs to know the evaluee's effort, since ethically and professionally we are required to offer suggestions and make decisions that directly affect people's lives. We are called on by employers to assist them in the reemployment process, by attorneys for expert testimony, by insurance companies who want cost-effective treatment and positive outcomes, and by physicians who are ultimately responsible for the decision to release the injured worker to work and with what restrictions.

The topic of MVE is identified in the literature as far back as 1954 (Bectol, 1954). Research on this topic is ongoing, and this area of practice needs further study. Significant research and clinical focus have been directed toward identifying the injured worker who is magnifying his or her symptoms through tests of MVE. In 1972, Donald B. Chaffin and his colleagues, from their attempts to reduce high injury rates among workers in strenuous jobs requiring frequent lifting, pushing, and pulling, advised a method of isometric strength testing for preemployment screening (cited in Ogden-Niemeyer & Jacobs, 1989). These tests were found to be reliable, with a coefficient of variation (CV) for repetitive trials between 10 percent and 13 percent (Ogden-Niemeyer & Jacobs, 1989). A coefficient of variation is a standard deviation of the test and retest scores divided by the mean, multiplied by 100. Static strength testing combined with coefficients of variation was the hallmark of the more objective methods of determining effort. Equipment such as the Isometric Strength Testing Unit (ISTU) produced by Ergometrics and the Force Gauge Platform devised by Keith Blankenship, PT, became avail-

able. The Jamar Dynamometer, utilizing CVs, also became widely used. Ogden-Niemeyer and Jacobs (1989, p. 101) point out that

> the rationale for maximum voluntary effort is based on a number of assumptions. The first assumption is that, given an inherently reliable procedure where body posture, individual joint angles, and muscles are carefully controlled, individuals giving maximum effort during an assessment of strength will show a high level of reliability and low variance during closely spaced serial trials. The second assumption is that the individual who is magnifying dysfunction consciously or unconsciously will not give maximum effort during physical testing. The third is that the lack of maximum effort is associated with inconsistency or unreliability of performance.

Multiple literature sources traditionally list 15 percent as the cutoff point for MVE. That is, if enough CVs are greater than 15 percent, submaximal effort is suspected. Recent research is challenging this concept (Robinson et al., 1993). Robinson and colleagues showed that classification rates had unacceptably large errors, with 69 percent of submaximal efforts being classified as maximal with the traditional 15 percent cutoff. They also reported that the currently practiced method of using a low number of repetitions to calculate CVs may result in very unstable measures. Currently many facilities and evaluation systems (e.g., Blankenship, Key, Ergos, Maximum Voluntary Effort Protocol) rely at least partially, if not heavily, on using CVs to determine MVE. Further confirmatory research in this area seems to be warranted; however, it should be noted that most of the research supports CVs as a method of determining submaximal effort. The literature reveals other methods for determining MVE. Bell-shaped curves were first described by Stokes in 1983. He proposed that using a five-position dynamometer, a modified bell-shaped curve represents a maximal effort. Additionally, flattened curves were demonstrated in conjunction with electromyography (EMG) in the 1993 literature by Hoffmaster and associates. Coefficients of variation with the dynamometer on multiple trials are also frequently used as another indicator of MVE.

Incidentally, Bectol (1954) described the beginnings of using CVs. This method was formally described in 1988 in an excellent article by Leonard Matheson entitled, "How do you know he tried his best? The reliability crisis in industrial rehabilitation." This concept was developed into a specific set of protocols, as described by Barren and coworkers (1992). They suggested that a baseline of 14 sets of 20 would fall below the CV standardized cutoff point to determine the trial as a maximum effort on the Baltimore Therapeutic Equipment (BTE). The BTE is an upper extremity work simulator that can measure static strength of the upper extremities.

In 1988, King and Berryhill described a method for comparing the BTE with the dynamometer. They stated "no assumption of validity and subsequent maximum voluntary effort should be made solely on the position of the hand on the dynamometer test" (i.e., bell-shaped curves) (p. 207). In this study, King and Berryhill showed a positive correlation between the BTE Work Simulator and the Jamar Dynamometer.

The Rapid Exchange of Grip (REG) test was described by Hildreth and colleagues (1989) for assessing MVE. Utilizing a hand grip dynamometer on position two is recommended. The evaluee then switches hands rapidly while exerting maximum effort. If the REG decreases, the effort is considered valid; if it increases, lack of MVE is suspected. From this author's experience, increase of 100 percent or more in grip strength has been demonstrated with rapid exchange of grip. The theory is that when REG is done quickly, the evaluee has less cortical control, and a truer assessment of strength is measured.

Distraction tests are also used in assessing MVE. As Blankenship (1989, p. 506) indicates,

these are tests which are performed while the patient is aware that the test is being performed, and performed again when the patient is not aware that the test is being performed. A passed distraction test results when the response to both tests is the same. A failed distraction test results when one result is recorded when the patient is aware that the test is being performed and a different result is recorded when the patient is not aware it is being performed.

An example of this is when the evaluee is told that he or she is going on a "walking test," and the evaluee stops approximately 20 feet after going out the front door, claiming that low back pain prevents further walking. If later during the FCE, the evaluee walks twice the original distance during the carrying test, then this would be a failed distraction test. The idea is that during the carrying test, the evaluee and his or her accompanying symptoms are focused on the 5-lb weight. Logically, the individual would not be able to carry the 5-lb weight farther than he or she is able to walk unencumbered. Blankenship (1989) cites another important example, the straight leg test. Since most chronic patients are aware that the straight leg raises should be limited and produce pain when performed in the supine test position, that result usually occurs. But they are not aware that the same results should occur while performing a manual muscle test of the quadriceps in the seated position while the hips are at approximately 80 degrees of flexion and the knee fully extended. In this position, with the client holding onto the front edge of the table so that he or she cannot lean backward, the leg is being raised to what would be comparable to a 60- to 80-degree straight leg raise. Significant differences in the results indicate that the patient is trying to control the results of the test. It should be noted that Blankenship (1989) describes in great detail additional validity criteria.

For elaboration in this area, see the section on abnormal illness behavior in this chapter.

Force curves with dynamic testing are also available for validity criteria. Torque curves and range of motion are available for consistency, and thorough training is available through the manufacturers (e.g., Cybex, Biodex, and Medex). This equipment is more fully described in the computerized test section of this chapter.

The central theme of the MVE testing is that no one test should be used to determine MVE— not pain drawings, elevated CVs, stocking anesthesia of the lower extremity, or even inconsistent SLR with distraction. Although all of these tests are signs of suspected lack of effort, a combination of tests is ideal. But what is the critical number of tests failed before the therapist can identify the effort as submaximal? Everyone would probably agree that more is better. In the changing field of health care, multiple-day evaluations may be a thing of the past. In our experience, the ability to do 2-day FCEs representing 8 to 12 hours of testing and being reimbursed appropriately is gone. Therefore, it becomes imperative to assess the situation in 1 to 2 hours to see if the evaluee is giving full effort. The luxury of observing consistency over days, making careful detailed analysis of behavior and function and how they relate to the diagnosis, is gone. Now the therapist must perform provocative tests that require the proper response from the injured worker to assess the level of effort.

Assessing validity must start with informed consent. The evaluee must know that his or her effort and physical function will be assessed. As stated previously, the client is told verbally and in writing that consistency of effort and MVE will be assessed throughout the evaluation. Be wary of the individual who makes a production of how much pain he or she is in but reports that he or she is here to "do my best." Such individuals may further state that "I have always tried hard at everything I do," as evidenced by his or her prior line of work, number of working years, number of hours per day, and other supporting evidence. As Blankenship (1994, p.430) suggests, be wary of the evaluee who reports high pain yet continues testing:

From a logical position, a person expressing high pain for which there is an organic basis would not agree to go through with an FCE which would cause further pain and possible re-injury. Therefore a person reporting a high pain level but who agrees to be subjected to an FCE must not be feeling much pain, or they would refuse to participate.

Excellent continuing education courses are available from multiple sources (e.g., Matheson Associates; Keith Blankenship and Duwane Saunders; and Karen Schultz-Johnson provide valuable information and may be reached at (714) 836-1224, (800) 248-8846, and (800) 654-8357, respectively). It is also recommended that for the uninitiated therapist in this field, following set procedures is perhaps best. Using set procedures with respected research behind their methods is advantageous in providing a high level of care, and it can be defended during a deposition for a litigated case. Using established procedures also minimizes the clinician's liability exposure. Therapists performing FCEs are commonly required to give depositions supporting the validity and reliability of the testing measures, as well as information regarding the client's performance during the testing.

If the evaluee is giving full effort, then the rest of the FCE is used to develop a level of restrictions and identify specific activities the client may be restricted from or may need to avoid. If, however, the test results are invalid and the initial portion of the FCE represents submaximal effort, a decision must be made. The therapist may choose to complete the evaluation to give a minimum amount of activity that the client can tolerate or may choose to terminate the test entirely and report the results to the physician or carrier. In some cases, it is advisable to discuss the findings of less-than-full effort with the evaluee. This should be done on a case-by-case basis, assessing the client's psychological strength and ability to handle this type of information. It is possible that with certain individuals, a change of behavior will occur, especially when the issue is discussed in a nonthreatening way. If a decision has been made to discuss the less-than-full effort findings with the injured worker, the therapist may go about it using language such as "perhaps you were distracted and the results indicate less than full effort. Would you like to attempt some of the tests again?" It is necessary that the therapist develop rapport with the individual to be tested. It has been reported that decreased fear helps the evaluee to give more consistent responses on objective testing.

In summary, the therapist observes, evaluates, documents, analyzes, and gives objective findings. If the results are inconsistent with maximum effort, therapists may instruct and give guidance to the client in an effort to attain full effort.

The state of the art of MVE is gaining the cooperation and appropriate responses from the client. The state of the science is collecting and analyzing the data with the current research in mind. The state of the "guess" is what the future research holds for determining MVE.

FUNCTIONAL CAPACITY EVALUATION SYSTEMS

Blankenship System

According to a personal communication by Blankenship (1994),

The Blankenship System of Functional Capacity Evaluations is a computerized system for evaluating the effect that any pathology has on an injured workers ability to work. The entire evaluation pro-cess is based on the bibliography of over 150 published articles which increases the credibility of legal testimony by the user. There are over 150 validity criteria in the evaluation process to help determine if the patient is responding to answers accurately and exerting good effort. The evaluation can be performed with a non-computerized system or computerized system. The computerized system includes report writing software which totally automates the entire process. This evaluation takes three to four hours.

Key Method

The Key Method was developed in 1980 by physical therapist Glenda Key in an attempt to objectively measure the capability of injured workers and their abilities to perform work. The Key Method of whole-body assessment is a standardized, computerized, objective evaluation tool used for return-to-work decisions and assessment. It can be used with any injury, such as "musculoskeletal, neurological, repetitive trauma, and others" (Miller, 1994, personal communication). Over 27 functional tests typically can be used in the 4-hour assessment. These procedures measure weight lifting, pushing and pulling, carrying, work day tolerance, sitting, standing, upper extremity function, and walking tolerance, as well as posture consistency and inconsistency and four levels of participation. The Key Method names four levels of validity: 1) valid (safe); 2) conditionally valid (underworking); 3) conditionally invalid (overworking); and 4) invalid (manipulator). The manufacturer reports that over 600 providers used the Key Method in the United States, the United Kingdom, Australia, and Canada and that their computerized system was built on the principles of whole-body functioning, return-to-work capabilities, standardized protocols, and functionally based outcomes. A picture of the system is included (Fig. 20–4).

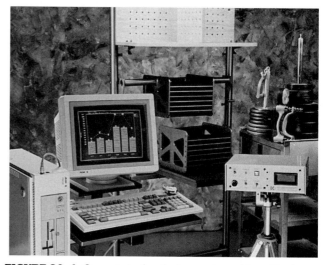

FIGURE 20–4. Computerized evaluation equipment from Key Assessment.

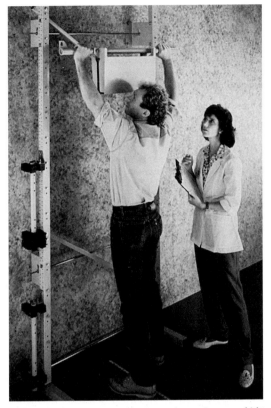

FIGURE 20–5. West II testing equipment for evaluation of lifting and lowering to various heights.

STANDARDIZED TESTING

Work Evaluations Systems Technologies II

The Work Evaluations Systems Technologies II (WEST II) equipment line provides the therapist with work simulators that may be used in preplacement or preemployment screening, work evaluation, work hardening, and performance of FCEs. The equipment's use is designed to address the conservative evaluation of dynamic lifting, range of motion, upper extremity strength, fatigue tolerance, and hand tool use in a safe clinical environment. The WEST equipment may be used to evaluate injuries of the upper extremities, back, neck, hand, and all the physical functions involving dynamic lifting. A picture of the WEST II is included (Fig. 20–5), and a standardization manual is available from the manufacturer.

EPIC Lift Capacity Test

The EPIC Lift Capacity (ELC) Test is an outgrowth of the WEST standard evaluation. Both tests were developed by Leonard M. Matheson. The ELC is a progressive isoinertial test that is composed of six subtests and is used to evaluate lift capacity across a broad spectrum of disability groups. This group of tests can measure occasional lifting and frequent lifting throughout a range of 12 inches off the floor to shoulder height. The client's experience of "how heavy the box feels" is used to help gauge lifting ability. Recently, a multisite study involving 65 ELC evaluators and 318 subjects in the United States and Canada was completed. The study demonstrated that

1. The ELC has an excellent interrater reliability, ranging from $r = 0.80$ to $r = 0.93$.
2. In addition to the primary variable under study, which was maximal acceptable weight, variables such as rating of perceived load, maximal heart rate, and heart rate increase are consistent over time.
3. Body mass is closely related to maximum acceptable weight, while age and resting heart rate make a significant but less important contribution.
4. The quotient of maximum acceptable weight divided by the body mass (termed relative acceptable weight) is normally distributed and provides a good index of lift capacity within each gender (normative data for females aged 18 through 29 years are depicted in Table 20–1).
5. Age stratification of the relative acceptable weight variable is appropriate, reflecting cross-sectional age differences, and will become more refined as the database increases in size.
6. Aerobic fitness, as indicated by resting heart rate, makes a small but significant contribution to lift capacity, especially with frequent lift tasks.

TABLE 20–1.							
NORMS FOR HEALTHY FEMALES IN TERMS OF RELATIVE ACCEPTABLE WEIGHT ACROSS SIX ELC SUBTESTS							
Age	Percentile	Test #1	Test #2	Test #3	Test #4	Test #5	Test #6
18 to 29 y (n = 96)	90	0.444*	0.593	0.433	0.357	0.480	0.368
	75	0.372	0.504	0.364	0.305	0.414	0.317
	50	0.315	0.390	0.308	0.261	0.322	0.250
	25	0.268	0.319	0.260	0.201	0.260	0.196
	10	0.211	0.261	0.208	0.171	0.192	0.159

*Maximum acceptable weight divided by body mass.

7. Cross-sectional age differences in lift capacity were found. If these represent actual age changes and lift capacity, the results of this research suggest that such changes may be the result of the combined effects of distribution of the musculoskeletal and cardiovascular systems with age. This can be studied through the ELC lift capacity test in a longitudinal or cross-sequential design.

8. The ELC can be used to evaluate adequacy for job demands as depicted by the U.S. Department Physical Demand Characteristics Support System. The ELC is an inexpensive procedure that does not require commercial equipment; however, several companies have been licensed to use the patented protocol. An example of the EPIC test device is seen in Figure 20–6.

Hand Tool Dexterity Test

The Hand Tool Dexterity Test was constructed to provide a measure of efficiency using regular mechanics tools, as this type of skill is important in a wide variety of jobs. This test attempts to measure manipulative skill independent of intellectual factors. "The essence of the examination procedure is to measure the ability of the examinee to perform manual tasks required" (Bennett, 1981, p. 3). This test is ideal as part of a functional evaluation due to the ease of administration in scoring, and no reading ability is required of the examinee. The score is the total amount of time it takes to remove 12 nuts and

bolts from the left upright and mount them on the right. The time begins when the examinee picks up the first wrench and ends when the last bolt has been tightened.

Norms have been established for industrial and educational groups, male job applicants in a southern plant, male adults at a vocational guidance center, airline engine mechanics, apprentice welders in a steel company, electric maintenance workers, employees and applicants in a manufacturing company, boys in a vocational high school, and high school drop-outs in a metropolitan center. Both the reliability and the validity of the Hand Tool Dexterity Test have been established.

Purdue Pegboard

The Purdue Pegboard measures dexterity for two types of activity, one involving gross movements of the hands, fingers, and arms and the other, primarily fingertip dexterity. It was initially designed to help select employees for assembly packing and other industrial and assembly jobs. The Purdue Pegboard is used increasingly by rehabilitation agencies as an assessment tool and is used frequently in the FCE and work hardening settings due to the low cost and ease of administration and scoring. The Purdue Pegboard was standardized after testing thousands of employees in a wide variety of industrial jobs. However, it is recommended that the Purdue Pegboard test be validated locally, as jobs that have the same titles often differ significantly from employer to employer. Test, retest reliabilities for single trial scores ranged from 0.60 to 0.76, and according to the Spearman Brown formula, the three trial scores estimated range was 0.82 to 0.91 (Tiffin, 1987).

Minnesota Rate of Manipulation

The Minnesota Rate of Manipulation was designed to give employers an instrument that would improve the efficiency of personnel selection for jobs that required arm and hand dexterity. As stated in the Examiner Manual of the Minnesota Rate of Manipulation (1969, p. 95),

The first two tests of the series (the placing test and the turning test) are the most widely used. The other three (the displacing test, the one hand turning and placing test and the two hand turning and placing test) vary in difficulty; however, these three may be better predictors of success in certain situations. All five of the tests have moderate inter-correlations indicating that related though somewhat different information is attained from each.

Each test requires that the examinee place blocks into the holes of a board in some specific manner. Incidentally, as was noted in the 1957 edition, the test may also reveal personality characteristics of the examinee, including atti-

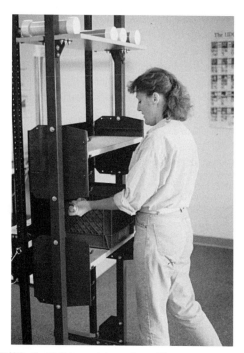

FIGURE 20–6. ELC is used to evaluate lift capacity across a broad spectrum of disability groups.

tude, coordination, precision, nervousness, poise, assurance, and ability to follow instructions. These characteristics are not tangible enough to yield norms, but the evaluators can incorporate their observations into the overall functional evaluation.

In 1943, the reliability was determined on the four tests by correlating time on the first and second trials and correcting with the Spearman Brown formula. The reliability ranged from 0.87 to 0.94 on two-trial reliability and from 0.93 to 0.97 on four-trial reliability.

In the scope of FCEs, the Minnesota Rate of Manipulation is frequently used for clients with hand injuries to assess movement patterns, speed, increased symptomology, and overall ability to manipulate objects. The Minnesota Rate of Manipulation results can be used to help assess a person's ability to reach for and finger objects, as defined in *The Dictionary of Occupational Titles* (Field & Field, 1988).

VALPAR Component Work Samples

The VALPAR Component Work Samples (VCWS) were first introduced in 1974 and were designed for use in the field of vocational evaluation. They have since been used in millions of evaluations all over the world and these work samples have become the standard-setting vocational evaluation tools. Over the years, the work samples have been widely used among other health-related disciplines, including physical therapy, occupational therapy, functional capacity evaluations, and work hardening programs. "A work sample is a defined work activity involving tasks, materials and tools that are similar to those in an actual job or occupation. It is used to appraise an individual's physical and mental abilities, interests and other characteristics" (Wright, cited in Christopherson & Hayes, 1992, p. 1). The VCWS has 21 individual work samples. Each is unique and has its own special advantages, but they all have several qualities in common that make them particularly useful in the FCE and work hardening settings. VALPAR work samples are criterion-referenced instruments, and the focus is not on how individuals compare with others but on whether they can perform certain tasks. The work samples were designed to simulate work factors that are required in thousands of specific jobs but not actually to simulate specific jobs. The work samples are rated in terms of which factors they require and in terms of the number of factors they each require. To establish this, VALPAR used the most prevalent system of job classification, the fourth edition of the U.S. Department of Labor's *Dictionary of Occupational Titles* (Field & Field, 1988, revised in 1991) and the U.S. Department of Labor's *The Handbook for Analyzing Jobs* (1972, revised in 1991), as well as other related documents. Work samples frequently used in the FCE and work hardening setting are

- VCWS-1, Small Tool, which helps assess the ability of an individual to work with small tools and parts

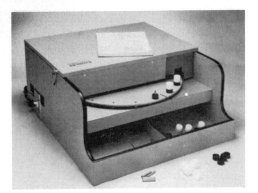

FIGURE 20–7. VCWS 8 (VALPAR) "Simulated Assembly," used to assess the ability to perform repetitive assembly work.

in small confined spaces. The VCWS-4, Upper Extremity Range of Motion, assesses upper extremity range of motion and endurance involving shoulders, upper arms, forearms, elbows, wrists, hands, and fingers; the work simulates light to sedentary work; assesses reaching, handling, fingering, feeling and ability to see; and requires motor coordination and finger and manual dexterity.

- VCWS-5, -6, and -7 are used to assess physical capacities associated with clerical jobs.
- VCWS-8, The Simulated Assembly (Fig. 20–7), is used for job simulation to assess upper and lower extremity function and trunk tolerance, as well as standing tolerance and bimanual dexterity. This particular work sample has also been described as a good teaching device, as it provides a sense of accomplishment. Because this task is so absorbing, it is good for revealing inconsistencies between a client's perceived limitations and his or her actual ability.
- VCWS-9, Whole Body Range of Motion (Fig. 20–8), des information that is useful in examining consistency of client performance; this work sample simu-

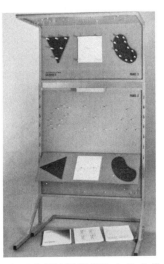

FIGURE 20–8. VCWS 9 (VALPAR) "Whole Body Range of Motion," assesses whole body range of motion, agility, and stamina.

lates light work and assesses a client's ability to balance, stoop, kneel, crouch, reach, handle, finger, feel, and see. It also assesses whole body range of motion, agility, and stamina through gross body movements.

- VCWS-14, Integrated Peer Performance, provides information relevant to the assessment of a variety of capacities, including sitting tolerance, the use of arms, ability to pinch, and sensation. Secondary characteristics typically revealed by this work sample include various work-related social skills, the ability to follow instruction, concentration, motivation, communication skills, the ability to cooperate with others, and self-confidence.

- VCWS-19, Dynamic Physical Capacity, is a work sample designed to simulate the work tasks of a shipping clerk. The client must read invoices, locate a shipping carton, remove the carton from a shelf, pack the carton correctly, weigh it, and place it in a simulated shipping and receiving area. The work sample allows the evaluator to observe the client's ability to follow instructions, physical stamina, concentration, motivation, communication skills, decision making, frustration control, and self-confidence. The VCWS-201 is a physical capacity and mobility screening evaluation, and the sample is designed specifically to be a nonmedical screening of the 17 physical demand factors of The Department of Labor (climbing, balancing, stooping, kneeling, crouching, crawling, walking, standing, talking, lifting, reaching, handling, fingering, feeling, pushing, pulling, and seeing).

The VALPAR Corporation has a publication entitled *VALPAR Component Work Samples, uses in allied health* (Christopherson & Hayes, 1992), which thoroughly explains each of the work samples. This can be obtained by contacting VALPAR International Corporation, P.O. Box 5767, Tucson, AZ, 85703.

COMPUTERIZED TESTING (ISOMETRIC, ISOINERTIONAL, AND ISOKINETIC)

Static Strength Testing

Evaluation of strength is usually an extremely important part of the FCE. Assessment of strength can be very specific. One can measure a specific muscle or muscle group (e.g., pinch strength after carpal tunnel release) or more general function (e.g., in functional assessment, lifting from waist to shoulder height). Lifting involves many muscle groups and, if functionally related to the job, is important to evaluate.

Assessment of strength can be done utilizing three frameworks of assessment. As Isernhagen (1988) points

out, strength testing "measures a person's abilities to exert forces in functional situations: static (isometric), dynamic and psychophysical tests." Examples of dynamic testing equipment include tools manufactured by Lido, Cybex, and Biodex, as well as the BTE. Psychophysical tests, as described by Snook and associates (1970) and others, provide information about a specific task, such as lifting. This type of testing provides information based on the fact that lifting is a function of more than pure strength. In fact, this type of testing demonstrates that a person's lifting ability (or any other ability) is determined by a combination of judgment and motivational, perceptual, and physical abilities. An example of this type of test is the ELC, as described previously under "Standardized Testing."

Isometric Testing

Isometric testing is one form of strength testing generally regarded as safe to administer and reliable. It should not be the only method of strength testing during an FCE. The therapist would not be able to predict how a hand can use a pair of pliers by just dynamometer testing, as he or she would not be able to predict how well a plumber could install a commode using an isometric lifting device. In general terms, static assessments are very useful. The National Institute of Occupational Safety and Health (NIOSH) recommended in 1981 that strength testing be employed on a preemployment basis. Much research on static testing has been done as a component of preemployment and postoffer screening processes. Static test equipment is typically less expensive than isokinetic or isodynamic equipment.

As described by Chaffin and others (1972), isometric strength testing involves exertion of a force in a given posture against a fixed resistance. The exertion is measured hydraulically (dynamometer), mechanically (spring gauge), or electrically (load cell) and is compared with the strength requirements of a job. The height of the measuring device when measuring lifting can be adjusted to simulate a certain job. The width of the dynamometer can also be adjusted to simulate the width of a tool for gripping to measure position-specific strength. Recently, these devices have been combined with computers to be able to make the measurements more accurate. An advantage of most of these systems is that a CV is usually computed for the therapist as well. Consequently, measures of MVE are available, which are very accurate, simultaneous with the needed information of static strength. Most static lifting devices are also easily adjusted to a height to measure the injured worker's pushing and pulling ability.

Static strength testing is not without drawbacks. As Isernhagen (1988, p. 99) points out,

isometric lifts traditionally test only in one geometric plane of movement whereas normal human function normally cuts across three planes. Second, it tests strength in only one position devoid of joint movement. This does not allow for the dynamic changes in posture, joint loading, and muscle length/tension ratios that accompany functional activity . . .

On the other hand, Chaffin and coworkers (1972) note that if the worker is able to isometrically exert a force that is double the maximum force required on a person's job, then he or she is in a lower risk category for developing a back injury ("understressed"). If the worker produces a force between the actual force on the job and twice the force on the job, he or she is rated "considerably stressed." If the worker cannot isometrically exert the amount that the job requires, he or she is considered "overly stressed." Workers in the overly and considerably stressed category showed back injury and severity rates two to three times those in the understressed groups (Chaffin et al., 1972). The ISTU (Fig. 20–9) is a good example of static strength testing equipment. This unit is adjustable, and strength can be assessed in the arm, leg or squat, and torso lifting positions. Static pushing and pulling can also be assessed with the ISTU. The strength tests are all performed as a sustained voluntary isometric exertion for 5 seconds. The average exertion by the worker during the final 3 seconds is registered, as well as the peak value during the 5-second time interval. At least three successive lifts are performed, with a reasonable rest period (30 seconds) between trials generally being used. Coefficients of variation can then be utilized to assess MVE on this type of testing. If a specific lifting height is known to correlate with the worker's job duties, so much the better. To minimize variations due to motivational factors of the client, these instructions are recommended by Chaffin and colleagues (1972):

1. Instructions to the evaluee are to be objective with no emotional appeal

2. The worker is to increase exertion during the first 2 seconds, then hold steady for 3 seconds more
3. Other influences on performance (e.g., noise or spectators) are to be minimized
4. The worker should be informed of any risk inherent in the testing procedure
5. The worker should be informed of how the data will be used
6. The worker should be advised of his or her general performance in positive terms but not be given specific values to compare with other participants
7. Workers should not be coerced to perform tests; i.e., the person tested should be allowed to discontinue participation at any time without malice

Strength testing is particularly germane to FCEs. Mayer and Gatchel (1988) note that patients with back injuries who received a comprehensive treatment program in an interdisciplinary setting (physical or occupational therapy, psychological counseling, medical treatment, and rehabilitation counseling) achieved an 85 percent success in return-to-work rates, whereas the nontreatment group achieved a 45 percent successful return-to-work rate. Similar numbers were obtained in a 2-year follow-up study. Strength training and job-oriented postures were an integral part of this program. In their program, Mayer and colleagues (1985) used both isokinetic strength trunk testing and isometric lifting capacity evaluations. They note that following treatment, their patients developed capacities that surpassed those in the general non–back-injured population. This statement perhaps points out the biggest advantage of isometric testing; it is well researched, giving excellent validity and reliability data. A picture of the ISTU, which is available from Ergometrics, is in Figure 20–9. This equipment is currently available linked to a computer, giving MVE information as well as documenting force curves. Force curves are the amount of force plotted versus time. Analyzing these force curves is an additional way of assessing MVE.

The Baltimore Therapeutic Equipment Work Simulator

The BTE Work Simulator is a computerized treatment and evaluation device for use in a variety of rehabilitation clinics. The system consists of three major components: an electric/mechanical exercise head that provides variable resistance, a control panel that provides options for selecting the type and amount of resistance desired, and a computer system to monitor sessions and collect data. The Work Simulator's attachments (currently over 20) are versatile enough to reproduce all motions needed to simulate almost any job, activity, or activity of daily living function. The system is fairly simple, and most patients can be taught how to operate it with minimal supervision.

Over 2400 BTE Work Simulators are in use around the

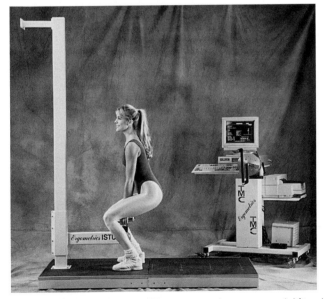

FIGURE 20–9. ISTU, adjustable, isometric (no movement) lifting/pulling/pushing computerized equipment.

world. They are used in many types of rehabilitation, including industrial, orthopedic, cardiac and pulmonary, and upper extremity. The Work Simulator's uses in the evaluation procedures are also well documented. Studies have been published describing the Simulator's uses in consistency of effort testing, standardized upper extremity strength testing, and FCEs. The following research has been completed on the BTE: Several studies have tested the reliability and validity collected from the system. Reliability coefficients have been recorded from 0.913 to 0.998, showing high reliability. Studies by King and Berryhill (1988) and Matheson (1989) have focused on the use of the BTE in the assessment of MVE. Studies by Williams (1991), Schultz-Johnson (1987), and others have discussed the Work Simulator's application to FCE and work hardening. Studies by Anderson (1990) and Berlin and Vermette (1985) have focused on the development of normative data for standardized tests performed on the Work Simulator. In our opinion, this equipment is state of the art in regard to upper extremity evaluation and is very useful for validity testing (Fig. 20–10).

Trunk Testing

There are several ways of testing strength. Some manufacturers use isometric, isoinertial, and isokinetic torque values to measure strength. Most of the reasearch has been done with isokinetics, which is discussed here.

The use of the isokinetic machine for trunk testing became very popular in the 1980s as new technology increased. Many studies have been done, and the equipment has been shown to be reliable (Friedlander et al., 1991). Normally, specific trunk testing equipment is not used in the FCE; however, some valuable information could be gained if it is available. Many argue about whether trunk testing equipment realistically measures patient function (i.e., ability to return to work), which is needed in the FCE report. Mayer and associates (1989) found that isolated trunk extension strength paralleled lifting capacity. On the other hand, many practitioners believe that actual dynamic lifting is a better assessment for lifting capacity (Blankenship, 1989). Few, if any, practioners use trunk testing equipment as a sole testing device to determine function.

In the sagittal plane, trunk extension musculature consists primarily of the erector spinae, gluteus maximus, and hamstrings. Often, the lumbar paraspinals get injured because the primary movers (the glutei) get fatigued or the client was in an awkward position and the secondary movers (the lumbar paraspinals) had to be used instead. Trunk flexor musculature consists of the rectus abdominis, obliqus externus abdominis, and iliopsoas (Smith et al., 1985), and rotation in the axial plane is primarily performed by the contralateral abdominal oblique (Mayer et al., 1985).

Several studies give some general principles that can be useful in assessing a patient's torque curves. Mayer and colleagues (1989) found that postoperative patients had profound deficits in true lumbar mobility and isolated trunk extension. Lumbar motion was 50 percent to 60 percent of normals, and trunk strength values were between 50 percent and 60 percent of gender-specific normative values (Mayer et al., 1989). In other studies, patients with chronic low back pain had decreased values and showed greater variability than normals. Patients also showed a more rapid decline in torque values as the velocity increased (Mayer et al., 1985; Smidt et al., 1983). Studies have also revealed that female patients and normals show 66 to 75 percent of the total trunk strength of male patients and normals (Mayer, et al., 1985; Smith et al., 1985). Another study showed that for peak abdominal and back extensor strength, the range of superiority of men over women was 39 to 57 percent, and the range of superiority of normals over patients with chronic low back pain was 48 to 82 percent (Smidt et al., 1983). Studies also indicate that while men have greater trunk strength, women demonstrate endurance equal to or greater than that of men (Langrana & Lee, 1984; Smidt et al., 1983). Also, greater discrepancies were found between patients and controls for women than for men (Mayer et al., 1985). It was also found that age and gender tend to change peak torque values (Langrana & Lee, 1984; Smith et al., 1985). In comparing trunk flexors and extensors, some studies demonstrated that the abdominals were more susceptible

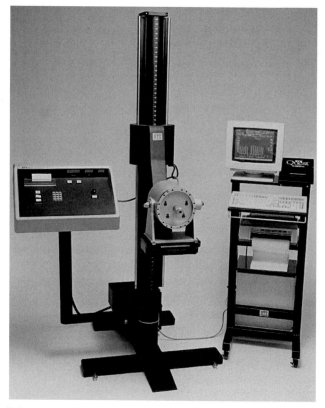

FIGURE 20–10. BTE, computerized treatment and evaluation device for use in a variety of rehabilitation clinics. Note the excellent adjustability.

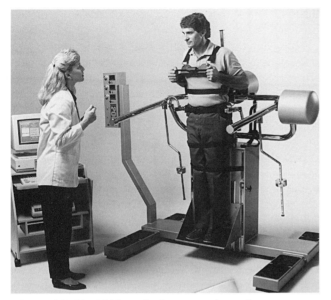

FIGURE 20–11. B200 is a lumbar testing device that can measure isometric and isotonic, torque, velocity, and range of motion.

to fatigue than back extensors in patients and normals (Langrana & Lee, 1984; Smidt et al., 1983) and that in patients with low back pain, the most substantial strength deficit was in trunk extensors (Mayer et al., 1985).

Patient positioning is one of many factors that can cause discrepancies in trunk torque (strength). One study found that the iliopsoas doubled flexor strength when the patient was tested in standing (Langrana & Lee, 1984). Also, if the pelvis is not stabilized adequately, lumbar paraspinal strength cannot be differentiated from the glutei, which are functionally much stronger muscles.

Variability in force output can be secondary to submaximal effort, which is also a factor in the substantial strength deficits found (Mayer et al., 1985). This lowered effort can have two main causes: 1) fear of injury intensified by psychological factors and 2) conscious effort to mislead (Mayer et al., 1985). One of the uses of a trunk testing machine during an FCE is visual observation of torque curves. Many manufacturers support that inconsistency of the shape and quality of curves with several trials can show an uncooperative subject (Jones et al., 1988). However, Hazard and associates (1988) demonstrated that intercurve variability can distinguish maximal from submaximal isokinetic effort only 70 to 90 percent of the time in normal subjects. This article stated that visual technique is subjective and that inexperienced subjects could produce consistent curves inadvertently while exerting submaximal effort. Although some argue about the accuracy of these data, they still can be useful when used in combination with other results of MVE testing.

Many trunk testing machines are on the market. In this section, only three are reviewed, but manufacturers are more than happy to give a prospective buyer ample information as well as research articles. Most of the

research presented so far has to do with isokinetics; however, the Isostation B200 (Fig. 20–11) is a lumbar testing device that can measure isometric and isotonic torque, velocity, and range of motion. The unique parameter of this machine is that it collects this information in all three cardinal planes simultaneously, which gives the therapist the opportunity to look at muscular substitutional tendencies of the measured plane. For example, if dynamic flexion and extension torque were being measured, once the data had been entered and stored, a therapist may enter the other two planes and observe any activity occurring as well (Geril, 1994, personal communication). Extensive research by many different researchers also has been done using this machine, and it has been the subject of many reliability and validity studies. These studies have shown good values for reproducibility for normal subjects for isometric torque and dynamic performance parameters (Gomez et al., 1991); however, the B200 showed poor reproductivity for range of motion measurements (Dillard et al., 1991), which the company recognizes as well.

MedX (Fig. 20–12) manufactures another machine that can measure trunk extension. This was invented by Arthur Jones, who developed the Nautilus fitness equipment. Much research has been done using this machine in several areas of the United States, and dramatic increases in lumbar paraspinal strength have been recorded after rehabilitation (Jones, 1993). The MedX machine isolates the lumbar paraspinals by anchoring the pelvis very carefully. This decreases the effect of the glutei. Testing on the MedX is that of maximal isometric effort through a series of seven points throughout the lumbar range of motion, which researchers say is approximately 72 degrees. A free booklet can be obtained from the MedX Corporation (Jones, 1993), which gives ample information regarding rehabilitation and testing procedures.

The Lido Back (Fig. 20–13) attachment is a good example of what several manufacturers are doing to make back testing available to clinics who already own an isokinetic device for extremity testing. This makes an easily affordable answer for the clinic; however, pelvic stabilization might be difficult compared with that using a machine that measures only low back musculature.

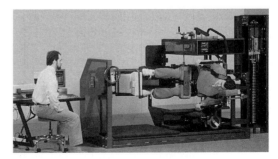

FIGURE 20–12. MedX, Primarily intended for clinical research. This version of the lumbar extension machine provides both testing and exercises when rotated into the lateral position.

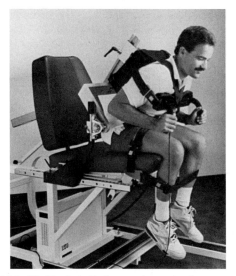

FIGURE 20–13. The Lido Back, an isokinetic lumbar assessment and exercise machine.

For the new user of these types of machines, the computerization and complexity of knobs, belts, braces, and manufacturers' claims can be overwhelming. It is important to remember that none of these pieces of equipment give job-specific data (unless it is the injured worker's real job to sit in one of these pieces of equipment as a product tester).

ASSESSMENT OF ABNORMAL ILLNESS BEHAVIOR

At this point in the evaluation process is the optimal time to perform additional tests for abnormal illness behavior. When dealing with clients who are involved in a social renumeration system as a result of their injury or illness (i.e., workers' compensation, personal injury compensation, or long-term disability), a phenomenon sometimes occurs in which the client's perceived disability exceeds the objective medical pathology. This phenomenon has been identified as inappropriate illness behavior (Blankenship, 1989), abnormal illness behavior (Pelowski, cited in Ogden-Niemeyer & Jacobs, 1989), and symptom magnification syndrome (Matheson, 1990; Isernhagen, 1988). In the past, the terms *conversion* or *somatization disorder*, *functional overlay*, *secondary gain*, *malingering*, *nonorganic pain*, *hypochondriases*, and *hysterical neurosis* also were used.

Assessment of abnormal illness behavior is a complex task requiring clinical observation, psychometric testing, and physical or functional testing. In the realm of functional capacity evaluation and work hardening programs, an interdisciplinary team made up of a physical or occupational therapist, a psychologist, and a vocational specialist typically address the abnormal illness behaviors. Unless

addressed, these behaviors will prolong or even prohibit a successful return to work.

Waddell and others (1980) named five types of nonorganic signs for which to test patients who may require further psychosocial evaluation. The five types of physical signs are tenderness, simulation, distraction, regional reaction, and overreaction. A positive finding of three or more of the five types is clinically significant of abnormal illness behavior. Isolated positive signs are ignored. Tenderness should be related to physical disease and should be localized to a particular skeletal or neuromuscular structure. A positive sign would be if the skin is tender to light touch over a wide area around the lumbar spine or the patient complains of deep tenderness, again over a wide area that often extends to a thoracic spine, sacrum, or pelvis.

Two simulation tests give the patient the impression that an examination is being carried out when it is not. If the patient reports pain during these tests, a nonorganic symptom is suggested. The first is the axial loading test, which has a positive result if the client reports low back pain with gentle vertical compression over the client's skull. The axial rotation test has a positive result if low back pain is reported when the shoulders and pelvis are passively rotated together in the same plane. Waddell and colleagues (1980) caution the examiner that in the presence of nerve root irritation, leg pain may be produced, and the results of this test should not be considered positive for symptom exaggeration.

The third physical sign is tested by the distraction test. This is performed while the client's attention is distracted, and then the test must be "non-painful, non-emotional and non-surprising" (Waddell et al., 1980, p. 119). One way is simple observation throughout the entire examination by watching for inconsistencies in movement while another body part is being tested. One of the best distraction tests is the straight leg test described earlier, in which the examiner is looking for inconsistencies when the test is performed in supine and later in the sitting position.

The fourth physical sign involves regional disturbances, i.e., the patient reports and demonstrates weakness or sensory disturbances that diverge from accepted neuroanatomy. For example, the patient may demonstrate on formal manual muscle testing a partial cogwheel, "giving away" of several muscle groups, that differs from neuroanatomy findings (Waddell et al., 1980). Sensory changes for a positive test result would fit a global rather than a dermatomal pattern. Of course, the examiner must be aware of the patient's medical history, which may include spinal stenosis or multiple levels of spinal surgeries, both of which could present with multiple levels of weakness or sensory disturbance.

The last physical sign, overreaction, is demonstrated by disproportionate verbalization, facial expression, muscle tension, collapsing, or sweating. The examiner should be very careful to minimize his or her own emotional reactions while evaluating the patient, since certain emotional responses from the evaluator may increase the reactions of the patient. It must be reiterated that for the results of the Waddell Test to be positive, three or more of the five signs must be significant.

It is important to note that no specific tests can identify a person's motivation to remain in a sick role. This must be deduced from all of the information gathered by the trained professionals. Gatchel (cited in Blankenship, 1989) identified behaviors he called **"red flags,"** which include

1. The patient agitating the other patients with behavior disruptive to the treatment milieu
2. No work plan or changing work plan
3. The patient receiving or applying for Social Security or long-term disability
4. Opposition to presence of psychologist or refusal to fill out forms or answer questions
5. Florid psychosis
6. Significant neuropsychologic or cognitive deficits
7. Excessive anger at individuals involved in the case
8. Current substance abuse
9. Family resistant to patient recovery or return to work
10. Patient with young children at home or short-term work history done primarily for financial reasons
11. Continual complaints about facility, staff, and program accommodations rather than willingness to deal with physical and psychological issues
12. Patient's continual lateness to activities and other cases of noncompliance with excuses that do not check out
13. Patient's continuing to focus on pain complaints in counseling sessions rather than dealing with psychological issues

Identifying these characteristics in a client indicates that a psychological work-up must be done to identify predisposing factors for the behavior and to initiate a plan of action that includes a return to work as soon as possible.

The following are descriptions of assessment tools used to help identify abnormal illness behavior that can readily be adapted to an acute treatment setting as well as to work hardening programs.

Minnesota Multiphasic Personality Inventory

The Minnesota Multiphasic Personality Inventory (MMPI) is one of the oldest and most frequently used means of psychological assessment. When administered to chronic pain patients, a pattern of elevation has been reported on the clinical scales of Hysteria (Hy) and Hypochondriasis (Hs), with a normal Depression (D) scale (Mayer & Gatchel, 1988; Ogden-Neimeyer & Jacobs 1988; Ransford et al., 1976). This is reported as the "conversion v" and is generally thought to identify clients who magnify their symptoms and at the same time are at best ambivalent regarding their reported limitations. Barnett (cited in Mayer & Gatchel, 1988) evaluated changes in MMPI profiles before and after functional restoration treatment and identified a significant decrease in the posttreatment Hy and Hs scales when looking at average profile scores. The MMPI is a 550-item paper and pencil test administered under the supervision of a psychologist and can be scored electronically.

Numeric Pain Rating Scale

The purpose of the numeric pain rating scale is to obtain a subjective, self-reported, quantitative rating of pain that allows the client to change his or her rating based on the previously known score. The client is asked to rate his or her present level of pain on Borg's 0 to 10+ scale, with 0 being no pain at all and 10+ being maximal or emergency pain. The client is then asked to use the same scale to rate his or her pain at its best and worst over the past 30 days. The number that the client chooses is his or her score. A pain rating of 0 would indicate no pain and no external indications of pain. A person with a 0 pain rating would be a nonsymptom exaggerator. Patients reporting low pain from 1 to 2 are typically not symptom exaggerators and are often able to return to work. A person who has a moderate pain rating of 3 to 5 typically has movement patterns that are notably slower and are definitely observable to a therapist. Before any physical activity, 3 is considered to be a moderate pain rating, but after aggressive activities, 3 may be considered a low pain rating. Before any physical activity, 5 is considered a high pain rating, but after aggressive physical activity, 5 is considered a moderate pain rating for the purposes of classifying symptom exaggeration. Therefore, after an FCE, a pain rating of 5 may not be viewed as symptom exaggeration. A rating of 6 to 10 is categorized as a high pain rating, and this level represents severe impairment or symptom exaggerating behavior. Symptom exaggerators generally rate their pain in this region, and most commonly their pain rating before FCE is 6 or 7. It is important to note that the movement patterns of the patients do not correlate with the high pain rating, and the patient may attempt to simulate painful movement patterns but cannot do so consistently. A pain rating of 10+ represents overt symptom exaggeration when reported as pain while resting, before the FCE has begun, or even after mild activity. Patients with a pain level of 10+ secondary to organic impairment would be hospitalized and not in a clinic seeking treatment on an outpatient basis and definitely would not be in a clinic to begin a functional capacity evaluation. Overt symptom exaggerators report a 10+ level and demonstrate normal movement patterns, which is impossible with a level of impairment necessary to cause a 10+ pain level (Blankenship, 1994).

McGill Pain Questionnaire

The McGill Pain Questionnaire consists primarily of three major classes of word descriptors, which are categorized into 20 groups used to describe a patient's subjective pain experience. Clients are instructed to chose one word from each group that presently describes their pain, but only if one of the words in the group applies to them. A Pain Rating Index is obtained by adding the numeric value of all the words chosen from the 20 groups. Four groups are used; group 1 to 10 describes sensory aspects of the pain; group 11 to 15 describes the affective aspect of the pain; group 16 describes the overall subjective intensity of the pain; and group 17 to 20 contains miscellaneous descriptive words. Another score is given for the number of words chosen (NWC), as well as a score for the present pain intensity (PPI). The McGill Questionnaire is easy to administer, and research has shown it to be a reliable and consistent measure of a client's change after a procedure or a series of procedures has been completed. This is advantageous in the work hardening setting to determine if the client experiences improvement (Melzak, 1975, 1987).

The Millon Behavioral Health Inventory

The Millon Behavioral Health Inventory (MBHI) is a relatively new assessment tool that was adapted by Gatchel and others (1986) at the University of Texas Health Science Center to determine its usefulness in evaluating potentially effective psychological predictors of therapeutic outcome. The MBHI is a 150-question true or false self-report inventory based on 20 clinical scales that reflect medically related concerns. The scales are introversion, inhibited, cooperative, sociable, confident, forceful, respectable, sensitive, chronic tension, recent stress, premorbid pessimism, future despair, social alienation, somatic anxiety, allergic inclinations, gastrointestinal susceptibility, cardiovascular tendency, pain treatment responsivity, life threat reactivity, and emotional vulnerability. The MBHI is still too new to assess its reliability; however, Mayer and Gatchel (1988) report that the inventory is useful in their overall assessment of low back pain patients, and they did find a number of scales clinically meaningful. For example, patients who scored low on the cooperative style scale and high on the sensitive scale demonstrated poor outcome in a functional restoration program. The patient scoring high on the cooperative and sociable scales demonstrated an excellent outcome.

One advantage of the MBHI is that it is perceived as less threatening than the MMPI because it includes questions related to medical care and it takes significantly less time (approximately 20 minutes) to complete.

The Beck Depression Inventory

The Beck Depression Inventory (BDI) was originally developed by Beck and colleagues (1961) as a means of assessing the cognitive components of depression. The BDI consists of 21 self-report items focusing on common manifestations of depression, such as sleep disturbance, sexual dysfunction, and weight change. A study by Beck and others (1961) indicates that the BDI was able to discriminate among groups of people with depression and reflect the changes in the intensity of the depression over time, thus establishing validity and reliability. The BDI is a simple psychological test that patients can complete in a few minutes. Administering it before, during, and after work hardening programs can track progression and the effects of treatment. Pharmacologic treatment of depression can encourage patient motivation and compliance with therapy and has become increasingly popular for the treatment of chronic pain.

The Owestry Low Back Pain Disability Questionnaire

The Owestry is a self-rating scale that illustrates the degree of functional impairment a patient is experiencing. The questionnaire consists of 10 questions regarding pain intensity, personal care, lifting, walking, sitting, standing, sleeping, sex life, social life, and traveling. The patient chooses one of six statements in each question that most accurately describes his or her experienced limitations. The questionnaire takes 3.5 to 5 minutes to complete and about 1 minute to score. The highest possible value for each section is five, and the score is obtained by adding the value for each section and dividing the total by 50; the quotient is expressed as a percentage. A score of 0 to 20 percent represents minimal disability, 20 to 40 percent, moderate disability, 40 to 60 percent, severe disability, 60 to 80 percent, crippled, and 80 to 100 percent, bed bound or exaggerating symptoms (Fairbanks et al., 1980). Blankenship's (1994) criteria, based on research on the work-injured population, are 0 to 29 percent, Low (non–symptom exaggeration); 30 to 39 percent, Equivocal; 40 to 100 percent, High (significant impairment or symptom exaggeration). As with other assessment tools, if the demonstrated function is significantly better than the reported function, symptom magnification syndrome and abnormal illness behavior may be present. "The questionnaire is a valid indicator of disability if its score closely reflects the patient's observed disability and symptoms" (Fairbanks et al., 1980, p. 271).

The Owestry is an effective clinical tool that requires a minimum amount of time in which to assess the patient's perceived disability. It is also helpful in assessing the effectiveness of rehabilitation programs.

Dallas Pain Questionnaire

The Dallas Pain Questionnaire (DPQ) by Lawlis and others (1989) is another self-report questionnaire designed to assess the amount of chronic spine pain that affects four aspects called factors of a patient's life. There are 16 questions, 7 related to interference of daily activities, 3 to anxiety and depression, 3 to work and leisure, and 3 to social interests. The sections are answered by marking a 10-cm visual analog scale rated from 0 to 100th percentile, normal being 0, and the worst being the 100th percentile. To score the DPQ, count the divisions on the visual analog scale starting with 0 with the first division on the left. The number of the division the patient chooses is the score for that section. Then add the total score for all sections for each factor and multiply that score by the designated multiplier for each factor. The 50th percentile is the decided significant interference factor. Three profiles that predict outcome in terms of type of treatment that is appropriate are 1) medical treatment alone when factors 1 and 2 are greater than the 50th percentile and factors 3 and 4 are less than the 50th percentile; 2) behavioral treatment as the primary intervention when factors 3 and 4 are greater than the 50th percentile and factors 1 and 2 are less than the 50th percentile; and 3) combined medical and behavioral intervention when all four factors are greater than the 50th percentile.

The primary disadvantage of the DPQ is that it is a relatively new scale and needs more research substantiation (Lawlis et al., 1989).

The Millon Visual Analog Scale

The Millon Visual Analog Scale (MVAS) is another self-report assessment that describes back pain and its impact on several areas of function. There are 15 items that are marked from highest to lowest on a 10-cm line. The highest possible score is 50, and the lowest is 0.

The visual analog scales are desirable because of the high degree of reproducability and the opportunity for nonverbal expression. This assessment can also be used in the work hardening setting to assess the patient's report of symptom improvement (Ogden-Neimeyer & Jacobs, 1989).

MATERIALS HANDLING

The Dictionary of Occupational Titles (Field & Field, 1988) is published by the U.S. Department of Labor and lists jobs and their characteristics. It is recommended that the FCE measure physical activities as described in this book for legal and practical implications. Physical demands reports are a way of describing the physical activities that a job requires. Each job listed is described by different factors, such as lifting, carrying, and pushing or pulling. In this section, each physical demand to be tested is described. Some areas have very specific ways to be tested, while others can be tested in several different ways. The most important idea for the examiner to keep in mind is to measure the physical demand that *The Dictionary of Occupational Titles* defines.

The five degrees of physical demands ("Factor #1": lifting, carrying, and pushing or pulling) are as follows:

- Sedentary work: Lifting 10 lb maximum and occasionally lifting or carrying such articles as dockets, ledgers, and small tools. Although a sedentary job is defined as one that involves sitting, a certain amount of walking and standing is often necessary in carrying out job duties. Jobs are sedentary if walking and standing are required only occasionally and other sedentary criteria are met.
- Light work: Lifting 20 lb maximum with frequent lifting or carrying of objects weighing up to 10 lb. Although the weight lifted may be only a negligible amount, a job falls in this category when it requires walking or standing to a significant degree or pushing and pulling of arm or leg controls.
- Medium work: Lifting 50 lb maximum, with frequent lifting or carrying of objects weighing up to 25 lb.
- Heavy work: Lifting 100 lb maximum, with frequent lifting or carrying of objects weighing up to 50 lb.
- Very heavy work: Lifting objects in excess of 100 lb, with frequent lifting or carrying objects weighing 50 lb or more.

The Dictionary of Occupational Titles (Field & Field, 1988) also uses the terms *occasional, frequent,* and *constant* to refer to the frequency of exerting of force. This includes any physical activity. Blankenship (1989), Snook and colleagues (1970), and *The Dictionary of Occupational Titles* (Field & Field, 1988) have published charts that give ways of extrapolating data after they have been obtained from maximum lifts. This can be very helpful when attempting to predict the patient's endurance during an 8-hour day (Blankenship, 1989). If frequent lifting is a targeted job task, then specific evaluation of frequent lifting can be done using the ELC or the WEST II, as previously described. As the patient performs the different physical demands, care must be given to his or her body mechanics; improper techniques, such as excessive backward bending or jerking with lifting, are considered reasons to terminate the test by the examiner. The test can also be terminated if the patient states that his or her pain is increasing or has other problems. To reduce risk of injury, explain to the patient very carefully each procedure and that he or she should stop testing if any increase in pain occurs. Blankenship, before material handling testing, gives very specific instructions in written form and has the patient sign a

TABLE 20–2

DEFINITIONS AND ASSESSMENTS OF PHYSICAL DEMANDS OF OCCUPATIONAL TASKS

Formal *Dictionary of Occupational Titles* Definitions	Assessment of Physical Demands
Lifting: Raising or lowering an object from one level to another (included upward pulling)	Floor to waist (Fig. 20–14) Lift from bottle handles, deep squat to standing 12 in to waist: (Fig. 20–15) This lift places stress primarily on the low back muscles; lift from 12 in handles to standing Waist to shoulder: (Fig. 20–16) Patient lifts from 12 in handles at waist height and laterally moves so that hands go to a level at shoulder height Shoulder to overhead: (Fig. 20–17) Hands grasp box in a pronated position at shoulder level and patient lifts box 8 to 10 in overhead while side-stepping
Carrying: Transporting an object, usually holding it in the hands or arms or on the shoulder (Fig. 20–18)	At waist height, carrying should be performed with a 14 in box for any distance (15 ft); weights are added until the test is terminated
Pushing: Exerting force on an object so that the object moves away from the force (including jerking) (Fig. 20–19)	Pushing any type of "sled" for a distance (e.g., 25 ft) with the handle approximately 36 in from the floor (this will make comparison with Snook's data easier), which should be measured with a dynamometer; the torso should be straight or in slight kyphosis; add approximately 25 lb of weight with each repetition, which increases pushing force approximately 10 lb (Blankenship, 1989)
Pulling: Exerting force on an object so that the object moves toward the force (including jerking) (Fig. 20–20)	Pull with any type of sled for 7 to 10 ft using a dynamometer to measure force; for longer distance, workers tend to push instead of pull
Climbing: Ascending or descending ladders, stairs, scaffolding, ramps, poles, and the like, using the feet and legs or hands and arms (not pictured)	Normally, this is tested using stairs or ladder, depending on the job description of the worker; evaluator can use stairs, a single step, stairmaster, ladder, or versiclimber Five flights of stairs up and down at a steady pace gives an "occasional" *Dictionary of Occupational Titles* rating (Blankenship, 1989)
Bending or stooping: Bending the body downward and forward by bending the spine at the waist	Evaluator may want to choose either static or repetitive bending, depending on the patient's job
Kneeling: Bending the legs at the knees to come to rest on the knee or knees	Patient places one or both knees on the floor for approximately 2 min
Crouching or squatting: Bending the body downward and forward by bending the legs and spine	Patient may squat wth both feet flat or on metatarsal head, or he or she may sit on one heel with the other foot flat; occasional frequency is documented when the patient can hold this position for 2 min; patient can perform functional activities while in this position if evaluator desires
Crawling: Moving about on the hands and knees or hands and feet	Patient crawls nonstop for a distance or may stay confined to a small area and perform dexterity or assembling tasks
Reaching: Extending the hands and arms in any direction	Can be divided into overhead and forward reaching and also static and repetition; the patient can work statistically for 5 minutes or perform 25 repetitive reaches; the patient can be performing a functional activity or any kind of activity
Handling: Seizing, holding, grasping, turning, or otherwise working with the fingers primarily (rather than with the whole hand or arms, as in handling)	Handling can be assessed best by using standardized testing such as the Minnesota Rate of Manipulation, VALPAR Simulated Assembly, or others
Feeling: Perceiving such attributes of objects and materials as size, shape, temperature, or texture by means of receptors in the skin, particularly those of the fingertips	Fingering can be assessed by using standardized tests such as the Craford Small Parts Test, Purdue Pegboard Test, Jebsen Taylor Hand Function Test, or others (in part from Blankenshp, 1989)
Talking: Expressing or exchanging ideas by means of the spoken word **Hearing:** Perceiving the nature of sounds by the ear **Seeing:** Obtaining impressions through the eyes of the shape, size, distance, motion, color, or other characteristics of objects; the major visual functions are 1) acuity—far and near, 2) depth perception, 3) field of vision, 4) accommodation, and 5) color vision; the functions are defined as follows: 1. Acuity, far—clarity of vision at 20 ft or more Acuity, near—clarity of vision at 20 in or less 2. Depth perception—three-dimensional vision; the ability to judge distance and space relationships so as to see objects where and as they actually are 3. Field of vision—the area that can be seen up and down or to the right or left while the eyes are fixed on a given point 4. Accommodation—adjustment of the lens of the eye to bring an object into sharp focus; this item is especially important when doing near-point work at varying distances from the eye 5. Color vision—the ability to identify and distinguish colors	Talking, hearing, or seeing, although necessary components for most jobs, are usually not formally addressed during an FCE; the loss of these functions may be described in functional terms and noted in their impact on ability; however, formal assessment of talking, seeing, and hearing is best assessed by other professionals

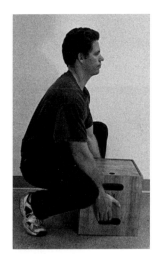

FIGURE 20–14. Lifting from the floor.

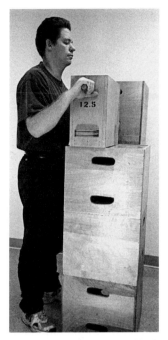

FIGURE 20–16. Lifting to shoulder height.

consent form as well. When adding weight, Blankenship teaches therapists to ask the patient very simply, "Would you like to try another weight?" (Blankenship, 1989, p. 10.20). This decreases possible injury and legal liability and can promote greater participation from symptom magnifiers by giving them control of their environment. Blankenship does not recommend coaching the patient during the FCE. Any test can be terminated 1) on the patient's request, 2) when the pain begins to increase, 3) when the patient successfully completes the test, or 4) at the evaluator's discretion.

Whether the patient lifts with a lordosis or kyphosis is determined by the examiner. Some therapists have the opinion that the patient should lift the way they prefer, and others believe that the patient should be shown the correct way to lift during the FCE; however, all therapists agree that the patient should never be allowed to perform a test in such a way that would cause injury. Documentation should

include not only numeric scores but also reasons why that test was terminated. Table 20–2 gives the activity, *The Dictionary of Occupational Titles* (Field & Field, 1988) definition, a description of each physical demand test, and the frequency of exertion (Figs. 20–14 to 20–20). Many tests can be changed at the discretion of the evaluator.

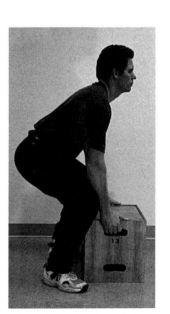

FIGURE 20–15. Lifting from 12 inches off the floor to waist height; note the neutral pelvis.

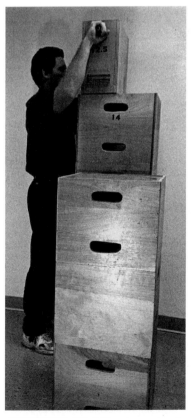

FIGURE 20–17. Lifting to overhead.

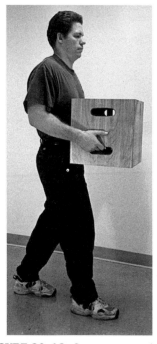

FIGURE 20–18. Carrying at waist level.

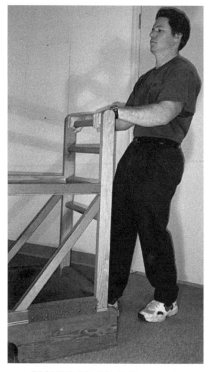

FIGURE 20–20. Pulling a sled.

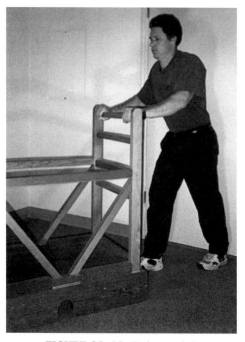

FIGURE 20–19. Pushing a sled.

SUMMARY

This chapter has provided an in-depth review of work assessment related to the industrially injured population. This population can be difficult to evaluate and treat for numerous psychological, social, vocational, and physical reasons. The therapist responsible for treatment and assessment of the injured worker must be aware of all of these factors to provide appropriate intervention.

The new graduate and the experienced therapist alike should have special training in performing FCEs because of the legal implications with this type of assessment. The therapist who takes on this responsibility must be prepared to give depositions and to provide expert testimony in court.

APPENDIX A

Case Study of Mr. C.

TIMELINE FROM DATE OF INJURY TO SUCCESSFUL RETURN TO WORK

Client:	30-year-old white male, smoker, second marriage, 11th grade education, family history positive for worker compensation injury's and litigation
6/90	Began working as sales route driver—classified medium work
6/7/91	Date of injury, 1 year after hire
6/7/91	Seen by neurologist, and diagnostics ordered:
	Diagnostics—magnetic resonance imaging, lumbosacral x-ray films, electromyography, nerve conductive study; electromyography suggestive of mild irritability of S-1 root
	Diagnosis—moderately severe myofascial injury
6/91 to 10/91	Referred for acute physical therapy
8/91	Thermogram—consistent with myofascial injury; no other abnormality
9/18/91	Therapist recommended FCE, work hardening, client contacted and reported he needed a second opinion
12/9/91	Independent medical evaluation with physiatrist, recommended FCE, work hardening and vocational evaluation
1/9 & 1/14/92	Vocational evaluation
1/20/92	FCE
2/4/92	Client returned to physician following FCE
2/92	Client attempted return to work—too painful to work
3/3/92	Return to physician
3/10/92	Rehabilitation counselor assigned
3/17/92	Return to physician
3/20/92	Return to physician
3/25 to 5/1/92	Client in work hardening
5/1/92	Discharged from work hardening
5/11/92	Client returned to work
5/15/92	Visit to physician for follow-up
6/1/92	Client successfully working
6/1/92	Return visit to physician for follow-up
7/1/92	Client successfully working
7/30/92	Impairment rating 3.5 percent
8/1/92	Client successfully working

CASE STUDY

Mr. C. is a 30-year-old white male who had a 1-year work history as a route driver at the time his injury occurred. His diagnosis was moderately severe myofascial injury. Diagnostic tests, including magnetic resonance imaging (MRI), EMG, nerve conduction studies (NCS), and lumbar spine films, were all within normal limits. According to the *Dictionary of Occupational Titles* (Field & Field, 1988), Mr. C.'s position as route driver was rated as medium work with the physical demands of reaching and handling and talking and hearing. The client reported working 56 to 60 hours in a 7-day work week. He reported working on commission making money per case of drinks that he sold. After his injury, he received $420.00 biweekly from worker's compensation. He stated that he had an attorney "on stand-by," and initially rehabilitation counseling was not assigned to him. Mr. C. reported that his truck was loaded incorrectly, and the product he was selling fell against the door. When he tried to open the door, he was injured. Mr. C. did have a history of difficulty with his

501

supervisor as well as a reported feeling that he could not go back to work for that company. Mr. C. was currently married to his second wife, who had also previously been injured on her job, with subsequent litigation. The client reported that his father and brother-in-law had also sustained totally disabling work injuries. Mr. C. had five children, three with his present wife and two from the previous marriage, who did not live with him. Mr. C. did pay child support for the two children who did not live with him. He reported having lost two cars owing to financial difficulties since the injury. He stated that a typical day for him included watching television and sometimes babysitting. He stated that around the house he occasionally did dishes and laundry and that since his accident, he was unable to participate in the hobbies of dancing, horseback riding, and sports. He did state that he was able to coach a children's football team; however, he did that with his physician's permission.

The client had an 11th grade education and reportedly was working on his General Education Degree. His past job experience included working for a landscaping firm as both a laborer and a maintenance superintendent and also route driving for another wholesale company. The client reported that someone else had been hired to take his place at his job, and that light-duty jobs were not available. He felt as though he had been terminated from his position and he wanted to consider retraining if he could be trained for a job with a good salary. The client also reported that he could not imagine who would hire someone with a back injury such as his.

After intervention of work hardening, Mr. C. successfully returned to work with his same employer doing the same job. This is a clear-cut case of the physician, injured worker, insurance adjustor, and work hardening teams all interacting to ensure a successful outcome.

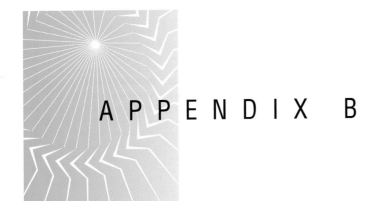

APPENDIX B

WORK CAPACITY CHECKLIST

Client's Name _____Bob R._____#380_____

Note: Assuming an 8 hour workday, OCCASIONALLY means that activity may be performed 1%-33% of the time during the workday. FREQUENTLY means 34%-66%, and CONTINUOUSLY means 67%-100%.

****

1. In an 8 hour workday, client can: (circle full capacity for each activity)   COMMENTS
   TOTAL AT ONE TIME
   A) Sit   (1) 2   3   4   5   6   7   8 (hrs)
   B) Stand   1 (2) 3   4   5   6   7   8 (hrs)
   C) Walk   1 (2) 3   4   5   6   7   8 (hrs)
   D) Drive, per client report   (1) 2   3   4   5   6   7   8 (hrs)

   TOTAL DURING ENTIRE 8 HOUR DAY
   A) Sit   1   2   3   4 (5) 6   7   8 (hrs)
   B) Stand   1   2   3   4   5   6   7 (8)(hrs)
   C) Walk   1   2   3   4   5   6   7 (8)(hrs)
   D) Drive, per client report   1   2   3   4 (5) 6   7   8 (hrs)

2. Client can lift:

		Continuously	Frequently	Occasionally	Never	
A) 1-10 lbs.	(Sedentary)	[ ]	[ ]	[ ]	[ ]	Max observed
B) 11-20 lbs.	(Light)	[ ]	[ ]	[ ]	[ ]	waist level lift: 50 lbs.
C) 21-50 lbs.	(Medium)	[ ]	[X] 30 lb.	[X]	[ ]	
D) 51-100 lbs.	(Heavy)	[ ]	[ ]	[ ]	[ ]	
E) 101+ lbs.	(Very Heavy)	[ ]	[ ]	[ ]	[ ]	

3. Client can carry:

		Continuously	Frequently	Occasionally	Never	
A) 1-10 lbs.	(Sedentary)	[ ]	[ ]	[ ]	[ ]	Maximum observed in
B) 11-20 lbs.	(Light)	[ ]	[ ]	[ ]	[ ]	right hand: 35 lbs.
C) 21-50 lbs.	(Medium)	[ ]	[ ]	[X]	[ ]	left hand: 35 lbs.
D) 51-100 lbs.	(Heavy)	[ ]	[ ]	[ ]	[ ]	both hands: 40 lbs.
E) 101+ lbs.	(Very Heavy)	[ ]	[ ]	[ ]	[ ]	

4. Client can use hands for repetitive action such as:

	SIMPLE GRASPING	PUSHING & PULLING OF ARM CONTROLS	FINE MANIPULATION
A) Right	[X] Yes [ ] No	[X] Yes [ ] No	[X] Yes [ ] No
B) Left	[X] Yes [ ] No	[X] Yes [ ] No	[X] Yes [ ] No

5. Client is able to:

	Continuously	Frequently	Occasionally	Never
A) Stoop/Bend	[ ]	[X]	[ ]	[ ]
B) Squat	[ ]	[X]	[ ]	[ ]
C) Crawl	[ ]	[ ]	[X]	[ ]
D) Climb	[ ]	[X]	[ ]	[ ]
E) Reach	[ ]	[X]	[ ]	[ ]
F) Push	[ ]	[ ]	[X]	[ ]
G) Pull	[ ]	[ ]	[X]	[ ]

6. Restriction of activities involving:

	None	Mild	Moderate	Total	Not Determined
A) Unprotected heights	[ ]	[ ]	[X]	[ ]	[ ]
B) Being around moving machinery	[X]	[ ]	[ ]	[ ]	[ ]
C) Exposure to dust, fumes, gases	[ ]	[ ]	[ ]	[ ]	[X]
D) Changes in temperature, humidity	[ ]	[ ]	[ ]	[ ]	[X]

7. Comments: _____
   _____

8. Form completed by ___Bruce A. Mueller, OTR/L, C.H.T.___ Date: ___June 20, 1993___

Physician's Recommendation

9. Client can work now: ___Yes ___No Part Time (Hrs/Days) _____ Full Time _____ RTW _____

10. Physician's Signature _____ Date: _____

Physical Restoration Center of Gainesville
2706 SW 34th Street * Gainesville, FL 32608 * (904) 336-6830 * (904) 336-6910 FAX

PHYSICAL RESTORATION CENTERS
of Florida

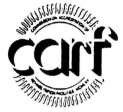

SUMMARY OF INTERDISCIPLINARY FUNCTIONAL CAPACITY EVALUATION

Client: Bob R.
PRC Case # 380
SS#: 000-00-0000
DOI: 2/14/93
Employer: Moo-Cow Farms
Occupation: Driver/delivery route
Diagnosis: Thoracic/lumbar strain

Date and time of Testing:
June 20, 1993
8:00 am until 12 noon
Ins. Carrier: Claims A Plenty
Physician: Dr. J.
DOB: 3/15/72
Date Last Worked: Presently working
with a 40-pound restriction

The following is a summary of the objective findings of the Interdisciplinary Functional Capacity Evaluation. The evaluators were Bruce A. Mueller, OTR/L, C.H.T., and Ellen Adams, M.A., C.R.C., C.C.M.

Validity: The client demonstrated consistent and maximal effort throughout the functional capacity evaluation, as evidenced by passing 88% of the validity criteria assessed (36 of 41).

Interdisciplinary Team Recommendations: The following recommendations have been made by the team:

1. Release this client to full duty with guidelines as listed on the enclosed Work Capacity Checklist.

Referral Questions

No specific questions were posed by the referral source. Questions identified by the Interdisciplinary Team include

1. **Can the client return to his same job?** Yes. The client demonstrates the appropriate physical abilities to comply with the physical demands of his previous job functions with Moo-Cow Farms as a delivery route driver.

2. **At what physical demand level can the client be released?** Medium. Medium work is defined by the U.S. Department of Labor Guidelines as lifting 50 pounds maximum with frequent lifting and/or carrying of objects weighing up to 25 pounds. His occasional carry is 40 pounds with two hands and 35 pounds with either hand. He can lift 50 pounds occasionally from the floor to waist height. He can frequently lift 30 pounds from floor to waist level.

3. **Is the client likely to benefit from further services?** No.

Vocational/Psychosocial Summary

Mr. R. reports that he is employed by Moo-Cow Farms and has been since August 10, 1992. He was involved in a work-related motor vehicle accident on February 14, 1994. The client reports he continues to work for Moo-Cow Farms, and at this time he is working as a trainer for milk delivery people. At the time he was injured, he was a milk delivery person. The client reports that he works from 3:30 am to 5:00 or 6:00 pm approximately 60 to 70 hours per week 5 days a week. He reports that prior to his injury he worked on commission, but now he receives an hourly rate. The client reports that prior to his injury, he grossed approximately $600 per week; now he is grossing $400 per week. The client does not have an attorney, and he does not have a rehabilitation counselor or nurse working with him.

Mr. R. states that to perform his job, he must drive a truck and deliver milk and butter to schools, hospitals, nursing homes, and restaurants. He reports using a milk hook, a hand truck, a computer, and a work truck. He reports lifting and carrying 40 pounds in one hand and 80 pounds in both hands and pushing and pulling over 240 pounds. He also reports having to stoop, bend, squat, kneel, crawl, climb ladders, climb stairs, twist, walk on uneven ground, reach above shoulder height, reach at shoulder height, and reach below shoulder height to perform his job duties. The client reported that the most difficult part of his job was dealing with mad customers. He states that he did get along well with his coworkers and his bosses, and he continues to do so.

The client is 23 years old, he has a 12th grade education, and he has special training as a certified machinist and has a class A commercial driver's license. He has a past work history that includes being a dock supervisor for a transportation company, where he drove a fork lift, supervised three other employees, and dispatched drivers for the trucking company. He also has a past history working in construction making custom cabinets. Mr. R. is married. He reports that his wife is a full-time student in a respiratory therapy program. He reports that at this time his living situation is such that he and his wife are able to meet their expenses. He reports that for the last year, since his marriage, he has lived on some property that belongs to his grandfather. He reports having to maintain the property and having to pay utility bills to live there. The client reports that he does have a current driver's license and dependable transportation. He reports he was ticketed for the accident and that he went to driving school to have the points removed from his license.

The client was asked what he does for fun, and he reported that he does not have much time to do fun activities because he works so much. He stated that his hobbies and interests were old cars and boating. He reports spending his days off working or fixing things that break down. He reports that around the house he does most everything including cooking, cleaning, and vacuuming; however, he reports some diminished activity.

The client reports that he is being told by his employer that as soon as he is physically able to return to driving the truck, he will be allowed to do that. The client, however, stated he is fearful of returning to driving a truck for fear he will have a muscle spasm that could cause him to have another accident. He reports that his position as a trainer is secure at this time, and that there is no pressure for him to return to driving.

Medical History: A thorough review of records provided from the treating physicians was performed by the interdisciplinary team.

Client's Diagnosis: Thoracic/lumbar strain.

Surgeries: None.

Pain Behaviors: The client does not appear to present with inappropriate illness behaviors. This is reinforced with his low scores on Waddell Signs of +2/5, a low score on appropriate pain inventories. He also does not improve his range of motion or performance via distraction throughout the evaluation.

Pain drawing and pain rating were performed both pre- and posttesting. Prior to the testing, the client rated his pain as a 3.5 on a 0 to 10 scale. After the testing, the client rated his pain as a 4.5. His area of discomfort did not change, nor did indicated pain levels increase in intensity. These areas are the low thoracic and upper lumbar spine.

Musculoskeletal Evaluation

Trunk ROM:

Forward bending	85°
Extension	12°
Right side bend	27°
Left side bend	30°

Motor, Sensory, and DTRs: Intact, brisk, and symmetric.

Flexibility: He is within normal limits in hamstring length; however, his hip flexors are mildly restricted, eliciting some back pain. His right piriformis complex is restricted at approximately 30° IR at the hip. The left is within normal limits.

SLR: He exhibits a 90° SLR in sitting bilaterally. He demonstrates a 45° SLR left and a 67° SLR right in the supine position.

Special Tests: He has a decreased left pelvic shear with some pain elicited. He also presents with an apparent posterior rotation of the right ilium causing him some discomfort with flexion of the right hip.

Tests Administered

1. *Grip Strength:* Grip strength was tested using a Jamar dynamometer and measured in pounds. Five level grips were taken to observe for a bell-shaped curve, suggestive of full effort. Coefficients of variation were calculated on these measurements. A CV less than 15% is indicative of full effort. Mathiowetz norms for this client's age and gender were recorded.

Results: The average right hand grip strength on the second setting was 123.3 pounds; the average left hand grip strength was 106.3 pounds. Mathiowetz norms are 121.0 pounds on the right and 104.5 pounds on the left. Coefficient of variation results were below 15% on 9 of 10 calculated.

2. *Computerized Testing, Isometric Strength Test Unit:* The ISTU is designed to quantify a person's ability to lift, push, or pull in various postures. This procedure has been recommended by NIOSH. The client was asked to repeat each position for three or more attempts to produce data for calculation of CV. The CV is less than 10% in a valid test.

    Arm lift: Average of 48.1 pounds
                      Coefficient of variation 10.0%
    High/near lift: Average of 75.2 pounds
                      Coefficient of variation 14.2%
    High/far lift: Average of 64.7 pounds
                      Coefficient of variation 3.24%
    Pull task: Average of 90.8 pounds
                      Coefficient of variation 6.31%
    Leg lift: Average of 97.7 pounds
                      Coefficient of variation 13.5%

  Comments: His values for dynamic lifting as extrapolated from static strength testing are as follows:
    Shoulder lift: Expected 40 pounds, 30 pounds for validity
    Front carry: Expected 42.3 pounds, 31.7 pounds for validity
    Leg lift: Expected 54.0 pounds, 32.4 pounds for validity
    Pull task: Expected 68.0 pounds, 51.5 pounds for validity
    Overhead lift: Expected 46.3 pounds, 43.7 pounds for validity

3. *Computerized Testing, Baltimore Therapeutic Equipment:* The BTE Work Simulator is designed to simulate upper extremity motions required during performance of job tasks. Tool attachments were selected to simulate motions appropriate to the client's functional use. A coefficient of variation less than 15% is indicative of full effort.

  The right is 0.8% of the left on tool #162. Coefficient of variation, right, 3.1%; left, 4.8%.

  The client was evaluated using the BTE to assess isometric strength. The following BTE attachments were used to test supination and pronation and pushing and pulling ability: 302, 504. Coefficient of variation results were below 15% on eight of eight calculated.

4. *Purdue Pegboard Test:* This test measures the dexterity needed for potential employees to perform jobs such as assembly work, packing, or machine operation. Tip pinch dexterity and the ability to reach when seated at a table height were assessed. The client completed three 1-minute trials following the Purdue Pegboard Assembly protocol. He completed an average of 36 assemblies. This places him in the high-speed trainable or good category for fine motor and assembly tasks using the hands.

5. *Repetitive Squats:* The client completed 20 full nonsupported squats.

6. *Dynamic One-Repetition Activities:* This test indicates the maximum weight an individual can handle one to four times in 8 hours. Results;
    Floor to waist level lift: 50 pound occasional maximum accepted with a 30 pound frequent lift demonstrated; exertion factor −3
    Waist level to shoulder lift: 30 pound occasional maximum accepted
    Waist level to overhead level lift: 25 pound occasional maximum accepted with a 20 pound frequent lift demonstrated; exertion factor −1
  Comments: His exertion factors of −3 and −1 are indicative of good correlation in his perception of effort as compared with increase of his heart rate measured on the Borg rating of perceived exertion scale.

7. *Push/pull:* The client was asked to push and pull a nonwheeled sled over carpet 150 feet each direction. He demonstrated the ability to push with 47.5 pounds force and pull with 50.0 pounds force. This translates into a moderate task for pushing and pulling.

8. *Prolonged Sitting:* 30 to 45 minutes per client report.

9. *Prolonged Standing:* 2 hours observed.

10. *One-Handed Carry:* The client was asked to carry the maximum amount of weight tolerable in the right hand for a distance of 150 feet. The client was then asked to repeat this test with the left hand. Right hand: 35 pounds. Left hand: 35 pounds.

11. *Two-Handed Carry:* The client was asked to carry the maximum tolerable weight in both hands for a total distance of 150 feet. Forty pounds were tolerated.

12. *Repetitive Reach:* This reach was performed at a waist level with unweighted upper extremities. The client was requested to continue with this bilateral repetitive reaching activity for 8 minutes. Overhead reaching was completed for 8 minutes with 192 repetitions.

13. *Sustained Reach:* This reach was performed at a waist level, shoulder level, or overhead level with unweighted upper extremities. The client was asked to complete an 8-minute test time. Overhead level reaching for 8 minutes was completed.

14. *Crawling:* The client was asked to complete a 1-minute trial of crawling on the mat. He was able to do this, and this places him in the occasional category for crawling.

15. *Kneeling:* The client was asked to kneel and then stand upright on carpet for one repetition. The client was able to do this.

16. *Stair Climbing:* The client was asked to complete five flights of 11 steps, both ascending and descending. He completed the task in 1 minute and 18 seconds, with a pretest heart rate of 82, posttest of 123, and a recovery rate of 96. He completed a total of 110 steps, placing him in the frequent category for stair or ladder negotiation.

17. *Balance:* The client was asked to walk the 5.5-inch balance beam over a 1-minute trial. He used an ankle with an occasional hip strategy throughout the test. This would give him some minimal to moderate restrictions for working in unprotected heights.

Tests Deferred by the Evaluator: None.

Tests Declined by the Client: None.

Thank you for allowing us to assist in the care of this client. Ellen Adams, M.A., C.R.C., C.C.M., completed the Vocational Psychosocial Summary and coauthored the referral questions and recommendations. If we can be of any further assistance, please feel free to call us at (904) 336-6830. Any further written reports can be forwarded on request.

Sincerely,

_____

Bruce A. Mueller, OTR/L, C.H.T.
BAM/EA/pjp
cc: Physician
   Insurance Company

APPENDIX C

Physician and Attorney Comments on Functional Capacity Evaluation

Included are two comments on the usefulness of FCE, one by a physician and the other from an attorney who usually represents the insurance company in workers' compensation litigation.

Work assessment, as indicated earlier, is best done in an interdisciplinary team approach. Many professionals utilize functional capacity evaluations within the scope of their participation not only of treating but also of evaluating the patient.

PHYSICIAN STATEMENT

The confusion in medical, legal, employer, and administrative circles regarding the difference between disability and impairment is well known to those who work in the occupational medicine community. Now, add to this the additional confusion created by the use of information gained by functional capacity testing of claimants.

Historically, physicians have been required by administrative bodies to provide an opinion based on the medical findings and diagnosis of what the patient was "restricted" from doing, primarily for the occupational setting but also for general physical activities. This opinion has traditionally been provided at the judgment of the physician based on the training and experience of the physician. Such a system has been fraught with a lack of objectivity.

An opinion regarding restriction of physical activity obtained in this manner from a physician (scientist) was in most cases, however, not really based on any scientific principles, not obtained in an objective manner, and not supported by any valid medical evidence. In reality, an opinion based in this manner provided no real functional value to the claimant, except to meet statutory and administrative requirements. With the evolution of physical or functional capacity testing of injured workers, the problems of lack of objectivity in determining "restrictions" at a first glance would have appeared to have been resolved. Unfortunately, new problems with use and misuse of information obtained in this manner became evident. To understand this new problem, let us look back at the concept of "restriction." A restriction on the activity of the patient was supposed to be set by the physician based on the medical findings, diagnosis, and prognosis. As discussed previously, this determination has been historically inconsistent, unscientific, arbitrary, and not truly objective. In most cases, restrictions were set only because of administrative requirements to establish that a "disability" existed so that a claim of injury could be adjudicated.

With the advent of functional capacity testing, in most instances we can generate objective, scientific data and truly measure the really important question of "what can the patient do, what can the patient not do" after being permanently injured. But was the information obtained by functional capacity testing really providing the physician with a tool to set "restrictions"' based on the effects of the occupational injury? The answer to this question is at the heart of the problem. The functional capacity test evaluates the physical capacity of the whole person. The physical capacity of the whole person is affected by many variables, only one of which is the occupational injury in question. In addition, the general health, congenital conditions, prior injuries, physical build, motivation, and, probably, age and sex all contribute to some extent to the performance of the patient on functional capacity testing.

Functional testing in reality determines the ability of the claimant to perform on standardized tests and equipment, then extrapolates this information to provide a summary or estimate of the patient's general physical capacity. If valid, testing determines the limits of the claimant's physical performance, at least on the day of the testing. It thus can provide us [physicians] with the limits of the abilities or performance of the claimant. However, the concept of limits or limitations of ability determined by functional capacity testing is not the same as the concept of restrictions on activities that are set by physicians. If the role of the occupational physician is to set restrictions based solely on an industrial injury or condition, use of functional capacity testing to set such restriction is truly not appropriate. The FCE is providing us with information that is not exactly congruent with the concept of restrictions. If functional capacity testing is providing us with the physical ability or limitations of a claimant's abilities, then why are these data used to determine what restrictions should be placed on a claimant? Practically, this method, despite its limits, is probably giving us the closest objective approximation that we can get at this stage of the evolution of functional testing because there is currently no other reliable method for determining restrictions on function objectively.

The compensation system demands of the medical provider a statement or opinion of the effect of an injury on function. The provider [physician] has a duty to set restrictions that fit the diagnosis but must use the best means available for making this determination. Currently, the FCE is the only objective method available to determine function of the claimant. This type of testing is not cheap, however, and cost-containment strategies may prohibit the use of FCEs to only the more complex and difficult cases.

When an FCE is performed, validity criteria need to be considered to assess the patient's motivation to provide best performance during the testing process. If validity criteria are not met yet there is evidence of injury and organic disease, the physician must then rely on judgment and experience in establishing appropriate restrictions for the nature of the injury and physical condition of the patient. If a concomitant somatization disorder [DSM III diagnosis] has an effect on function, the use of FCE is even more difficult in establishing restrictions on a claimant's activities. Again, the physician must rely on judgment and experience in setting appropriate restrictions for the diagnosis, which is in this case not only physical but also crosses into the realm of psychological.

—OREGON K. HUNTER, MD, BOARD CERTIFIED PHYSIATRIST

ATTORNEY STATEMENT

From the workers' compensation defense prospective, FCEs and work hardening programs are, in my opinion, separate. The FCE is critical to the determination of whether a claimant is able to return to some type of physical activity that might be combined with a job description to indicate to the judge of compensation claims that the claimant is not completely disabled and retains some wage earning capacity. It is also very important in the FCE that accurate notes be kept to determine at a later date, in either deposition testimony or trial testimony, whether it appeared that the client was putting forth a full effort during the functional evaluation. I have seen many cases in which there will be notations that the claimant appear to have inconsistent results or even incomprehensible results from a FCE. These types of notations are very helpful to the judge in determining whether the claimant is or is not able to return to work.

The work hardening program is very important in a different way. Once it appears from a FCE that there may be a position in the work environment that the claimant may successfully complete, the work hardening program seems to help him or her get back into the flow of activity. Many of these claimants have been sitting around for a significant period of time, and just the physical and mental deconditioning make it difficult for them to return to more than a full schedule. Work hardening helps the claimant get over this hump and return to the work place. Again, notations in the file concerning efforts are very important to help the judge determine whether the claimant was in fact seeking to participate willingly or not.

—JAMES H. MCCARTY, JR., ESQUIRE, DEFENSE ATTORNEY
[ATTORNEY FOR THE INSURED]

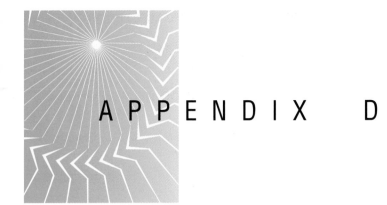

APPENDIX   D

PHYSICAL RESTORATION CENTERS
of Florida

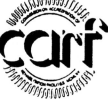

WELCOME

In order to get to know more about you, we would like you to answer these questions. This information will be very helpful to us through all phases of your treatment/evaluation. Thank you for your cooperation.

....

_____
Date

NAME: _____

WHAT DOCTOR(S) ARE CURRENTLY TREATING YOU FOR YOUR INJURY? _____

_____

WHO HAS TREATED YOU FOR THIS IN THE PAST? _____

_____

HAVE YOU REACHED MMI? _____

DO YOU HAVE AN IMPAIRED RATING? _____

HAVE YOU BEEN IN PHYSICAL THERAPY? Yes _____ No _____ AT THIS TIME? _____

IF YES, WITH WHOM _____

HAVE YOU EVER RECEIVED PSYCHOLOGICAL SERVICES? _____

PLACE OF EMPLOYEMENT WHERE INJURED: _____

DATE YOU BEGAN WORKING: _____

DATE OF ACCIDENT/INJURY: _____

LAST DATE YOU WORKED ANYWHERE: _____

ARE YOU ON JOB SEARCH? _____ HOW LONG? _____

WHAT IS/WAS YOUR JOB TITLE: _____

WHO IS/WAS YOUR WORK SUPERVISOR: _____

WHAT ARE/WERE YOUR WORK HOURS: _____

HOW MANY HOURS PER WEEK DO/DID YOU WORK: _____

ANNUAL/HOURLY SALARY WHILE WORKING: _____

PRESENT SALARY FROM WORKERS' COMP: _____

DO YOU HAVE AN ATTORNEY? _____ Yes _____ No

NAME: _____

WHEN DID YOU RETAIN THIS ATTORNEY? _____

DO YOU HAVE A REHABILITATION COUNSELOR/NURSE? _____ Yes _____ No

NAME: _____

PLEASE DESCRIBE YOUR JOB AS IF YOU WERE TELLING SOMEONE WHO KNEW NOTHING ABOUT THE WORK YOU DO:

_____

_____

_____

PLEASE LIST THE TYPE OF MACHINES, TOOLS, AND EQUIPMENT YOU USE/USED:

_____

_____

WHILE WORKING, HOW MUCH WEIGHT DO YOU THINK YOU HAD TO LIFT/CARRY?

WITH ONE HAND: _____ WITH BOTH HANDS: _____

HOW MUCH WEIGHT DO/DID YOU HAVE TO PUSH/PULL? _____

IN YOUR JOB, DO/DID YOU HAVE TO:

STOOP	_____	CLIMB STAIRS	_____
BEND	_____	TWIST	_____
SQUAT	_____	WALK ON UNEVEN GROUND	_____
KNEEL	_____	REACH ABOVE SHOULDERS	_____
CRAWL	_____	REACH AT SHOULDERS HEIGHT	_____
CLIMB LADDERS	_____	REACH BELOW SHOULDERS	_____

WHAT PARTS OF YOUR JOB MAKE/MADE YOU FEEL GOOD ABOUT YOURSELF?

_____

_____

_____

WHAT IS/WAS THE MOST DIFFICULT PART OF YOUR JOB?

_____

_____

DO/DID YOUR COWORKERS AND BOSS GET ALONG WITH YOU? (EXPLAIN)

_____

_____

WHAT DO YOU THINK NEEDS TO HAPPEN FOR YOU TO BE ABLE TO RETURN TO WORK?

_____

_____

_____

PLEASE LIST ANY OTHER JOBS YOU HAVE HELD IN THE PAST:

YEAR: _____   JOB TITLE: _____

YEAR: _____   JOB TITLE: _____

YEAR: _____   JOB TITLE: _____

YEAR: _____   JOB TITLE: _____

HAVE YOU SERVED IN THE MILITARY? _____

BRANCH: _____   RANK AT DISCHARGE: _____

ARE YOU CURRENTLY MARRIED: _____ Yes _____ No;   DIVORCED: _____ Yes _____ No;

SINGLE: _____ Yes _____ No;   WIDOWED: _____ Yes _____ No;   LIVE-IN RELATIONSHIP: _____ Yes _____ No

DOES YOUR SPOUSE/PARTNER HAVE A JOB? _____ Yes _____ No

IF YES, WHAT DOES HE/SHE DO? _____

HOW OLD ARE YOU? _____ HOW MANY CHILDREN DO YOU HAVE? _____

AGES: _____

DO YOU KNOW ANYONE ON SOCIAL SECURITY DISABILITY/WORKERS' COMPENSATION AT THIS

TIME? _____ Yes _____ No

ARE YOU ABLE TO MEET YOUR MONTHLY EXPENSES? _____

DO YOU HAVE ANY UNUSUAL EXPENSES? _____

_____

DO YOU SMOKE: _____ Yes _____ No   PACKS PER DAY: _____

HOW LONG HAVE YOU SMOKED? _____

DO YOU DRINK? _____ Yes _____ No   HOW OFTEN: _____

WHAT KIND OF ALCOHOL DO YOU DRINK? _____

DO YOU HAVE A CURRENT DRIVER'S LICENSE? Yes _____ No _____

DO YOU HAVE DEPENDABLE TRANSPORTATION? _____ Yes _____ No

WHAT DO YOU DO FOR FUN? (EXAMPLES: HOBBIES, INTERESTS):

_____

_____

HOW DO YOU SPEND YOUR DAY? _____

_____

_____

WHAT HOUSEHOLD TASKS DO YOU PERFORM? _____

_____

IS THIS MORE OR LESS THAN BEFORE YOUR INJURY? _____

WHAT IS THE HIGHEST GRADE IN SCHOOL THAT YOU COMPLETED? _____

WERE YOU IN REGULAR OR SPECIAL CLASSES? _____

DO YOU HAVE ANY SPECIAL TRAINING, LICENSES, OR DEGREES?

_____

_____

PLEASE LIST ANY COMMENTS THAT WOULD HELP US TO GET TO KNOW YOU OR BETTER UNDERSTAND YOUR SITUATION:

_____

_____

_____

_____

_____

_____

_____

THANK YOU FOR YOUR COOPERATION.

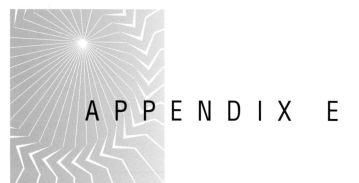

A P P E N D I X E

The ACHIEVEMENT CENTER
HCA Health Florida Regional Medical Center

PHYSICAL ABILITIES ASSESSMENT

Patient: _____ Physician: _____

Job Title: _____ Employer: _____

Job Duties: _____

Symptom Level: 1 2 3 4 5 6 7 8 9 10   Location: _____

Functional Job Activities, as defined by patient:
Total hours in a repetitive 8-hour work day   Break every _____ min/hr.
(Circle most appropriate)

Driving/sitting	1 2 3 4 5 6 7 8	Walking:	1 2 3 4 5 6 7 8
Squatting/kneeling:	1 2 3 4 5 6 7 8	Carrying:	1 2 3 4 5 6 7 8
Pushing/pulling:	1 2 3 4 5 6 7 8	Bending:	1 2 3 4 5 6 7 8
Standing:	1 2 3 4 5 6 7 8	Climbing:	1 2 3 4 5 6 7 8

Lift: _____ lbs. What is the heaviest item lifted? _____

Aerobic Endurance: A 10-minute treadmill walk to patient tolerance beginning at 1.0 mph and increasing every 30 seconds up to 3.5 mph. No grade change. Record time (minutes) and mph.

Dynamic Activities: Check appropriate category—occasionally means @ 2–5 hrs./day, no restrictions means continuously or @ 6–8 hrs./day.

	No Restrictions	**Frequently**	**Occasionally**	**Never**
Repetitive Bending: (slight knee bend, 10″ from chair; return to start position)	2 min; PP	1 min; PP	1–2 min; UMP	<1 min; UMP
Static Kneeling: (choice of kneeling position)	2 min; PP	1 min; PP	1–2 min; UMP	<1 min; UMP
Dynamic Squatting: (5 sec. squat, 10 sec. stand)	2 min; PP	1 min; PP	1–2 min; UMP	<1 min; UMP
Carrying: (13# box plus weights)	50 ft.; 50# max.	50 ft.; 30#	50 ft.; 20#	25 ft.; 10#
Overhead Reaching: (2# wt., elbow extension, alternate UE)	L & R full FL	1/2 full FL	shldr. level	<shldr. level
Climbing:	3 min; 15 flts.	2 min; 10 flts.	1 min; 5 flts.	<1 min; <5 flts.

PP = proper posture   UMP = unable to maintain proper posture

(WEST)

7022 NW 10TH PL, GAINESVILLE, FL 32605, PH (904) 333-4715

(MIDTOWN)

620 NW 16th AVE, GAINESVILLE, FL 32601, PH (904) 375-6559

Grip Strength: R _____ lbs., L _____ lbs.   **Pinch Strength:** R _____ lbs., L _____ lbs.

Static Push: _____ lbs.   **Static Pull:** _____ lbs.

Maximum Lift: **Floor to waist:** _____ lbs.
(using a 13-lb. box)   (hand hold must be at bottom of box)
    29″ table to waist: _____ lbs.

    Waist to shoulder: _____ lbs.
    (use hands as height marker)
    Waist to overhead: _____ lbs.
    (hand position must be overhead)

Observations:
Body Mechanics: Good Fair   Poor
(provide instructions during PAA)

Functional Endurance: Good Fair   Poor

Effort: Good Fair   Poor

Recommend Work Category: Dictionary of Occupational Titles, Vol II, U.S. Department of Labor, pp. 654–655, 1965.

Sedentary Work: 10 lbs. or less maximum and occasional lifting of objects 5 lbs. or less; minimal walking required.

Light Work: 20 lbs. maximum, with frequent lifting of 10 lbs. or less; some sitting and standing, pushing and pulling.

Medium Work: 50 lbs. maximum, 25 lbs. frequently.

Heavy Work: Lifting 100 lbs. max. with frequent lifting of objects to 50 lbs.

Very Heavy Work: Lifting objects more than 100 lbs., frequent lifting of objects 50 lbs. or more.

No Restrictions: Complies fully with present job description.

    Full Time _____   **Part Time** _____
COMMENTS:

_____

_____

_____

_____

_____

_____

_____

_____

_____

_____

Physician Signature: _____   **Date:** _____

Physical Therapist Signature: _____   **Date:** _____

GLOSSARY

Coefficients of variation—A ratio expression of the standard deviation and the mean in terms of a percentage; it has no units of measurement. A high percentage would indicate considerable variability.

Disability—An alteration, expressed in nonmedical terms, of an individual's capability to meet personal, social, or occupational demands or to meet statutory or regulatory requirements. The gap between what the individual is required to do and what he or she is able to do.

Electromyography—The recording and study of the intrinsic electric properties of skeletal muscle by means of surface or needle electrodes to determine whether the muscle is contracting.

Ergonomics—The branch of science and technology that includes what is known and theorized about human behavioral and biologic characteristics that can be validly applied to the specification, design, evaluation, operation, and maintenance of products and systems to enhance safe, effective, and satisfying use by individuals, groups, and organizations.

Functional capacity evaluation (FCE)—The objective determination of the claimant's ability to participate in activities within the work setting that require bending, lifting, pushing, pulling, balance, reaching, climbing, stooping, standing tolerance, sitting tolerance, eye-hand-foot coordination, manual and finger dexterity, and physical endurance. It may include the broader identification of existing impairments in speech, hearing, or vision and the behavioral observations including, but not limited to, memory, attention span, and frustration tolerance.

Impairment—An alteration, expressed in medical terms, of an individual's health status. That which is wrong with the health of an individual.

Inclometer—A device measuring the angle of a slope or inclined plane.

Independent medical examination—A physician who is not the treating physician conducts a physical evaluation and records review in order to provide an injured worker and the insurance carrier an opinion of the worker's condition.

Insurance adjustor—One who makes any adjustment or settlement, or who determines amount of a claim, as a claim against an insurance company. A representation of the insurer who seems to determine the extent of the firm's liability for loss when a claim is submitted. A person who acts for the insurance company or the insured in the determination and settlement of claims.

Interdisciplinary—An approach to client management that requires the integration of a core team from multiple disciplines, which, on an ongoing basis, assesses, plans, and implements a complex rehabilitation program for functional restoration. It differs significantly from an approach in which multiple disciplines are available as needed but function independently of one another to address isolated, clearly defined problems.

Isoinertional—The velocity is not controlled, but mass is held constant.

Isokinetic—The velocity is constant, while the force exerted is allowed to vary.

Isometric—The velocity is zero. Exercises consisting of voluntary muscle contractions, with no joint motion being elicited.

Kyphosis—A convex backward curvature of the spine.

Lordosis—Hollow back; anteroposterior curvature of the spine.

Prevocational evaluation—Evaluation of activities of daily living, educational abilities, and physical capabilities and deficits as required for participation in vocational activity or evaluation.

Psychophysical tests—A psychophysical test is a test in which the person being evaluated determines the acceptable results based on his or her response to external stimuli. The testee selects the appropriate forces based on level of exertion, anxiety ("I'm afraid of increasing my pain"), pain ("This weight increased my pain"), and biomechanical load.

Rehabilitation counselor—A person with a Bachelor's or Master's degree in rehabilitation counseling. May hold national certification as a Certified Rehabilitation Counselor (CRC). Often works as case manager with the industrially injured.

Reliability—Degree to which a test produces the same results on repeated administration.

Secondary gain—An advantage occurring after an accident or injury, such as financial benefit or increase in attention from spouse or family member.

Somatization disorder—Characterized by recurrent, multiple somatic complaints of several years duration. Complaints are usually dramatic but vague.

Torque—The torque or moment of force is the product of a force times the perpendicular distance from its line of action to the axis of motion. Torque is the expression of the effectiveness of a force in turning a lever system.

Validity—Statistical term; the degree to which a given measure indicates the quality or attribute it attempts to measure.

Vocational evaluation—Assessment of all factors (medical, psychological, educational, social, environmental, cultural, and vocational) that affect successful employment.

Workers' Compensation Act—The state statutes that provide for fixed awards to employees or their dependents in case of employment-related accidents and diseases, dispensing with proof or negligence and legal actions.

Work evaluation—Evaluation of vocational strengths and weaknesses through utilization of work (real or simulated).

Work hardening program—A highly structured, goal-oriented, and individualized program that provides transition between acute care and return to work, while addressing the issues of productivity, safety, physical tolerance, and work behavior. Services should be delivered in specific areas of expertise by registered, certified, licensed, or degreed personnel or should be performed substantially in their presence and should be provided on a regular continuing basis. Work hardening programs use real or simulated work activities in a relevant work environment.

Work sample evaluation—Sample of actual job tasks or a mock-up of actual tasks to determine the client's job skills and abilities.

REFERENCES

American College of Sports Medicine. (1991). *Guidelines for exercise testing and prescription* (4th ed.). Philadelphia: Lea & Febiger.
American Medical Association. (1988). *Guides to the evaluation of permanent impairment* (3rd ed.). Chicago: American Medical Association.
Anderson, P. A. (1990). Normative study of grip and wrist flexion strength employing a BTE Work Simulator. *Journal of Hand Surgery, 15A*(3), 420–425.

Barren, N., Gant, A., Nq, F., Slover, P., Wall, J., & Rash, G. (1992). The validity of the ERIC maximal voluntary effort protocol in distinguishing maximal from submaximal effort on the Baltimore Therapeutic Equipment work simulator. *National Association of Rehabilitation Professionals in the Private Sector Journal and News, 7*(6), 223–228.

Beck A., Ward C., Mendelson M., Mock, J., & Erbaugh, J. (1961). An inventory for measuring depression. *Archives of General Psychiatry, 4*, 53–61.

Bectol, C. O. (1954). Grip test use of dynometry with adjustable handle spacing. *Journal of Bone and Joint Surgery, 36A, 832.*

Bennett, G. K. (1981). *Hand tool dexterity test: Manual.* San Diego, CA: The Psychological Corporation. U.S.A., Harcourt Brace Jovanovich.

Benson, H. (1987). Lumbar spine. In D. J. Magee (Ed.), *Orthopedic physical assessment* (p. 77). Philadelphia: W. B. Saunders Company.

Berlin, S., & Vermette, J. (1985). An exploratory study of work simulator norms for grip and wrist flexion. *Vocational Evaluation and Work Adjustment Bulletin, Summer*, 61–68.

Blankenship, K. L. (1994). *The Blankenship System: Functional Capacity Evaluation. The procedure manual.* Macon, GA: Blankenship Corporation. Panaprint, Inc.

Blankenship, K. L. (1989). *Industrial rehabilitation* (3rd ed.). Macon, GA: American Therapeutics.

Borg, G. (1982). Psychological basis of perceived exertion. *Medicine and Science in Sports and Exercise, 14*, 377–381.

Chaffin, D. B. (1975). Ergonomics, guide for the assessment of human static strength. *American Industrial Hygiene Association Journal, July*, 505–511.

Chaffin, D. B., Herrin, D. F., Keysehing, W., & Foulke, J. A. (1972). Pre-employment strength testing in selecting workers for material handling jobs. Bethesda, MD: *NIOSH* contact no. CDD 99-74-62.

Christopherson, B. B., & Hayes, P. D. (1992). *VALPAR* component work samples: Uses in allied health. Tucson, AZ: VALPAR International Corporation.

Dillard, J., Trafimow, J., Anderson, G. B. J., & Cronin, K. (1991). Motion of the lumbar spine: Reliability of two measurement techniques. *Spine, 16*(3), 321–324.

Fairbanks J., Couper J., Davies J., & O'Brien, J. (1980). The Questry low back pain disability questionnaire. *Physiotherapy, 66*(8), 271–273.

Field, J. E., & Field, T. F. (1988). The classification of jobs according to worker trait factors. *Dictionary of Occupational Titles* (4th ed.). Athens, GA: Elliot and Fitzpatrick.

Friedlander, A. L., Block, J. E., Byl, N. N., Stubbs, H. A., Sasowsky, H. S., & Genant, H. K. (1991). Isokinetic limb and trunk muscle performance testing. *Journal of Orthopedic and Sports Physical Therapy, 14*(5), 220–224.

Gatchel R., Mayer T., Capra P., & Barnett J. (1986). Millon Behavioral Health Inventory: In predicting physical function in patients with low back pain. *Archives of Physical Medicine and Rehabilitation, 67*, 879–882.

Golding, L. A., Myers, C. R., & Sinning, W. E. (Eds.). (1989). *Y's way to physical fitness* (3rd ed.). Champaign, IL: Human Kinetics Publishers.

Gomez, T., Beach, G., Cooke, C., Hrudey, W., & Goyert, P. (1991). Normative database for trunk range of motion, strength, velocity, and endurance with the isostation B-200 lumbar dynamometer. *Spine, 16*, 15–21.

Hanson, C. S., & Walker, K. F. (1992). The history of work in physical dysfunction. *American Journal of Occupational Therapy, 46*(1), 56–62.

Harvey-Krefting L. (1985). The concept of work in occupational therapy: A historical review. *American Journal of Occupational Therapy, 39*(5), 301–307.

Hazard, R. G., Reid, S., & Fenwick, J. (1988). Isokinetic trunk and lifting strength measurements: Variability as an indicator of effort. *Spine, 13*(1), 54–58.

Hildreth, D. H., Briedenbach, W. C., Lister, G. D., & Hodges, A. D. (1989). Detection of submaximal effort by use of the rapid exchange grip. *Journal of Hand Surgery, 14*(A), 742–745.

Hoffmaster, E., Lech, R., & Niebuhr, B. R. (1993). Consistency of sincere and feigned grip exertions with repeated testing. *Journal of Occupational Medicine, 35*(8), 788–794.

Holmes, D. (1985). The role of the occupational therapist work evaluator. *American Journal of Occupational Therapy, 39*(5), 308–313.

Isernhagen, S. J. (1988). Work injury: Management and prevention. Gaithersburg, MD: Aspen Publishers.

Jones, A. (1993). *The lumbar spine, the cervical spine and the knee.* Ocala, FL: MedX.

Jones, A., Pollock, M., Graves, J., Fulton, M., Jones, W., MacMillan, M., Baldwin, D. D., & Cirulli, J. (1988). *The lumbar spine.* Santa Barbara, CA: Sequoia Communications.

Keeley, J., Mayer, T. G., Cox, R., Gatchel, R. J., Smith, J., & Mooney, V. (1986). Quantification of lumbar function. Part 5: Reliability of range of motion measures in the sagittal plane and an in vivo torso rotation measurement technique. *Spine, 11*(1), 31–35.

King, J. W., & Berryhill, B. H. (1988). A comparison of two static grip testing methods and its clinical applications, a preliminary study. *Journal of Hand Therapy, 1*(5), 204–208.

Kuhn, T. S. (1970). *The structure of scientific revolution.* Chicago: Chicago University Press.

Langrana, N. A., & Lee, C. K. (1984). Isokinetic evaluation of trunk muscles. *Spine, 9*(2), 171–175.

Lawlis, G., Cuencas, R., Selby, D., & McCoy, C. (1989). The development of the Dallas pain questionaire: An assessment of the impact of spinal pain on behavior. *Spine, 14*(5), 511–516.

Marshall, E. (1985). Looking back. *American Journal of Occupational Therapy, 39*(5), 297–300.

Matheson, L. N. (1988). How do you know that he tried his best? The reliability crisis in industrial rehabilitation. *Industrial Rehabilitation Quarterly*, (1), 1, 11, 12.

Matheson, L. N. (1989). Use of the BTE work simulator to screen for symptom magnification syndrome. *Industrial Rehabilitation Quarterly, 2*(2), 5–28.

Matheson, L. N. (1990). Symptom magnification syndrome: A modern tragedy and its treatment. *Industrial Rehabilitation Quarterly, 3*(3), 5–23.

Mayer, T. G., & Gatchel, R. J. (1988). *Functional restoration for spinal disorders: The sports medicine approach.* Philadelphia: Lea & Febiger.

Mayer, T. G., Gatchel, R. J., Kishino, N., Keeley, J., Capra, P., Mayer, H., Barnett, J., & Mooney, V. (1985). Objective assessment of spine function following industrial injury: A prospective study with comparison group and one-year follow-up. *Spine, 10*, 482–493.

Mayer, T. G., Mooney, V., Gatchel, R. J., Barnes, D., Terry, A., Smith, S., & Mayer, H. (1989). Quantifying postoperative deficits of physical function following spinal surgery. *Clinical Orthopedics and Related Research, 244*, 147–157.

Mayer, T. G., Smith, S. S., Keeley, J., & Mooney, V. (1985). Quantification of lumbar function. Part 2: Sagittal plane trunk strength in chronic low-back pain patients. *Spine, 10*(8), 765–772.

Mayer, T. G., Smith, S. S., Kondraske, G., Gatchel, R. J., Carmichael, T. W., & Mooney, V. (1985). Quantification of lumbar function. Part 3: Preliminary data on isokinetic torso rotation testing with myoelectric spectral analysis in normal and low-back pain subjects. *Spine, 10*, 912.

McNeill, T., Sinkora, G., & Leavitt, F. (1986). Psychologic classification of low back pain patients: A prognostic tool. *Spine, 11*(9), 955–959.

Melzack, R. (1975). The McGill pain questionnaire: Major properties and scoring. *Pain, 1*, 272–299.

Melzack, R. (1987). The short-form McGill pain questionnaire. *Pain, 30*, 191–197.

The Minnesota Rate of Manipulation Tests. (1969). Minneapolis, MN, American Guidance Service, Inc.

National Institute for Occupational Safety and Health. (1981). Work practices guide for manual lifting. Department of Health and Human Services Publication No. 81–122 Cincinnati, OH, Centers for Disease Control.

Ogden-Neimeyer L., & Jacobs K. (1989). *Work hardening: State of the art*, Thorofare, NJ: Slack, Inc.

Ransford, A., Cairns, D., & Money, V. (1976). The pain drawing as an aid to the psychologic evaluation of patients with low back pain. *Spine, 1*(2), 128–134.

Robinson, M. E., Geisser, M. E., Hanson, C. S., & O'Conner, P. D. (1993). Detecting submaximal efforts in grip strength and testing with the coefficient of variation. *Journal of Occupational Rehabilitation, 3*(1), 45–50.

Schultz-Johnson, K. (1987). Assesment of the upper extremity—Injured persons' return to work potential. *Journal of Hand Surgery, 12*(A), 950–957.

Smidt, G., Herring, T., Amendsen, L., Rogers, M., Russell, A., & Lehmann, T. (1983). Assessment of abdominals and back extension function. *Spine, 8*(2), 211–219.

Smith, S. S., Mayer, T. G., Gatchel, R. J., & Becker, T. J. (1985). Quantification of lumbar function. Part 1: Isometric and multispeed isokinetic trunk strength measures in sagittal and axial planes in normal subjects. *Spine, 10,* 912.

Snook, S. H., Irvine, C. H., & Bass, S. F. (1970) Maximum weights and workloads acceptable to male industrial workers. *American Industrial Hygiene Association Journal, 31,* 579–586.

Stokes, H. M. (1983). The seriously uninjured hand: Weakness of grip. *Journal of Occupational Medicine, 25,* 638–684.

Tiffin, J. (1987). *Purdue pegboard examiners manual.* Serence Research Associates: USA.

Uden, A., Astrom M., & Bergenuddtt, H. (1988). Pain drawings in chronic back pain. *Spine, 13*(4), 389–392.

U.S. Department of Labor. (1972). Handbook for Analyzing Jobs. Superintendent of Documents, US Government Printing Office, Washington, D.C. 20402.

Velozo, C. A. (1993). Work evaluations: Critique of the state of the art of functional assessment of work. *American Journal of Occupational Therapy, 47*(3), 203–209.

Waddell, G., Main, C., Morris, E., DiPaola, M., & Gray, L. (1984). Chronic low back pain, psychologic distress, and illness behavior. *Spine, 9*(2), 209–213.

Waddell, G., McCulloch, J. A., Kummel, E., & Venner, R. M. (1980). Nonorganic physical signs in low-back pain. *Spine, 5*(2), 117–125.

Waddell, G., Pilowsky, I., & Bond, M., (1989). Clinical assessment of and interpretation of abnormal illness behavior in low back pain. *Pain, 39,* 41–53.

Wegg, L. S. (1960). The essentials of work evaluation. *American Journal of Occupational Therapy, 14,* 65–69.

Williams, K. (1991). Functional capacity evaluation of the upper extremity. *Work, 1*(3), 48–64.

An Assessment Summary

In the health care arena of the late 1990s and early 21st century, rehabilitation has a major role since the emphasis of health care is increasingly on functional improvement, the ultimate goal of rehabilitation. Appropriate assessment is a major key to efficient and effective rehabilitation for the wide variety of patients or clients with whom occupational therapists and physical therapists are concerned. Since efficient and cost-effective but quality rehabilitation is mandated for the future, it is imperative that occupational therapists and physical therapists are able to demonstrate through accurate assessment the progress and increasing function of their clients. *Assessment in Occupational Therapy and Physical Therapy* has provided in one volume information from the experts on all aspects of this assessment process. Although contributors have primarily been drawn from the professions of the title, the expertise of other health professionals who are also concerned with increase in function has been included to illustrate the need for interdisciplinary cooperation throughout the client assessment process.

Because of the increasing time constraints in many health service settings, time for assessment is declining. Assessment of activities of daily living (self care, gait, home management, community activities, and work skills) may be the only feasible formal assessment allowed. However, knowledgeable rehabilitation professionals must be able to integrate the component assessments with the more obviously functional ones to obtain the information base necessary for effective intervention. Such dual-function instruments have been discussed in parts of Chapters 8 and 12. Furthermore, since initial assessment time may be limited, therapists are increasingly needing to mesh vital component assessments simultaneously with the treatment process. The thorough understanding of component assessment provided in Unit Two of *Assessment in Occupational Therapy and Physical Therapy* provides the therapist of the future with the in-depth information about component assessment necessary for integrated performance.

Because of continuing medical advances, people are living longer, and infant survival rate is higher. Thus, a greater proportion of the therapist's assessment involves instruments geared specifically to the geriatric population and a larger proportion of assessment also involves children. Although there is obvious overlap with the assessment of adults, assessment of children and elders requires the special considerations that have been elucidated in the age-related assessment portion of this book.

In conclusion, *Assessment in Occupational Therapy and Physical Therapy* has dealt in a comprehensive and rigorous fashion with all aspects of the assessment process vital to the roles these professions currently hold and will be assuming in the future changing health scene. Although much of the information has been directed toward advanced clinical assessment, the book has also included materials of value to the researcher in the rehabilitation fields. Thus, Dr. Brunt and I anticipate that this book will be of considerable use both for direct patient intervention and for research purposes.

JULIA VAN DEUSEN

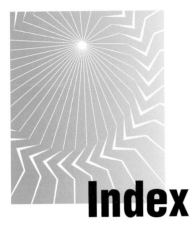

Index

Note: Page numbers in *italics* refer to illustrations; page numbers followed by t refer to tables.